Oral Cancer

Diagnosis, Management,
and Rehabilitation

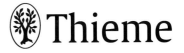

Oral Cancer

Diagnosis, Management, and Rehabilitation

John W. Werning, M.D., D.M.D.
Assistant Professor
Department of Otolaryngology
University of Florida
Gainesville, Florida

Thieme Medical Publishers
New York • Stuttgart

Thieme Medical Publishers, Inc.
333 Seventh Ave.
New York, NY 10001

Thieme and the author would like to thank the following sponsors for their financial support of production of this book:

LifeCell Corporation (Branchburg, NJ)
MedImmune Oncology, Inc.
MGI Pharma, Inc.
Daiichi Pharmaceutical Corporation
Straumann USA, LLC
Walter Lorenz Surgical
Varian Medical Systems, Inc.
Karl Storz Endoscopy
Medtronic Xomed, Inc.

Consulting Editor: Esther Gumpert
Managing Editor: J. Owen Zurhellen
Vice President, Production and Electronic Publishing: Anne T. Vinnicombe
Production Editor: Grace R. Caputo, Dovetail Content Solutions
Illustrator: Anthony M. Pazos
Associate Marketing Manager: Verena Diem
Sales Director: Ross Lumpkin
Chief Financial Officer: Peter van Woerden
President: Brian D. Scanlan
Compositor: Techset Composition Ltd.
Printer: The Maple Vail Book Manufacturing Group

Cover: Artist's rendition of a hemimandibulectomy (*left*) and a maxillectomy (*right*) as they were performed in 1912 at Massachusetts General Hospital. General anesthesia was achieved by the administration of ether through rubber nanopharyngeal tubes (originally described by Crile) that were inserted into either side of the nose. From Scudder CL. Tumors of the Jaws. Philadelphia: WB Saunders, 1912:296, 310. Used with permission.

Library of Congress Cataloging-in-Publication Data

Oral cancer: diagnosis, management, and rehabilitation/edited by John W. Werning.
    p.; cm.
  Includes bibliographical references.
  ISBN 978-1-58890-309-9—ISBN 978-3-13-135811-0
1. Mouth—Cancer. I. Werning, John W.
  [DNLM: 1. Mouth Neoplasms—diagnosis. 2. Mouth
  Neoplasms—rehabilitation. 3. Mouth Neoplasms—therapy. WU 280 O632 2007]
  RC280.M6O683 2007
  616.99'431—dc22   2007003216

Important note: Medical knowledge is ever-changing. As new research and clinical experience broaden our knowledge, changes in treatment and drug therapy may be required. The authors and editors of the material herein have consulted sources believed to be reliable in their efforts to provide information that is complete and in accord with the standards accepted at the time of publication. However, in view of the possibility of human error by the authors, editors, or publisher of the work herein or changes in medical knowledge, neither the authors, editors, nor publisher, nor any other party who has been involved in the preparation of this work, warrants that the information contained herein is in every respect accurate or complete, and they are not responsible for any errors or omissions or for the results obtained from use of such information. Readers are encouraged to confirm the information contained herein with other sources. For example, readers are advised to check the product information sheet included in the package of each drug they plan to administer to be certain that the information contained in this publication is accurate and that changes have not been made in the recommended dose or in the contraindications for administration. This recommendation is of particular importance in connection with new or infrequently used drugs.

Some of the product names, patents, and registered designs referred to in this book are in fact registered trademarks or proprietary names even though specific reference to this fact is not always made in the text. Therefore, the appearance of a name without designation as proprietary is not to be construed as a representation by the publisher that it is in the public domain.

5 4 3 2 1

The Americas ISBN: 978-1-58890-309-9
Rest of World ISBN: 978-3 13 135811 0

I dedicate this textbook to my wife and best friend, Valerie, and to my children, Corrianne and Noah, for their enduring love, patience, and support, as well as to my parents, John and Marcia Werning, for their love and unwavering support of my goals.

Contents

Foreword

The management of squamous cell carcinoma of the upper aerodigestive tract has evolved significantly during the past two decades. For patients with carcinoma of the oropharynx, hypopharynx, or larynx, functional organ preservation through the application of nonsurgical modalities has become the overarching principle of treatment, as the quest for therapies that provide significant survival benefit continues.

In contrast, surgery remains the primary treatment for patients with cancer of the oral cavity and has been demonstrated to provide better disease control and functional outcome than nonsurgical methods. Some 40 years ago, it was established that definitive radiation for squamous cell carcinoma of the oral cavity was associated with an unacceptable incidence of severe fibrosis, xerostomia, and osteoradionecrosis of the jaws. Contemporary methods of reconstruction introduced in the late 1980s permitted transfer of vascularized soft tissue and bone to reconstruct the tongue, floor of the mouth, and mandible with a high degree of success and acceptable functional outcome. Reliable free tissue transfer provided the oncologic surgeon with the latitude to resect tumors with adequate margins, knowing that advanced reconstruction would provide restoration of form and function and well-vascularized tissues that could better withstand postoperative radiotherapy. It is likely that the combination of better surgical resection—guided by contemporary imaging to more accurately assess the local extension of oral cavity tumors—and advanced reconstruction has contributed to the improved survival witnessed in these patients over the past decade.

Oral Cancer: Diagnosis, Management, and Rehabilitation is an important addition to the existing textbooks devoted to head and neck oncology. Editor John Werning, M.D., D.M.D., sought contributions from an expert field of clinicians to produce a textbook firmly advocating the multidisciplinary approach to cancer treatment that will afford patients the optimal chance for cure. Clearly articulated is the concept that comprehensive therapy will provide a high degree of tumor control and cosmetic and functional restoration. Dr. Werning has assembled in logical progression the key information necessary for the diagnostic evaluation, staging, and treatment of patients with oral cavity cancer.

Oral Cancer begins with a discussion of epidemiology and the molecular events that are precursors to invasive cancer, providing an understanding of the molecular biology of oral cancer progression that is critical to developing risk assessment models and identifying targets for new therapies. On this broad foundation, subsequent chapters provide an in-depth discussion of patterns of disease progression and a comprehensive management approach for the oral cavity subsites. The chapters focusing on cancer treatment are written in tandem by Dr. Werning, a head and neck surgical oncologist, and his University of Florida colleague, noted radiation oncologist William M. Mendenhall, and provide a comprehensive multidisciplinary management philosophy. Their approach leads to a consistency that is elusive with many multiauthored texts.

A key element in the treatment of patients with oral cancer is state-of-the-art reconstruction, and leaders in the field have contributed site-specific chapters covering the reconstructive options that are time tested and effective for restoring form and function. Appropriately, prosthetic rehabilitation, implantology, and speech and swallowing rehabilitation are covered in depth and serve as an adjunct to the chapters on therapy and surgical reconstruction. The textbook appropriately concludes with a discussion of future directions in cancer therapy, novel therapeutics that are on the horizon, and options for managing treatment sequelae that can significantly affect a patient's quality of life.

Oral Cancer: Diagnosis, Management, and Rehabilitation is an important new resource for the multidisciplinary team dedicated to the care of patients with oral cancer. Its comprehensive coverage of oral cancer prevention, diagnosis, therapy, reconstruction, and rehabilitation will assist providers in improving both therapeutic outcome and patient quality of life.

Randal S. Weber, M.D., F.A.C.S.
Chairman, Department of Head and Neck Surgery
Hubert L. and Olive Stringer Distinguished
Professor in Cancer Research
Professor of Radiation Oncology
University of Texas M. D. Anderson Cancer Center
Houston, Texas

Preface

The management of head and neck cancer is inherently multidisciplinary—that is, optimal outcomes are usually achieved through collaboration among clinicians from several disciplines, including radiology, pathology, dentistry, surgical oncology, radiation oncology, and medical oncology. Consequently, most head and neck cancer textbooks are compilations of chapters that have been written by contributors from several fields of specialization. Unfortunately, while the intent of such a textbook is to provide the reader with a multidisciplinary management perspective, the final offering is more frequently a collection of topical overviews from each author's viewpoint. The big picture becomes "lost in translation," and the reader is left to assimilate fragmented pieces of insightful information into his or her own treatment philosophy.

Oral Cancer: Diagnosis, Management, and Rehabilitation departs from this formulaic approach by interweaving the insights provided by each contributor into a unified management philosophy that is both multidisciplinary and evidence-based. These two concepts are interdependent on each other: The coordination of treatment between various disciplines is facilitated by knowledge of the best current evidence, and implementation of effective evidence-based treatment often requires interdisciplinary collaboration. Accordingly, the various evidence-based diagnoses and treatment recommendations offered by each author have been consolidated into a single multidisciplinary perspective that, I believe, supplies the reader with a different educational paradigm that will engender a more standardized approach to the management of oral cancer.

Over the past decade, most of the observed improvements in survival and quality of life for patients who have undergone treatment for head and neck cancer are the product of medical and scientific progress that has been more incremental than exponential and more evolutionary than revolutionary. In the absence of research that leads to revelatory scientific knowledge or a paradigmatic shift in treatment philosophy, the establishment of a unified evidence-based management philosophy would seem to afford the head and neck cancer field with the best opportunity to improve the quality of care.

It is my hope that *Oral Cancer: Diagnosis, Management, and Rehabilitation* provides readers with a more sophisticated appreciation for the complexities and nuances of oral cancer management, increases their knowledge and technical skills, and facilitates meaningful communication between each member of the multidisciplinary head and neck cancer team so that our patients may ultimately benefit by having improved chances for cure and enhanced quality of life.

◆ Acknowledgments

It is with heartfelt appreciation that I thank:

- Anthony Maniglia, Harvey Tucker, and David Stepnick from the University Hospitals of Cleveland for encouraging me to pursue a career in head and neck surgical oncology.
- Helmuth Goepfert, Robert Byers, Gary Clayman, David Callender, Ann Gillenwater, Eduardo Diaz, Jeffrey Myers, and Susan Eicher from the The University of Texas M. D. Anderson Cancer Center for transforming me into a head and neck surgical oncologist.
- William Mendenhall and Nicholas Cassisi for their continued professional support and mentorship.
- Patrick Antonelli for being a supportive chairman and colleague.

I am grateful to J. Owen Zurhellen and Esther Gumpert, the editors at Thieme, for their assistance and guidance, and to artist Anthony M. Pazos, for his creative talents and unique ability to convert the essence of a conversation into a work of art. Angela Prevatt Black generously offered her expertise by assisting me with the photographic editing process. Finally, I am deeply indebted to Sharon Milton-Simmons for her invaluable assistance with the completion of this textbook. Her steadfast devotion to and enthusiasm for this project have been immeasurable.

John W. Werning, M.D., D.M.D.

Contributors

James J. Abrahams, M.D.
Professor
Diagnostic Radiology and
  Surgery
Yale University School of
  Medicine
New Haven, Connecticut

Robert Amdur, M.D.
Professor and Interim Chair
Department of Radiation
  Oncology
University of Florida
Gainesville, Florida

**Richard E. Anderson,
  M.D., F.A.C.P.**
Chairman-CEO
The Doctors Company
Napa, California

Jeffrey A. Bennett, M.D.
Assistant Professor
Department of Radiology
University of Florida
Gainesville, Florida

**Daniel Buchbinder,
  D.M.D., M.D.**
Chief, Division of Maxillofacial
  Surgery
Department of Otolaryngology
Continuum Cancer Centers of
  New York
New York, New York

Michael E. Budd, M.D.
Resident, Plastic Surgery
University of California
Aesthetic and Plastic Surgery
  Institute
Orange, California

Mark S. Chambers, D.M.D., M.S.
Associate Professor
Department of Head and
  Neck Surgery
The University of Texas
  M. D. Anderson Cancer Center
Houston, Texas

Douglas B. Chepeha, M.D.
Associate Professor
Department of Otolaryngology–
  Head and Neck Surgery
University of Michigan Hospitals
Ann Arbor Michigan

Parminder Deol, M.D.
Fellow, Neuroradiology
Yale University School of Medicine
New Haven, Connecticut

**M. Franklin Dolwick,
  D.M.D., Ph.D.**
Professor and Director, Division of
  Oral and Maxillofacial Surgery
Department of Oral and
  Maxillofacial Surgery and
  Diagnostic Sciences
University of Florida
Gainesville, Florida

Gregory R. D. Evans, M.D.
Professor
Department of Surgery and the
  Center for Biomedical
  Engineering
Chief, Division of Plastic Surgery
University of California, Irvine
Irvine, California

Caroline E. Fife, M.D.
Chairman
Memorial Hermann Center
  for Wound Healing
Memorial Hermann Hospital
Houston, Texas

Neal D. Futran, M.D., D.M.D.
Professor and Director, Head
  and Neck Services
Department of Otolaryngology–
  Head and Neck Surgery
University of Washington
Seattle, Washington

Adam S. Garden, M.D.
Professor of Radiation Oncology
Medical Director, Head and
  Neck Center
Department of Radiation
  Oncology
The University of Texas
  M. D. Anderson Cancer Center
Houston, Texas

Leslie Gartner, Ph.D.
Professor
Department of Biomedical Sciences
Baltimore College of Dental
  Surgery
University of Maryland, Baltimore
Baltimore, Maryland

Peter J. Gerngross, D.D.S., M.S.
Maxillofacial Prosthodontist
Michael E. DeBakey VA Medical
  Center
Houston, Texas

Ann Gillenwater, M.D.
Associate Professor
Department of Head and Neck
  Surgery
The University of Texas
  M. D. Anderson Cancer Center
Houston, Texas

Maura L. Gillison, M.D., Ph.D.
Assistant Professor
Sidney Kimmel Comprehensive
  Cancer Center
The Johns Hopkins University
Baltimore, Maryland

Henry A. Gremillion, D.D.S.
Professor and Director
Parker E. Mahan Facial Pain Center
Department of Orthodontics
University of Florida College
  of Dentistry
Gainesville, Florida

Patrick J. Gullane, M.B., F.R.C.S.C., F.A.C.S., F.R.A.C.S. (hon.)
Professor and Chair
Department of Otolaryngology–
  Head and Neck Surgery
University of Toronto
Toronto General Hospital
Toronto, Ontario, Canada

James L. Hiatt, Ph.D.
Professor Emeritus
Department of Biomedical
  Sciences
Baltimore College of Dental
  Surgery
University of Maryland,
  Baltimore
Baltimore, Maryland

Russell W. Hinerman, M.D.
Associate Professor
Department of Radiation Oncology
University of Florida
Gainesville, Florida

Mark E. Izzard, M.B.B.S., F.R.A.C.S.
Head and Neck Surgeon
Auckland City Hospital
Auckland, New Zealand

Sanjay R. Jain, M.D., Ph.D.
Staff Physician
Division of Hematology and Oncology
Beth Israel Deaconess Medical
  Center
Boston, Massachusetts

Fadlo R. Khuri, M.D.
Professor of Hematology, Oncology,
  Medicine, Pharmacology and
  Otolaryngology
Blomeyer Chair in Translational
  Cancer Research
Associate Director, Clinical and
  Translational Research
Chief Medical Officer, Winship
  Cancer Institute
Emory University School of
  Medicine
Atlanta, Georgia

Edward S. Kim, M.D.
Assistant Professor
Thoracic/Head and Neck Medical
  Oncology
The University of Texas
  M. D. Anderson Cancer Center
Houston, Texas

Christopher D. Lansford, M.D.
Clinical Assistant Professor
University of Illinois,
  Urbana-Champaign
Carle Clinic Association
Department of Otolaryngology–
  Head and Neck Surgery
Urbana, Illinois

James C. Lemon, D.D.S.
Professor
Department of Head and
  Neck Surgery
The University of Texas
  M. D. Anderson Cancer Center
Houston, Texas

Jan S. Lewin, Ph.D., M.S.
Associate Professor
Department of Head and
  Neck Surgery
The University of Texas
  M. D. Anderson Cancer Center
Houston, Texas

Kristen Lloyd, M.D.
Resident
Department of Radiology
Emory University School of
  Medicine
Atlanta, Georgia

William M. Lydiatt, M.D.
Associate Professor
Department of Otolaryngology–
  Head and Neck Surgery
University of Nebraska Medical
  Center
Omaha, Nebraska

Ellen F. Manzullo, M.D., F.A.C.P.
Professor
Department of General Internal
  Medicine
The University of Texas
  M. D. Anderson Cancer Center
Houston, Texas

Jack W. Martin, D.D.S., M.S.
Professor and Chief
Section of Oncologic Dentistry
  and Prosthodontics
Department of Head and
  Neck Surgery
The University of Texas
  M. D. Anderson Cancer Center
Houston, Texas

William M. Mendenhall, M.D.
Professor
Department of Radiation Oncology
University of Florida
Gainesville, Florida

Jeffrey S. Moyer, M.D.
Assistant Professor
Department of Otolaryngology–
  Head and Neck Surgery
University of Michigan Hospitals
Ann Arbor, Michigan

Susan Müller, D.M.D., M.S.
Associate Professor
Department of Otolaryngology–
  Head and Neck Surgery, and
Department of Pathology
  and Laboratory Medicine
Emory University School
  of Medicine
Atlanta, Georgia

Peter Neligan, M.D.
Wharton Chair in Reconstructive
  Plastic Surgery
Professor and Chair
Division of Plastic Surgery
University of Toronto
Toronto General Hospital
Toronto, Ontario, Canada

Alyssa G. Rieber, M.D.
Fellow
Division of Cancer Medicine
The University of Texas
  M. D. Anderson Cancer
  Center
Houston, Texas

Hugo St. Hilaire, D.D.S., M.D.
Fellow
Division of Plastic and
  Reconstructive Surgery
Department of Surgery
Louisiana State University
New Orleans, Louisiana

Pamela L. Sandow, D.M.D.
Clinical Associate Professor
Department of Oral and
  Maxillofacial Surgery and
  Diagnostic Sciences
University of Florida
Gainesville, Florida

Erich M. Sturgis, M.D., M.P.H.
Associate Professor
Department of Head and
  Neck Surgery
The University of Texas
  M. D. Anderson Cancer Center
Houston, Texas

Theodoros N. Teknos, M.D.
Associate Professor
Department of Otolaryngology–
  Head and Neck Surgery
University of Michigan Hospitals
Ann Arbor, Michigan

Kevin Rand Torske, D.D.S., M.S.
Commander, United States Navy
Central Identification
  Laboratory
Joint POW/MIA Accounting
  Command
Hickam Air Force Base, Hawaii

Douglas B. Villaret, M.D.
Associate Professor
Department of Otolaryngology
University of Florida
Gainesville, Florida

Qingyi Wei, M.D., Ph.D.
Professor
Department of Epidemiology
The University of Texas
  M. D. Anderson Cancer Center
Houston, Texas

**John W. Werning, M.D.,
  D.M.D.**
Assistant Professor
Department of Otolaryngology
University of Florida
Gainesville, Florida

1

Epidemiology of Oral Cancer

Erich M. Sturgis and
Qingyi Wei

Although head and neck cancer is relatively rare in the United States, it is a common disease entity in some parts of the developing world. In the United States, the vast majority of head and neck malignancies are squamous cell carcinomas of the upper aerodigestive tract (i.e., the oral cavity, oro- and hypopharynx, and the larynx).[1] Because the epidemiologies of oral cavity cancer, pharyngeal cancer, and laryngeal cancer are so similar, these sites are often discussed as a single entity, squamous cell carcinoma of the head and neck (SCCHN). This chapter discusses oral cavity carcinomas (OCCs) as part of the entity of SCCHN and provides more specific information on OCC, as available. Approximately 90% of SCCHN occurs as a result of the use of tobacco or alcohol.[2-5] Emerging information suggests that, in addition to tobacco and alcohol use, an individual's genetic background and environmental exposures may increase the risk of SCCHN. Ultimately, public health initiatives must strive to prevent these malignancies by reducing the use of tobacco and alcohol, discovering other causative agents and persuading the public to avoid them, and identifying genetically susceptible individuals.

◆ Descriptive Epidemiology

Incidence

Approximately 19,400 new cases of OCC, 8300 new cases of pharyngeal cancer, and 9500 new cases of laryngeal cancer were diagnosed in 2003 (**Fig. 1–1**).[6] Head and neck cancers account for approximately 3% of all new cancer cases (excluding basal and squamous cell carcinomas of the skin)

in the United States, annually.[6] Since 1985, the annual absolute incidence of OCC and pharyngeal cancer has been approximately 21,000 and 9000 new cases, respectively; however, the number of newly diagnosed cases of laryngeal cancer has steadily declined from 12,600 in 1993 to only 9500 new cases in 2003 (**Fig. 1–1**).[6-8]

In the United States, approximately one in three OCCs and pharyngeal cancers and one in five laryngeal cancers occur in women.[6] The incidence of OCC and pharyngeal cancer is twice as high in men, and the incidence of laryngeal cancer is greater than three times more frequent in men than in women.[8] From the mid-1980s to 1999, the incidence rate (age-adjusted to the 2000 U.S. standard) for both OCCs and pharyngeal cancer in men steadily declined to 15.2/100,000. However, this rate was relatively stable in women during the same period.[8] Although black and white women have similar rates of OCC and pharyngeal cancer, black men have a 30% higher rate than white men, and Hispanics manifest the lowest rates.[8]

The median age at diagnosis for SCCHN is approximately 60 years, but the incidence of these cancers in young adults (age <40 years) appears to be increasing.[9-13] This increase has not been apparent in African Americans, and carcinoma of the tongue appears to account for most of the increased incidence.[1-13]

Although head and neck cancer is relatively rare in the United States, it is the fifth most common cancer worldwide.[14,15] In some regions of the world, head and neck cancers are the most common malignancies found in men. For example, in 1990 south-central Asia, home to one fifth of the world's population, there were approximately 76,800 new cases of OCC, which composed 8% of all cancers and 11% of all cancers occurring in men.[14] Although 77% of head

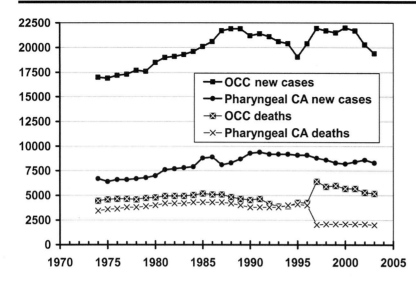

Figure 1–1   Incidence and mortality of oral cavity carcinomas and pharyngeal cancer in the United States.

and neck cancers in south-central Asia are OCCs and pharyngeal (excluding nasopharyngeal) cancers, laryngeal cancers and nasopharyngeal cancers account for a much higher percentage of head and neck malignancies in other regions of the world. For example, in southern and eastern Europe, approximately 40% of all head and neck cancers are laryngeal cancers. In China, nasopharyngeal cancer accounts for 55% of all head and neck cancers, and in Southeast Asia, nasopharyngeal cancer accounts for 70% of all head and neck cancers.[14]

Prevalence

In 1998, there were 219,175 individuals with a history of OCC or pharyngeal cancer in the United States.[8] As expected, the sex distribution of these prevalence figures reflects the sex distribution of the incident cases. However, African Americans accounted for only 7.9% of the prevalent OCCs and pharyngeal cancers, which probably reflects the poorer overall survival of African Americans diagnosed with OCC. African Americans have survival rates for OCC and pharyngeal cancer that are approximately 20% worse than those for Caucasians for the past 25 years.[6,8] The discrepancy in survival between Caucasians and African Americans has remained relatively constant over the past three decades, and survival has not improved for either group during that time period.[6,8]

Worldwide, head and neck cancer is the third most prevalent cancer after breast and colorectal cancers, accounting for 7% of the 22.4 million individuals with cancer (excluding nonmelanoma skin cancer).[15] Of the approximate 1.6 million individuals with head and neck cancer, 707,100 have OCC and 248,800 have oro- or hypopharyngeal cancer.[15]

Mortality

In the United States, it was expected that 11,000 individuals would die from head and neck cancer in 2003, including 5200 from OCC and 2000 from pharyngeal cancer (**Fig. 1–1**).[6] However, head and neck cancer accounts for less than 2% of all cancer deaths in the United States annually.[6] Although less than half the number of people

died from pharyngeal cancer in 2003 as in 1983, the number of deaths from OCC during the same time period has not declined (**Fig. 1–1**).[6,7]

In the United States, the ratio of males to females that die from head and neck cancer is similar to the incidence of these cancers in both groups.[6] The age-adjusted mortality rates for OCC and pharyngeal cancer have steadily declined over the past two decades.[8] African Americans have higher OCC and pharyngeal cancer mortality rates than whites (**Fig. 1–2**),[8] whereas Hispanics have the lowest mortality rates.[8] The discrepancy in mortality between African-American males and white males is the fourth highest among all types of cancer in the United States.[16]

Worldwide, head and neck cancer accounts for 333,400 deaths annually (127,900 due to OCC and 78,700 due to oro- or hypopharyngeal cancers).[15] As with other cancer sites, the mortality to incidence ratio for head and neck cancers is much higher in developing countries for both men and women than in the United States, probably because of the better survival for these cancers in the United States.[15]

◆ Risk Factors

Tobacco Use

Tobacco has a linear dose–response carcinogenic effect in which duration is more important than the intensity of exposure. The major carcinogenic activity of cigarette smoke resides in the particulate (tar) fraction, which contains a complex mixture of interacting cancer initiators, promoters, and co-carcinogens. In the late 1950s, a landmark case-control study by Dr. Ernst Wynder established the link between tobacco use and OCC.[17] This was followed a year later by a cohort study of more than 180,000 men that revealed a higher risk of death due to SCCHN in cigarette smokers than in men who never smoked.[18] These studies also showed elevated risks for SCCHN death in cigar and pipe smokers. In 1964, the Advisory Committee to the Surgeon General of the Public Health Service published its

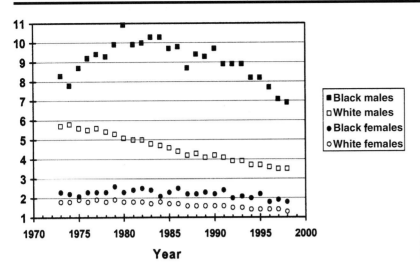

Figure 1–2 Oral cavity carcinomas and pharyngeal cancer mortality rates, age-adjusted to the 1970 United States standard.

report linking smoking to cancer, which was based on many of Doll and Hill's criteria for disease causality.[19,20] Because of its small sample size and short follow-up time, Doll and Hill's classic cohort study of more than 40,000 British physicians showed only a borderline increase in risk of SCCHN related to smoking.[19] However, multiple independent investigations over the past 40 years have confirmed Doll and Hill's criteria demonstrating a link between SCCHN and tobacco smoking.[2–5,17,18,21–24] Most importantly, the strength and consistency of the association between smoking and SCCHN have been demonstrated in numerous case-control and cohort studies with statistically significant relative risk or odds ratios in the 3- to 12-fold range. Furthermore, these studies consistently showed a dose–response effect, with an increased risk of SCCHN that was related to the duration and frequency of smoking, and a decrease in risk that was related to the length of time since tobacco use had been terminated.[2–5,21,22,25] Other mucosal malignancies of the head and neck such as nasopharyngeal carcinoma and sinonasal malignancies have a weaker association with tobacco use.[26] The strength of the association between tobacco use and SCCHN as well as the biologic plausibility of the well-established tobacco-induced carcinogenesis model have established tobacco as the chief etiologic agent in SCCHN.

Although the risk of bronchogenic carcinoma appears to be less significant for cigar and pipe smokers than for cigarette smokers, these forms of tobacco use are also clearly associated with an increased risk of OCC[2,3,5,17,25,27] (reviewed in Baker et al[28]). The pooling of saliva containing carcinogens in low areas of the mouth may account for the frequent occurrence of oral carcinomas along the lateral and ventral surfaces of the tongue and in the floor of the mouth.[29] Smokeless tobacco use has also been associated with OCC.[29–32] Some have suggested that the type of smokeless tobacco may be related to the risk of developing cancer,[33] and some studies from Scandinavia have found that the use of Swedish snuff did not elevate the risk of OCC.[34,35] Smokeless tobacco users and pipe smokers who frequently position the quid or pipe stem in the same place often develop carcinomas and dysplasias at that site, which suggests that physical and thermal trauma may contribute to OCC.

In the United States, smoking rates have declined since the Surgeon General's warning in 1964.[36] Between 1965 and 1999, the proportion of the U.S. adult population that smoked decreased from 42.4% to only 23.5%. Although the reduction in cigarette smoking over the last three decades has been much greater in men, the rate of current cigarette use remains higher in men (25.7%) than in women (21.5%). In addition, 40.8% of Native Americans continue to smoke.[36,37] Other concerns include the increasing rates of cigarette smoking among high-school seniors and the dramatic increase in the number of new cigar users in the last decade.[36,37] Sharp increases in smokeless tobacco use have also been implicated in the rise of OCC mortality rates among young people.[9–13,38]

Although smoking rates are declining in industrialized countries, they are rising in the developing world, where four fifths of the world's population resides. The striking variations in head and neck cancer sites and incidence seen among different regional, cultural, and demographic groups are due in large part to differences in the use of tobacco and other substances.[2,31] Smokeless tobacco and similar products are frequently used in parts of Asia and Africa.[30,31,33,39] Most tobacco consumed in India is in the form of unregulated tobacco products. Bidis (hand-rolled, filterless tobacco cigarettes produced at home, mainly by millions of poor women and children) account for at least 40% of all tobacco consumed in India.[40] Other common tobacco products in India include hookah (traditional water pipe), chutta (clumps of tobacco smoked with the lighted end inside of the mouth), mishri (a powdered tobacco rubbed on the gums), and various other forms of smokeless tobacco products.[40,41] Furthermore, pano (a mixture of betel leaf, lime, catechu, and areca nut) is commonly chewed in India, either mixed with tobacco or alone, and is a strong risk factor independent of tobacco use for carcinoma of the oral cavity.[39,42]

Alcohol Use

Tobacco is not the only factor in the complex causality equation of these cancers. Alcohol, another etiologic agent for risk of SCCHN, is an important promoter of carcinogenesis and contributes to at least 75% of SCCHNs.[2] Furthermore, alcohol appears to result in an increase in risk of developing SCCHN that is independent of tobacco use.[2-5,17,22] Studies attempting to correlate the type of alcoholic beverage with specific cancer risks have had conflicting results, and most investigators believe that ethanol itself is the main causative factor.[2,3,5,17,22,43] Nevertheless, the major clinical significance of alcohol consumption appears to be that it potentiates the carcinogenic effect of tobacco at every level of tobacco use, although this effect is most striking at the highest levels of alcohol use. The magnitude of the effect is at least additive, but may be multiplicative for certain SCCHN subsites and at the highest levels of exposure.[2-5,21,22] Mate, a nonalcoholic tea-like beverage that is brewed in South America, has also been linked to SCCHN after adjustment for smoking.[44]

Genetic Susceptibility

The predominant risk factor for SCCHN is a history of exposure to tobacco and alcohol. However, because only a fraction of smokers and drinkers develop cancer, variations in genetic susceptibility may be equally important in the etiology of SCCHN. That SCCHN has a genetic component has also been supported by large family studies demonstrating a three- to eightfold increased risk of SCCHN in the first-degree relatives of patients with SCCHN.[45-48] Furthermore, there is molecular epidemiologic evidence for genetic susceptibility in SCCHN patients.[49] Emerging data from several case-control phenotypic and genotypic studies support the hypothesis that genetic susceptibility plays an important role in the etiology of SCCHN. According to this hypothesis, inherited differences in the efficiency of carcinogen-metabolizing systems, DNA repair systems, or cell-cycle control/apoptosis systems influence an individual's risk for tobacco-induced cancers. Identifying such at-risk individuals in the general population, by use of these biomarker assays, would substantially improve primary prevention, early detection, and secondary prevention strategies.

Infectious Agents

Although it has been suggested that various infectious agents play a role in head and neck carcinogenesis, only Epstein-Barr virus (EBV) and human papillomavirus (HPV) can be implicated as etiologic agents in head and neck carcinogenesis based on current scientific evidence. EBV infection appears to be associated with most nasopharyngeal carcinomas.[50-54] HPV (most commonly type 16) infection is associated with approximately 50% of oropharyngeal carcinomas, but HPV does not appear to play a major role in OCC[55-57] (reviewed in Gillison et al[58]). HPV infection may also be involved in the etiology of squamous cell carcinomas arising in the sinonasal tract.[59] Although herpes simplex virus infection has been suggested as a risk factor for OCC,[60] this connection has not been confirmed.

Environmental Tobacco Smoke

A recent high-profile legal case in Australia brought significant attention to the risk of SCCHN from exposure to environmental tobacco. In May 2001, the New South Wales Supreme Court ruled that a 62-year-old nonsmoker's SCCHN was associated with long-term exposure to environmental tobacco smoke in her job as a bar attendant, and imposed liability on her employer.[61,62] The results of two case-control studies were used to support the court's finding. In a study of 173 cases of SCCHN and 176 cancer-free controls, environmental tobacco smoke was associated with a more than twofold increased risk of SCCHN, and a dose–response relationship was also observed.[63] In a separate investigation of 44 nonsmokers with SCCHN and 132 cancer-free nonsmoker controls, environmental tobacco smoke was associated with a significantly increased risk for SCCHN [odds ratio (OR) = 5.34], especially for women (OR = 8.00) and for those reporting exposure at work (OR = 10.16).[64]

Marijuana

Marijuana smoke has four times more tar and 50% more benzopyrene and aromatic hydrocarbons than does tobacco smoke. Although anecdotal evidence has long suggested that marijuana use is a risk factor for SCCHN, few studies have found direct evidence that marijuana is an etiologic factor for SCCHN because most marijuana users also use tobacco and alcohol.[65,66] A recent case-control study demonstrated a cigarette-adjusted risk for SCCHN of 2.6 [95% confidence interval (CI) 1.1–6.6] associated with marijuana use, and evidence for a dose–response relationship.[67] However, a large retrospective cohort of 64,855 members of a health-maintenance organization found no association between marijuana use and tobacco-related cancers.[68]

Diet

Epidemiologic evidence from traditional case-control studies has suggested that diets high in animal fats and low in fruits and vegetables may increase the risk for SCCHN.[69-72] Winn and colleagues[69] found that the risk of oral and pharyngeal cancer in women is inversely related to their consumption of fresh fruits and vegetables. Similarly, in a study of 871 individuals with oral and pharyngeal cancer and 979 cancer-free controls, McLaughlin et al[70] noted an inverse relationship between fruit intake and the risk of oral and pharyngeal cancer. More recently, European and U.S. studies have confirmed the protective effects of fruits and vegetables and the risk of animal fat consumption after adjustment for smoking and alcohol use.[72,73] Several case-control studies have correlated consumption of salted fish with increased risk of nasopharyngeal carcinoma, perhaps because of the high nitrosamine content of preserved foods such as salted fish.[74,75]

There is some evidence that vitamin A and beta-carotene are responsible for the protective effect of diets high in fruits and vegetables, and deficiencies in carotenoids appear to be a risk factor for SCCHN and lung cancers.[70] It is not known, however, which of the more than 500 carotenoids are protective, what chemical interactions occur, or what protective role other micronutrients in carotenoid-rich foods may play. Others have found that high intake of vitamins C and E is also protective.[69,70] Dietary intake is frequently difficult to assess and validate; in particular, it is often difficult to determine the constituent nutrients of specific foods. Further studies are needed to more precisely define the relationship between dietary intake and serum levels of the various carotenoid components. It may be impossible to determine which of the vast array of compounds is most beneficial, and controlling for other dietary variables and confounding risk factors has remained a difficult methodologic problem. Further confounding this situation, smoking has been associated with reduced dietary intake and serum levels of carotenoids. Despite these issues, prospective and retrospective nutritional (serum and dietary) epidemiologic studies have provided important clues about the development and prevention of oral cancer.

Occupation

Although occupational exposures probably play a minor role in the development of SCCHN, they are major risk factors for malignancies of the sinonasal region.[76] The most important exposures occur in the metalworking and refining, woodworking, and leather/textile industries.[76-78] Although asbestos has been implicated as a risk factor for laryngeal cancer, some of the evidence does not support this association.[79,80]

Radiation

No strong association has been demonstrated between exposure to ionizing radiation and the development of SCCHN. However, squamous carcinomas of the lip are associated with ultraviolet radiation exposure. Furthermore, gamma irradiation is associated with thyroid cancers, sarcomas of the head and neck, and salivary gland malignancies, including paranasal sinus cancers. Therapeutic irradiation of head and neck malignancies does not appear to induce second primary squamous carcinomas of the aerodigestive tract, but it is associated with an increased risk for sarcoma of the head and neck.[81] This is a particular concern for children who have received therapeutic irradiation. Furthermore, environmental, medical diagnostic, and therapeutic irradiation of the head and neck are all significantly associated with salivary gland malignancies.[82,83] These studies revealed a significant dose–response relationship, with risk increasing with dose, and mucoepidermoid carcinomas appear to be the most common radiation-induced malignancy.[82,83] In the past, the use of radium for painting watch dials and the use of Thoratrast, a previously used contrast agent in sinonasal imaging, were associated with increased risk of paranasal sinus malignancies.

Air Pollution

Although recent evidence suggests that fine particulate and sulfur oxide air pollution is a risk factor for lung cancer,[84] most studies exploring air pollution as a risk factor for SCCHN have focused on measurements of indoor exposures. Indoor air pollution has been classified into four categories: emissions of combustion, chemical vapors, radiation gases, and biologic contaminants.[85] In a case-control study from Brazil that included 784 individuals with

SCCHN and 1568 controls, the use of wood stoves for cooking or heating was associated with a significantly increased risk for SCCHN (crude OR = 2.68, 95% CI 2.17–3.31).[86] After adjusting for tobacco and alcohol consumption, the risk of SCCHN associated with wood stove use remained significant (adjusted OR = 2.39, 95% CI 1.88–3.05), as it did after further adjustment for other potential confounders. Furthermore, these risks were consistent across all SCCHN sites (oral cavity, pharynx, and larynx). The authors concluded that 32% of SCCHNs in Brazil may be due to wood stove use. In an earlier study from Brazil that included 232 incident patients with oral cancer and 464 cancer-free individuals, wood stove use was associated with a significant increase in risk for OCC (crude OR = 2.4, 95% CI 1.6–3.5), and this risk was stable after multivariate adjustment for tobacco and alcohol (adjusted OR = 2.5, 95% CI 1.6–3.9).[87] Incident patients with OCC were matched to cancer-free hospital controls by age, sex, and trimester of hospital admission, and questionnaire-based interviews with all subjects were used to obtain exposure information. A German case-control study of 369 subjects with OCC, pharyngeal cancer, or laryngeal cancer, and 1476 matched control subjects showed that both heating and cooking with fossil fuels significantly increase the risk for all three cancers.[88]

However, these risk estimates were not consistently stable after adjustment for tobacco and alcohol consumption. Long-term exposure to outdoor air pollution (both automotive and industrial) did not increase risk.[88] These studies demonstrated that indoor air pollution due to combustion of fossil fuels is an independent and important risk factor for SCCHN in certain parts of the world. Although there is little evidence that other indoor contaminants are risk factors for SCCHN, occupational studies have suggested that indoor exposure to radon gas or volatile chemicals may also increase the risk for SCCHN. Regardless, indoor air pollution is a significant problem in much of the developing world, where indoor stoves using organic or fossil fuels are the primary method of cooking and heating. Not only are these exposures probably risk factors for SCCHN, but they also increase the risk of paranasal sinus cancer, lung cancer, chronic pulmonary disease, and childhood illness.[89,90]

◆ Conclusion

In 2003, there were approximately 20,000 new cases of OCC and 5000 deaths from OCC in the United States.[6] Although OCC annually accounts for only 1.5% of all new cancer cases and less than 1% of all cancer deaths in the United States,[6] it is much more common in certain regions of the world such as south-central Asia. OCC is largely a preventable disease, because tobacco and alcohol are the primary etiologic agents. This assertion is supported by the declining incidence and mortality of OCC and pharyngeal cancer in the United States over the past two decades, which is partly attributable to public anti-tobacco efforts. The impact of anti-tobacco campaigns, however, has slowly occurred. Although smoking rates in the United States began to plateau and eventually decline in the 1960s, the rates of oral and pharyngeal cancer did not decrease until

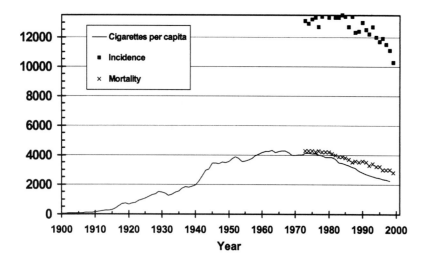

Figure 1–3 Per capita consumption of cigarettes in the United States, and U.S. incidence and mortality rates for oral cavity carcinomas and pharyngeal cancer per 100 million, age-adjusted to the United States 2000 standard.

the mid-1980s (**Fig. 1–3**).[36] Because OCC is a major problem in south-central Asia and other areas of the developing world, aggressive anti-tobacco efforts must be strengthened in these regions. An investment in prevention will help to alleviate future costs to these already overburdened economies and health care systems. Further research into other potential etiologic factors (including genetic susceptibility) will also help to refine prevention strategies. In the United States, disparities in incidence and mortality of OCC in men and African Americans indicate that additional efforts at prevention, early detection, and treatment are imperative in these populations.

References

1. Funk GF, Karnell LH, Robinson RA, Zhen WK, Trask DK, Hoffman HT. Presentation, treatment, and outcome of oral cavity cancer: a national cancer database report. Head Neck 2002;24:165–180

2. Blot WJ, McLaughlin JK, Winn DM, et al. Smoking and drinking in relation to oral and pharyngeal cancer. Cancer Res 1988;48:3282–3287

3. Franceschi S, Talamini R, Barra S, et al. Smoking and drinking in relation to cancers of the oral cavity, pharynx, larynx, and esophagus in Northern Italy. Cancer Res 1990;50:6502–6507

4. Franceschi S, Levi F, La Vecchia C, et al. Comparison of the effect of smoking and alcohol drinking between oral and pharyngeal cancer. Int J Cancer 1999;83:1–4

5. Merletti F, Boffetta P, Ciccone G, Mashberg A, Terracini B. Role of tobacco and alcoholic beverages in the etiology of cancer of the oral cavity/oropharynx in Torino, Italy. Cancer Res 1989;49:4919–4924

6. Jemal A, Murray T, Samuels A, Ghafoor A, Ward E, Thun M. Cancer statistics, 2003. CA Cancer J Clin 2003;53:5–26

7. Silverberg E. Cancer statistics, 1985. CA Cancer J Clin 1985;35:19–35

8. Cancer Statistics Review SEER, 1973–1999. http://seer.cancer.gov/, 2003

9. Shemen LJ, Klotz J, Schottenfeld D, Strong EW. Increase of tongue cancer in young men. JAMA 1984;252:1857

10. Depue RH. Rising mortality from cancer of the tongue in young white males. N Engl J Med 1986;315:647

11. Schantz SP, Byers RM, Goepfert H. Tobacco and cancer of the tongue in young adults. JAMA 1988;259:1943–1944

12. Myers JN, Elkins T, Roberts D, Byers RM. Squamous cell carcinoma of the tongue in young adults: increasing incidence and factors that predict treatment outcomes. Otolaryngol Head Neck Surg 2000;122:44–51

13. Schantz SP, Yu GP. Head and neck cancer incidence trends in young Americans, 1973–1997, with a special analysis for tongue cancer. Arch Otolaryngol Head Neck Surg 2002;128:268–274

14. Parkin DM, Pisani P, Ferlay J. Estimates of the worldwide incidence of 25 major cancers in 1990. Int J Cancer 1999;80:827–841

15. Parkin DM, Bray F, Ferlay J, Pisani P. Estimating the world cancer burden: Globocan 2000. Int J Cancer 2001;94:153–156

16. Ghafoor A, Jemal A, Cokkinides V, et al. Cancer statistics for African Americans. CA Cancer J Clin 2002;52:326–341

17. Wynder EL, Bross IJ, Feldman RM. A study of the etiological factors in cancer of the mouth. Cancer 1957;10:1300–1323

18. Hammond EC, Horn D. Smoking and death rates—report on forty-four months of follow-up of 187,783 men. JAMA 1958;166:1294–1308

19. Doll R, Hill AB. Lung cancer and other causes of death in relation to smoking: a second report on the mortality of British doctors. BMJ 1956;2:1071–1081

20. Smoking and Health. Report of the Advisory Committee to the Surgeon General of the Public Health Service. Washington, DC: U.S. Department of Health, Education, and Welfare, 1964

21. Falk RT, Pickle LW, Brown LM, Mason TJ, Buffler PA, Fraumeni JF. Effect of smoking and alcohol consumption on laryngeal cancer risk in coastal Texas. Cancer Res 1989;49:4024–4029

22. Schlecht NF, Franco EL, Pintos J, et al. Interaction between tobacco and alcohol consumption and the risk of cancers of the upper aerodigestive tract in Brazil. Am J Epidemiol 1999;150:1129–1137

23. Cattaruzza MS, Maisonneuve P, Boyle P. Epidemiology of laryngeal cancer. Eur J Cancer B Oral Oncol 1996;32B:293–305

24. La Vecchia C, Tavani A, Franceschi S, Levi F, Corrao G, Negri E. Epidemiology and prevention of oral cancer. Oral Oncol 1997;33:302–312

25. Schlecht NF, Franco EL, Pintos J, Kowalski LP. Effect of smoking cessation and tobacco type on the risk of cancers of the upper aerodigestive tract in Brazil. Epidemiology 1999;10:412–418

26. Zhu K, Levine RS, Brann EA, Hall HI, Caplan LS, Gnepp DR. Case-control study evaluating the homogeneity and heterogeneity of risk factors between sinonasal and nasopharyngeal cancers. Int J Cancer 2002;99:119–123

27. Iribarren C, Tekawa IS, Sidney S, Friedman GD. Effect of cigar smoking on the risk of cardiovascular disease, chronic obstructive pulmonary disease, and cancer in men. N Engl J Med 1999;340:1773–1780

28. Baker F, Ainsworth SR, Dye JT, et al. Health risks associated with cigar smoking. JAMA 2000;284:735–740

29. Moore C, Catlin D. Anatomic origins and locations of oral cancer. Am J Surg 1967;114:510–513

30. Rao DN, Ganesh B, Rao RS, Desai PB. Risk assessment of tobacco, alcohol and diet in oral cancer—a case-control study. Int J Cancer 1994;58:469–473

31. Scully C, Bedi R. Ethnicity and oral cancer. Lancet Oncol 2000;1:37–42

32. Winn DM. Smokeless tobacco and cancer: the epidemiologic evidence. CA Cancer J Clin 1988;38:236–243

33. Idris AM, Ibrahim SO, Vasstrand EN, et al. The Swedish snus and the Sudanese toombak: are they different? Oral Oncol 1998;34:558–566

34. Lewin F, Norell SE, Johansson H, et al. Smoking tobacco, oral snuff, and alcohol in the etiology of squamous cell carcinoma of the head and neck: a population-based case-referent study in Sweden. Cancer 1998;82:1367–1375

35. Schildt EB, Eriksson M, Hardell L, Magnuson A. Oral snuff, smoking habits and alcohol consumption in relation to oral cancer in a Swedish case-control study. Int J Cancer 1998;77:341–346

36. Centers for Disease Control and Prevention. Tobacco use—United States, 1900–1999. MMWR Morb Mortal Wkly Rep 1999;48:986–993

37. Centers for Disease Control and Prevention. Cigarette smoking among adults—United States, 1999. MMWR Morb Mortal Wkly Rep 2001;50:869–873

38. Marwick C. Increasing use of chewing tobacco, especially among younger persons, alarms surgeon general. JAMA 1993;269:195

39. Merchant A, Husain SSM, Hosain M, et al. Paan without tobacco: an independent risk factor for oral cancer. Int J Cancer 2000;86:128–131

40. Shimkhada R, Peabody JW. Tobacco control in India. Bull World Health Organ 2003;81:48–52

41. Zolty B. Country profiles: India. In: Lopez A, ed. Tobacco or Health: A Global Status Report. Geneva: WHO Reg Publ Eur Ser, 1997;414–417

42. Brandwein-Gensler M, Hille JJ. Behind the cover: the guthka story. Arch Otolaryngol Head Neck Surg 2003;129:699–700

43. Kabat GC, Wynder EL. Type of alcoholic beverage and oral cancer. Int J Cancer 1989;43:190–194

44. Goldenberg D, Golz A, Joachims HZ. The beverage mate: a risk factor for cancer of the head and neck. Head Neck 2003;25:595–601

45. Goldgar DE, Easton DF, Cannon-Albright LA, Skolnick MH. Systematic population-based assessment of cancer risk in first-degree relatives of cancer probands. J Natl Cancer Inst 1994;86:1600–1608

46. Foulkes WD, Brunet JS, Kowalski LP, Narod SA, Franco EL. Family history of cancer is a risk factor for squamous cell carcinoma of the head and neck in Brazil: a case-control study. Int J Cancer 1995;63:769–773

47. Copper MP, Jovanovic A, Nauta JJ, et al. Role of genetic factors in the etiology of squamous cell carcinoma of the head and neck. Arch Otolaryngol Head Neck Surg 1995;121:157–160

48. Foulkes WD, Brunet JS, Sieh W, et al. Familial risks of squamous cell carcinoma of the head and neck: retrospective case-control study. BMJ 1996;313:716–721

49. Sturgis EM, Wei Q. Genetic susceptibility—molecular epidemiology of head and neck cancer. Curr Opin Oncol 2002;14:310–317

50. Henle W, Henle G, Ho HC, et al. Antibodies to Epstein-Barr virus in nasopharyngeal carcinoma, other head and neck neoplasms, and control groups. J Natl Cancer Inst 1970;44:225–231

51. Pearson GR, Weiland LH, Neel HB, et al. Application of Epstein-Barr virus (EBV) serology to the diagnosis of North American nasopharyngeal carcinoma. Cancer 1983;51:260–268

52. Feinmesser R, Miyazaki I, Cheung R, Freeman JL, Noyek AM, Dosch HM. Diagnosis of nasopharyngeal carcinoma by DNA amplification of tissue obtained by fine-needle aspiration. N Engl J Med 1992;326:17–21

53. Zong YS, Sham JS, Ng MH, et al. Immunoglobulin A against viral capsid antigen of Epstein-Barr virus and indirect mirror examination of the nasopharynx in the detection of asymptomatic nasopharyngeal carcinoma. Cancer 1992;69:3–7

54. Chien YC, Chen JY, Liu MY, et al. Serologic markers of Epstein-Barr virus infection and nasopharyngeal carcinoma in Taiwanese men. N Engl J Med 2001;345:1877–1882

55. Mork J, Lie AK, Glattre E, et al. Human papilloma virus infection as a risk factor for squamous-cell carcinoma of the head and neck. N Engl J Med 2001;344:1125–1131

56. Schwartz SM, Daling JR, Doody DR, et al. Oral cancer risk in relation to sexual history and evidence of human papillomavirus infection. J Natl Cancer Inst 1998;90:1626–1636

57. Strome SE, Savva A, Brissett AE, et al. Squamous cell carcinoma of the tonsils: a molecular analysis of HPV associations. Clin Cancer Res 2002;8:1093–1100

58. Gillison ML, Koch WM, Capone RB, et al. Evidence for a causal association between human papillomavirus and a subset of head and neck cancers. J Natl Cancer Inst 2000;92:709–720

59. Dictor M, Johnson A. Association of inverted sinonasal papilloma with non-sinonasal head-and-neck carcinoma. Int J Cancer 2000;85:811–814

60. Maden C, Beckmann AM, Thomas DB, et al. Human papillomaviruses, herpes simplex viruses, and the risk of oral cancer in men. Am J Epidemiol 1992;135:1093–1102

61. Loff B, Cordner S. Passive smoking test case wins in Australia. Lancet 2001;357:1511

62. Chapman S. Australian bar worker wins payout in passive smoking case. BMJ 2001;322:1139

63. Zhang ZF, Morgenstern H, Spitz MR, et al. Environmental tobacco smoking, mutagen sensitivity, and head and neck squamous cell carcinoma. Cancer Epidemiol Biomarkers Prev 2000;9:1043–1049

64. Tan E-H, Adelstein DJ, Droughton MLT, Van Kirk MA, Lavertu P. Squamous cell head and neck cancer in nonsmokers. Am J Clin Oncol 1997;20:146–150

65. Donald PJ. Marijuana smoking—possible cause of head and neck carcinoma in young patients. Otolaryngol Head Neck Surg 1986;94:517–521

66. Caplan GA, Brigham BA. Marijuana smoking and carcinoma of the tongue; is there an association? Cancer 1990;66:1005–1006

67. Zhang ZF, Morgenstern H, Spitz MR, et al. Marijuana use and increased risk of squamous cell carcinoma of the head and neck. Cancer Epidemiol Biomarkers Prev 1999;8:1071–1078

68. Sidney S, Quesenberry CP, Friedman GD, Tekawa IS. Marijuana use and cancer incidence (California, United States). Cancer Causes Control 1997;8:722–728

69. Winn DM, Ziegler RG, Pickle LW, Gridley G, Blot WJ, Hoover RN. Diet in the etiology of oral and pharyngeal cancer among women from the southern United States. Cancer Res 1984;44:1216–1222

70. McLaughlin JK, Gridley G, Block G, et al. Dietary factors in oral and pharyngeal cancer. J Natl Cancer Inst 1988;80:1237–1243

71. Zheng W, Blot WJ, Shu XO, et al. Diet and other risk factors for laryngeal cancer in Shanghai, China. Am J Epidemiol 1992;136:178–191

72. Levi F, Pasche C, LaVecchia C, Lucchini F, Franceschi S, Monnier P. Food groups and risk of oral and pharyngeal cancer. Int J Cancer 1998;77:705–709

73. Schantz SP, Zhang ZF, Spitz MS, Sun M, Hsu TC. Genetic susceptibility to head and neck cancer: interaction between nutrition and mutagen sensitivity. Laryngoscope 1997;107:765–781

74. Ning JP, Yu MC, Wang QS, Henderson BE. Consumption of salted fish and other risk factors for nasopharyngeal carcinoma (NPC) in Tianjiin, a low-risk region for NPC in the People's Republic of China. J Natl Cancer Inst 1990;82:291–296

75. Farrow DC, Vaughan TL, Berwick M, Lynch CF, Swanson GM, Lyon JL. Diet and nasopharyngeal cancer in a low-risk population. Int J Cancer 1998;78:675–679

76. Mannetje A, Kogevinas M, Luce D, et al. Sinonasal cancer, occupation, and tobacco smoking in European women and men. Am J Ind Med 1999;36:101–107

77. Luce D, Gerin M, Morcet JF, Leclerc A. Sinonasal cancer and occupational exposure to textile dust. Am J Ind Med 1997;32:205–210

78. Holt GR. Sinonasal neoplasms and inhaled air toxics. Otolaryngol Head Neck Surg 1994;111:12–14

79. Straif K, Keil U, Taeger D, et al. Exposure to nitrosamines, carbon black, asbestos, and talc and mortality from stomach, lung, and laryngeal cancer in a cohort of rubber workers. Am J Epidemiol 2000;152:297–306

80. Browne K, Gee JB. Asbestos exposure and laryngeal cancer. Ann Occup Hyg 2000;44:239–250

81. Ko JY, Chen CL, Lui LT, Hsu MM. Radiation-induced malignant fibrous histiocytoma in patients with nasopharyngeal carcinoma. Arch Otolaryngol Head Neck Surg 1996;122:535–538

82. Saku T, Hayashi Y, Takahara O, et al. Salivary gland tumors among atomic bomb survivors, 1950–1987. Cancer 1997;79:1465–1475

83. Preston-Martin S, Thomas DC, White SC, Cohen D. Prior exposure to medical and dental X-rays related to tumors of the parotid gland. J Natl Cancer Inst 1988;80:943–949

84. Pope CA, Burnett RT, Thun MJ, et al. Lung cancer, cardiopulmonary mortality, and long-term exposure to fine particulate air pollution. JAMA 2002;287:1132–1141

85. Chen BH, Hong MR, Pandey MR, Smith KR. Indoor air pollution in developing countries. World Health Stat Q 1990;43:127–138

86. Pintos J, Franco EL, Kowalski LP, Oliveira BV, Curado MP. Use of wood stoves and risk of cancers of the upper aerodigestive tract: a case-control study. Int J Epidemiol 1998;27:936–940

87. Franco EL, Kowalski LP, Oliveira BV, et al. Risk factors for oral cancer in Brazil: a case-control study. Int J Cancer 1989;43:992–1000

88. Dietz A, Senneweld E, Maier H. Indoor air pollution by emissions of fossil fuel single stoves: possibly a hitherto underrated risk factor in the development of carcinomas in the head and neck. Otolaryngol Head Neck Surg 1995;112:308–315

89. Zheng W, Blot WJ, Shu X-O, et al. A population-based case-control study of cancers of the nasal cavity and paranasal sinuses in Shanghai. Int J Cancer 1992;52:557–561

90. Bruce N, Perez-Padilla R, Albalak R. Indoor air pollution in developing countries: a major environmental and public health challenge. Bull World Health Organ 2000;78:1078–1092

2

Oral Precancer

Susan Müller

Leukoplakia and erythroplakia are two well-known precancerous lesions of the oral cavity. Oral precancer has been defined as morphologically altered tissue in which cancer is more likely to occur than in its apparently normal counterpart.[1] The development of these lesions and potential malignant transformation is probably due to a number of factors. Predicting which lesions will progress to squamous cell carcinoma is problematic and under investigation. Although most oral squamous cell carcinomas are associated with a precursor lesion, some cases apparently arise from clinically normal mucosa.[2] The transformation of a clinically and histologically benign leukoplakia to cancer can last for years, and on average occurs 2.5 years after initial presentation.

Compounding the difficulty in treating oral precancer, the grade of epithelial dysplasia may not be proportional to the risk of malignant transformation. The search for predictive risk markers to assess malignant potential still requires much research before they could be used routinely in diagnosis.[3]

◆ Oral Precancer

Leukoplakia

Oral leukoplakia, as defined by the World Health Organization (WHO) is a clinical white patch or plaque that cannot be rubbed or scraped off and cannot be given another specific diagnostic name.[1] Hence, the term *leukoplakia* is a term of exclusion of other oral entities that can present as white plaques or patches. These include frictional keratoses such as chronic tongue or cheek biting, hyperplastic candidiasis, nicotina stomatitis, lichen planus, lichenoid lesions, hairy leukoplakia, and tobacco pouch keratosis.

Leukoplakia is unusual in patients under 30 years of age, and is usually encountered in the fifth through seventh decade of life. Generally, leukoplakia is more common in men than in women, however the reported male/female ratios vary considerably. The prevalence of oral leukoplakia demonstrates geographic differences and ranges from 0.4 to 11.7% (**Table 2–1**).[4–36] The wide variation noted is most likely due to cultural differences in diet, tobacco smoking, chewing of tobacco/betel quid use, and alcohol.[37] Another reason for the wide disparity could be how leukoplakia was defined in the earlier studies, and may include frictional keratosis and nicotine stomatitis. In 1987, Axéll[38] outlined guidelines on the classification of leukoplakia that most subsequent studies have utilized. When only European and North American studies are evaluated, the prevalence rate of oral leukoplakia is 2.0%. This prevalence rate has been relatively unchanged over the past 30 years.

The premalignant potential of oral leukoplakia has been recognized since the mid–nineteenth century. The long-term behavior of oral leukoplakia is unknown, but malignant transformation has been well documented. Published malignant transformation rates range from 0.13 to 17.5% (**Table 2–2**).[39–54] This wide variation in reported transformation rates may be due to factors such as length of follow-up, location of leukoplakia, dietary factors, and tobacco usage. Although these studies provide good documentation of the precancerous nature of leukoplakia, they are limited due to lack of uniformity in design. Recently, there have been proposals to develop uniform reporting of leukoplakia utilizing

Table 2–1 Studies on the Prevalence of Oral Leukoplakia

Author	Year	Country	Number of Persons Examined	Population Type	Prevalence (%)
Gerry et al[4]	1952	Guatemala	2,004	Rural	0.4
Bruszt[5]	1962	Hungary	5,613	Rural	3.6
Kovács[6]	1962	Hungary	500	Urban	2.0
Atkinson et al[7]	1964	New Guinea	3,996	Rural	8.1
Pindborg et al[8–10]	1965–1966	India	30,000	Rural/urban	1.5–3.3
Zachariah et al[11]	1966	India	5,000	Urban	2.4
Pindborg et al[12]	1968	New Guinea	1,255	Rural	4.6
Bánóczy et al[13]	1969	Hungary	16,332	Rural	0.57
Mehta et al[14]	1969	India	50,915	Rural	1.7
Jussawala and Rajpal[15]	1969	India	40,000	Rural	7.0
Wahi and Mital[16]	1970	India	7,286	Rural	5.2
Ross and Gross[17]	1971	U.S.	11,884	Urban	2.8
Gangadharan and Paymaster[18]	1971	India	203,249	Hospital patients	7.0
Mehta[19]	1972	India	4,734	Urban police	3.5
Srivastava[20]	1973	India	8,428	Urban/suburban	2.8
Sonkodi and Toth[21]	1974	Hungary	1,071	Urban	1.2
Axéll[22,23]	1975, 1976	Sweden	20,333	Urban	3.6
Silverman et al[24]	1976	India	57,518	Urban	11.7
Wilsch et al[25]	1978	Germany	4,000	Urban	2.2
Lay et al[26]	1982	Burma	6,000	Rural	1.7
Zachariah and Pindborg[27]	1985	India	24,000	Suburban	2.0
Bouquot and Gorlin[28]	1986	U.S.	23,616	Urban/rural	2.9
Hogewind and van der Waal[29]	1988	Netherlands	1,000	Urban	1.4*
Ikeda et al[30]	1991	Japan	3,131	Urban	2.5
Bánóczy and Rigo[31]	1991	Hungary	7,820	Rural	1.3
Ikeda et al[32]	1995	Cambodia	1,319	Rural	1.3
Schepman et al[33]	1996	Netherlands	1,000	Urban	0.6*
Reichart and Kohn[34]	1996	Germany	1,000	Urban	0.9*
Kovač-Kovačič and Skalerič[35]	2000	Slovenia	1,609	Urban	3.1
Reichart[36]	2000	Germany	2,022	Urban	1.2
			Total 546,635		**Mean** 3.03

*More than 50% of population younger than 40 years old.

specific diagnostic criteria including appearance, size, and histologic grade.[55] Using such a system in future studies may reflect a more accurate malignant transformation rate.

Oral leukoplakia is generally divided into two subtypes: homogeneous and nonhomogeneous. A homogeneous leukoplakia is a uniformly white lesion that has a smooth or corrugated surface (**Figs. 2–1** and **2–2**). An early stage of homogeneous leukoplakia, sometimes referred to as pre-leukoplakia, exhibits a thin, white or gray plaque that may be translucent. This lesion is potentially reversible, but can progress laterally and become thickened with keratin, acquiring the typical white appearance. The

Table 2–2 Malignant Transformation Rates of Leukoplakia

Author	Year	Country	Sample Size	Observation Period (Years)	Malignant Transformation (%)
Škach et al[39]	1960	Czechoslovakia	71	3–6	1.4
Mela and Mongini[40]	1966	Italy	141	11	3.5
Einhorn and Wersäll[41]	1967	Sweden	782	20	4.0
Pindborg et al[42]	1968	Denmark	248	3–9	4.4
Silverman and Rosen[43]	1968	U.S.	117	1–11	6.0
Kramer[44]	1969	U.K.	187	1–16	4.8
Roed-Petersen[45]	1971	Denmark	331	12	3.6
Mehta et al[46]	1972	India	117	10	0.9
Silverman et al[47]	1976	India	4,762	2	0.13
Maerker and Burkhardt[48]	1978	Germany	200	5.5	11.0
Gupta et al[49]	1980	India	360	7	0.3
Gupta et al[49]	1980	India	410	7	2.2
Silverman et al[50]	1984	U.S.	257	7.2	17.5
Hodgewind et al[51]	1989	Netherlands	84	8	3.6
Lumerman et al[52]	1995	U.S.	44	0.5–6.5	13.8
Schepman et al[53]	1998	Netherlands	166	1–30	12.0
Shiu et al[54]	2000	Taiwan	435	0.1–10	13.5

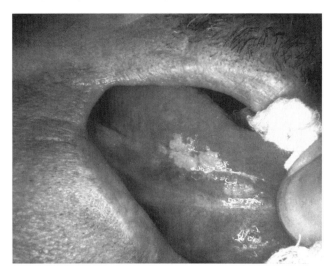

Figure 2–1 Homogeneous leukoplakia of the lateral border of the tongue. Biopsy revealed hyperkeratosis with moderate dysplasia.

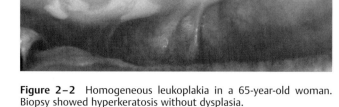

Figure 2–2 Homogeneous leukoplakia in a 65-year-old woman. Biopsy showed hyperkeratosis without dysplasia.

lesion can become corrugated in appearance with a leathery feeling. Again, this lesion may regress, remain stable, or progress.

The nonhomogeneous leukoplakias include nodular leukoplakia, speckled leukoplakia, and proliferative verrucous leukoplakia (**Figs. 2–3** and **2–4**). Although the nonhomogeneous subtype is rarer than the homogeneous subtype, it is much more worrisome, exhibiting a greater degree of epithelial dysplasia.[50,56]

The clinical appearance of leukoplakia, particularly the nonhomogeneous type, is not a reliable indicator of biologic behavior. Microscopic findings can range from a benign keratosis ("leukokeratosis") to an early infiltrating squamous cell carcinoma. Because of the varied histopathologic findings, the term *leukoplakia* should never be used as a pathologic term.

Homogeneous leukoplakias can exhibit either hyperparakeratosis or hyperorthokeratosis, and both can be seen at times in the same lesion (**Figs. 2–4** and **2–5**). Epithelial

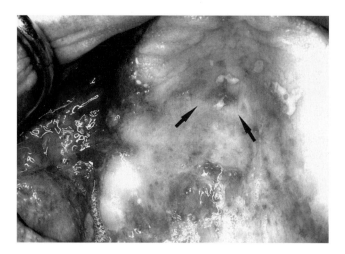

Figure 2–3 Nonhomogeneous or speckled leukoplakia of the palate. Biopsy of the erythroplakic area (*arrows*) revealed severe epithelial dysplasia.

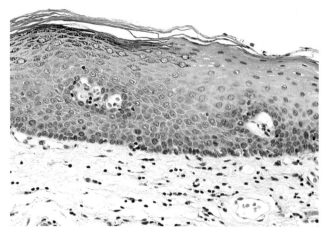

Figure 2–4 Biopsy from a leukoplakia showing a transition from orthokeratinized (*left side*) to parakeratinized (*right side*) epithelium without dysplasia.

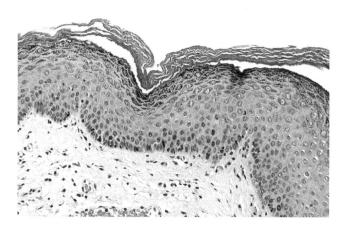

Figure 2–5 Mild dysplasia with marked orthokeratosis.

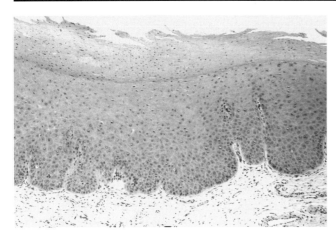

Figure 2–6 Moderate dysplasia exhibiting epithelial hyperplasia and marked parakeratosis.

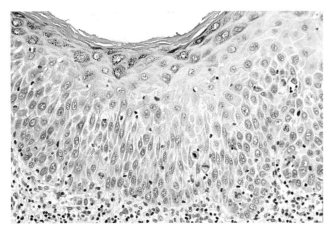

Figure 2–7 Moderate dysplasia showing mitoses in the lower half of the epithelium. Lymphocytes are noted in the superficial lamina propria as well as migrating through the epithelium.

hyperplasia, or acanthosis can also be seen when parakeratosis is present (**Fig. 2–6**). Occasional lymphocytes may be observed in the superficial lamina propria (**Fig. 2–7**).

The nonhomogeneous leukoplakias exhibit a wider range of microscopic features. Irregular keratosis, atrophic epithelium, and increased inflammatory cells are often observed. The inflammatory cells often migrate through the epithelium forming microabcesses. Aided by a periodic acid-Schiff (PAS) stain, candidal hyphae or spores can sometimes be seen in these inflamed areas. Histologic findings of epithelial dysplasia are more common in nonhomogeneous leukoplakia than in homogeneous leukoplakia.

Grading of epithelial dysplasia is somewhat subjective, particularly in the mild and moderate categories. Nevertheless, the WHO has defined the histologic features associated with epithelial dysplasia as follows[1]:

1. Loss of polarity of the basal cells
2. The presence of more than one layer having a basaloid appearance
3. Drop-shaped rete-ridges
4. Increased nuclear/cytoplasmic ratio
5. Enlarged nucleoli
6. Nuclear hyperchromatism
7. Increased number of mitotic figures
8. Abnormal mitotic figures
9. The presence of mitotic figures in the superficial half of the epithelium
10. Cellular and nuclear pleomorphism
11. Irregular epithelial stratification
12. Loss of cellular cohesion
13. Keratinization of single cells or cell groups in the stratum spinosum

The risk of malignant transformation of a dysplastic lesion is generally considered greater than a nondysplastic lesion. However, some dysplastic lesions can remain clinically unchanged, whereas carcinoma can develop in nondysplastic leukoplakia. Gupta et al,[49] in a 7-year observation period in an Indian population, documented that 60% of dysplastic leukoplakic lesions remained clinically unchanged or showed partial to complete regression. In contrast, 7% of the dysplastic lesions progress to cancer. Future research

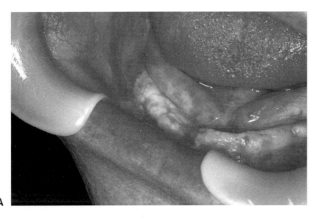

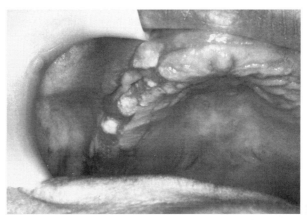

Figure 2–8 (**A,B**) Proliferative verrucous leukoplakia in a 63-year-old woman with a history of cigarette smoking. The patient has not smoked in 20 years. Focal leukoplakia has been noted for greater than 10 years. The leukoplakia involves the edentulous mandibular and maxillary alveolus and the buccal mucosa.

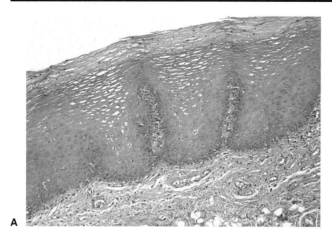

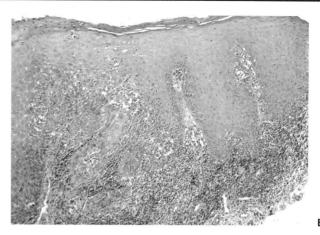

Figure 2–9 **(A)** Biopsy from the lower alveolus from patient in Figure 2–8. There is hyperparakeratosis and acanthosis but no epithelial dysplasia. **(B)** The biopsy from the upper alveolus demonstrates microinvasive squamous cell carcinoma. Note the prominent lymphocytic infiltrate in the lamina propria.

into the molecular basis of leukoplakia may help determine which markers are strong predictors of malignant transformation.

Clinical location and the incidence of dysplasia in oral leukoplakia have also been noted. Although two thirds of oral leukoplakia occurs at the lip vermilion, buccal mucosa, and gingiva, the sites with the highest risk for dysplasia are the lateral and ventral tongue, floor of mouth, and lower lip. These sites account for greater than 90% of all oral leukoplakias with dysplasia or carcinoma.[28,57]

A unique type of nonhomogeneous leukoplakia, termed *proliferative verrucous leukoplakia*, was first reported in 1985.[58] Characteristically the lesions grow slowly but continue to spread over one to two decades or even longer. The lesions become multifocal and typically have a verrucal or exophytic appearance (**Fig. 2–8**). Because of the slow development of this disease, proliferative verrucous leukoplakia is a diagnosis made retrospectively. Microscopically, biopsied lesions can range from hyperkeratosis to verrucous hyperplasia to dysplasia to verrucous carcinoma or squamous cell carcinoma (**Fig. 2–9**). The reported malignant transformation rate in proliferative verrucous leukoplakia has ranged from 70 to 93%.[58–60] The sites in which malignancies occur in proliferative verrucous leukoplakia also differ from traditional oral cancer. The gingiva, alveolus, and buccal mucosa are commonly involved. The typical risk factors for oral cancer seem less associated with proliferative verrucous leukoplakia. The patients are typically older, with an equal number of men and women affected, and tobacco history involving approximately 50% of patients. Treatment for proliferative verrucous leukoplakia is unsatisfactory. Multiple recurrences are usually encountered with this disease with a relentless progression to carcinoma.

Tobacco is the single most important etiologic factor in the development of leukoplakia. Anywhere from 70 to 90% of patients with leukoplakias have tobacco smoking histories.[61] Many of these leukoplakias either partially or completely regress after smoking cessation.

Another tobacco-related keratotic change is nicotine stomatitis (smoker's palate). The palate becomes thickened with papular elevations with a red center that represents

the inflamed salivary gland ducts (**Fig. 2–10**). This feature is mostly associated with pipe smoking, but can also be seen in cigar and cigarette smokers and is proportional to the frequency of the smoking habit. The clinical findings are thought to be due to the heat generated by the pipestem. This is not considered to be premalignant and is completely reversible after the tobacco habit is discontinued.

In some countries, reverse smoking is practiced. The lit end of the cigarette or cigar is placed in the mouth. A result of the intense high heat generated is known as reverse smoker's palate and, unlike nicotina stomatitis, this is associated with an increase in malignant transformation.

Smokeless tobacco keratosis is another tobacco-related mucosal alteration. These lesions usually occur in the buccal or labial mucosa where the tobacco is held and usually is completely reversible after the product is discontinued (**Fig. 2–11**).[62] The clinical presentation can range from a thin, translucent wrinkling of the mucosa to more thickened hyperkeratotic lesions with fissures and folds.[63] The clinical presentation usually correlates with the type of

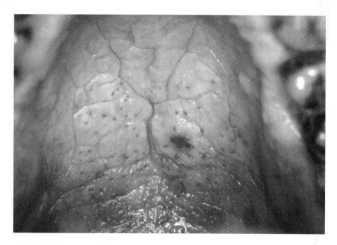

Figure 2–10   Nicotine stomatitis in a 58-year-old pipe smoker. The red spots on the palate represent the inflamed orifices of the minor salivary glands.

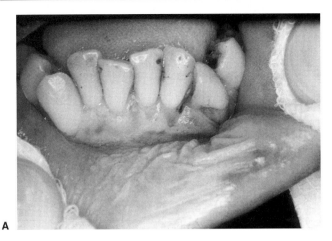

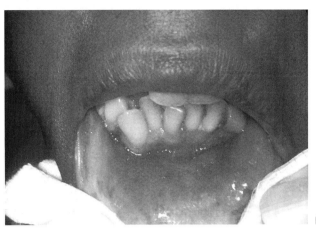

A | **B**

Figure 2–11 **(A)** A 35-year-old woman with a longer than 10-year history of smokeless tobacco use. The anterior labial mucosa has a corrugated appearance with thickened keratotic folds. **(B)** Four

weeks after discontinuing the smokeless tobacco the labial mucosa has returned to normal.

tobacco, the frequency of use, and length of time the product is used. There are different forms of smokeless tobacco. Chewing tobacco is air-cured tobacco that is shredded and treated with flavoring agents. Moist snuff is air-cured or fire-cured and then finely cut. Snuff is generally fermented in the United States. Swedish snuff, also called snus, is nonfermented. Dry snuff is fire-cured tobacco that is pulverized into a powder. Women, particularly in parts of the southern United States, typically use dry snuff.

Most biopsies of smokeless tobacco keratoses show hyperkeratosis with typical chevron keratinization (**Fig. 2–12**).[64] Dysplasia is uncommon and when encountered is usually mild. The risk of developing oral cancer is relatively low with chewing tobacco and the moist form of smokeless tobacco.[65] There have been reported cases of long-term users of smokeless tobacco (>40 years) developing squamous cell carcinoma. These users usually have been women who used dry snuff for long periods of time. Cancer usually develops in the buccal mucosa or alveolar ridge, corresponding to the site where the product was placed. Unlike

oral cancer development in patients with a positive history of smoking tobacco, a prolonged period of exposure to the smokeless tobacco usually occurs before carcinomatous transformation. In one study by Wray and McGuirt,[66] of 128 patients who used smokeless tobacco and developed oral cancer, 78% had a greater than 40-year history of smokeless tobacco use.

Erythroplakia

Considered to be a red analogue of leukoplakia, *erythroplakia* is a clinical term used to describe a red patch or plaque on the oral mucosa that cannot be diagnosed clinically or pathologically as any other condition. Benign inflammatory conditions including erythematous candidiasis may clinically mimic erythroplakia and must be ruled out. Erythroplakia usually appears as a well-demarcated red plaque with a soft, velvety texture. The lesion often is asymptomatic, although some patients complain of burning after ingesting certain foods.

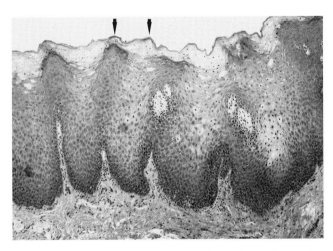

Figure 2–12 Biopsy of a smokeless tobacco keratosis showing marked parakeratosis with chevron keratinization (*arrows*). Epithelial hyperplasia is present, but no dysplasia is seen.

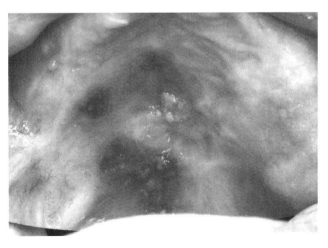

Figure 2–13 Erythroleukoplakia of the hard and soft palate. A biopsy of the erythroplakic component showed severe dysplasia.

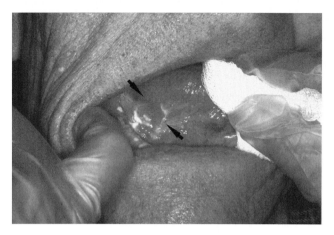

Figure 2–14 Erythroleukoplakia of the posterior lateral border of the tongue. A biopsy revealed carcinoma-in-situ.

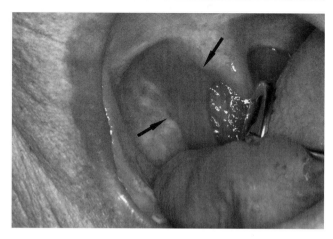

Figure 2–15 Erythroplasia of the tonsillar pillar. A biopsy revealed carcinoma-in-situ.

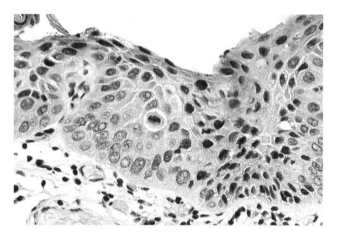

Figure 2–16 Severe dysplasia. There is atrophic epithelium with cellular pleomorphism, nuclear hyperchromasia, and mitoses.

Erythroplakia is more commonly found in men over the age of 50. Erythroplakia is most often noticed in the floor of mouth, lateral and ventral tongue, soft palate,

tonsillar pillar, and retromolar trigone (**Figs. 2–13, 2–14, and 2–15**). Although erythroplakia is significantly less common than oral leukoplakia, it is more likely to show dysplasia or carcinoma. In one study by Shafer and Waldron,[67] only 58 cases of erythroplakia were identified in 65,359 biopsy specimens compared with 3360 cases of oral leukoplakia. Significantly, all cases of erythroplakia demonstrated microscopic evidence of dysplasia, carcinoma-in-situ, or invasive carcinoma. Mashberg et al[68] evaluated 158 cases of early oral cancer. An erythroplakic component was noted in 92% of the cases; 62% of the cases, in addition to erythroplasia, had a leukoplakic component; only 2.5% presented as leukoplakia. These data emphasize the malignant potential of erythroplakia. Biopsy of a mixed erythroleukoplakia, therefore, should always include the red component.

Microscopically, erythroplakia often demonstrates varying degrees of dysplasia and epithelial atrophy (**Figs. 2–16 and 2–17**). The surface usually lacks keratinization, correlating with the red clinical appearance. The lamina propria often exhibits prominent vascularity and a chronic inflammatory infiltrate.

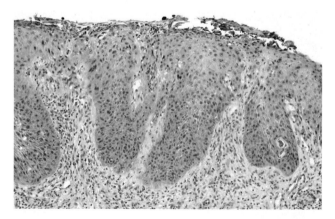

Figure 2–17 Carcinoma-in-situ. Note the lack of a keratinized surface that corresponds to the clinically red appearance of the lesion.

◆ Oral Precancerous Conditions

Oral Submucous Fibrosis

In India and Southeast Asia, the use of betel quid, nass, mawa, and many other substances is strongly related to the development of oral cancer. Although rare in Western countries, it is seen in immigrants from these countries. Oral submucous fibrosis is a chronic, irreversible disease that usually involves the buccal mucosa, but may affect the entire oral cavity as well as the oropharynx. Initially, the earliest symptom of oral submucous fibrosis is a burning sensation while eating spicy foods. This progresses to blanching of the mucosa, hardening, and the presence of fibrous bands with limited mouth opening.

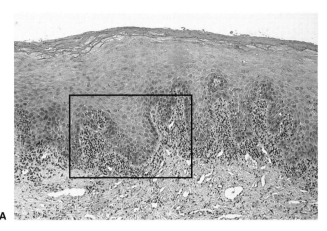 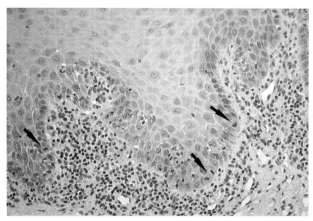

Figure 2–18 A biopsy taken from a white plaque on the buccal mucosa in a 37-year-old woman, which shows lichenoid dysplasia exhibiting a band-like inflammatory cell infiltrate and epithelial hyperplasia. **(B)** On higher power, the inflammatory infiltrate is composed of plasma cells and lymphocytes. There is migration of the inflammatory cells through the epithelium, and an abnormal maturation sequence is observed.

The precancerous nature of submucous fibrosis was first noted by Paymaster and subsequently confirmed by Pindborg.[69] In one study, a 7.6% malignant transformation rate was observed over a 17-year period.[70]

The pathogenesis of submucous fibrosis is considered multifactorial but is strongly related to the areca nut, which is a component of betel quid (pan). Typically pan is a betel leaf (*Piper betel*) onto which slaked lime is smeared and wrapped with areca nut (the fruit of the areca palm tree). Additional ingredients are added according to regional preferences, including tobacco, catechu, aniseed, and cardamon. Chewing the betel nut releases an active alkaloid, arecoline. This alkaloid has been shown to stimulate fibroblasts to increase collagen production in vitro. Other studies have linked fibroblast stimulation to the enzyme lysl oxidase, a metalloenzyme of copper, which is released when chewing areca nut. Again, it must be stressed that there are multiple components that must interact to result in submucous fibrosis. These include a genetic component, immunologic process, and nutritional deficiencies such as iron deficiency anemia and vitamin B complex deficiency.

In recent years, the reported age distribution of submucous fibrosis has shifted to a younger population, with more than 70% of cases occurring in patients less than 35 years of age.[71] This sudden increase in younger patients is thought to be related to commercially available products, pan masala and gutkha. Gutkha is a combination of powdered areca nut, tobacco, lime, preservatives, and flavoring agents, including chocolate, which can appeal to children. These products have been heavily marketed throughout India and other south Asian countries.

The microscopic features of submucous fibrosis are characterized by epithelial atrophy, and diffuse hyalinization of the lamina propria with a marked decrease of ground substance and vascularity. Epithelial dysplasia can be seen especially in biopsies taken from erythroplakic lesions or from nonhealing ulcers. The underlying skeletal muscle may show atrophy.

Treatment of the disease depends on severity. Intralesional injections of steroid and interferon-γ along with topical application of hyaluronidase have been used to improve mouth movements.[72] Surgical intervention is required in patients with severe trismus.

Oral Lichen Planus

The relationship between oral lichen planus and oral squamous cell carcinoma is controversial. In some cases reported malignant transformation of lichen planus was not based on any histological studies and anecdotal at best. Krutchkoff et al[73] reviewed 222 published cases and accepted only 15 cases with adequate documentation of malignant transformation. Other authors have found a 1.2% rate of oral cancer development over a 5.6-year observation period in patients with lichen planus.[74] This is not significantly greater than one would see in the general population. Possible explanations as to the presence of oral cancer in patients with oral lichen planus are that the mucosal alteration seen in lichen planus makes it more susceptible to carcinogens, or that the carcinoma could coincidentally occur in the site of lichen planus.[75] The erosive form and the plaque type of oral lichen planus can be difficult to distinguish from leukoplakia or erythroleukoplakia.

An erroneous initial histologic diagnosis may also play a role in evaluating the malignant potential of lichen planus. Distinguishing lichenoid reactions, lichenoid dysplasia, and lichen planus can be challenging. Krutchkoff and Eisenberg[76] have outlined strict histologic criteria to distinguish these entities. Often lichenoid dysplasia exhibits a band-like inflammatory cell infiltrate that can appear histologically similar to lichen planus (**Fig. 2–18**). On closer examination, the inflammatory infiltrate of lichenoid dysplasia is typically mixed, whereas in lichen planus it is typically composed of lymphocytes and occasional plasma cells. Importantly, dysplasia should never be seen in lichen planus, and therefore should preclude a diagnosis of lichen planus.

◆ Conclusion

Most clinicians rely on visual inspection as the initial method of screening for precancerous lesions of the oral cavity. Accordingly, mucosal abnormalities such as erythroplakia or nonhomogeneous forms of leukoplakia must be recognized as lesions that have an increased risk of progressing to invasive squamous carcinoma. At the same time, the indefinite correlation that exists between gross appearance, microscopic features, and biologic behavior limits our ability to consistently select those lesions that require biopsy or ablation. This shortcoming underscores the need to develop better screening techniques that are able to characterize the biologic aggressiveness of a particular oral mucosal lesion and its potential for malignant transformation.

References

1. Kramer IR, Lucas RB, Pindborg JJ, Sobin LH. Center for Oral Precancerous Lesions: definition of leukoplakia and related lesions: an aid to studies on oral precancer. Oral Surg Oral Med Oral Pathol 1978;45:518–539

2. van der Waal I, Shepman KP, van der Meij EH, Smeele LE. Oral leukoplakia: a clinicopathologic review. Oral Oncol 1997;33:291–301

3. Warnakulasuriya S. Lack of molecular markers to predict malignant potential of oral precancer. J Pathol 2000;190:407–409

4. Gerry RG, Smith ST, Calton ML. The oral characteristics of Guamians including the effects of betel chewing on the oral tissues. Oral Surg Oral Med Oral Pathol 1952;5:762–781

5. Bruszt P. Stomato-oncological screening tests in 7 villages of the Baia and Bacsalmas district. Magy Onkol 1962;6:28–33

6. Kovács G. Die moderne diagnostik und therapie von prablastomatosen der mundhohle. Ther Hung 1962;10:1–3

7. Atkinson L, Chester IC, Smith FG, et al. Oral cancer in New Guinea: a study in demography and etiology. Cancer 1964;17:1289–1298

8. Pindborg JJ, Kalapessi HK, Kale SA, et al. Frequency of oral leukoplakias and related conditions among 10,000 Bombayites. J All India Dent Assoc 1965;37:228–229

9. Pindborg JJ, Chawla TN, Misra RK, et al. Frequency of oral carcinoma, leukoplakia, leukoedema, leukokeratosis, submucous fibrosis and lichen planus in 10,000 Indians in Lucknow, Uttar Pradesh, India. J Dent Res 1965;44:615–618

10. Pindborg JJ, Rhatt M, Devanath KE, et al. Frequency of oral white lesions among 10,000 individuals in Bangalore, South India. Indian J Med Sci 1966;20:349–352

11. Zachariah J, Matthew B, Varma NAR, et al. Frequency of oral mucosal lesions among 5,000 individuals in Trivandrum, South India. J All India Dent Assoc 1966;38:290–294

12. Pindborg JJ, Barmes OD, Roed-Petersen B. Epidemiology and histology of oral leukoplakia and leukoedema among Papuans and New Guineans. Cancer 1968;22:379–384

13. Bánóczy J, Radnai T, Remenyi I. Modszertani tapasztalataink Dunakeszi es Felsogod, lakossagan vegzett stomato-onkologiai szurovizsgalatok alapjan. Fogorv Sz 1969;62:118–122

14. Mehta FS, Pindborg JJ, Gupta PC, et al. Epidemiologic and histologic study of oral cancer and leukoplakia in 57,518 industrial workers in Gujaret, India. Cancer 1969;24:832–849

15. Jussawala DJ, Rajpal RN. Leukoplakia: Proceedings of the Symposium on Precancer. Bulletin No. 39. New Dehli: National Institute of Sciences of India, 1969:19–27

16. Wahi PN, Mital VP, Lahiri B, et al. Epidemiological study of precancerous lesions of the oral cavity: a preliminary report. Indian J Med Res 1970;58:1362–1391

17. Ross NM, Gross E. Oral Findings based on an automated multiphasic health screening program. J Oral Med 1971;26:21–26

18. Gangadharan P, Paymaster JC. Leukoplakia and epidemiologic study of 1504 cases observed at the Tata Memorial Hospital, Bombay, India. Br J Cancer 1971;25:657–668

19. Mehta FS. Oral leukoplakia in relation to tobacco habits: a ten-year follow-up study of Bombay policemen. Oral Surg Oral Med Oral Pathol 1972;34:426–433

20. Srivastava YC. Oral leukoplakia. Int Surg 1973;58:614–618

21. Sonkodi I, Toth K. Szegedi textilipari munkasok stomato-onkologiai vizsgalata. Fogorv Sz 1974;67:165–169

22. Axéll T. A preliminary report on prevalence of oral mucosal lesions in a Swedish population. Community Dent Oral Epidemiol 1975;3:143–145

23. Axéll T. A prevalence study of oral mucosal lesions in an adult Swedish population. Odontol Revy 1976;27(suppl 36):1–103

24. Silverman S, Bhargava K, Mani N, et al. Malignant transformation and natural history of oral leukoplakia in 57,518 industrial workers of Gujaret, India. Cancer 1976;38:1790–1795

25. Wilsch L, Hornstein OP, Bruning H, et al. Orale Leukopkien II. Ergebnisse einer 1 jahrigen poliklinischen pilostudie. Dtsch Zahnarztl Z 1978;33:132–142

26. Lay KM, Sein K, Myint A, et al. Epidemiologic study of 6,000 villagers of oral precancerous lesions in Bihigynn: preliminary report. Community Dent Oral Epidemiol 1982;10:152–155

27. Zachariah J, Pindborg JJ. Oral precancer. In: Barnes L, ed. Surgical Pathology of the Head and Neck. New York: Marcel Dekker, 1985:282

28. Bouquot JE, Gorlin RJ. Leukoplakia, lichen planus, and other oral keratoses in 23,616 white Americans over the age of 35 years. Oral Surg Oral Med Oral Pathol 1986;61:373–381

29. Hogewind WFC, van der Waal I. Prevalence study of oral leukoplakia in a selected population of 1000 patients for the Netherlands. Community Dent Oral Epidemiol 1988;16:302–305

30. Ikeda N, Ishii T, Lida S, Kawai T. Epidemiological study of oral leukoplakia based on mass screening for oral mucosal diseases in a selected Japanese population. Community Dent Oral Epidemiol 1991;19:160–163

31. Bánóczy J, Rigo O. Prevalence study of oral precancerous lesions within a complex screening system in Hungary. Community Dent Oral Epidemiol 1991;19:265–267

32. Ikeda N, Handa Y, Khim SP, et al. Prevalence study of oral mucosa lesions in a selected Cambodian population. Community Dent Oral Epidemiol 1995;23:49–54

33. Schepman KP, van der Meij EH, Smeele LE, van der Waal I. Prevalence study of oral white lesions with special reference to a new definition of oral leucoplakia. Eur J Cancer B Oral Oncol 1996;32B:416–419

34. Reichart PA, Kohn H. Prevalence of oral leukoplakia in 1000 Berliners. Oral Dis 1996;2:291–294

35. Kovač-Kovačič M, Skalerič U. The prevalence of oral mucosal lesions in a population in Ljubljana, Slovenia. J Oral Pathol Med 2000;29:331–335

36. Reichart PA. Oral mucosal lesions in a representative cross-sectional study of aging Germans. Community Dent Oral Epidemiol 2000;28:390–398

37. Reichart PA. Identification of risk groups for oral precancer and cancer and preventive measures. Clin Oral Investig 2001;5:207–213

38. Axéll T. Occurrence of leukoplakia and some other oral white lesions among 20333 adult Swedish people. Community Dent Oral Epidemiol 1987;15:46–51

39. Škach M, Svoboda O, Kubát K. A note on the question of leukoplakia [in Czech, English summary]. Acta Univ Carol [Med] (Praha) 1960;10:276–277 (Med Suppl)

40. Mela F, Mongini F. Contributo cafistico allo studio delle leuchoplachie orali [English summary]. Minerva Stomatol 1966;15:502–507

41. Einhorn J, Wersäll J. Incidence of oral carcinoma in patients with leukoplakia of the oral mucosa. Cancer 1967;20:2184–2193

42. Pindborg JJ, Jolst O, Renstrup G, Roed-Petersen B. Studies in oral leukoplakia: a preliminary report on the period prevalence of malignant transformation in leukoplakia based on a follow-up study of 248 patients. J Am Dent Assoc 1968;78:767–771

43. Silverman S, Rosen RD. Observations on the clinical characteristics and natural history of oral leukoplakias. J Am Dent Assoc 1968;76:772–776

44. Kramer IRH. Precancerous conditions of oral mucosa: a computer aided study. Ann R Coll Surg Engl 1969;45:340–356

45. Roed-Petersen B. Cancer development in oral leukoplakia: follow-up of 331 patients [abstract]. J Dent Res 1971;50:711

46. Mehta FS, Shroff BC, Gupta PC, et al. Oral leukoplakia in relation to tobacco habits. Oral Surg Oral Med Oral Pathol 1972;34:426–433

47. Silverman S, Bhargava K, Mani N, et al. Malignant transformation and natural history of oral leukoplakia in 57,518 industrial workers of Gujaret, India. Cancer 1976;38:1790–1795

48. Maerker R, Burkhardt A. Klinik der oralen leukoplakien und prakanzerosen. Retrospektive studie on 200 patienten. Dtsch Z Mund Kiefer Gesichtschir 1978;2:206–220

49. Gupta PC, Mehta FS, Daftary DK, et al. Incidence rate of oral cancer and natural history or oral precancerous lesions in a 10 year follow-up study of Indian villagers. Community Dent Oral Epidemiol 1980;8:287–333

50. Silverman S, Gorsky M, Lozada F. Oral leukoplakia and malignant transformation. A follow-up study of 257 patients. Cancer 1984;53:563–568

51. Hodgewind WFC, van der Kwast WAM, van der Waal I. Oral leukoplakia with emphasis on malignant transformation. J Craniomaxillofac Surg 1989;17:128–133

52. Lumerman H, Freedman P, Kerpel S. Oral epithelial dysplasia and the development of invasive squamous cell carcinoma. Oral Surg Oral Med Oral Pathol Oral Radiol Endod 1995;79:321–329

53. Schepman KP, van der Meij EH, Smeele LE, van der Waal I. Malignant transformation of oral leukoplakia: a follow-up study of a hospital-based population of 166 patients with oral leukoplakia from The Netherlands. Oral Oncol 1998;34:270–275

54. Shiu MN, Chen THH, Chang SH, Hahn LJ. Risk factors for leukoplakia and malignant transformation to oral carcinoma: a leukoplakia cohort in Taiwan. Br J Cancer 2000;82:1871–1874

55. van der Waal I, Axéll T. Oral leukoplakia: a proposal for uniform reporting. Oral Oncol 2002;38:521–526

56. Gupta PC, Bhonsle RB, Murti PR, et al. An epidemiologic assessment of cancer risk in oral precancerous lesions in India with special reference to nodular leukoplakia. Cancer 1989;63:2247–2252

57. Waldron CA, Schafer WG. Leukoplakia revisited: a clinico-pathologic study of 3256 oral leukoplakias. Cancer 1975;36:1386–1392

58. Hansen LS, Olson JA, Silverman S. Proliferative verrucous leukoplakia. Oral Surg Oral Med Oral Pathol 1985;60:285–298

59. Silverman S, Gorsky M. Proliferative verrucous leukoplakia. Oral Surg Oral Med Oral Pathol Oral Radiol Endod 1997;84:154–157

60. Seyer BA, Muller S. Predictive factors for the development of squamous cell carcinoma in proliferative verrucous leukoplakia: distinction from conventional oral squamous cell carcinoma [abstract]. Mod Pathol 2001;14:154A

61. Bouquot JE, Whitaker SB. Oral leukoplakia-rationale for diagnosis and prognosis of its clinical subtypes or "phases." Quintessence Int 1994;25:133–140

62. Martin GC, Brown JP, Eifler CW, Houston GD. Oral leukoplakia status six weeks after cessation of smokeless tobacco use. J Am Dent Assoc 1999;130:945–954

63. Kaugars GE, Riley WT, Brandt RB, et al. The prevalence of oral lesions in smokeless tobacco users and an evaluation of risk factors. Cancer 1992;70:2579–2585

64. Smith JF, Mincer HA, Hopkins KP, et al. Snuff-dipper's lesion. A cytological study in a large population. Arch Otolaryngol 1970; 92:450–456

65. Rodu B, Cole P. Smokeless tobacco use and cancer of the upper respiratory tract. Oral Surg Oral Med Oral Pathol Oral Radiol Endod 2002;93:511–515

66. Wray A, McGuirt F. Smokeless tobacco usage associated with oral carcinoma. Arch Otolaryngol Head Neck Surg 1993;119:929–933

67. Shafer WG, Waldron CA. Erythroplakia of the oral cavity. Cancer 1975;36:1436–1445

68. Mashberg A, Morrissey JB, Garfinkel L. A study of the appearance of early asymptomatic oral squamous cell carcinoma. Cancer 1973;32:1436–1445

69. Pindborg JJ. Is submucous fibrosis a precancerous condition in the oral cavity? Int Dent J 1972;22:474–480

70. Murti PR, Bhonsle RB, Pindborg JJ, et al. Malignant transformation rate in oral submucous fibrosis over a 17-year period. Community Dent Oral Epidemiol 1985;13:340–341

71. Gupta PC. Mouth cancer in India: a new epidemic? J Indian Med Assoc 1999;97:370–373

72. Haque MF, Meghji S, Nazir R, Harris M. Interferon gamma (IFN-gamma) may reverse oral submucous fibrosis. J Oral Pathol Med 2001;30:12–21

73. Krutchkoff DJ, Cutler L, Laskowski S. Oral lichen planus: the evidence regarding potential malignant transformation. J Oral Pathol 1978;7:1–7

74. Silverman S, Gorsky M, Lozado-Nur F. A prospective follow-up study of 570 patients with oral lichen planus: persistence, remission, and malignant association. Oral Surg Oral Med Oral Pathol 1985;60:30–34

75. Lo Muzio L, Mignogna MD, Favia G, et al. The possible association between oral lichen planus and oral squamous cell carcinoma: a clinical evaluation on 14 cases and a review of the literature. Oral Oncol 1998;34:239–246

76. Krutchkoff DJ, Eisenberg E. Lichenoid dysplasia: a distinct histopathologic entity. Oral Surg Oral Med Oral Pathol 1985;60:308–315

3

Malignant Lesions of the Oral Cavity

Kevin Rand Torske

Squamous epithelium is the primary surface structure of the skin, lips, and mucous membranes of the oral cavity, and 86 to 95% of head and neck malignancy originates from this tissue.[1-3] This chapter discusses the clinical and surgical pathologic features of oral squamous cell carcinoma and its histologic variants. In addition, malignancies of the minor salivary glands and mucosal melanoma are discussed.

◆ Squamous Cell Carcinoma

Clinical Pathology

The following discussion is a general overview of the clinical features of oral squamous cell carcinoma. Detailed description of cancer within specific anatomical sites is presented in subsequent chapters.

Leukoplakia, Erythroplakia, and Erythroleukoplakia. *Leukoplakia* is a clinical term meaning "white patch." This term relates only to the clinical appearance of the lesion and is not a true pathologic diagnosis. The white clinical appearance is due to increased thickness of the keratin layer of the epithelium. Histologically, leukoplakia may range from simple hyperkeratosis (thickening of the epithelial keratin layer), to epithelial dysplasia, to an early stage of an invasive carcinoma. Leukoplakic carcinomas may appear flat and uniform, granular, or nodular, and are usually early cases that have not yet produced a mass lesion or ulcer.

Erythroplakia is a clinical term meaning "red patch." The red clinical appearance is due to a reduction in epithelial thickness or overt lack of a keratinized layer, which permits visualization of the underlying vascular connective tissue.

Areas of redness are more concerning for malignant change, as they may indicate that the epithelial cells are too genetically altered to produce a keratinized layer. Lesions may be entirely erythroplakic or a combination of red and white (*erythroleukoplakic*).

Although most oral cavity squamous cell carcinomas begin as a red-white patch, this classic presentation is eventually destroyed by a developing exophytic or endophytic mass. However, cancer diagnosed in the floor of the mouth, soft palate, alveolar mucosa, or gingiva is commonly within this stage of development (**Fig. 3–1**).

Exophytic Lesions. Exophytic carcinomas are mass-forming lesions, and may be nodular, fungating, papillary, or verruciform in appearance. The color may vary from red to white, depending on the amount of keratinization of the epithelial surface. Also, due to fibrosis of the underlying connective tissue in response to tumor invasion, the mass may feel hard (*indurated*). In addition, if the cancer has spread into the underlying musculature or bone, the mass may feel fixed to the surrounding tissues. This presentation is common within the buccal mucosa and lateral border of the tongue (**Fig. 3–2**).

Endophytic Lesions. Endophytic carcinomas are mainly ulcerative. This is due to the carcinomatous epithelium's inability to create a stable and intact structural unit. Carcinomas of this type display a depressed, irregularly shaped, ulcerated central zone with a "rolled" border (**Fig. 3–3**). The rolled border is created when the tumor invades downward and laterally, thereby pulling the epithelial edges that are adjacent to the ulcer. Carcinomas of the lower lip, floor of the mouth, hard palate, and lateral border of the tongue

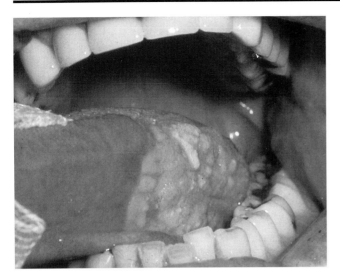

Figure 3–1 Squamous cell carcinoma of the lateral border of the tongue. This example is mostly leukoplakic in appearance.

frequently appear endophytic. This appearance is not unique to squamous cell carcinoma, however, as fungal infections, tuberculosis, tertiary syphilis, necrotizing sialometaplasia, traumatic ulcers, Wegener's granulomatosis, and Crohn's disease may all present with similar oral findings.

Histopathology

Squamous cell carcinoma is defined as an invasive malignant neoplasm with squamous epithelial origin and differentiation. Characteristics such as keratin formation and intercellular bridges are classically present. Origination from dysplastic (premalignant) surface epithelium is common, although not all epithelial dysplasias progress to invasive disease.[2] The epithelial basement membrane is destroyed, with invasion of the subepithelial connective tissue by sheets, cords, islands, or individual squamous cells. The neoplasm may progress to involve deeper structures such as adipose tissue, muscle, vascular spaces (both lymphatic and blood), or bone. Neural invasion may occur with the tumor tracking up or down the neural bundle. A tumor

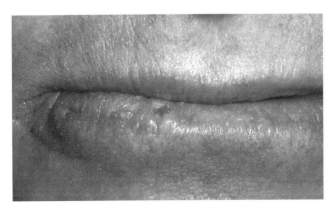

Figure 3–3 Squamous cell carcinoma of the lower lip. Note the rolled borders and central ulceration just lateral to the midline. (Courtesy of Dr. Robert Foss.)

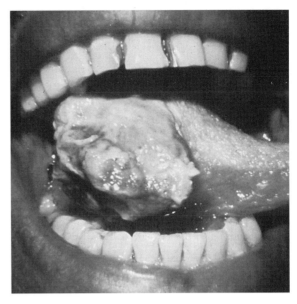

Figure 3–2 Squamous cell carcinoma of the lateral border of the tongue. This example is a large, irregular exophytic mass with surface necrosis.

may be termed *superficially invasive* if only very minimal invasion into the underlying connective tissue is observed. The stroma surrounding the infiltrative epithelial islands commonly displays a moderately dense mixed inflammatory infiltrate.

The neoplastic tissue displays structural resemblance to squamous epithelium. However, there is a considerable range of histologic appearances. The degree to which the neoplasm histologically resembles the tissue of origin is termed *grade*. A *well-differentiated* (low-grade; grade 1) tumor closely mimics normal squamous epithelium. The tumor islands show relatively normal maturation with peripheral basal cells, a well-defined spinous layer, and central keratinization. Histologic features of malignancy, such as hyperchromaticity, enlarged nuclei, pleomorphism, increased amount of mitotic figures, atypical mitotic figures, individual cell keratinization, and necrosis, are at a minimum (**Fig. 3–4**). *Poorly differentiated* (high-grade; grade 3) tumors display meager resemblance to normal squamous epithelium. Keratin formation is rare or absent, and intercellular bridges are indistinct. The cytologic features of malignancy mentioned above are easily identified. *Anaplastic* or *undifferentiated* (grade 4) tumors lack squamous differentiation altogether, and immunohistochemical studies for the presence of cytokeratins may be required. A *moderately differentiated* (moderate or intermediate grade; grade 2) tumor will display characteristics in between that of well-differentiated and poorly differentiated (**Fig. 3–5**).[4] Eighty-three percent of squamous cell carcinomas occurring in the oral cavity or lips are well to moderately differentiated.[3]

Prognosis

Despite significant advances in treatment, the prognosis of oral squamous cell carcinoma has not significantly changed over time.[4–6] In general, age greater than 35 years, male

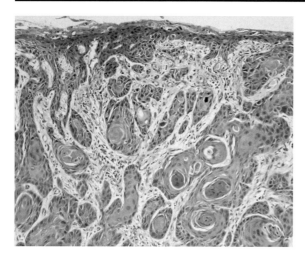

Figure 3–4 Well-differentiated squamous cell carcinoma. The surface displays full-thickness cytologic changes. Numerous variably sized nests of malignant squamous epithelium are invading the underlying connective tissues. Note the central keratinization within many of the islands.

gender, and African-American race all portend a poorer prognosis.[3] Although the location and stage of the neoplasm play the most significant role in the prognosis, the histologic grade of oral cancer does have general prognostic value. Well-differentiated tumors have a better prognosis overall than poorly differentiated, with a lower probability of lymph node metastasis.[7,8] Five-year survival rates of 40%, 26%, and 12% are reported for well-differentiated, moderately differentiated, and poorly differentiated tumors, respectively.[9] The correlation of grade with tumor behavior is not absolute, however, and the subjective nature of grading, the quality and amount of biopsy material, and the use of different grading schemes all complicate this analysis.

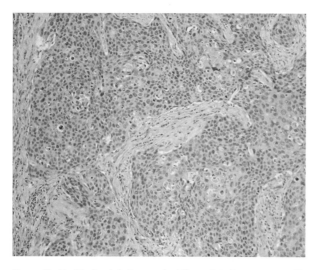

Figure 3–5 Moderately to poorly differentiated squamous cell carcinoma. Areas with moderate differentiation show more voluminous cytoplasm and individual cell keratinization. Poorly differentiated cells are mostly polygonal, hyperchromatic, and with a higher nuclear/cytoplasmic ratio.

Other histologic factors besides tumor grade may affect prognosis. Perineural invasion has been reported to be associated with a higher likelihood of cervical lymph node metastasis.[10,11] Histologic tumor thickness beyond 6 mm has also been shown to correlate with cervical metastatic spread.[12] However, the analysis of vascular invasion and tumor necrosis does not add any prognostic value beyond that of the histologic grade.

Many studies have sought to elaborate the prognostic significance of different molecular factors, some of which include DNA ploidy, p53, p27, K_i-67, proliferating cell nuclear antigen (PCNA), argyrophilic nucleolar organizer regions (AgNORs, erbB, *ras*, cyclin D1, and loss of chromosomal heterozygosity (LOH). Although a detailed description of the molecular pathology of each marker is beyond the scope of this chapter, some conclusions can be drawn from the literature. Nondiploid tumors have been associated with a higher likelihood of cervical lymph node metastases and therefore a poorer prognosis.[7,13–15] Other molecular factors that have been shown to correlate with a poor prognosis include decreased expression of p27, LOH on chromosome 3p, and high expression of cyclin D1 or AgNORs.[16–24] p53 has received a tremendous amount of attention, and although results are conflicting, the majority of studies have failed to indicate p53 overexpression as a prognostic factor within the oral cavity.[4,25,26] Conflicting research also has been presented in regard to the significance of erb-B and the proliferation markers PCNA and K_i-67.[4,26] It is hoped that further investigation of the individual or interactive roles of these molecular factors will lead to an increased understanding of their prognostic value.

◆ Variants of Squamous Cell Carcinoma

There are many histologic and clinical variants of squamous cell carcinoma that affect the oral cavity. Verrucous carcinoma, spindle cell carcinoma, basaloid squamous cell carcinoma, adenosquamous cell carcinoma, papillary squamous cell carcinoma, adenoid squamous cell carcinoma, and lymphoepithelial carcinoma have all been described. As the latter forms have not been well elucidated or are debatable as true varieties, only verrucous, spindle cell, and basaloid squamous carcinomas will be discussed here.

Verrucous Carcinoma

Clinical Pathology

Verrucous carcinoma within the oral cavity was first described by Ackerman[27] in 1948. Lesions tend to arise in a setting of clinical leukoplakia and eventually transform into a diffuse, gray-white, well-demarcated, thick plaque with an exophytic papillary or verrucous surface texture.[28–31] It is usually painless and slow growing, and therefore relatively innocuous. Its significance lies in its relentless growth, local blunt penetration into contiguous structures (cheek, periosteum, or underlying bone), and the potential for eventual transformation into conventional squamous cell carcinoma (**Fig. 3–6**).[32]

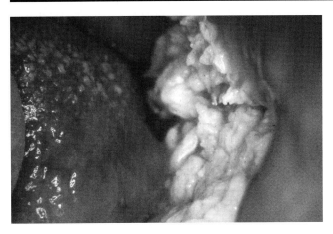

Figure 3–6 Verrucous carcinoma. This extensive lesion on the left buccal mucosa displays multiple exophytic projections. This white appearance is due to the abundant keratin on the epithelial surface. (Courtesy of Dr. Robert Goode.)

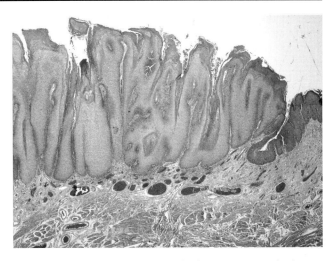

Figure 3–7 Verrucous carcinoma. This low-power view displays an abrupt transition from the relatively normal epithelium to verrucous carcinoma at the right side of the photomicrograph. Note the large, papillary folds of epithelium with abundant surface keratinization, parakeratin "crypting," and a blunt pushing inferior border.

Verrucous carcinoma represents approximately 2% of all cases of oral cancer, and occurs annually in one to three of every million persons.[3,32–34] Males are affected more often than females, with the incidence increasing over age 55 years. In descending order, the most common areas affected by this disease are the buccal mucosa, gingiva/alveolus, oral vestibule, and palate.[3,35] Patients may present with clinically enlarged cervical lymph nodes, normally corresponding to inflammatory or reactive changes (see below).[28]

Histopathology

Verrucous carcinoma is characterized by an epithelial proliferation with a papillary-to-verrucous architectural pattern and a broadly based "pushing" margin.[27,28,34] An abrupt transition between adjacent normal-appearing epithelium and the neoplasm may be present. A thick keratin layer covers the surface of the lesion, and parakeratin crypting is common. The rete ridges appear large, bulbous, and blunt. Importantly, the basement membrane is intact. The broad-based margin, however, may bluntly push its way deeper into the connective tissues, attach to the periosteum, and lead to erosion and destruction of the underlying bone.[28] The underlying connective tissue commonly displays a variably dense lymphoplasmacytic infiltrate (**Fig. 3–7**).

One of the most significant features is an overall lack of cytomorphologic features of malignancy, with bland, relatively normal squamous epithelial maturation. Mitotic figures are rare and relegated to the basilar or suprabasilar areas. The overall cell size is slightly increased, with enlargement of the nucleus and more abundant cytoplasm. Intercellular bridges in the spinous layer are easily identified (**Fig. 3–8**).

The primary distinguishing features of verrucous carcinoma from squamous cell carcinoma are an intact basement membrane, lack of invasion into the underlying connective tissues, large bulbous rete ridges, and bland cytomorphology. However, complete and thorough examination of the biopsy must be performed, as verrucous carcinoma may focally

transition into conventional invasive squamous cell carcinoma with a resultant change in clinical behavior and prognosis.[32]

Prognosis

Verrucous carcinoma is a relatively indolent malignancy, carrying a much better prognosis than traditional squamous cell carcinoma. Verrucous carcinoma is best treated by complete and thorough surgical excision, which has historically achieved a 74 to 90% cure rate. However, the recurrence potential is high, ranging from 26 to 70%, and multiple recurrences are common. As the basement membrane is

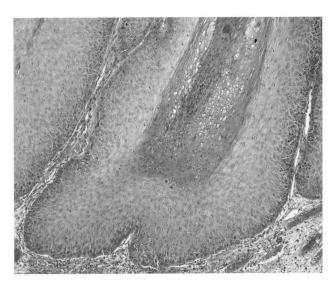

Figure 3–8 Verrucous carcinoma. This high-power view demonstrates relatively normal squamous epithelial maturation, a blunt rete ridge, and parakeratin crypting. Significant epithelial dysplasia is not identified in a true verrucous carcinoma and if present should signify early transformation into a squamous cell carcinoma.

not penetrated in verrucous carcinoma, it does not have the ability to metastasize. Eventual transformation into conventional squamous cell carcinoma is possible, however, and therefore long-term follow-up is required.[28,34,35]

Spindle Cell (Sarcomatoid) Carcinoma

Clinical Pathology

Spindle cell (sarcomatoid) carcinoma (SCSC) is a biphasic or monophasic neoplasm composed of squamous cell carcinoma (either in situ or invasive) and a malignant spindle-cell population.[36–38] The average presentation is in the sixth or seventh decade with a male predilection.[39] Similar to conventional squamous cell carcinoma, tobacco plays a large part in the pathogenesis of these lesions. Prior history of irradiation to the tumor site has also been cited as a predisposing factor.[38,40]

Spindle cell carcinoma occurs predominantly in the upper aerodigestive tract, with the larynx and oral cavity most commonly affected.[36,38] Although any intraoral site may be involved, SCSC tends to present in the lower lip, lateral posterior tongue, or alveolar ridge (**Fig. 3–9**). Spindle cell carcinoma typically appears as a polypoid mass, a rather unique feature of this form of epithelial cancer. The polypoid presentation is especially common in the larynx. However, it may also clinically resemble other forms of squamous cell carcinoma, presenting as a fungating nodular mass or an endophytic ulcerative condition.[40] Depending on the location of the tumor, clinical complaints may include hoarseness, pain, burning sensation, dyspnea, dysphagia, loose teeth, swelling, or a nonhealing ulcer.

Histopathology

Spindle cell sarcomatoid carcinoma is commonly a biphasic neoplasm with conventional squamous epithelial dysplasia or carcinoma and pleomorphic spindle cells.[37,41,42] As the surface is often ulcerated, the dysplastic or frankly malignant epithelial areas may be scant to nonexistent.[37,39] This is especially true in small incisional biopsies. Locating the epithelial component may require extensive sampling, and is most consistently identified at the base of the lesion, at the advancing margins, or the nonulcerated areas (**Fig. 3–10**).[36,38]

Spindle cells often compose the bulk of the lesion and may be arranged in fascicular, whorled, storiform, herringbone, or haphazard architectural patterns. The spindle cells demonstrate mild-to-moderate pleomorphism with variable mitotic activity. They may blend with or "drop off" the overlying epithelium, a feature that may be helpful in clarifying the epithelial nature of the disease. The neoplasm may mimic sarcomas such as malignant fibrous histiocytoma, fibrosarcoma, or leiomyosarcoma, or other entities such as amelanotic melanoma, nodular fasciitis or fibromatosis. Other confounding presentations may include the presence of multinucleated giant cells, osteosarcoma, or chondrosarcoma-like areas.[36,38,42] Immunohistochemistry and electron microscopy demonstrates spindle cells with epithelial, "transitional," and mesenchymal characteristics, which may add to the diagnostic confusion.[43,44]

Prognosis

The prognosis for SCSC within the oral cavity is worse than that of the larynx.[41,42] One possibility for this dissimilarity in prognosis is differences in the depth of invasion. Laryngeal tumors tend to be exophytic and polypoid, with the bulk of the tumor being superficial and confined within the polyp. Intraoral neoplasms are frequently more bulky or ulcerative with tumor invasion into the underlying minor salivary glands, skeletal muscle, or bone. This feature of deep invasion has been found to be of significant prognostic importance.[40] Patients whose lesions developed secondary to radiotherapy also demonstrate a worse prognosis. Otherwise,

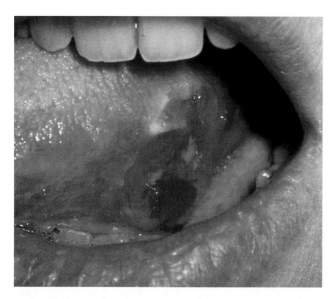

Figure 3–9 Spindle cell (sarcomatoid) carcinoma of the lateral border of the tongue. A large area of ulceration is surrounded by areas of erythroplakia. (Courtesy of Dr. Esther Childers.)

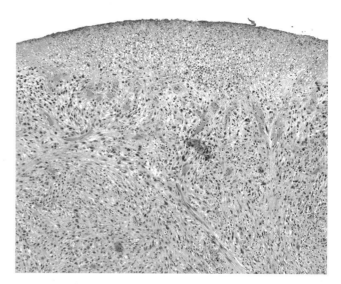

Figure 3–10 Spindle cell (sarcomatoid) carcinoma. Surface ulceration is a common histologic finding and traditional squamous cell carcinoma may be scant or absent. The bulk of the lesion is composed of malignant spindle cells displaying significant pleomorphism and hyperchromaticity.

the prognosis is similar to that for high-grade squamous cell carcinoma in the same location, with possible distant metastatic spread to lung, skin, or bone.

Basaloid Squamous Cell Carcinoma

Clinical Pathology

Basaloid squamous cell carcinoma (BSCC) is a rare, aggressive, biphasic variant of squamous cell carcinoma consisting of a high-grade basaloid epithelial proliferation and traditional squamous cell carcinoma or epithelial dysplasia.[45-48] It has a tendency to originate within the base of the tongue, hypopharynx (pyriform sinus), tonsillar mucosa, and supraglottic larynx. Intraoral sites include the floor of mouth, palate, buccal mucosa, retromolar pad, and gingiva.[49-54]

Etiologic and demographic factors are similar to those of conventional squamous cell carcinoma, although tumors within the oral cavity are almost equally distributed between the two genders.[45,47,54-56] The tumors are often large and deeply invasive at initial presentation. Multifocality, either initially or during the course of the disease, may be seen.[55] Patients also commonly present at a high initial stage, with almost 70% of patients having cervical metastasis or distant spread. Presenting symptoms may include pain, dysphagia, weight loss, or cough.[57]

Histopathology

Basaloid squamous cell carcinoma is a biphasic epithelial malignancy with conventional squamous cell carcinoma (invasive or in situ) and undifferentiated basaloid cells.[45,47,53,58] There may be an abrupt transition between the two elements, which is usually just below the overlying mucosa. As with spindle cell (sarcomatoid) carcinoma, the conventional squamous component may be scant.

The basaloid cells are small, with scant cytoplasm and hyperchromatic nuclei, with or without nucleoli. They are usually closely apposed to the surface mucosa and may be in nests, solid sheets, or festoon, cribriform, pseudoglandular, or trabecular growth patterns. A brisk mitotic rate is common, and comedonecrosis within the tumor lobules is a characteristic feature. The tumor lobules may demonstrate peripheral palisading of the basaloid cells (**Fig. 3–11**). Other characteristic features include small cyst-like areas containing mucinous material and hyalinization of the stroma with microcyst formation. The tumor may be extensively invasive into nerves, vascular channels, soft tissue, or adjacent bone. An associated spindle cell carcinoma has also been reported in the literature.[59]

Prognosis

There has been much debate within the literature about whether BSCC is truly a more aggressive malignancy than conventional SCC when matched for tumor location, patient age, and clinical stage.[45,47,48,60] One study found that, when compared with squamous cell carcinoma in the

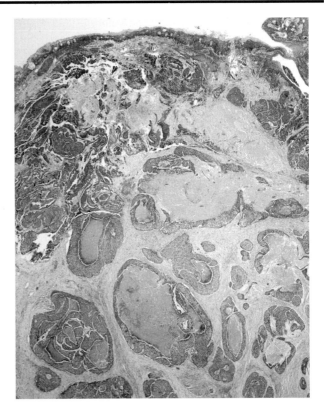

Figure 3–11 Basaloid squamous cell carcinoma. This low-power view shows epithelial surface dysplasia and variably sized nests and trabeculae. Note the large islands deep within the tumor displaying central necrosis (comedonecrosis).

floor of the mouth, BSCC within the same location showed a higher incidence of recurrence, metastasis, and mortality, with a shorted mean survival time.[49] Regardless, as the patients tend to present late in the course of their disease, prognosis is uniformly poor. In addition, as this tumor may exhibit multifocal presentation and carries a high recurrence rate, long-term follow-up is required.

◆ Cancer of the Minor Salivary Glands

Although squamous cell carcinoma makes up the vast majority of malignancies within the oral cavity, other forms of malignancy exist. Cancer of the minor salivary glands is a well-documented occurrence, and as a group makes up the second most common type of primary intraoral cancer.[3]

Minor salivary gland malignancies make up 46 to 49% of the total number of malignant neoplasms that affect the salivary glands.[61-64] In addition, about half of all neoplasms that originate from the minor salivary glands are malignant. Site-specific differences do occur, with those within the upper lip typically being benign, whereas those in the tongue, floor of mouth, and retromolar trigone are more frequently malignant. A majority of malignant intraoral salivary gland neoplasms occur in the hard palate, which is the only oral site where the incidence of minor salivary gland neoplasms approximates squamous cell carcinoma.[3,65]

Table 3–1 Malignancies Involving the Minor Salivary Glands

Mucoepidermoid carcinoma
Polymorphous low-grade adenocarcinoma
Adenoid cystic carcinoma
Adenocarcinoma, not otherwise specified
Acinic cell adenocarcinoma
Clear cell adenocarcinoma
Carcinoma ex pleomorphic adenoma
Cystadenocarcinoma

Multiple forms of malignancy originate from the minor salivary glands (**Table 3–1**), consisting primarily of mucoepidermoid carcinoma, polymorphous low-grade adenocarcinoma and adenoid cystic carcinoma.[63,64,66,67] Adenocarcinoma, not otherwise specified, is also a frequently identified form of cancer. Although many other types of salivary gland malignancy exist, they are rare in the minor salivary glands and thus are not discussed here.

Staging for malignancies of the minor salivary glands is identical to that of intraoral squamous cell carcinoma. See Chapter 7 for a detailed account.

Mucoepidermoid Carcinoma

Clinical Pathology

Mucoepidermoid carcinoma (MEC) is the most common malignancy involving the intraoral minor salivary glands. Although practically any age may be affected, it is generally seen in the fifth to sixth decade, with an average age of 43 years. It is the most common salivary gland malignancy in childhood, typically occurring between the ages of 11 and 16. Females are affected slightly more commonly than males. The palate is by far the most frequently affected site, followed by the buccal mucosa, tongue, lower lip, floor of mouth, vestibule, and tonsillar areas.

Many intraoral mucoepidermoid carcinomas are asymptomatic and discovered during routine evaluation. A painless, slow-growing mass is the most common complaint. Patient awareness of this mass occurs on average 1.5 years before diagnosis. Some may persist for long periods of time, only to become worrisome after recent accelerated growth. Pain or paresthesia is unusual, and tends to be associated with high-grade neoplasms or those with intrabony spread (**Fig. 3–12**) The lesions may be blue, red, purple, or magenta, and may mimic vascular proliferations or mucoceles. The surface is typically smooth, although granular and papillary presentations may occur. The neoplasms may be fluctuant or firm and seldom attain size greater than 5 cm. A mucous draining sinus tract may be present.[63,67–70]

Histopathology

Mucoepidermoid carcinoma is an epithelial malignancy composed of multiple cells types and architectural patterns. Common to all MECs is the mucocyte, which may be seen singly, in nests, or within the wall of cystic or ductal structures. They are oval to polygonal in shape, have a peripherally

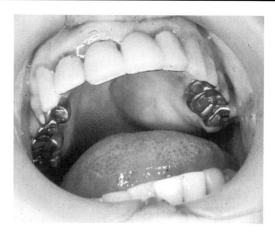

Figure 3–12 Mucoepidermoid carcinoma. Hard palate swelling that appears smooth and nonulcerated. This is a typical appearance for low-grade lesions.

located nucleus, and have abundant bluish cytoplasm. Although all MECs contain mucocytes, these cells are not pathognomonic of this disease as they may be seen in several other salivary gland neoplasms. Other cell types include epidermoid (squamoid), clear, and "intermediate." Architectural patterns may include cystic, solid, and nested arrangements (**Fig. 3–13**).

Primary mucoepidermoid carcinomas are given a histologic grade. Although many grading schemes have been proffered, the one designed by Auclair and colleagues[68] has demonstrated good reproducibility and correlation with prognosis (**Table 3–2**). This weighted scale is dependent on features such as the amount of intracystic component, perineural invasion, tumor necrosis, number of mitoses, and cellular anaplasia. Low-grade tumors are primarily cystic, cytologically bland, with low numbers of mitotic figures and infrequent necrosis or neural invasion. Mucocytes may

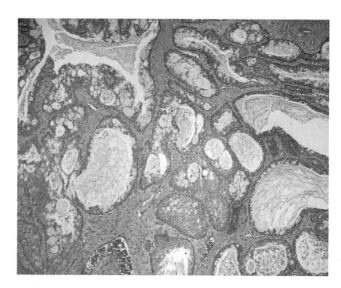

Figure 3–13 Mucoepidermoid carcinoma. The low-power view demonstrates numerous variably sized cysts and solid nests of epithelial cells. The walls of the cysts contain numerous mucocytes with voluminous clear cytoplasm.

Table 3–2 Histologic Grading of Mucoepidermoid Carcinoma

Parameter	Point Value
Intracystic component <20%	+2
Neural invasion present	+2
Necrosis present	+3
Four or more mitoses per 10 high-powered fields	+3
Anaplasia	+4
Grade	**Total Point Score**
Low	0–4
Intermediate	5–6
High	7 or more

From Auclair PL, Goode RK, Ellis GL. Mucoepidermoid carcinoma of intraoral salivary glands: evaluation and application of grading criteria in 143 cases. Cancer 1992;69:2021–2030, with permission.

be abundant. High-grade tumors are frequently more solid, necrotic, and cytologically anaplastic with numerous mitoses. Mucocytes may be rare.

Prognosis

Prognosis depends on adequacy of excision, tumor grade, and clinical stage. A recurrence rate of 7 to 13% has been reported if tumor-free margins are achieved.[68,71] However, 50% of low- to intermediate-grade neoplasms and 80% of high-grade lesions recurred if margins were positive for tumor.[72] Recurrence tends to occur within the first year after therapy. However, as recurrences have been reported as late as 22 years after treatment, long-term follow-up is required.[68]

Low-grade tumors of the minor salivary glands metastasize to regional lymph nodes in approximately 2.5% of cases, and the 5-year survival rate is 90 to 100%. Intermediate- and high-grade lesions have a greater tendency to recur and metastasize, with high-grade lesions metastasizing in 80% of cases.[69] Almost all patients who perish of the disease have regional or distant metastases. Distant sites may include the lung, skeletal bone, and brain.

Histologic grade and tumor stage are interrelated yet independent factors in prognosis. Low-grade neoplasms are less aggressive than high-grade tumors regardless of clinical stage, and stage I patients have better survival than stage III or IV regardless of histologic grade.[73] Better survival is seen among female patients and those who are younger. Patients older than 60 years have a poorer prognosis irrespective of other factors.[74] MEC in the base of tongue has a worse prognosis than when affecting other minor salivary gland sites.

Polymorphous Low-Grade Adenocarcinoma

Clinical Pathology

Polymorphous low-grade adenocarcinoma (PLGA) is a relatively recently described malignancy that is almost exclusively relegated to the intraoral minor salivary glands.[75–77] It is the second most common minor salivary gland malignancy.[67] Females are affected almost twice as often as males, with an average age at presentation of 58 years. As opposed to mucoepidermoid carcinoma, PLGA is almost

never encountered in the first or second decade of life. The palate is by far the most affected site, followed by the buccal mucosa, lips, alveolar ridge, and retromolar trigone.

Polymorphous low-grade adenocarcinoma presents as a slowly enlarging mass lesion in a majority of patients. Rare complaints of pain, bleeding, or ulceration may be noted. An ill-fitting denture may be the initial presenting symptom, whereas several PLGAs may be discovered incidentally during routine examination. As this malignancy behaves in a relatively indolent fashion, the average duration of signs or symptoms is quite long, being reported as 27 months.[75]

Histopathology

Polymorphous low-grade adenocarcinoma is characterized by numerous architectural patterns but limited cytologic variations. It tends to be well circumscribed but unencapsulated. Architecturally, cords and trabeculae, solid nests, and tubular/duct-like structures are commonly identified. Other patterns may include cribriform, microcystic, fascicular, papillary, and single-file chains. A targetoid arrangement is classic, with swirls of neoplastic cells surrounding a central nidus, typically a peripheral nerve. Perineural invasion is identified in a vast majority of PLGAs and is a characteristic feature of this disease. Infiltration into the surrounding minor salivary glands or connective tissues is common, although extension into the overlying epithelium is rare (**Fig. 3–14**).

Although multiple architectural patterns may be present, the cells are relatively uniform. They are round to polygonal and of small to medium size. Nuclear morphology is bland, with limited to absent pleomorphism. The nuclei are round to oval in shape with evenly dispersed chromatin and small-to-nonexistent nucleoli. Mitoses are uncommon and never atypical. Necrosis, when present, is very limited. The cells may be set within a hyalinized or mucohyaline

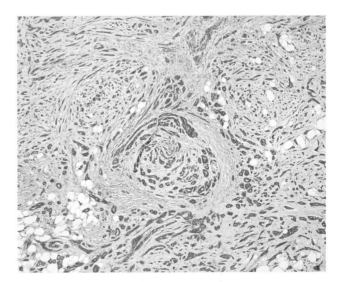

Figure 3–14 Polymorphous low-grade adenocarcinoma. This low-power view shows numerous small duct-like structures, trabeculae, and small nests of epithelial cells. A targetoid pattern is present with swirls of cells surrounding a central nidus. Tumor cells are infiltrating the fat and connective tissue.

background, simulating a pleomorphic adenoma. However, the myxochondroid stroma of a pleomorphic adenoma is not a feature of PLGA.[75–77]

Prognosis

A 9 to 17% recurrence rate for PLGA has been noted.[75,78] The range of time for recurrence is very broad (1 to 24 years), with an average of just over 7 years.[76] Female gender and palatal location are associated with higher recurrence. Most recurrences are controlled by additional surgical treatment. Lymph node metastasis is rare. Distant metastasis is also uncommon, though it has been reported in the lung, skeletal bone, and skin.

Polymorphous low-grade adenocarcinoma is a relatively nonaggressive malignancy with an excellent prognosis, and it only rarely causes a patient's demise. Distant metastasis seems to be the only factor influencing the outcome of the disease. The presence of recurrences, the location of the tumor, tumor size, cervical metastases, patient age, or tumor invasion of bone have not been shown to alter survival. High-grade transformation by the tumor has been reported, but this also has not proven to alter prognosis.[79,80]

Adenoid Cystic Carcinoma

Clinical Pathology

Adenoid cystic carcinoma (ACC) is overall the third most common minor salivary gland malignancy.[81] It is seen in a wide age range, being noted from the first through the ninth decades, with the average seen in the middle of the sixth decade of life.[65,82] Females are affected equal to, or slightly more often than, males.[81,82]

The palate is by far the most frequently involved site, followed distantly by the posterior tongue, buccal mucosa, lips, floor of mouth, and retromolar trigone area. A slow-growing swelling or mass is the most common presenting symptom. Pain or mucosal surface ulceration may be present at the later stages of development. Invasion into adjacent bone may occur, necessitating radiographic evaluation (**Fig. 3–15**). Regional lymph node metastasis is uncommon for this neoplasm (6 to 8%), whereas distant spread is more frequent, seen in 3 to 8% of patients during initial presentation and 40 to 55% overall.[82–87]

Histopathology

Adenoid cystic carcinoma consists primarily of three architectural patterns and two cell types. The three patterns include tubular, cribriform, and solid. The tubular pattern consists of small tubules or duct-like structures set within a hyalinized background. The cribriform pattern consists of variably sized islands of tumor punctuated by well-formed round spaces imparting a Swiss-cheese appearance. The solid pattern portrays solid sheets or nests of tumor cells without spaces or ductal structures. True ductal lumina may be evident, especially notable in the tubular pattern. ACC may be limited to any one pattern, although most

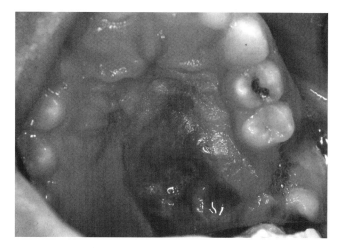

Figure 3–15   Adenoid cystic carcinoma. A large ulcerated swelling is present in the mid-to-posterior hard palate. (Courtesy of Dr. Chris Fielding.)

display a variety (**Fig. 3–16**). If the solid pattern represents greater than 30% of the neoplasm, it is considered the predominant pattern for prognostic purposes.[88,89]

Ductal epithelial and myoepithelial cells are present within ACCs. The vast majority of the cells are myoepithelial, being small to medium-sized with scant, typically clear cytoplasm. The nuclei are hyperchromatic and round to angular in morphology. Larger cells with prominent nucleoli are seen in the solid pattern. Mitoses are rare in the cribriform and tubular patterns, but commonly numerous and atypical in the solid portions. The ductal cells are polygonal with eosinophilic cytoplasm and are usually surrounded by the myoepithelial cells. Perineural invasion is very common in adenoid cystic carcinoma. Necrosis is most often identified in the solid areas.

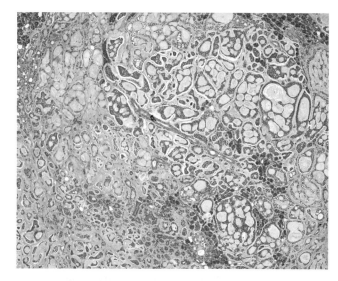

Figure 3–16   Adenoid cystic carcinoma. Low-power view of a diffusely infiltrative malignancy with tubular, trabecular, and cribriform growth patterns. Amorphous hyaline material surrounds the islands and is present within the lumina.

Prognosis

Recurrence rate is higher than for any other minor salivary gland malignant neoplasm, with reports being anywhere from 53 to 62%.[90,91] Most recurrences occur within the first 5 years, although local failure as long as 20 years after initial treatment is possible.[85]

Adenoid cystic carcinoma has a deceptively high 5-year survival rate, ranging from 38 to 89%.[92,93] However, ACC is known for late distant metastatic spread, most commonly to the lungs, skeletal bone, brain, liver, thyroid, or spleen, leading to a 10-year survival of 29 to 67%. The average time from diagnosis to distant spread is 37 months, with a range from 0 to 112 months.[82] Negative factors influencing mortality include a large tumor size, solid architectural pattern, perineural invasion, invasion into bone, positive surgical margins, and lymph node or distant metastases.[94] An improved prognosis is seen with a tubular or cribriform histologic pattern.[65]

◆ Mucosal Melanoma

Mucosal melanoma of the head and neck represents approximately 0.4 to 1.8% of all melanomas.[95,96] The sinonasal region and oral cavity are by far the most commonly affected regions, with about equal distribution between the two sites.[95] The following discussion focuses on those lesions involving the oral cavity.

Clinical Pathology

Oral mucosal melanoma makes up approximately 0.5% of all oral malignancies.[97] As the oral cavity may also harbor metastases from another site, it is important to rule out a distant primary before accepting the disease as originating within the mouth.[98]

Oral melanoma is often asymptomatic, with 16% of lesions discovered incidentally.[99] Pain, ulceration, bleeding, loose teeth, ill-fitting dentures, or nodular growth may occur, with an average clinical duration of 1 to 5 months.[100] A preexisting macular pigmented lesion (melanosis) is present in 30 to 50% of patients. This may last for many years before a mass lesion develops.[101–103] Color variations include black, gray, purple, red, or white, with pigmentation being uniform or irregular (**Fig. 3–17**). Multifocal presentation is seen in 22%.[99]

The palate is the most common site for oral melanoma, representing 42% of the lesions. The alveolus, lips, and buccal mucosa are also affected. In contrast to squamous cell carcinoma, the tongue and floor of mouth are only rarely involved.[101,104] Overall, males slightly outnumber females with an average age of presentation being in the middle of the sixth decade.[99,105,106]

Histopathology

Melanoma may present with multiple cytomorphologies and architectural patterns. The malignant melanocytic population may be relegated to the epithelium (in-situ pattern),

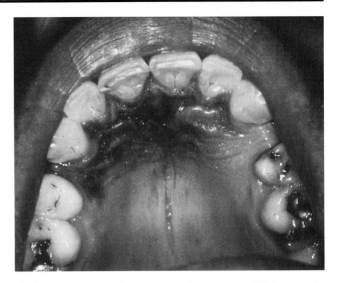

Figure 3–17 Mucosal melanoma. This pigmented lesion on the anterior hard palate is asymmetric, with ill-defined, irregular borders and an uneven color density. All of these features are in keeping with melanoma.

completely within the underlying connective tissues (invasive pattern), or a combination of the two. In the in-situ pattern, there is an increased amount of irregular melanocytes that may be unevenly distributed at the epithelial/connective tissue interface, or less commonly found in small nests. The nuclei are hyperchromatic and pleomorphic, and mitotic figures may be identified. The invasive pattern consists of spindled, epithelioid, plasmacytoid, or anaplastic cells within the lamina propria. Mitoses are common and may be atypical. Alveolar, nested, solid, desmoplastic, or diffuse architectural growth patterns may be observed. Melanin is present in approximately 90% of the lesions; the remaining lesions are amelanotic (**Fig. 3–18**). S-100

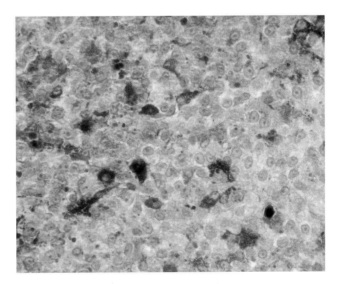

Figure 3–18 Melanoma. This high-power view demonstrates sheets of fairly monotonous epithelioid cells with large nuclei and prominent nucleoli. Many of the cells contain granular pigmented material consistent with melanin. This tissue strongly expressed S-100 and HMB-45.

is generally strongly and diffusely reactive in all melanomas. HMB-45 may be reactive in the epithelioid cells, whereas it is regularly nonreactive in the spindled cells. Melan-A and tyrosinase may also decorate the malignant melanocytes.

Staging

No American Joint Committee on Cancer (AJCC) tumor, node, and metastasis (TNM) staging system exists for oral mucosal melanoma. Currently three basic stages are recognized: stage I, localized disease; stage II, regional lymph node metastasis; and stage III, distant metastasis. Oral mucosal melanoma tends to be diagnosed late in its disease course, with 25 to 48% of patients presenting with nodal disease (stage II), and approximately 6 to 14% harboring distant metastases (stage III).[96,99,100] The lung and brain are the most common sites of distant spread.

Prognosis

Oral mucosal melanoma carries a very poor prognosis. Although an inherent biologic aggressiveness may play a role, the poor prognosis is usually related to late diagnosis and high clinical stage.[104,107] The prognosis of oral melanoma is related to stage at presentation. The presence of distant metastasis (stage III) is the most compelling factor, followed by nodal metastasis. Patients with nodal disease experience an 18-month median life expectancy, whereas those without are extended to 46 months.[99,100] Other aspects influencing survival include tumor thickness greater than 5 mm, invasion or erosion of bone, and vascular invasion.[108] Location of the melanoma also has an effect, where those located in the alveolus/gingiva have a slightly greater 5-year survival rate and median survival time (18% and 46 months) than palatal lesions (11% and 22 months). The overall 5-year survival is 12 to 15% with a median of 18 to 25 months.[97,101,108]

After surgical excision, local failure occurs in 50% of the cases. Local failure has not been shown to statistically alter survival; however, it is related to distant metastatic spread. Distant failure occurs in approximately 67% of patients, and 89% of patients with distant metastasis displayed local recurrences.[109] Regional nodal failure occurs in approximately 36 to 42% of patients.[99,110] However, this was not found to be statistically significant in relation to overall prognosis.

◆ Conclusion

This chapter provided a brief overview of the large and very complex topic of oral cavity malignant neoplasms. As the vast majority of types of oral malignancies have been well elucidated in the literature, current research is concentrating on the molecular and genetic characteristics of the various diseases. With time, the molecular pathogenesis of each neoplasm may be determined, and subsequent chemotherapeutic agents directed at specific genetic targets may greatly assist in treatment. Presently, however, complete surgical excision is the treatment of choice for all of the entities discussed, and clinical cure is best achieved with adequate initial surgical intervention.

References

1. Ostman J, Anneroth G, Gustafsson H. Malignant oral tumors in Sweden 1960–1989—an epidemiologic study. Eur J Cancer B Oral Oncol 1995;31B:106–112

2. Sugerman PB, Savage NW. Current concepts in oral cancer. Aust Dent J 1999;44:147–156

3. Funk GF, Karnell LH, Robinson RA, Zhen WK, Trask DK, Hoffman HT. Presentation, treatment, and outcome of oral cavity cancer: a National Cancer Data Base report. Head Neck 2002;24:165–180

4. Tralongo V, Rodolico V, Luciani A. Prognostic factors in oral squamous cell carcinoma: a review of the literature. Anticancer Res 1999;19:3503–3510

5. Prince S, Bailey BMW. Squamous carcinoma of the tongue: review. Br J Oral Maxillofac Surg 1999;37:164–174

6. Cancer Statistics Review SEER, 1975–2000. Oral Cavity and Pharynx Cancer (Invasive). National Cancer Institute, 2003

7. Klijanienko J, El-Naggar A, De Braund F. Tumor vascularization, mitotic index, histopathologic grade, and DNA ploidy in the assessment of 114 head and neck squamous cell carcinomas. Cancer 1995;75:1649–1656

8. Hibbert J, Marks NJ, Winter PJH. Prognostic factors in oral carcinoma and their relation to clinical staging. Clin Otolaryngol 1983;8:197–203

9. Henk L. Malignant Tumors of the Oral Cavity. London: Edward Arnold, 1985

10. Frierson HF, Cooper PH. Prognostic factors in squamous cell carcinoma of the lower lip. Hum Pathol 1986;17:346–354

11. Byers RM, O'Brien CJ, Waxler J. The therapeutic and prognostic implications of nerve invasion in cancer of the lower lip. Int J Radiat Oncol Biol Physiol 1978;4:215–219

12. Daniele E, Rodolico V, Leonardi V. Prognosis in lower lip squamous cell carcinoma: assessment of tumor factors. Pathol Res Pract 1998;194:319–324

13. Hemmer J, Schon E, Kreidler J. Prognostic implications of DNA ploidy in squamous cell carcinomas of the tongue assessed by flow cytometry. J Cancer Res Clin Oncol 1990;116:83–86

14. Tytor M, Franzen G, Olofsson J. DNA pattern in oral cavity carcinomas in relation to clinical stage and histologic grading. Pathol Res Pract 1987;182:202–206

15. Baretton G, Li X, Stoll C. Prognostic significance of DNA ploidy in oral squamous cell carcinomas: a retrospective flow and image cytometric study with comparison of DNA ploidy in excisional biopsy specimens and resection specimens, primary tumors, and lymph node metastases. Oral Surg Oral Med Oral Pathol Oral Radiol Endod 1995;79:68–76

16. Migaldi M, Criscuolo M, Zunarelli E. p120 and AgNOR nucleolar protein expression. Oral Surg Oral Med Oral Pathol Oral Radiol Endod 1998;85:189–196

17. Sano K, Takahashi H, Fujita S. Prognostic implication of silver binding nucleolar organizer regions (AgNORs) in oral squamous cell carcinoma. J Oral Pathol Med 1991;20:53–56

18. Teixeira G, Antonangelo L, Kowalski L. Argyrophilic nucleolar organizer regions staining is useful in predicting recurrence-free interval in oral tongue and floor of mouth squamous cell carcinoma. Am J Surg 1996;172:684–688

19. Michalides RJ, van Veelen NM, Kristel PM, et al. Overexpression of cyclin D1 indicates a poor prognosis in squamous cell carcinoma of the head and neck. Arch Otolaryngol Head Neck Surg 1997;123:497–502

20. Wang X, Pavelic ZP, Li YQ, et al. Amplification and overexpression of cyclin D1 gene in head and neck squamous cell carcinoma. Clin Mol Pathol 1995;48:256–259

21. Partridge M, Emilion G, Langdon JD. LOH at 3p correlates with a poor survival in oral squamous cell carcinoma. Br J Cancer 1996;73:366–371

22. Field JK, Tsiriyotis C, Zoumpourlis V. Allele loss on chromosome 3 in squamous cell carcinoma of the head and neck correlates with poor clinical prognostic indicators. Int J Oncol 1994;4:543–549

23. Venkatesan TK, Kuropkat C, Caldarelli DD. Prognostic significance of p27 expression in carcinoma of the oral cavity and oropharynx. Laryngoscope 1999;109:1329–1333

24. Mineta H, Miura K, Suzuki I. Low p27 expression correlates with poor prognosis for patients with oral tongue squamous cell carcinoma. Cancer 1999;85:1011–1017

25. Nylander K, Dabelsteen E, Hall PA. The p53 molecule and its prognostic role in squamous cell carcinomas of the head and neck. J Oral Pathol Med 2000;29:413–425

26. Bankfalvi A, Piffko J. Prognostic and predictive factors in oral cancer: the role of the invasive tumor front. J Oral Pathol Med 2000;29: 291–298

27. Ackerman LV. Verrucous carcinoma of the oral cavity. Surgery 1948;23:670–678

28. Batsakis JG, Hybels R, Crissman JD. The pathology of head and neck tumors: verrucous carcinoma, part 15. Head Neck Surg 1982;5:29–38

29. Sciubba JJ. Oral cancer: the importance of early diagnosis and treatment. Am J Clin Dermatol 2001;2:239–251

30. Neville BW, Day TA. Oral cancer and precancerous lesions. CA Cancer J Clin 2002;52:195–215

31. Summerlin DJ. Precancerous and cancerous lesions of the oral cavity. Dermatol Clin 1996;14:205–223

32. Schwartz RA. Verrucous carcinoma of the skin and mucosa. J Am Acad Dermatol 1995;32:1–21

33. Bouquot JE. Oral verrucous carcinoma, incidence in two U.S. populations. Oral Surg Oral Med Oral Pathol Oral Radiol Endod 1998;86:318–324

34. Florin EH, Kolbusz RV. Verrucous carcinoma of the oral cavity. Int J Dermatol 1994;33:618–622

35. McDonald JS, Crissman JD, Gluckman JL. Verrucous carcinoma of the oral cavity. Head Neck Surg 1982;5:22–28

36. Thompson LD, Wieneke JA, Miettinen M. Spindle cell (sarcomatoid) carcinomas of the larynx: a clinicopathologic study of 187 cases. Am J Surg Pathol 2002;26:153–170

37. Zarbo RJ, Crissman JD, Venkat H. Spindle-cell carcinoma of the upper aerodigestive tract mucosa. Am J Surg Pathol 1986;10: 741–753

38. Ellis GL, Corio RL. Spindle cell carcinoma of the oral cavity: a clinicopathologic assessment of 59 cases. Oral Surg Oral Med Oral Pathol 1980;50:523–534

39. Ellis GL, Langloss JM, Heffner DK. Spindle-cell carcinoma of the aerodigestive tract. Am J Surg Pathol 1987;11:335–342

40. Leventon GS, Evans HL. Sarcomatoid squamous cell carcinoma of the mucous membranes of the head and neck. Cancer 1981; 48:994–1003

41. Batsakis JG, Saurez P. Sarcomatoid carcinomas of the upper aerodigestive tracts. Adv Anat Pathol 2000;7:282–293

42. Batsakis JG, Rice DH, Howard DR. The pathology of head and neck tumors: spindle cell lesions (sarcomatoid carcinomas, nodular fasciitis, and fibrosarcoma). Head Neck Surg 1982;4:499–513

43. Battifora H. Spindle cell carcinoma: ultrastructural evidence of squamous origin and collagen production by tumor cells. Cancer 1976;37:2275–2282

44. Weidner N. Sarcomatoid carcinoma of the upper aerodigestive tract. Semin Diagn Pathol 1987;4:157–168

45. Wain SL, Kier R, Vollmer RT. Basaloid-squamous carcinoma of the tongue, hypopharynx, and larynx: report of ten cases. Hum Pathol 1986;17:1158–1166

46. Barnes L, Ferlito A, Altavilla G. Basaloid squamous cell carcinoma of the head and neck: clinicopathologic features and differential diagnosis. Ann Otol Rhinol Laryngol 1996;105:75–82

47. Banks ER, Frierson HF, Mills SE. Basaloid squamous cell carcinoma of the head and neck: a clinicopathologic and immunohistochemical study of 40 cases. Am J Surg Pathol 1992;16:939–946

48. Luna MA, El-Naggar A, Parichatikanond P. Basaloid squamous carcinoma of the upper aerodigestive tract: clinicopathologic and DNA flow cytometric analysis. Cancer 1990;66:537–542

49. Coppola D, Catalano E, Tang CK. Basaloid squamous cell carcinoma of the floor of mouth. Cancer 1993;72:2299–2305

50. Campman SC, Gandour-Edwards RF, Sykes JM. Basaloid squamous carcinoma of the head and neck: report of a case in the floor of the mouth. Arch Pathol Lab Med 1994;118:1229–1232

51. Hellquist HB, Dahl F, Karlsson MG. Basaloid squamous cell carcinoma of the palate. Histopathology 1994;25:178–180

52. Lovejoy HM, Matthews BL. Basaloid squamous carcinoma of the palate. Otolaryngol Head Neck Surg 1992;106:159–162

53. Coletta RD, Cotrim P, Almeida OP. Basaloid squamous cell carcinoma of oral cavity: a histologic and immunohistochemical study. Oral Oncol 2002;38:723–729

54. Ide F, Shimoyama T, Horie N. Basaloid squamous cell carcinoma of the oral mucosa: a new case and review of 45 cases in the literature. Oral Oncol 2002;38:120–124

55. Ferlito A, Altavilla G, Rinaldo A. Basaloid squamous cell carcinoma of the larynx and hypopharynx. Ann Otol Rhinol Laryngol 1997; 106:1024–1035

56. Raslan WF, Barnes L, Krause JR. Basaloid squamous cell carcinoma of the head and neck: a clinicopathologic and flow cytometric study of 10 new cases with review of the English literature. Am J Otolaryngol 1994;15:204–211

57. Paulino AF, Singh B, Shah JP. Basaloid squamous cell carcinoma of the head and neck. Laryngoscope 2000;110:1479–1482

58. Wieneke JA, Thompson LD, Wenig BM. Basaloid squamous cell carcinoma of the sinonasal tract. Cancer 1999;85:841–854

59. Muller S, Barnes L. Basaloid squamous cell carcinoma of the head and neck with a spindle cell component. Arch Pathol Lab Med 1995;119:181–182

60. Winzenburg SM, Niehans GA, George E. Basaloid squamous cell carcinoma: a clinical comparison of two histologic types with poorly differentiated squamous cell carcinoma. Otolaryngol Head Neck Surg 1998;119:471–475

61. Eveson JW, Cawson RA. Tumors of the minor salivary glands: a demographic study of 336 cases. J Oral Pathol 1985;14:500–509

62. Seifert G, Miehlke A, Haubrich J. Diseases of the Salivary Glands: Pathology, Diagnosis, Treatment, Facial Nerve Surgery. New York: George Thieme Verlag, 1986

63. Auclair PL, Ellis GL, Gnepp DR, et al. Salivary Gland Neoplasms: General Considerations. In: Ellis GL, Auclair PL, Gnepp DR, eds. Surgical Pathology of the Salivary Glands. Philadelphia: WB Saunders, 1991:135–164

64. Ellis GL, Auclair PL. Atlas of Tumor Pathology: Tumors of the Salivary Glands. Armed Forces Institute of Pathology, 1996:203–216

65. Witt RL. Adenoid cystic carcinoma of the minor salivary glands. Ear Nose Throat J 1991;70:218–222

66. 66. Neely MM, Rohrer MD, Young SK. Tumors of minor salivary glands and the analysis of 106 cases. Okla Dent Assoc J 1996;Spring:50–52

67. Waldron CA, El-Mofty SK, Gnepp DR. Tumors of the intraoral minor salivary glands: a demographic and histologic study of 426 cases. Oral Surg Oral Med Oral Pathol 1988;66:323–333

68. Auclair PL, Goode RK, Ellis GL. Mucoepidermoid carcinoma of intraoral salivary glands: evaluation and application of grading criteria in 143 cases. Cancer 1992;69:2021–2030

69. Auclair PL, Ellis GL. Mucoepidermoid carcinoma. In: Ellis GL, Auclair PL, Gnepp DR, eds. Surgical Pathology of the Salivary Glands. Philadelphia: WB Saunders, 1991:269–298

70. Luna MA, Batsakis JG, El-Naggar A. Salivary gland tumors in children. Ann Otol Rhinol Laryngol 1991;100:869–871

71. Melrose RJ, Abrams AM, Howell FV. Mucoepidermoid tumors of the intraoral minor salivary glands: a clinicopathologic study of 54 cases. J Oral Pathol 1973;2:314–325

72. Healey WV, Perzin KH, Smith L. Mucoepidermoid carcinoma of salivary gland origin: Classification, clinical pathologic correlation, and results of treatment. Cancer 1970;26:368–388

73. Nascimento AG, Amaral AL, Prado LA. Mucoepidermoid carcinoma of salivary glands. Head Neck Surg 1986;8:409–417

74. O'Brien CJ, Soong SJ, Herrera GA. Malignant salivary gland tumors: analysis of prognostic factors and survival. Head Neck Surg 1986;9:82–92

75. Castle JT, Thompson LDR, Frommelt RA. Polymorphous low-grade adenocarcinoma. Cancer 1999;86:207–219

76. Evans HL, Luna MA. Polymorphous low-grade adenocarcinoma: a study of 40 cases with long term follow-up and an evaluation of the importance of papillary areas. Am J Surg Pathol 2000;24:1319–1328

77. Perez-Ordonez B, Linkov I, Huvos AG. Polymorphous low-grade adenocarcinoma of minor salivary glands: a study of 17 cases with emphasis on cell differentiation. Histopathology 1998;32:521–529

78. Vincent SD, Hammond HL, Finkelstein MW. Clinical and therapeutic features of polymorphous low-grade adenocarcinoma. Oral Surg Oral Med Oral Pathol 1994;77:41–47

79. Simpson RH, Reis-Filho JS, Pereira EM. Polymorphous low-grade adenocarcinoma of the salivary glans with transformation to high-grade carcinoma. Histopathology 2002;41:250–259

80. Pelkey TJ, Mills SE. Histologic transformation of polymorphous low-grade adenocarcinoma of salivary gland. Am J Clin Pathol 1999;111:785–791

81. Tomich CE. Adenoid cystic carcinoma. In: Ellis GL, Auclair PL, Gnepp DR, eds. Surgical Pathology of the Salivary Glands. Philadelphia: WB Saunders, 1991:333–349

82. van der Wal JE, Becking AG, Snow GB. Distant metastases of adenoid cystic carcinoma of the salivary glands and the value of diagnostic examinations during follow-up. Head Neck 2002;24:779–783

83. Huang M, Ma D, Sun K. Factors influencing survival rate in adenoid cystic carcinoma of the salivary glands. Int J Oral Maxillofac Surg 1997;26:435–439

84. Spiro RH, Huvos AG. Stage means more than grade in adenoid cystic carcinoma. Am J Surg 1992;164:623–628

85. Garden AS, Weber RS, Morrison WH. The influence of positive margins and nerve invasion in adenoid cystic carcinoma of the head and neck treated with surgery and radiation. Int J Radiat Oncol Biol Phys 1995;32:619–626

86. Spiro RH. Distant metastasis in adenoid cystic carcinoma of salivary origin. Am J Surg 1997;174:495–498

87. Warren CJ, Gnepp DR, Rosenblum BN. Adenoid cystic carcinoma metastasizing before detection of the primary lesion. South Med J 1989;82:1277–1280

88. Szanto PA, Luna MA, Tortoledo ME. Histologic grading of adenoid cystic carcinoma of the salivary glands. Cancer 1984;54:1062–1069

89. Nascimento AG, Amaral AL, Prado LA. Adenoid cystic carcinoma of salivary glands. Cancer 1986;57:312–319

90. Shingaki S, Saito R, Kawasaki T. Adenoid cystic carcinoma of the major and minor salivary glands: a clinicopathologic study of 17 cases. J Maxillofac Surg 1986;14:53–56

91. Beckhardt RN, Weber RS, Zane R. Minor salivary gland tumors of the palate: clinical and pathologic correlates of outcome. Laryngoscope 1995;105:1155–1160

92. Fordice J, Kershaw C, El-Naggar AK. Adenoid cystic carcinoma of the head and neck: predictors of morbidity and mortality. Arch Otolaryngol Head Neck Surg 1999;125:149–152

93. Sur RK, Donde B, Levin V. Adenoid cystic carcinoma of the salivary glands: a review of 10 years. Laryngoscope 1997;107:1276–1280

94. Vrielinck LJG, Ostyn F, van Damme B. The significance of perineural spread in adenoid cystic carcinoma of the major and minor salivary glands. Int J Oral Maxillofac Surg 1988;17:190–193

95. Batsakis JG, Suarez P, El-Naggar AK. Mucosal melanomas of the head and neck. Ann Otol Rhinol Laryngol 1998;107:626–630

96. Batsakis JG, Suarez P. Mucosal melanomas: a review. Adv Anat Pathol 2000;7:167–180

97. Hicks MJ, Flaitz CM. Oral mucosal melanoma: epidemiology and pathobiology. Oral Oncol 2000;36:152–169

98. Patton LL, Brahim JS, Baker AR. Metastatic malignant melanoma of the oral cavity: a retrospective study. Oral Surg Oral Med Oral Pathol 1994;78:51–56

99. Patel SG, Prasad ML, Escrig M. Primary mucosal malignant melanoma of the head and neck. Head Neck 2002;24:247–257

100. Pandey M, Mathew A, Iype EM. Primary malignant mucosal melanoma of the head and neck region: pooled analysis of 60 published cases from India and review of the literature. Eur J Cancer Prev 2002;11:3–10

101. Manolidis S, Donald PJ. Malignant mucosal melanoma of the head and neck. Cancer 1997;80:1373–1386

102. Batsakis JG, Regezi JA, Solomon AR. The pathology of head and neck tumors: mucosal melanomas. Head Neck Surg 1982;4:404–418

103. Regezi JA, Hayward JR, Pickens TN. Superficial melanomas of the oral mucous membranes. Oral Surg Oral Med Oral Pathol 1978;45:730–740

104. Barker BF, Carpenter WM, Daniels TE. Oral mucosal melanomas: The WESTOP Banff workshop proceedings. Oral Surg Oral Med Oral Pathol Oral Radiol Endod 1997;83:672–679

105. Manganaro AM, Hammond HL, Dalton MJ. Oral melanoma. Oral Surg Oral Med Oral Pathol Oral Radiol Endod 1995;80:670–676

106. Snow GB, van der Waal I. Mucosal melanomas of the head and neck. Otolaryngol Clin North Am 1986;19:537–547

107. Umeda M, Komatsubara H, Shibuya Y. Premalignant melanocytic dysplasia and malignant melanoma of the oral mucosa. Oral Oncol 2002;38:714–722

108. Rapini RP, Golitz LE, Greer RO. Primary malignant melanoma of the oral cavity. Cancer 1985;55:1543–1551

109. Stern SJ, Guillamondegui OM. Mucosal melanoma of the head and neck. Head Neck 1991;13:22–27

110. Nandapalan V, Roland NJ, Helliwell TR. Mucosal melanoma of the head and neck. Clin Otolaryngol 1998;23:107–116

4

Evaluation of Oral Premalignant Lesions

Ann Gillenwater

Most oral cancer patients present with advanced disease, and treatment for these patients is more complex, more expensive, and less successful than interventions for early-stage disease. Therefore, advances in early detection and diagnosis should have a substantial impact on survival rates, functional outcome and quality of life scores, and cost of care measures. Exposure of oral mucosa to carcinogenic agents, such as those contained in tobacco and alcohol, initiates the multistep process of carcinogenesis. The resultant progression of neoplastic changes, from normal to dysplasia and finally to invasive cancer, occurs variably over the course of months to several years. This premalignant phase provides us with an opportunity to detect, diagnose, treat, and potentially reverse neoplastic changes prior to the development of invasive carcinoma. Early detection and treatment of neoplastic cells before they have had the opportunity to invade into the underlying tissue or to metastasize has the potential to improve quality of life and survival rates. This chapter reviews the clinical and molecular features of premalignant lesions of the oral mucosa, and discusses several approaches to the diagnosis and management of these lesions.

◆ Transformation of Normal Oral Mucosa to Invasive Carcinoma

Oral Carcinogenesis Progression Model

Like other solid tumors, oral cancers are thought to arise from the clonal outgrowth of viable cells with persistent, accumulated genetic damage.[1] The progression model of epithelial carcinogenesis suggests that there is a sustained,

stepwise accumulation of mutations, resulting in transition of normal mucosa to dysplasia to invasive carcinoma over time.[2,3] Research efforts focused on unraveling the mechanisms of oral carcinogenesis have identified specific mutations that occur during these transitional steps.[3,4] These mutations often involve inactivation of tumor suppressor genes or activation of proto-oncogenes. Future diagnostic and therapeutic intervention during this process may be directed at preventing or reversing these specific molecular abnormalities.

Oral Premalignant Lesions

In some cases, the genetically damaged cells are clinically indistinguishable from normal oral mucosa, but genetic mutations frequently produce phenotypic changes that can be visually identified. Thus, some patients with premalignant changes in the oral mucosa may present with clinically apparent lesions. A premalignant lesion can be considered an area of morphologically or genetically altered tissue that is more likely than normal tissue to develop cancer. Well-recognized oral lesions and conditions that are associated with malignant potential include leukoplakia (a predominantly white lesion), erythroplakia (a predominantly reddish lesion), lichen planus, and submucous fibrosis.

Oral leukoplakia is defined as a white plaque that cannot be scraped off and that cannot be otherwise classified.[5] The term *leukoplakia*, reportedly first used in 1877,[5a] has generated both confusion and controversy; it is purely a clinical term, a diagnosis of exclusion, and it should not be used in histopathologic assessments of biopsy specimens. Many conditions, such as traumatic irritation, lichen planus, candida infections, severe dysplasia, and even carcinoma, can initially present as leukoplakia. Once a specific clinical or pathologic diagnosis is obtained, then the oral lesion is no longer considered leukoplakia. Leukoplakia that has an erythematous component is often termed erythroleukoplakia, speckled leukoplakia, or nonhomogeneous leukoplakia. Erythroplakia or erythroplasia describes predominantly reddish lesions, often velvety in texture, that have a high propensity for the presence of dysplasia and development of carcinoma.[6]

Over the years, oral premalignant lesions have been grouped into clinical categories. *Leukoplakia, erythroleukoplakia,* and *erythroplakia* are subjective, descriptive terms indicating the relative amounts of white versus reddish coloration. Homogeneous leukoplakia is characterized by a uniform, thin, smooth, predominantly white appearance without erythema or ulceration.[7,8] A nonhomogeneous leukoplakia is a lesion that is predominantly white or white and red (erythroleukoplakia) with an irregular texture. Nonhomogeneous leukoplakia can be exophytic, papillary, or even verrucous in texture and is often associated with pain or discomfort.[7] An unusual subtype of leukoplakia is proliferative verrucous leukoplakia (PVL),[9–11] which may initially present as a solitary homogeneous leukoplakia that on histopathologic assessment shows only hyperkeratosis without evidence of dysplasia. However, the leukoplakia typically recurs and relentlessly spreads to become diffuse, multifocal, and hyperkeratotic, with increasingly severe dysplasia and eventually carcinoma. In a long-term follow-up study of 54 patients with PVL, 70.3% of the patients developed squamous carcinoma in a mean of 7.7 years.[10]

Oral lichen planus is a chronic inflammatory disease of unknown etiology that occurs in 1 to 4% of the general population. Oral lichen planus is an autoimmune, T-cell–mediated condition resulting in accumulation of lymphocyte beneath basal keratinocytes and accelerated differentiation of the squamous epithelium with hyperkeratosis. Lesions most commonly occur on the buccal mucosa, tongue, gingiva, and lips. Relapses and remissions are characteristic. There are several well-documented clinical presentations of oral lichen planus. The reticular form, which usually presents as asymptomatic white lesions in a linear or lacy pattern, is the most common form. Erosive forms of oral lichen planus demonstrate erythema and ulceration with white striations at the periphery. Erosive lichen planus is often painful. Mild to moderate cases are treated with topical corticosteroids; severe cases may require systemic immunosuppression. Other topical agents such as tacrolimus and retinoids have also been used. The risk of malignant transformation of oral lichen planus lesions remains unclear, but estimates range from 0.5 to 3%.[12–14]

Formalized classification and staging systems for oral premalignant lesions have been proposed.[8,15,16] A staging system proposed by van der Waal et al is presented in **Table 4–1**.[16] The importance of adopting and consistently using a common staging system for oral premalignant lesions to facilitate uniform reporting cannot be overemphasized.

The prevalence of leukoplakia and other oral premalignant lesions has been hard to quantify. A 1988 review of 11 published studies found the prevalence of oral leukoplakia to range from 0.7 to 11.7%.[17] The prevalence varies based on the type of lesions included as "leukoplakia" and on the geographic area, socioeconomic class, racial/ethnic background, and age of the individuals surveyed.[18] In the United States, the prevalence of oral leukoplakia was reported to be 2.9% in 23,000 white subjects in 1986, whereas in a survey of 16,000 individuals published in 2003, the prevalence was found to be only 0.6% for males and 0.23% for females.[18,19] Some of the highest prevalence figures have been found in surveys of industrial workers in India.[20]

In general, the prevalence of leukoplakia increases with age and tobacco use. Reported risk factors for oral leukoplakia include use of tobacco, alcohol, and areca nut; dietary factors; and poor dental hygiene.[21,22] Dietrich et al[23] reported an analysis of risk factors for oral leukoplakia in 15,811 subjects enrolled in the U.S. National Health and Nutrition Survey. In this cohort, the most significant risk factor was tobacco use; other risk factors included diabetes, age, and socioeconomic status. Similarly, in a case-control study performed in Kerala, India, higher socioeconomic status, education, and income were associated with a decreased risk for development of oral leukoplakia and other oral premalignant lesions.[24] In addition, there have been reports of leukoplakia associated with the use of toothpaste or mouthwash containing sanguinaria, an herbal extract.[25–27] However, the relative risk of exposure to sanguinaria for the development of oral leukoplakia and malignant transformation requires further clarification.

Malignant Transformation

Leukoplakia, although benign by definition, is also associated with malignant transformation. The percentage of leukoplakic lesions, as well as other oral lesions, that progress to invasive carcinoma depends on various factors such as location within the oral cavity, clinical appearance (homogeneous versus heterogeneous), presence of dysplasia, demographic population assessed, and length of observation period. The rate of malignant transformation of leukoplakia reported in the literature varies between zero and 38%.[28–33] Silverman et al[32] studied 257 patients with oral leukoplakia for an average of 7.2 years and documented a 17.5% rate of subsequent malignant conversion. For those patients with histologic findings of dysplasia, the rate of malignant conversion at 8 years was 36.4%.

The annual rate of transformation for oral premalignant lesions allows for better comparison between different study populations by eliminating the discrepancies due to length of follow-up evaluation. The annual transformation rate for leukoplakia is generally reported as 1%, but in other studies was 2.9% or higher.[34] The mean duration of the intraepithelial phase of precancerous lesions of both the cervix and the oral cavity is approximately 11 to 12 years.[35] Two additional confounding factors hinder the ability to decipher patterns in transformation rates of oral premalignant lesions. First, areas of clinically normal mucosa can have histologic and genetic changes indicative of malignant progression.[36,37] Second, patients with oral leukoplakia not infrequently develop invasive carcinoma in a clinically normal-appearing oral cavity site that is distinct from the initial lesion(s). These factors, together with the high rates of multiple primary carcinomas in these patients, lends

Table 4–1 Classification and Staging System for Oral Leukoplakia (OLEP)

Classification or Stage	Definition
L (size of the leukoplakia)	
L_1	Size of single or multiple leukoplakias together ≤2 cm
L_2	Size of single or multiple leukoplakias together >2–4 cm
L_3	Size of single or multiple leukoplakias together >4 cm
L_x	Size not specified
P (pathology)	
P_0	No epithelial dysplasia (includes "no or perhaps mild epithelial dysplasia")
P_1	Distinct epithelial dysplasia (includes "mild to moderate" and "moderate to possibly severe" epithelial dysplasia)
P_x	Absence or presence of epithelial dysplasia not specified in the pathology report
Stage (OLEP staging system)	
I	L_1P_0
II	L_2P_0
III	L_3P_0 or $L_1L_2P_1$
IV	L_3P_1

From van der Waal I, Schepman, KP, van der Meij. A modified classification and staging system for oral leukoplakia. Oral Oncol 2000;36:264–266, with permission. Copyright © 2000, Elsevier.

credence to the theory of field cancerization proposed by Slaughter.[38] In these patients, the entire oropharyngeal and upper aerodigestive tract mucosal surface that is exposed to carcinogens (such as those in tobacco) sustains genetic damage and is at risk to develop other cancers.[38,39]

At present, there is no accepted method to predict an individual's risk of progression to invasive carcinoma from an oral premalignant lesion. The histologic finding of dysplasia is strongly associated with an increased rate of invasive cancer development.[32,40] In a large prospective study of oral leukoplakia patients conducted by Silverman et al,[32] 37 of 235 (15.7%) patients without dysplasia developed invasive cancer, compared with 8 of 22 (36.4%) patients with dysplasia. Similarly, in a study conducted in the Netherlands, there was a significantly higher risk of cancer development associated with leukoplakia lesions containing moderate or severe dysplasia compared with those without dysplasia.[34] Reflecting this, the staging system for oral leukoplakia presented in **Table 4–1** classifies lesions according to size and the presence or absence of dysplasia.[16]

However, it remains difficult to determine the frequency of dysplasia in oral leukoplakia lesions from the published literature. This is due to various factors, including differences in patient populations sampled in different series, variations in the clinical definition of leukoplakia, heterogeneity in the pathologic and molecular makeup within leukoplakia lesions leading to sampling errors, and lack of uniformity for diagnosing and classifying epithelial dysplasia. Given these limitations, the frequency of dysplasia within clinically apparent leukoplakic lesions most likely falls within the range of 5 to 25%.[6,41,42]

Extensive research efforts have focused on identifying clinical and molecular risk factors for malignant conversion of oral premalignant lesions. Some molecular biomarkers that show promise as potential diagnostic factors include DNA content and chromosome polysomy, loss of heterozygosity (LOH), nucleolar organizer regions, histo-blood group antigens, differentiation markers such as keratin, proliferation markers (such K_i-67), increased epidermal growth factor receptor (EGFR), decreased expression of RAR-β, p16, and p53.[40,43–50] Despite some promising preliminary

results, a reliable, validated marker or marker panel for providing clinically useful prognostic information has not been established. With the advent of high throughput genomic and proteonomic analysis techniques, we may soon see real advances toward a prognostically relevant molecular classification system.

◆ Diagnosis and Detection of Oral Premalignant Lesions

Oral cancer is an ideal tumor type to target for early detection and screening due to the easy accessibility of the oral cavity to physical examination, the presence of clinically apparent premalignant lesions, and an immense resource of trained dentists and health care providers who routinely inspect the oral cavity. Yet, many patients with oral cancer are not diagnosed until they have advanced disease. The failure to identify and diagnose premalignant and early cancerous oral lesions stems from several factors. These include a lack of public awareness of the signs, symptoms, and dangers of oral cancer, insufficient awareness and training of health care providers in oral cancer diagnosis, and the inherent difficulty in distinguishing the sometimes subtle changes associated with early neoplastic changes from the more common benign and inflammatory lesions.[51–55]

The standard method for oral cancer screening relies heavily on the clinical experience of the examiner to recognize suspicious lesions during physical examination. Although dentists and physicians frequently examine the oral cavity, most dentists have received cursory training in oral oncology, and physicians often have little experience or training in oral examination techniques.[57] Studies have documented that many dental and medical students and practitioners do not feel that they are adequately trained to detect and diagnose oral neoplasia, and many patients, including those in high-risk categories, do not routinely undergo oral examinations.[57–60] In addition, reports of community-based screening programs in various geographic sites around the world using visual oral examination have demonstrated variable levels of effectiveness.[61,62] In general, the detection yield of dysplasia and invasive carcinoma increases in screening programs that focus on high-risk populations. At this time, however, there is no conclusive evidence demonstrating that mass screening of the general population for oral cancer with visual examinations is an effective means to improve survival.[63,64]

The definitive diagnosis of oral dysplasia or invasive carcinoma requires a tissue biopsy and standard histopathologic review. Usually, a small incisional biopsy with a scalpel, scissors, or 3- to 4-mm punch instrument provides sufficient tissue to obtain a diagnosis. The wound can be left open, producing very little surrounding inflammation. Unless the lesion in question is quite small and can be completely excised with clear margins, excision should be attempted only by the specialist who will care for the patient long-term, to avoid complicating the staging and subsequent management of an invasive carcinoma. Because of the great variability in histologic findings within nonuniform lesions, the choice of biopsy site may affect the ultimate histologic diagnosis. It is therefore recommended that tissue be obtained from the area within the lesion that looks most worrisome.

Various adjuvant diagnostic aids have been proposed for use in diagnosis of oral lesions due to the difficulties in visual recognition and detection of the subtle mucosal changes that often accompany early oral neoplastic lesions. Vital staining with agents such as tolonium chloride (toluidine blue) has been used to improve recognition of early neoplastic lesions for many years. Tolonium chloride stains the perinuclear cisternae of DNA and RNA, and is preferentially taken up by dysplastic and malignant cells that contain higher quantities of these molecules.[65] Clinical trials have assessed the sensitivity, specificity, and positive and negative predictive ability of examinations using vital staining to identify oral neoplasia with varying results. Rosenberg and Cretin[66] performed a meta-analysis of studies using tolonium chloride for oral neoplasia identification, and found sensitivities ranging from 93.5 to 97.8%, and specificities ranging from 73.0 to 92.9%. A large multicenter study supported by Zila Biomedical (Phoenix, AZ) compared the ability to detect oral neoplasia using standard clinical examination and using a tolonium chloride rinse in 668 patients who had been previously treated for upper aerodigestive tract carcinoma.[67] In this study, 396 lesions were identified in 224 patients on the first clinical examination, 60 (15.2%) of which were thought to be suspicious, and on the second clinical examination, 185 lesions were identified in 92 patients, 36 (19.5%) of which were thought to be suspicious. This compares to the identification of 360 stained lesions in 197 patients after rinsing with tolonium chloride at the first visit, and 108 identified stained lesions in 74 patients during the second clinical visit. Thirty of 96 biopsies were diagnosed as carcinoma or carcinoma in situ; 29 of 30 positive biopsy sites stained positive with tolonium chloride, whereas only 12 were believed to be suspicious on standard clinical examination. Sixty-six lesions were identified histologically as "no carcinoma"; 60 of these stained with tolonium chloride and 21 were thought to be suspicious on clinical examination. Thus, using histologic evaluation as the gold standard, the sensitivity of standard clinical examination versus tolonium chloride rinse methods was reported

to be 40% and 96.7%, respectively. The positive predictive value was 36.4% and 32.6%, respectively. No data were provided regarding the sensitivity for diagnosis of oral dysplasia. This study, like previous studies, suggests that staining with vital dyes such as tolonium chloride may increase the sensitivity of visual examination by experienced examiners in high-risk patient populations. However, the use of vital staining in screening the general population is not recommended. Vital staining may be most useful for helping to identify the optimal site to perform an invasive biopsy in nonuniform lesions.

In a translational, correlative study to the above-mentioned multicenter clinical trial, Guo et al[68] analyzed a subset of 46 biopsies for genetic alterations. The 13 carcinoma, 11 carcinoma in situ/dysplasia, and 22 histologically normal samples were analyzed for LOH at 9p21, 3p21, and 17p13(TP53). Interestingly, all of the neoplastic cases and 13 of 22 (59%) histologically normal specimens had LOH in at least one tested marker. However, similar genetic changes were found in both tolonium chloride staining and nonstaining areas.[68]

Computer-assisted analysis of oral brush biopsy specimens, currently marketed under the trade name OralCDx (OraScan Laboratories, Suffern, NY), is another technology that may serve as an aid for detection and diagnosis of oral neoplasia. With this technique, a cytobrush, which reportedly enables the collection of cells from all epithelial layers, is used to obtain exfoliated cells from a questionable oral site. The specimen then undergoes computer-assisted analysis in a central laboratory, which is followed by standard cytologic evaluation if any abnormalities are detected on the initial screen. Results of a multicenter trial performed by academic dental specialists demonstrated impressive sensitivity rates. However, because only clinically suspicious lesions were biopsied, the false-negative rate using this technique could not be determined.[69] A study of 930 dentists and dental hygienists identified 93 benign-appearing oral lesions in 89 subjects. Computer-assisted analysis of these 93 lesions produced results of six atypical and one positive. Subsequent surgical biopsy and histopathologic assessment revealed that three of these seven lesions contained dysplasia. Again, none of the lesions identified as "negative" by computer analysis were biopsied. A report of four cases of false-negative brush biopsy results, in what are described as clinically obvious neoplastic lesions, reinforces the need for education and training of health care providers in oral cancer diagnosis and management.[70] Although further studies are needed, this technology appears to be a promising addition to facilitate oral diagnosis.

Another technology being marketed to assist in diagnosis of oral neoplasia is ViziLite (Zila Biomedical). This product is a kit containing a disposable chemiluminescent light and a raspberry-flavored 1% acetic acid mouth rinse. According to the company Web site (http://www.zila.com/assets/ppt2/frame.htm), the kit is designed to aid health care providers to visualize abnormal oral tissue. With this technique, patients rinse their mouths with the acetic acid prerinse for 1 minute, then the chemiluminescent light is activated, and the oral mucosa is examined in a dimly lit room. Under the blue light, normal tissue should appear dark, whereas abnormal areas will cause more reflection of the light and appear white. A small pilot study evaluating the visual appearance of oral lesions after an acetic acid wash under chemiluminescent illumination has been published.[71] Although the authors report that hyperkeratotic lesions, lesions with chronic inflammatory infiltrate, and areas with altered nuclear-cytoplasmic ratio strongly reflect the blue-white light and become clinically discernible, any benefit of this technology for the detection and diagnosis of oral neoplasia thus far remains unproved. Nevertheless, this technique appears promising and should be further investigated in clinical trials.

Several investigational approaches to detection and diagnosis of oral neoplasia are currently being evaluated. Optical technologies, such as fluorescence and reflectance spectroscopy, may provide an important new diagnostic tool to noninvasively identify and characterize early oral lesions. When tissue is illuminated, light photons are scattered, absorbed, reflected, and interact with molecules called fluorophores, which precipitates release of photons in a process termed fluorescence. Fluorescence spectroscopy is a technique to evaluate the physical and chemical properties of a substance by analyzing the intensity and character of the emitted fluorescent light. Reflected light is evaluated during reflectance spectroscopy. The spectroscopy systems used to obtain fluorescence spectra from oral mucosa consist of a monochromatic light source (either laser or lamp with appropriate filters to obtain specific wavelengths), an optical fiber probe, and a spectrometer and detector to record fluorescence intensities at specific wavelengths. Many groups have shown that fluorescence and reflectance spectroscopies are promising new technologies for the automated recognition of premalignant and malignant lesions in many sites.[72,73] Fluorescence spectra have been measured from normal and neoplastic oral areas in vivo using fiber optic probes in several small clinical series.[74–77] In general, the fluorescence intensity from normal mucosa is greater than that from abnormal mucosa. Computer-generated algorithms based on differences between the fluorescence spectra could discriminate normal mucosa from dysplastic and carcinomatous tissue with high sensitivity and specificity.[76–78] These optical approaches to oral diagnosis appear promising and should be further investigated.

◆ Management of Oral Premalignant Lesions

The management of patients with oral premalignant lesions is challenging and controversial. Management strategies for patients with oral leukoplakia can be categorized into three groups: close observation, medical therapies (i.e., chemoprevention), and surgical removal or ablation.[79] Most oral lesions described above are asymptomatic and do not hinder the patient's function. Therefore, the primary goal in managing these patients is to detect and prevent the development of oral cancer. Given that many, if not most, oral premalignant lesions never progress to malignancy, and that there is presently no reliable method to predict whether a given lesion will undergo malignant transformation, it is important that the health care provider carefully weigh the risks and potential morbidity of any therapeutic intervention against the potential benefits. Chemopreventive strategies (see Chapter 29) or other novel therapies such as those involving molecular targets (see Chapter 30), both of which remain investigational, may ultimately play an important role in the management of these lesions.

All patients with clinically apparent oral premalignant lesions such as leukoplakia should have routine oral examinations and should be counseled to avoid known risks factors for this malignancy, such as tobacco and alcohol. In addition, biopsy is usually indicated to assess for the presence of dysplasia or occult carcinoma. It should be emphasized, however, that a "negative" (i.e., nondysplastic) pathologic result does not exclude the possibility of dysplastic changes within the oral mucosa due to the presence of skip areas of dysplasia interspersed with histologically normal areas and the risk of sampling error, as well as the lack of uniformity among pathologists for diagnosing dysplasia.[16] Therefore, an understanding of the natural history of oral premalignant lesions and good clinical judgment remain key components in managing these patients.

◆ Conclusion

Recently, there have been several aggressive efforts to improve the diagnostic capabilities of clinicians for the detection of premalignant changes in the oral mucosa. An accurate, objective, and noninvasive method to determine the risk of malignant conversion of premalignant lesions is also needed. Researchers continue to search for reliable molecular biomarkers that are predictive of malignant conversion and aggressive behavior. Unfortunately, there remains no effective treatment for all patients with oral premalignant lesions once they have been diagnosed. It is hoped that clinical research into chemoprevention and other strategies to reverse the genetic damage sustained by premalignant cells will result in effective therapeutic options.

References

1. Bishop JM. Molecular themes in oncogenesis. Cell 1991;64:235–248
2. Vogelstein B, Fearon ER, Hamilton SR, et al. Genetic alterations during colorectal-tumor development. N Engl J Med 1988;319:525–532
3. Califano J, van der Riet P, Westra W, et al. Genetic progression model for head and neck cancer: implications for field cancerization. Cancer Res 1996;56:2488–2492
4. Lippman SM, Hong WK. Molecular markers of the risk of oral cancer. N Engl J Med 2001;344:1323–1326
5. "Leukoplakia," "keratosis," and intraepithelial squamous cell carcinoma of the head and neck. In: Batsakis JG, ed. Tumors of the Head and Neck: Clinical and Pathological Considerations. Baltimore: Williams & Wilkins, 1974:68–71

5a. Neville BW, Day TA. Oral cancer and precancerous lesions. CA Cancer J Clin 2002;52:195–215

6. Silverman S, ed. American Cancer Society Atlas of Clinical Oncology Oral Cancer, 5th ed. Hamilton, Ontario: BC Decker, 2003

7. van der Waal I, Schepman KP, van der Meij EH, Smeele LE. Oral leukoplakia: a clinicopathological review. Oral Oncol 1997;33:291–301

8. Axell T, Pindborg JJ, Smith CJ, van der Waal I. Oral white lesions with special reference to precancerous and tobacco-related lesions: conclusions of an international symposium held in Uppsala, Sweden, May 18–21 1994. International Collaborative Group on Oral White Lesions. J Oral Pathol Med 1996;25:49–54

9. Hansen LS, Olson JA, Silverman S Jr. Proliferative verrucous leukoplakia. A long-term study of thirty patients. Oral Surg Oral Med Oral Pathol 1985;60:285–298

10. Silverman S Jr, Gorsky M. Proliferative verrucous leukoplakia: a follow-up study of 54 cases. Oral Surg Oral Med Oral Pathol Oral Radiol Endod 1997;84:154–157

11. Batsakis JG, Suarez P, el-Naggar AK. Proliferative verrucous leukoplakia and its related lesions. Oral Oncol 1999;35:354–359

12. Silverman S Jr. Oral lichen planus: a potentially premalignant lesion. J Oral Maxillofac Surg 2000;58:1286–1288

13. Silverman S Jr, Gorsky M, Lozada-Nur F, Giannotti K. A prospective study of findings and management in 214 patients with oral lichen planus. Oral Surg Oral Med Oral Pathol 1991;72:665–670

14. van der Meij EH, Schepman KP, Smeele LE, van der Wal JE, Bezemer PD, van der Waal I. A review of the recent literature regarding malignant transformation of oral lichen planus. Oral Surg Oral Med Oral Pathol Oral Radiol Endod 1999;88:307–310

15. Schepman KP, van der Waal I. A proposal for a classification and staging system for oral leukoplakia: a preliminary study. Eur J Cancer B Oral Oncol 1995;31B:396–398

16. van der Waal I, Schepman KP, van der Meij EH. A modified classification and staging system for oral leukoplakia. Oral Oncol 2000;36:264–266

17. Hogewind WF, van der Waal I. Prevalence study of oral leukoplakia in a selected population of 1000 patients from the Netherlands. Community Dent Oral Epidemiol 1988;16:302–305

18. Scheifele C, Reichart PA, Dietrich T. Low prevalence of oral leukoplakia in a representative sample of the US population. Oral Oncol 2003;39:619–625

19. Bouquot JE, Gorlin RJ. Leukoplakia, lichen planus, and other oral keratoses in 23,616 white Americans over the age of 35 years. Oral Surg Oral Med Oral Pathol 1986;61:373–381

20. Silverman S, Bhargava K, Smith LW, Malaowalla AM. Malignant transformation and natural history of oral leukoplakia in 57,518 industrial workers of Gujarat, India. Cancer 1976;38:1790–1795

21. Zain RB. Cultural and dietary risk factors of oral cancer and precancer: a brief overview. Oral Oncol 2001;37:205–210

22. Reichart PA. Identification of risk groups for oral precancer and cancer and preventive measures. Clin Oral Investig 2001;5:207–213

23. Dietrich T, Reichart PA, Scheifele C. Clinical risk factors of oral leukoplakia in a representative sample of the US population. Oral Oncol 2004;40:158–163

24. Hashibe M, Jacob BJ, Thomas G, et al. Socioeconomic status, lifestyle factors and oral premalignant lesions. Oral Oncol 2003;39:664–671

25. Damm DD, Curran A, White DK, Drummond JF. Leukoplakia of the maxillary vestibule—an association with Viadent? Oral Surg Oral Med Oral Pathol Oral Radiol Endod 1999;87:61–66

26. Eversole LR, Eversole GM, Kopcik J. Sanguinaria-associated oral leukoplakia: comparison with other benign and dysplastic leukoplakic lesions. Oral Surg Oral Med Oral Pathol Oral Radiol Endod 2000;89:455–464

27. Mascarenhas AK, Allen CM, Loudon J. The association between Viadent use and oral leukoplakia. Epidemiology 2001;12:741–743

28. Scheifele C, Reichart PA. Is there a natural limit of the transformation rate of oral leukoplakia? Oral Oncol 2003;39:470–475

29. Einhorn J, Wersall J. Incidence of oral carcinoma in patients with leukoplakia of the oral mucosa. Cancer 1967;20:2189–2193

30. Pindborg JJ, Jolst O, Renstrup G, Roed-Petersen B. Studies in oral leukoplakia: a preliminary report on the period prevalence of malignant transformation in leukoplakia based on a follow-up study of 248 patients. J Am Dent Assoc 1968;76:767–771

31. Roed-Petersen B. Cancer development in oral leukoplakia: follow-up of 331 patients [abstract]. J Am Dent Assoc 1971;50:711

32. Silverman S Jr, Gorsky M, Lozada F. Oral leukoplakia and malignant transformation: a follow-up study of 257 patients. Cancer 1984;53:563–568

33. Saito T, Sugiura C, Hirai A, et al. Development of squamous cell carcinoma from pre-existent oral leukoplakia: with respect to treatment modality. Int J Oral Maxillofac Surg 2001;30:49–53

34. Schepman KP, van der Meij EH, Smeele LE, van der Waal I. Malignant transformation of oral leukoplakia: a follow-up study of a hospital-based population of 166 patients with oral leukoplakia from The Netherlands. Oral Oncol 1998;34:270–275

35. Kuffer R, Lombardi T. Premalignant lesions of the oral mucosa: a discussion about the place of oral intraepithelial neoplasia (OIN). Oral Oncol 2002;38:125–130

36. Brennan JA, Sidransky D. Molecular staging of head and neck squamous carcinoma. Cancer Metastasis Rev 1996;15:3–10

37. Incze J, Vaughan CW Jr, Lui P, Strong MS, Kulapaditharom B. Premalignant changes in normal appearing epithelium in patients with squamous cell carcinoma of the upper aerodigestive tract. Am J Surg 1982;144:401–405

38. Slaughter OP. Multicenter origin of intraoral carcinoma. Surgery 1946;20:133–146

39. Strong MS, Incze J, Vaughan CW. Field cancerization in the aerodigestive tract—its etiology, manifestation, and significance. J Otolaryngol 1984;13:1–6

40. Rosin MP, Cheng X, Poh C, et al. Use of allelic loss to predict malignant risk for low-grade oral epithelial dysplasia. Clin Cancer Res 2000;6:357–362

41. Banoczy J. Follow-up studies in oral leukoplakia. J Maxillofac Surg 1977;5:69–75

42. Waldron CA, Shafer WG. Leukoplakia revisited: a clinicopathologic study 3256 oral leukoplakias. Cancer 1975;36:1386–1392

43. Kim J, Shin DM, El-Naggar A, et al. Chromosome polysomy and histological characteristics in oral premalignant lesions. Cancer Epidemiol Biomarkers Prev 2001;10:319–325

44. Lee JJ, Hong WK, Hittelman WN, et al. Predicting cancer development in oral leukoplakia: ten years of translational research. Clin Cancer Res 2000;6:1702–1710

45. Mao L, Lee JS, Fan YH, et al. Frequent microsatellite alterations at chromosomes 9p21 and 3p14 in oral premalignant lesions and their value in cancer risk assessment. Nat Med 1996;2:682–685

46. Partridge M, Emilion G, Pateromichelakis S, A'Hern R, Phillips E, Langdon J. Allelic imbalance at chromosomal loci implicated in the pathogenesis of oral precancer, cumulative loss and its relationship with progression to cancer. Oral Oncol 1998;34:77–83

47. Xie X, Clausen OP, Sudbo J, Boysen M. Diagnostic and prognostic value of nucleolar organizer regions in normal epithelium, dysplasia, and squamous cell carcinoma of the oral cavity. Cancer 1997;79:2200–2208

48. Dabelsteen E. ABO blood group antigens in oral mucosa. What is new? J Oral Pathol Med 2002;31:65–70

49. Bloor BK, Seddon SV, Morgan PR. Gene expression of differentiation-specific keratins in oral epithelial dysplasia and squamous cell carcinoma. Oral Oncol 2001;37:251–261

50. Reibel J. Prognosis of oral pre-malignant lesions: significance of clinical, histopathological, and molecular biological characteristics. Crit Rev Oral Biol Med 2003;14:47–62

51. Warnakulasuriya KA, Harris CK, Scarrott DM, et al. An alarming lack of public awareness towards oral cancer. Br Dent J 1999;187:319–322

52. Horowitz AM, Nourjah P, Gift HCUS. Adult knowledge of risk factors and signs of oral cancers: 1990. J Am Dent Assoc 1995;126:39–45

53. Horowitz AM, Goodman HS, Yellowitz JA, Nourjah PA. The need for health promotion in oral cancer prevention and early detection. J Public Health Dent 1996;56:319–330

54. Ahluwalia KP, Yellowitz JA, Goodman HS, Horowitz AM. An assessment of oral cancer prevention curricula in U.S. medical schools. J Cancer Educ 1998;13:90–95

55. Rankin KV, Burznski NJ, Silverman S Jr, Scheetz JP. Cancer curricula in U.S. dental schools. J Cancer Educ 1999;14:8–12

56. Mashberg A. Diagnosis of early oral and oropharyngeal squamous carcinoma: obstacles and their amelioration. Oral Oncol 2000;36:253–255

57. Canto MT, Horowitz AM, Child WL. Views of oral cancer prevention and early detection: Maryland physicians. Oral Oncol 2002;38:373–377

58. Canto MT, Horowitz AM, Drury TF, Goodman HS. Maryland family physicians' knowledge, opinions and practices about oral cancer. Oral Oncol 2002;38:416–424

59. Clovis JB, Horowitz AM, Poel DH. Oral and pharyngeal cancer: knowledge and opinions of dentists in British Columbia and Nova Scotia. J Can Dent Assoc 2002;68:415–420

60. Rankin KV, Jones DL, McDaniel RK. Oral cancer education in dental schools: survey of Texas dental students. J Cancer Educ 1996;11:80–83

61. Sankaranarayanan R, Mathew B, Jacob BJ, et al. Early findings from a community-based, cluster-randomized, controlled oral cancer screening trial in Kerala, India. The Trivandrum Oral Cancer Screening Study Group. Cancer 2000;88:664–673

62. Clayman GL, Chamberlain RM, Lee JJ, Lippman SM, Hong WK. Screening at a health fair to identify subjects for an oral leukoplakia chemoprevention trial. J Cancer Educ 1995;10:88–90

63. Warnakulasuriya KA, Johnson NW. Strengths and weaknesses of screening programmes for oral malignancies and potentially malignant lesions. Eur J Cancer Prev 1996;5:93–98

64. Kujan O, Glenny AM, Duxbury AJ, Thakker N, Sloan P. Screening programmes for the early detection and prevention of oral cancer. Cochrane Database Syst Rev 2003; 4:CD004150

65. Herlin P, Marnay J, Jacob JH, Ollivier JM, Mandard AM. A study of the mechanism of the toluidine blue dye test. Endoscopy 1983;15:4–7

66. Rosenberg D, Cretin S. Use of meta-analysis to evaluate tolonium chloride in oral cancer screening. Oral Surg Oral Med Oral Pathol 1989;67:621–627

67. Epstein JB, Feldman R, Dolor RJ, Porter SR. The utility of tolonium chloride rinse in the diagnosis of recurrent or second primary cancers in patients with prior upper aerodigestive tract cancer. Head Neck 2003;25:911–921

68. Guo Z, Yamaguchi K, Sanchez-Cespedes M, Westra WH, Koch WM, Sidransky D. Allelic losses in OraTest-directed biopsies of patients with prior upper aerodigestive tract malignancy. Clin Cancer Res 2001;7:1963–1968

69. Sciubba JJ. Improving detection of precancerous and cancerous oral lesions. Computer-assisted analysis of the oral brush biopsy. U.S.

Collaborative OralCDx Study Group. J Am Dent Assoc 1999;130: 1445–1457

70. Potter TJ, Summerlin DJ, Campbell JH. Oral malignancies associated with negative transepithelial brush biopsy. J Oral Maxillofac Surg 2003;61:674–677

71. Huber MA, Bsoul SA, Terezhalmy GT. Acetic acid wash and chemiluminescent illumination as an adjunct to conventional oral soft tissue examination for the detection of dysplasia: a pilot study. Quintessence Int 2004;35:378–384

72. Wagnieres GA, Star WM, Wilson BC. In vivo fluorescence spectroscopy and imaging for oncological applications. Photochem Photobiol 1998;68:603–632

73. Ramanujam N. Fluorescence spectroscopy of neoplastic and non-neoplastic tissues. Neoplasia 2000;2:89–117

74. Schantz SP, Kolli V, Savage HE, et al. In vivo native cellular fluorescence and histological characteristics of head and neck cancer. Clin Cancer Res 1998;4:1177–1182

75. Kolli VR, Savage HE, Yao TJ, Schantz SP. Native cellular fluorescence of neoplastic upper aerodigestive mucosa. Arch Otolaryngol Head Neck Surg 1995;121:1287–1292

76. Dhingra JK, Perrault DF Jr, McMillan K, et al. Early diagnosis of upper aerodigestive tract cancer by autofluorescence. Arch Otolaryngol Head Neck Surg 1996;122:1181–1186

77. Gillenwater A, Jacob R, Ganeshappa R, et al. Noninvasive diagnosis of oral neoplasia based on fluorescence spectroscopy and native tissue autofluorescence. Arch Otolaryngol Head Neck Surg 1998;124:1251–1258

78. Heintzelman DL, Utzinger U, Fuchs H, et al. Optimal excitation wavelengths for in vivo detection of oral neoplasia using fluorescence spectroscopy. Photochem Photobiol 2000;72:103–113

79. Tradati N, Grigolat R, Calabrese L, et al. Oral leukoplakias: to treat or not? Oral Oncol 1997;33:317–321

5

Anatomic Considerations

Leslie Gartner,

James L. Hiatt,

John W. Werning, and

Kristen Lloyd

The evaluation and management of oral cancer and its sequelae are ideally undertaken by clinicians who have a sound working knowledge of the macroscopic and microscopic anatomy of the oral cavity. Radiographic interpretation and clinical evaluation that is performed with particular attention to anatomical nuances improves the accuracy of tumor staging and allows the clinician to devise anatomically precise surgical and radiotherapeutic treatment plans. An appreciation for anatomic variation and three-dimensional anatomic relationships also enables surgeons to perform surgical resections that minimize morbidity, facilitate reconstruction, and optimize postoperative function. This chapter focuses on those aspects of oral cavity anatomy that are particularly germane to clinicians who evaluate and manage patients with oral cancer, and is intended to complement other clinically relevant anatomic reviews that are provided elsewhere in this book.

Although numerous anatomic interconnections between the oral cavity and the adjacent oropharynx, face, nose, and paranasal sinuses exist, a comprehensive review of the anatomy of each adjacent region is impractical. For example, the oral cavity and oropharynx share arterial branches from the external carotid artery and neural contributions from the glossopharyngeal nerve. In this case, only the oral cavity contributions are discussed here since the focus of this book is limited to cancer of the oral cavity.

◆ The Oral Mucosa

The oral cavity, as defined by the American Joint Committee on Cancer (AJCC), "extends from the skin-vermilion junction of the lips to the junction of the hard and soft palate above and to the line of circumvallate papillae below."[1] The AJCC divides the mucosal surfaces of the oral cavity into the following eight areas or subsites (**Fig. 5–1**)[1]:

1. *Mucosal lip:* "The lip begins at the junction of the vermilion border with the skin and includes only the vermilion surface or that portion of the lip that comes into contact with the opposing lip. It is well defined into an upper and lower lip joined at the commissures of the mouth."
2. *Buccal mucosa:* "This includes all the membrane lining of the inner surface of the cheeks and lips from the line of contact of the opposing lips to the line of attachment of mucosa of the alveolar ridge (upper and lower) and pterygomandibular raphe."
3. *Lower alveolar ridge:* "This refers to the mucosa overlying the alveolar process of the mandible, which extends from the line of attachment of mucosa in the buccal gutter to the line of free mucosa of the floor of the mouth. Posteriorly it extends to the ascending ramus of the mandible."
4. *Upper alveolar ridge:* "This refers to the mucosa overlying the alveolar process of the maxilla, which extends from the line of attachment of mucosa in the upper gingival buccal gutter to the junction of the hard palate. Its posterior margin is the upper end of the pterygopalatine arch."
5. *Retromolar gingiva (retromolar trigone):* "This is the attached mucosa overlying the ascending ramus of the mandible from the level of the posterior surface of the last molar tooth to the apex superiorly, adjacent to the tuberosity of the maxilla."
6. *Floor of the mouth:* "This is a semilunar space over the mylohyoid and hyoglossus muscles, extending from the inner surface of the lower alveolar ridge to the

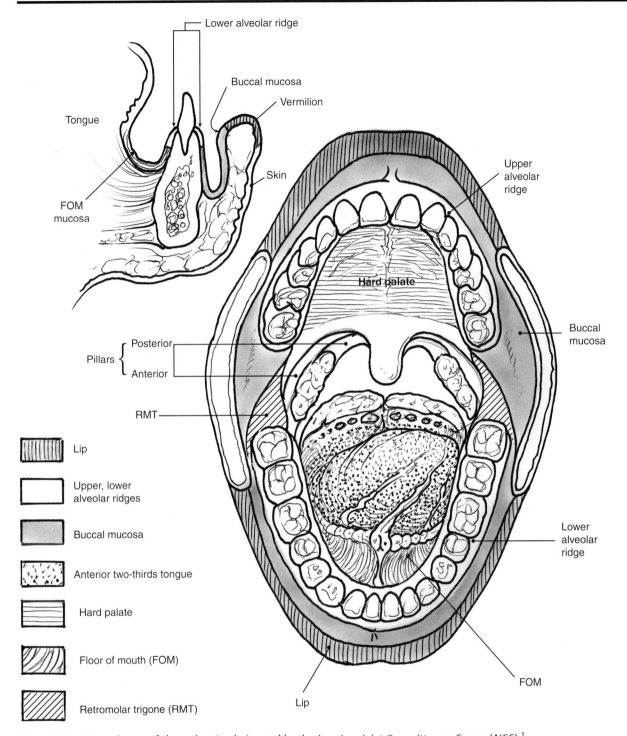

Figure 5–1 Mucosal areas of the oral cavity designated by the American Joint Committee on Cancer (AJCC).[1]

undersurface of the tongue. Its posterior boundary is the base of the anterior pillar of the tonsil. It is divided into two sides by the frenulum of the tongue and contains the ostia of the submaxillary and sublingual salivary glands."

7. *Hard palate:* "This is the semilunar area between the upper alveolar ridge and the mucous membrane covering the palatine process of the maxillary palatine bones. It extends from the inner surface of the superior alveolar ridge to the posterior edge of the palatine bone."

8. *Anterior two thirds of the tongue (oral tongue):* "This is the freely mobile portion of the tongue that extends anteriorly from the line of circumvallate papillae to the undersurface of the tongue at the junction of the floor of the mouth. It is composed of four areas: the tip, the lateral borders, the dorsum, and the undersurface (non-villous ventral surface of the tongue). The undersurface of the tongue is considered a separate category by the World Health Organization (WHO)."

Table 5–1 lists the relative percentage of cancer cases that arise from each oral cavity subsite according to the National Cancer Data Base (NCDB) and the U.S. Surveillance, Epidemiology, and End Results program (SEER).[2-4] The oral tongue is the most common location for oral cancer, and cancers of the oral tongue, floor of the mouth, and mucosal lip make up more than 70% of all oral cancers.

The oral mucosa is composed of a stratified squamous epithelium, the *oral epithelium*, and an underlying connective tissue layer, the subepithelial connective tissue or *lamina propria*. These are the analogues of the epidermis and dermis of the skin. In regions such as the buccal mucosa, lip, and parts of the hard palate, a submucosal layer of loose fatty or glandular connective tissue containing blood vessels and nerves separates the oral mucosa from underlying bone or muscle. In contrast, the oral mucosa overlying the alveolar ridges, retromolar region, and parts of the hard palate attaches directly to the periosteum of the underlying bone with no intervening submucosa, resulting in a firm immovable *mucoperiosteum*.[5] As much as 10% of the cell population of the oral epithelium is composed of cell types other than keratinocytes, and they include Langerhans' cells, Merkel cells, inflammatory cells such as lymphocytes, and melanocytes. Minor salivary glands, when present, are located within or immediately deep to the lamina propria.[5]

There are three main classifications of oral mucosa: *lining, masticatory,* and the *specialized mucosa* of the tongue dorsum (**Table 5–2**).[5] The movable oral mucosa covering the

Table 5–1 Percentage of Cancer Cases (All Histologic Types) Arising from Each Oral Cavity Subsite in the National Cancer Data Base (NCDB) and the U.S. Surveillance, Epidemiology, and End Results (SEER) Program[2-4]

Oral Cavity Subsite	NCDB (%)*	Rank	SEER (%)	Rank
Oral tongue	27.5	1	36.2	1
Floor of mouth	24.5	2	19.8	3
Mucosal lip	19.8	3	24.5	2
Retromolar gingiva	8.0	4	19.5†	4–8†
Hard palate	6.7	5		
Buccal mucosa	5.8	6		
Lower alveolar ridge	5.2	7		
Upper alveolar ridge	2.5	8		

*Lip cancer was not included in the NCDB compilation by Funk et al.[2] Hoffman et al[3] reported lip cancer data from the NCDB in a separate publication. The data from these two reports were combined to calculate the proportion of cancer cases at each of the eight subsites in the following manner: Cancer cases that were classified as arising from "mouth vestibule" or "other parts of mouth" were excluded from analysis since they are not considered primary tumor sites by the AJCC. There were 54,801 remaining cases of oral cavity cancer in the report by Funk et al that were used to calculate the proportion of cancers arising from each oral cavity site except for the lip. Hoffman et al reported a total of 51,764 cases of cancer arising from the oral cavity and lip, including 41,490 cases of oral cancer and 10,274 cases of lip cancer. The proportion derived for each oral cavity site from the data supplied by Funk et al was multiplied by 41,490 and divided by 51,764 to obtain the percentage of cancer cases arising from each oral cavity site, including the lip.
†Of 33,863 cases of oral cancer registered, 19.5% were classified as arising from "gum" or "other mouth." These cases are reported as one group that represents the cases from the five oral cavity sites that were not individually reported.[4]

undersurface of the tongue, floor of mouth, buccal regions, the inner aspect of the lips, and the alveolar processes up to its junction with the attached gingiva is termed the *lining mucosa*. The epithelium and lamina propria of the lining mucosa is thicker than that of the masticatory mucosa, resulting in its flexibility and deformability. The *masticatory mucosa* covers the hard palate, dorsal surface of the oral tongue, and gingivae, areas that are exposed to compressive and shear abrasive forces during mastication. The epithelium is moderately thick and keratinized (or parakeratinized), and the junction between the epithelium and the thick lamina propria is convoluted by numerous elongated papillae. The masticatory mucosa firmly binds to underlying structures by either of the following ways:

1. Direct attachment of the lamina propria to the periosteum of underlying bone, resulting in a mucoperiosteum. The mucosa is firmly "attached" by collagen fibers to the underlying periosteum to form the mucoperiosteum. The bundles of collagenous fibers, or *Sharpey's fibers*, extend from the lamina propria into the circumferential lamellae of the underlying bone.[5,6]
2. Indirectly attaching by a fibrous submucosa that is interspersed with areas of fat and glandular tissue in the lateral regions of the palate.[5]

The dorsal surface of the oral tongue is covered by the *specialized mucosa*, interspersed within the extensible masticatory mucosa that contains four different types of lingual papillae that have mechanical and sensory functions. The *circumvallate papillae* lie anterior to the V-shaped *sulcus terminalis*, which defines the anatomic boundary between the oral tongue and the tongue base. The anterior portion of the tongue is covered by numerous *filiform papillae,* which form an abrasive surface that functions as a masticatory mucosa by facilitating the compression and breakage of food between the tongue and the hard palate. The oral tongue also contains scattered taste-bud–containing *fungiform* and *foliate papillae.*[5]

It is important to appreciate that the AJCC description of these oral mucosal subsites deviates in some instances from the usual anatomic description of these regions. The lip, for example, has been defined as "only the vermilion surface or that portion of the lip that comes into contact with the opposing lip," since the etiology and epidemiology of lip cancer differs from malignancies of the labial vestibular mucosa.[1] Consequently, the buccal mucosa, as defined by the AJCC, also extends anteriorly to include the lining mucosa of the labial vestibule, more commonly referred to as the labial mucosa. The mucosa of the upper and lower alveolar ridge extends from "the line of attachment of mucosa in the upper gingival buccal gutter to the junction of the hard palate" and from "the line of attachment of mucosa in the buccal gutter to the line of free mucosa of the floor of the mouth," respectively.[1] Thus, the mucosa of the upper and lower alveolar ridges as defined by the AJCC begins at the mucogingival junction where the lining buccal mucosa meets the masticatory mucosa, or attached gingiva, overlying the alveolar ridges (**Fig. 5–2**). Similarly, the lining mucosa of the floor of the mouth terminates along the lingual mucogingival junction.

Table 5-2 Structure of the Mucosa in Different Regions of the Oral Cavity

Region of the Oral Cavity	Mucosa		
	Covering Epithelium	Lamina Propria	Submucosa
Lining mucosa			
Lips			
Vermilion zone	Thin, orthokeratinized	Numerous narrow papillae	Mucosa firmly attached to muscle, minor SG
Intermediate zone	Thin, parakeratinized	Long irregular papillae, collagen/elastin in CT	
Labial, buccal	Very thick, nonkeratinized	Long papillae, dense fibrous CT	Mucosa firmly attached to muscle by collagen and elastin, minor SG
Alveolar mucosa	Thin, nonkeratinized	Short papillae, many elastic fibers	Loose CT, elastic fibers attaching to periosteum, minor SG
Ventral tongue	Thin, nonkeratinized	Thin short papillae, few minor SG	Thin, irregular
Floor of mouth	Very thin, nonkeratinized	Short papillae	Loose CT, minor SG
Masticatory mucosa			
Gingiva	Thick, ortho/parakeratinized	Long papillae, dense CT	None, mucosa firmly attached by collagen to cementum and periosteum (mucoperiosteum)
Dorsal surface of tongue	Thick, keratinized and nonkeratinized	Long papillae, minor SG posteriorly	No distinct layer, mucosa bound to CT
Hard palate	Thick, ortho/parakeratinized	Long papillae, dense CT	Mucoperiosteum; fat and minor SG in CT where mucosa overlies lateral neurovascular bundle
Specialized mucosa			
Dorsal surface of tongue	Intraepithelial taste buds	Long papillae, minor SG posteriorly	No distinct layer; mucosa bound to CT

CT, connective tissue; SG, salivary gland.
Adapted from Squier CA, Hill MW. Oral mucosa. In: Ten Cate AR, ed. Oral Histology: Development, Structure, and Function, 4th ed. St. Louis: Mosby-Year Book, 1994:424, with permission.

◆ Salivary Glands

The paired parotid, submandibular and sublingual glands, and the minor salivary glands secrete saliva into the oral cavity via ducts that open into the oral cavity by piercing the oral mucosa. The *parotid duct* (Stensen's duct), first described by the Danish anatomist Niels Stensen, enters the oral cavity through the buccal mucosa. The *submandibular duct* (Wharton's duct), which was described by the English anatomist Thomas Wharton, opens into the floor of the mouth at the *sublingual papilla*. The main excretory duct of the *sublingual gland (duct of Bartholin)* and numerous smaller *sublingual ducts (ducts of Rivinus)* typically open into the floor of the mouth posterolateral to the sublingual papillae (**Fig. 5–3**). Between 600 and 1000 *minor salivary glands* are present throughout the oral cavity, with the exception of the gingiva and anterior hard palate, and empty into the oral cavity through numerous small ducts.[7] The major and minor salivary glands receive parasympathetic and sympathetic innervation. Parasympathetic stimulation produces more profuse watery secretions, whereas sympathetic stimulation results in less voluminous, thicker, mucous saliva.[8] Postganglionic sympathetic fibers from the superior cervical ganglion travel to major and minor salivary glands via the carotid plexus along branches of the external and internal carotid artery. For example, sympathetic fibers travel to the submandibular and sublingual glands via branches of the facial artery, whereas sympathetic that supply to many of the minor salivary glands of the maxillary region travel intracranially along with the internal carotid artery and eventually form part of the *nerve of the Vidian canal*. Parasympathetic innervation to the salivary glands is discussed in greater detail in the next section.

◆ Innervation of the Oral Cavity Region (see Table 5–3 on p. 43)

The oral cavity region receives its sensorimotor innervation via the trigeminal, facial, and hypoglossal nerves. Knowledge of the sensory innervation supplied by the trigeminal nerve

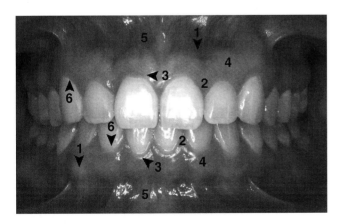

Figure 5–2 Surface anatomy of the gingiva: 1, mucogingival junction; 2, interdental papilla; 3, free gingiva; 4, attached gingiva; 5, alveolar mucosa; 6, gingival margin.

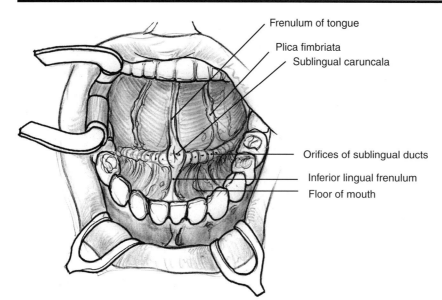

Frenulum of tongue
Plica fimbriata
Sublingual caruncala

Orifices of sublingual ducts

Inferior lingual frenulum
Floor of mouth

Figure 5–3 Surface anatomy of the anterior floor of the mouth.

provides the basis for evaluating neuropathic pain of the oral cavity and temporomandibular joint regions that may be attributable to oral cancer and its treatment. Furthermore, the clinical and radiographic evaluation of paresthesia or anesthesia that may be caused by retrograde, and rarely, anterograde perineural tumor invasion requires an understanding of the complex neural pathways that course between the oral cavity and the skull base. The anatomy of the maxillary and mandibular divisions of the trigeminal nerve is comprehensively reviewed because they play a central role in the innervation of the oral cavity, and a selective overview of facial nerve anatomy that directly pertains to oral cavity innervation is presented.

Maxillary Division of the Trigeminal Nerve (see Fig. 5–4 on p. 44)

The *maxillary division of the trigeminal nerve* is purely sensory and innervates the skin of the side of the nose, cheek, eyelids, middle of the face, nasopharynx, palate, tonsil, maxillary sinus, and the gingiva, teeth, and related structures of the maxillary arch. It enters the deep face via the *foramen rotundum* and passes through the *pterygopalatine fossa* where it becomes associated with the pterygopalatine ganglion. During its passage through this fossa, it provides a slender branch, the *posterior superior alveolar nerve*, which enters the deep face via the *pterygomaxillary fissure* and courses along the maxillary tuberosity. The majority of the fibers of the posterior superior alveolar nerve traverse the same named foramen to serve the three maxillary molars (but not the mesiobuccal root of the first molar), their supporting structures, and maxillary sinus, and also to form a dental plexus in association with the middle and anterior superior alveolar nerves, whereas those fibers that do not enter this foramen supply the mucous membranes of the cheek and the gingiva. The maxillary division leaves the pterygopalatine fossa via the *inferior orbital fissure* to gain entry into the floor of the orbit, where it becomes known as the *infraorbital nerve*, which continues

anteriorly in the infraorbital canal to enter the superficial face by way of the *infraorbital foramen*. Within the infraorbital canal, the *middle* and *anterior superior alveolar nerves* arise from the infraorbital nerve. The former innervates the maxillary sinus as well as the two maxillary premolars and the mesiobuccal root of the first maxillary molar, whereas the latter serves the canine and the incisors of the maxillary arch, the mucosa of the maxillary sinus, the floor of the nasal cavity, and the inferior meatus.

Some of the branches of the maxillary nerve that arise from it while in the pterygopalatine fossa also carry postganglionic parasympathetic fibers, belonging to the facial nerve because they originate in the pterygopalatine ganglion. These are secretomotor fibers destined for the lacrimal glands, minor salivary glands of the palate and mucosa of the cheeks, and glands of the nasal cavity. The maxillary nerve also gives off two *pterygopalatine nerves* within the pterygopalatine fossa that provide branches to the orbit, palate, nasal cavity, and pharynx via branches similarly named. The *orbital branches* serve not only the periorbita but also the sphenoidal and ethmoidal sinuses. The *greater palatine nerve* passes inferiorly within the pterygopalatine canal, where it bifurcates to form the greater and lesser palatine nerves, each leaving the canal through the same-named foramina (see **Fig. 5–5** on p. 44). The *greater palatine nerve* serves the hard palate and abutting soft palate, and travels anteriorly to communicate with the nasopalatine nerve. It also provides *posterior inferior nasal branches* to the inferior concha and the middle and inferior meatus. The *lesser palatine nerve* supplies the soft palate and adjoining areas and also receives sensory and postganglionic parasympathetic fibers, via the *nerve of the pterygoid canal* and the *greater petrosal nerve,* from the pterygopalatine ganglion.

The *posterior superior nasal branches* of the pterygopalatine nerves gain entry into the nasal cavity via the *sphenopalatine foramen*, located on the medial wall of the pterygopalatine fossa, and provide sensory fibers to the mucoperiosteum of the superior and middle conchae. Its

Table 5–3 Organization of the Cranial Nerves Supplying the Oral Cavity Region

Cranial Nerve	Branches	Fiber Components	Function
Trigeminal nerve (V)			
Maxillary division (V2)			
Pterygopalatine fossa			
	Zygomatic nerve	GSA, GVE from VII	Cutaneous sensation,
	Zygomaticotemporal		parasymp. to lacrimal
	Zygomaticofacial		
	Pterygopalatine nerves	GSA, GVE from VII	Mucosal sensation,
	Orbital branches		parasymp. to lacrimal,
	Nasal branch: nasopalatine		minor SG
	Palatine branches: greater,		
	lesser palatine		
	Posterior superior alveolar		
Infraorbital canal		GSA, GVE from VII	Mucosal
	Middle superior alveolar		sensation, parasymp.
	Anterior superior alveolar		to minor SG
Branches on the face		GSA	Mucocutaneous sensation
	Inferior palpebral		
	External nasal		
	Superior labial		
Mandibular division (V3)			
Main trunk			
	Meningeal	GSA	Meningeal sensation
	Medial pterygoid	SVE	Branchial motor to medial pterygoid,
			tensor tympani, tensor veli palatini
Anterior division			
	Masseteric	SVE	Branchial motor to
	Pterygoid branches		muscles of mastication
	Deep temporal nerves		
	Buccal (long buccal)	GSA, GVE from VII	Mucosal sensation, parasymp. to minor SG
Posterior division			
	Auriculotemporal	GSA, GVE from IX	Sensory (TMJ, skin)
			Parasymp. to parotid
	Lingual	GSA, SVA and GVE from VII	Mucosal sensation
			Taste
			Parasymp. to submandibular
			and sublingual glands
	Inferior alveolar		
	Mylohyoid	SVE	Branchial motor
	Dental branches	GSA	Sensation to pulp, periodontium
	Incisive	GSA	Sensation to pulp, periodontium
	Mental	GSA	Mucocutaneous sensation
Facial nerve (VII)			
	Parotid plexus	SVE	Branchial motor to muscles
			of facial expression
	Chorda tympani	SVA, GVE	Taste, parasymp. to
			submandibular, sublingual,
			and minor SG
	Nerve of the pterygoid canal	GSA, GVE	Mucosal sensation, parasymp.
	(gr. petrosal + deep petrosal)		from VII, sympathetic fibers
			from carotid plexus
Glossopharyngeal nerve (IX)	Lingual branches	GSA, SVA	Mucosal sensation, taste to
			sulcus terminalis and
			circumvallate papillae
Hypoglossal nerve (XII)		GSE	Motor to muscles of tongue

*Nerve branches to the oropharynx are not described.
GSA, general somatic afferent (pain, temperature, pressure, vibration, touch, proprioception, two-point discrimination); GVE, general visceral efferent (parasympathetic from cranial nerves, sympathetic from superior cervical ganglion); SVE, special visceral efferent (motor to striated muscles derived from branchial arches); SVA, special visceral afferent (taste, smell); GSE, general somatic efferent (motor innervation to muscles derived from myotomes); SG, salivary glands; CT, connective tissue.

longest branch is the *nasopalatine nerve* that grooves the nasal septum and leaves the nasal cavity through the incisive foramen, innervating the anterior teeth and primary palate, the triangular region whose three apices are the incisive papilla, and the space between the canine and lateral incisor of each side.

Mandibular Division of the Trigeminal Nerve (Fig. 5–4)

The sensory and motor components of the *mandibular division of the trigeminal nerve* leave the cranial vault via the *foramen ovale*, entering the deep face as two separate structures that

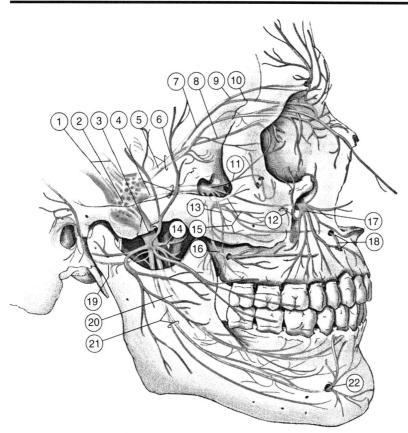

Figure 5–4 Distribution of the trigeminal nerve (1). The branches are as follows: 2, gasserian ganglion; 3, mandibular nerve and foramen ovale; 4, maxillary nerve and foramen rotundum; 5, ophthalmic nerve and superior orbital fissure; 6, nasociliary nerve; 7, frontal nerve; 8, lacrimal nerve; 9, supraorbital nerve; 10, supratrochlear nerve; 11, zygomatic nerve; 12, anterior superior alveolar branches; 13, posterior superior alveolar branches; 14, buccal nerve; 15, posterior nasal branches; 16, greater palatine nerve; 17, infraorbital nerve; 18, nasopalantine nerve; 19, auriculotemporal nerve; 20, lingual nerve; 21, inferior alveolar nerve; 22, mental nerve. (From Malamed SF. Anatomic considerations. In: Handbook of Local Anesthesia, 5th ed. New York: Elsevier, 2004:172, with permission.)

join to form a single, short trunk, from which two small branches arise. The two small branches are the *meningeal branch*, which reenters the cranial cavity via the *foramen spinosum*, and the *medial pterygoid branch*, which not only serves the muscle of the same name but also provides branches to the *tensor tympani* and the *tensor veli palatini muscles*. The short trunk then subdivides into a mostly sensory posterior division and a mostly motor anterior division.

The *anterior division of the mandibular nerve* provides branches that innervate the masseter, medial and lateral pterygoid muscles, as well as the temporalis muscle. The nerves to the temporalis are the *anterior* and *posterior deep temporal nerves* that pass between the superior and inferior heads of the lateral pterygoid and pierce the deep aspect of the temporalis. The sensory component of the anterior division, the *buccal nerve* (or *long buccal nerve)*, also passes between the two heads of the lateral pterygoid, and reaches the lateral surface of the buccinator muscle where it forms a plexus of nerves. Some of these fibers travel with branches of the facial nerve to supply sensory fibers to the skin of the cheek; others penetrate the buccinator to serve the buccal mucosa and gingiva.

The only motor branch of the *posterior division* is the *mylohyoid nerve* that originates from the *inferior alveolar nerve* just before it enters the mandibular foramen. The three sensory portions of the posterior division are the auriculotemporal, inferior alveolar, and lingual nerves. Shortly after the origin of the *auriculotemporal nerve* from the posterior division, it receives postganglionic parasympathetic fibers (*secretomotor*

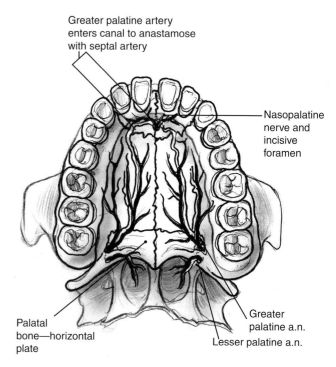

Greater palatine artery enters canal to anastamose with septal artery

Nasopalatine nerve and incisive foramen

Greater palatine a.n.

Lesser palatine a.n.

Palatal bone—horizontal plate

Figure 5–5 Arterial and sensory supply to the hard palate, provided by the pterygopalatine portion of the maxillary artery and the maxillary division of the trigeminal nerve, respectively.

fibers) from the glossopharyngeal nerve via the otic ganglion destined for the parotid gland. The auriculotemporal nerve continues deep to both the lateral pterygoid muscle and the parotid gland, reaches the narrow space between the ear and the temporomandibular joint, and travels cranially, accompanying the superficial temporal vessels. It serves the skin of the anterior region of the ear, the external ear canal, the temporomandibular joint, and supplies branches that travel with the facial nerve to supply sensory innervation to the face. It also provides sensation to the temple via its *superficial temporal branches*. Temporomandibular joint sensation is primarily from the auriculotemporal nerve with contributions from the masseteric and deep temporal nerves.[9,10] The *lingual nerve* originates from the posterior division deep to the lateral pterygoid muscle, and as it passes along the surface of the medial pterygoid muscle it receives preganglionic parasympathetic fibers, destined for the submandibular ganglion, as well as taste fibers from the *chorda tympani nerve*, a branch of the facial nerve. The *submandibular ganglion* is anatomically associated with but does not belong to the lingual nerve. Postganglionic parasympathetic fibers from the ganglion serve the submandibular gland, which they reach directly, as well as the sublingual gland, which they reach by traveling along with the lingual nerve. As the lingual nerve proceeds inferiorly in the deep face it lies medial to the *mandibular ramus*, then, as it proceeds anteriorly in the submandibular region, it lies medial to the *body of the mandible*, in close proximity to the *roots of the third molar*. As it approaches the lateral aspect of the tongue it is flanked by the submandibular gland and the hyoglossus muscle and courses anteriorly to reach the tip of the tongue, and is accompanied part of the way by the submandibular duct. The lingual nerve is responsible for supplying sensory fibers, as well as taste fibers from the chorda tympani, to the anterior two thirds of the tongue. It also supplies sensation to the lingual aspect of the mandibular gingiva and to the mucosa in the vicinity of the tongue.

The *inferior alveolar nerve* arises lateral to and, for a short distance, follows the path of the lingual nerve, passing medial to the ramus of the mandible and lateral to the *sphenomandibular ligament*. The inferior alveolar nerve gives off the *mylohyoid nerve*, then enters the *mandibular foramen*, and continues anteriorly within the *mandibular canal* where it provides sensory innervation to the mandibular teeth and adjacent supporting structures. While in the mandibular canal, it subdivides into mental and incisive nerves. The *mental nerve* exits the mandibular canal via the *mental foramen* to serve the skin and mucous membrane of the lower lip and the skin of the chin. The *incisive nerve* continues anteriorly within the mandibular canal to serve the anterior mandibular teeth and surrounding structures with sensory innervation.

There is a paucity of published research that characterizes the intraoral sensation provided by the trigeminal nerve. Recently, intraoral sensory thresholds were evaluated at four oral mucosal sites in 23 healthy volunteers to serve as baseline measurements that could be used to compare results following nonsensate and sensate flap reconstructions following oral cancer resection.[11] The mucosa of the lower lip and the lateral aspect of the tongue had the lowest sensory thresholds, whereas the buccal mucosa and central tongue demonstrated higher sensory thresholds.

Research pertaining to the impact of surgery and radiation therapy (RT) on intraoral sensation is also in its infancy, but initial findings demonstrate that treatment adversely impacts oral sensation. For example, a preliminary investigation that assessed intraoral sensation following RT for oral or pharyngeal cancer found that a dose of 64 Gy resulted in a significant deterioration of oral sensation 6 months after RT, an effect that persisted 1 year following treatment.[12]

The Facial Nerve

The *facial nerve* has two roots as it emerges from the brainstem: a larger motor root, and a smaller root containing special sensory fibers for taste and parasympathetic fibers, known as the *nervus intermedius*. The two roots enter the internal acoustic meatus, travel through the petrous temporal bone, within the facial canal, where they join each other at the *geniculate ganglion*, the sensory ganglion of the facial nerve. The motor nerve exits the skull via the *stylomastoid foramen* to innervate the muscles of facial expression, including the perioral musculature supplied by the zygomatic, buccal, and marginal mandibular branches.

Branches of the facial nerve that arise within the facial canal are the *greater petrosal nerve*, originating from the geniculate ganglion; the *chorda tympani nerve;* and the nerve to the stapedius muscle. Other branches arise from the facial nerve outside the stylomastoid foramen, and these serve the muscles of facial expression, scalp, and those controlling movement of the pinna of the ear, as well as supplying motor innervation to the platysma, posterior belly of the digastric, and stylohyoid muscles. General sensory fibers from the facial nerve along with the glossopharyngeal nerve serve the soft palate, external ear canal, and regions of the pharynx. The facial nerve also supplies taste fibers to the anterior two thirds of the tongue, as well as secretomotor fibers to the submandibular and sublingual glands via the chorda tympani and submandibular ganglion. Additionally, secretomotor fibers from the facial nerve via the pterygopalatine ganglion are destined for the palatine, nasal, and lacrimal glands, arriving at their destination via maxillary division branches of the trigeminal nerve.

The *greater petrosal nerve* arises from the *geniculate ganglion* and carries preganglionic parasympathetic and general sensory fibers. It passes through the *hiatus of the facial canal* to leave the cranial cavity and then enters the *pterygoid (Vidian) canal* accompanied by the *deep petrosal nerve*, postganglionic sympathetic fibers from the carotid plexus. The two nerves together are known as the *nerve of the pterygoid canal* (Vidian nerve); they join the *pterygopalatine ganglion* where only the preganglionic parasympathetic fibers synapse. Postganglionic parasympathetic fibers arising from the pterygopalatine ganglion are secretomotor fibers that travel with branches of the maxillary division of the trigeminal nerve, as discussed above, as do the general sensory fibers derived from the greater petrosal nerve. The pterygopalatine ganglion is synonymous with the *sphenopalatine ganglion* identified in some anatomic sources.

The *chorda tympani* arises from the facial nerve within the petrous portion of the temporal bone, passes in an arc-shaped path above the tympanic membrane, exits the tympanic cavity via the *petrotympanic fissure*, and leaves the skull at the spine of the sphenoid bone. It travels in the deep face to join the *lingual nerve,* and its function was described previously in the discussion of the *lingual nerve,* a branch of the mandibular division of the trigeminal nerve.

Glossopharyngeal Nerve

The *glossopharyngeal nerve* passes through the *jugular foramen* to exit the cranial vault. Within the foramen are the superior and inferior ganglia of the glossopharyngeal nerve, housing the soma of that nerve's sensory neurons. As the glossopharyngeal nerve leaves the jugular foramen it travels deep to the styloid process, follows the path of the *stylopharyngeus muscle,* which it supplies with motor innervation, and provides fibers to the *carotid sinus* and *carotid body* as well as to the *pharyngeal plexus.* The glossopharyngeal nerve then passes between the superior and inferior pharyngeal constrictors to enter the wall of the pharynx and supplies sensory fibers to the tonsils and posterior tongue as well as taste fibers to the circumvallate papillae. These fibers, which course anterior to the sulcus terminalis to innervate the posterior aspect of the oral tongue, are the only neural contribution to the oral cavity from the glossopharyngeal nerve.

Hypoglossal Nerve

The *hypoglossal nerve* leaves the cranial cavity via the same-named foramen to supply motor innervation to all of the muscles of the tongue with the exception of the palatoglossus. The hypoglossal nerve parallels the course of the *lingual artery* on its way to the tongue, but the nerve travels superficial to the hyoglossus muscle, whereas the artery passes deep to that muscle.

◆ Arterial Supply to Oral Cavity Region (Table 5–4; Fig. 5–6)

The arterial supply of the oral cavity region, which arises from the *ascending pharyngeal, lingual, facial,* and *maxillary branches of the external carotid artery,* is summarized in **Table 5–4**.[13–16] Although many regions of the oral cavity receive contributions from other arterial sources, the anatomy of the *maxillary artery,* which has a complex anatomic course that supplies numerous branches to the oral cavity region, is reviewed in detail.

Table 5–4 Arterial Blood Supply to the Oral Mucosa*

Region	External Carotid Branch	Via	Terminal Branch
Upper lip	Facial[13,14]		Superior labial
	Maxillary (3rd portion)		Infraorbital
Hard palate	Maxillary (3rd portion)	Descending palatine	Greater, lesser palatine
	Maxillary (3rd portion)	Sphenopalatine	Nasopalatine
	Facial		Ascending palatine
	Ascending pharyngeal		Palatine
Anterior upper alveolar ridge			
Labial aspect	Maxillary (3rd portion)	Infraorbital	ASA, MSA
Palatal aspect	Maxillary (3rd portion)	Descending palatine	Greater palatine
	Maxillary (3rd portion)	Sphenopalatine	Nasopalatine
Posterior upper alveolar ridge			
Buccal aspect	Maxillary (3rd portion)		PSA
	Maxillary (2nd portion)[15]		Buccal artery
Palatal aspect	Maxillary (3rd portion)	Descending palatine	Greater, lesser palatine
	Facial		Ascending palatine
Buccal mucosa			
Anterior to Stensen's duct	Facial		Superior, inferior labial[16]
Posterior to Stensen's duct	Maxillary (2nd portion)		Buccal[15,16]
Lower lip	Facial		Inferior labial
	Facial		Sublabial
	Facial		Submental
Anterior lower alveolar ridge			
Labial aspect	Maxillary (1st portion)	Inferior alveolar	Mental
Lingual aspect	Lingual		Sublingual
Posterior lower alveolar ridge			
Buccal aspect	Maxillary (1st portion)		Inferior alveolar
	Maxillary (2nd portion)[15]		Buccal
	Facial		Superior, inferior labial
Lingual aspect	Lingual		Sublingual
	Maxillary (1st portion)		Inferior alveolar
Oral tongue	Lingual		Sublingual, deep lingual
Floor of mouth	Lingual		Sublingual

*Primary arterial supply is described; some oral cavity regions are supplied by other arterial sources that are not listed.
ASA, anterior superior alveolar artery; MSA, middle superior alveolar artery; PSA, posterior superior alveolar artery; 1st portion, mandibular portion of maxillary artery; 2nd portion, pterygoid portion of maxillary artery; 3rd portion, pterygopalatine portion of maxillary artery.

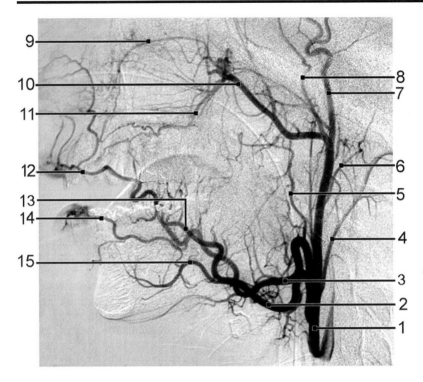

Figure 5–6 External carotid arteriogram, lateral projection: 1, external carotid artery; 2, facial artery; 3, lingual artery; 4, occipital artery; 5, ascending palatine artery; 6, posterior auricular artery; 7, superficial temporal artery; 8, middle meningeal artery; 9, infraorbital artery; 10, maxillary artery; 11, descending palatine artery; 12, superior labial artery; 13, deep lingual artery; 14, inferior labial artery; 15, sublingual artery. (From http://www.medcyclopaedia.com, reprinted with permission from GE Healthcare.)

Maxillary Artery (Fig. 5–6)

The *maxillary artery* arises within the substance of the parotid gland, passes anteriorly between the ramus of the mandible and the *sphenomandibular ligament*, proceeds along either the deep or superficial aspect of the *lateral pterygoid muscle*, and enters the *pterygopalatine fossa* by passing between the two heads of the lateral pterygoid and through the *pterygomaxillary fissure*. The maxillary artery is said to have three regions: mandibular, pterygoid, and pterygopalatine.

The *mandibular portion* of the maxillary artery lies deep to the ramus of the mandible and gives rise to the deep auricular, anterior tympanic, inferior alveolar, middle meningeal, and accessory meningeal arteries. The *deep auricular artery* is very small and passes medial to the temporomandibular joint that it supplies. The *anterior tympanic artery* arises near or in common with the deep auricular artery. It traverses the *petrotympanic fissure* to serve the tympanic membrane and adjacent regions. The *inferior alveolar artery* follows the course of and has branches that mirror the *inferior alveolar nerve* in the *mandibular canal*. Thus it provides the *mylohyoid artery* to the same named muscle just before its entry into the *mandibular foramen*. Within the mandibular canal it provides dental branches to the molar and premolar teeth, then divides to form the *incisive* and *mental arteries*. The former serves the canine and the incisors and the latter exits the mandibular canal via the mental foramen to vascularize the lower lip and chin. The *middle meningeal artery* originates just superior to the *inferior alveolar artery*. It passes superiorly, deep to the lateral pterygoid muscle, and just before it traverses the *foramen spinosum* to enter the cranial cavity, the artery is usually encircled by

the split *auriculotemporal nerve*. The *accessory meningeal artery* is inconstant; when present, it is anterior to and parallels the middle meningeal artery and enters the cranial cavity via the *foramen ovale*.

The *pterygoid portion* of the maxillary artery is bounded by the anterior and posterior borders of the lateral pterygoid muscle. Its branches include the deep temporal, pterygoid, masseteric, and buccal arteries. The *anterior* and *posterior* (and occasionally, *middle*) *deep temporal arteries* pass between the temporalis muscle, which they vascularize, and the temporal bone of the skull. The *pterygoid arteries* are very short and they serve the lateral and medial pterygoid muscles. The *masseteric artery* passes between the condylar and coronoid processes, through the *mandibular notch*, to pierce the deep aspect of the masseter muscle to vascularize it. The *buccal artery* parallels the buccal nerve as it passes between the two heads of the lateral pterygoid muscle to follow the anterior border of the tendon of the temporalis muscle on its way to the buccinator muscle, which it vascularizes along with the buccal mucosa.

The *pterygopalatine portion* of the maxillary artery passes through the *pterygomaxillary fissure* to enter the *pterygopalatine fossa*. Its branches include the posterior superior alveolar, infraorbital, descending palatine arteries, as well as the artery of the pterygoid canal, pharyngeal, and sphenopalatine arteries. The *posterior superior alveolar artery* arises from the maxillary artery just within the pterygomaxillary fissure; it accompanies the posterior superior alveolar nerve along the maxillary tuberosity to enter the posterior superior alveolar foramen to vascularize the three molars and two premolars and their respective gingivae as well as the maxillary sinus. The maxillary artery continues as the *infraorbital artery* as it enters the orbit by way of the inferior orbital fissure. It passes along the floor of the orbit, lying within the infraorbital groove, enters the infraorbital canal, and exits into the face via the infraorbital foramen. The infraorbital artery has several branches, the *orbital arteries*, which vascularize the lacrimal gland, inferior rectus and inferior oblique muscles; the *middle* and *anterior superior alveolar arteries*, which serve the canine and incisor teeth as well as their respective gingivae; and the *facial branches*, which provide vascular supply to the nose, lacrimal sac, and upper lip via their various subsidiaries. Continuing with other branches of the pterygopalatine portion, the *descending palatine artery* enters the pterygopalatine canal, where it bifurcates to form the greater and lesser palatine arteries. These vessels follow the same named nerves to leave the canal via the greater and lesser palatine foramina, respectively (**Fig. 5–5**). The *greater palatine artery* proceeds anteriorly to vascularize the mucosa of the hard palate as well as the lingual gingivae and anastomose with the *nasopalatine artery* within the confines of the *incisive canal*. The lesser palatine arteries serve the tonsil and the soft palate. The *artery of the pterygoid canal* is a small vessel that accompanies the *nerve of the pterygoid canal* and serves the pharynx, middle ear, eustachian tube, and sphenoidal sinus. The tiny *pharyngeal branch* traverses the pharyngeal canal and provides vascularization to the pharynx, sphenoid sinus, and auditory (eustachian) tube. The *sphenopalatine artery* leaves the pterygopalatine fossa via the *sphenopalatine foramen*, enters the nasal cavity, and branches into the *posterior septal* and *posterior lateral nasal branches* to serve the nasal cavity. The largest branch of the sphenopalatine artery is the *nasopalatine artery* that grooves the median nasal septum and enters the *incisive canal*, where it anastomoses with the *greater palatine artery*.

In general, most regions of the oral cavity are supplied by multiple arterial sources, limiting the risk of ischemia when flow through one of the feeding vessels is compromised. It is important, however, to appreciate the variations in arterial anatomy that can exist in the oral cavity region as well as the anatomic regions that are susceptible to vascular compromise. For example, cadaveric studies have documented marked variability of the arterial supply to the upper and lower lips.[14] In a study of 14 human cadavers that were subjected to intraarterial silicone rubber injection, bilateral *inferior labial arteries* were found in less than half of the cadavers, and end-to-end anastomosis between the inferior labial arteries was demonstrated in only 15% of the cadavers.[14] Moreover, the location, course, and dimensions of the inferior labial artery were not constant. These findings dispel the conventional anatomic teaching that these arteries create an anastomotic arch from one side to the other that lies along the border of the lip. Knowledge of these anatomic variants is critical for reconstruction of the oral commissure following cancer resection, because conventional anatomic teachings provide the foundation upon which lower lip reconstruction has been approached.

The oral region of the tongue (anterior two thirds of the tongue) has a rich blood supply that arises primarily from the paired *lingual arteries*. Although the oropharyngeal tongue base (posterior one third of the tongue) receives contributions from the facial artery and the oral tongue receives branches from the inferior alveolar and buccal branches of the maxillary artery, these contributions are relatively minor.[17] The midline raphe that divides the musculature of the tongue results in poor vascular crossover between the right and left sides, which makes each side of the oral tongue a vascular end organ.[17] This fibrous *lingual septum*, which is seen as a hypodense midline structure on computed tomography (CT) scans through the tongue, has been referred to as the *midline low-density plane*.[18] Although tongue viability is preserved following the ligation or disruption of one lingual artery, ligation of both lingual arteries likely results in necrosis of the entire tongue. A case report has documented maintenance of tongue viability following bilateral ligation, but the lingual arteries were disrupted several years apart, suggesting that the development of collateral circulation played a role.[19]

Our present understanding of the vascular supply of the maxilla has been refined by important research that establishes the biologic basis for orthognathic surgery. Bell and colleagues[20–22] observed wound healing following the performance of maxillary osteotomies on adult rhesus monkeys and demonstrated that down-fracture of the maxilla with complete mobilization, also known as the LeFort I osteotomy, can be accomplished with maintenance of adequate vascular supply as long as the maxilla remains attached to a broad soft tissue pedicle of the posterior palatal and buccal soft tissues. Subsequent prospective randomized research performed on patients undergoing LeFort I osteotomy was unable to document a significant decrease in maxillary gingival blood flow when both *descending palatine arteries* were ligated.[23] Although the descending palatine artery provides much of the blood supply to the maxilla through the *greater and lesser palatine arteries*, the maxilla also receives significant blood supply from other vessels that traverse the soft palate and the posterior buccal region.

Although some regions of the oral cavity receive multiple arterial contributions, an appreciation for the primary arterial supply to each of these areas can be exploited so that the viability of surrounding tissue is preserved following surgical resection and the number and quality of possible reconstructive options are maximized. Ink and lead oxide injections into catheterized arteries have elucidated the presence of relatively constant oral mucosal territories that are supplied by the buccal, inferior alveolar, labial, lingual, ascending palatine, and ascending pharyngeal arteries.[16] For example, the buccal mucosal surface posterior to the parotid duct orifice is consistently supplied by the *buccal artery*, a branch of the *pterygoid portion of the maxillary artery*, whereas the buccal mucosa anterior to the parotid duct orifice is supplied by the *superior* and *inferior labial arteries* that arise from the facial artery. These vascularized "territories" provide us with the anatomic basis for intraoral flap design using structures such as the tongue, buccal mucosa, and palate during oral cavity reconstruction.

The angiosome concept divides the body into multiple three-dimensional composite blocks of tissue supplied by particular source arteries.[24] The junctional zone between angiosomes is usually represented by anastomotic vessels that are considered "choke" anastomoses because the vessel caliber in the anastomotic region is reduced.

Angiosomes of the head and neck are usually connected by "choke" anastomoses with some exceptions. For example, the caliber of the anastomosis between the vertebral and the internal carotid system is not reduced, resulting in a "true anastomosis." In contrast, the junctional zone between the left and right sides of the tongue, hard palate, and posterior pharyngeal wall is nearly nonexistent and is formed predominantly by minute vessels. The choke vessels that link adjacent vascular territories are believed to regulate flow between angiosomes under normal circumstances and can increase in caliber when a decrease in vascular flow is detected. Indeed, surgically delayed flaps performed in two stages on dogs have shown that maximal arterial dilation occurs at the site of the "choke anastomosis," providing a biologic explanation for the use of surgical delay to improve flap survival.[25] The *buccinator muscle* and its overlying mucosa are at the anastomotic center of the facial and maxillary arteries, which explains why buccinator flaps that are pedicled on either artery can be reliably used for intraoral reconstruction. The temporalis, masseter, trapezius, and levator scapulae muscles are other examples of muscles that cross at least two angiosome territories and are useful in head and neck reconstruction.[17]

◆ Lymphatic Drainage of the Oral Cavity

The lymphatic drainage system of the oral cavity has recently been characterized using light and transmission electron microscopy and lymphographic dye injections.[26] The most peripheral lymphatic vessels are avalvular, endothelially lined *capillaries* with an intraluminal diameter of 30 to 50 μm that drain into valve-bearing *precollecting vessels* at the junction of the mucosa and submucosa. The precollecting vessels subsequently empty into *peripheral collecting vessels* that carry the lymph to the first lymph node station. The mucosa of the tongue, mandibular alveolar ridge, and floor of mouth drain into the lymphatics of the floor of the mouth, where some lymph vessels cross the midline. Collecting vessels in the anterior floor of mouth can drain into the *submental lymph nodes*. Occasionally, draining lymphatic vessels pass through the mylohyoid muscle into a *preglandular submandibular node*.[27] The ventral surface of the anterior oral tongue drains medially into the floor of the mouth and to the submandibular and upper jugular lymph nodes via five to seven collecting vessels that traverse between the *genioglossal muscles*. The lateral oral tongue and the posterior floor of the mouth drain to the upper jugular nodes.[26] Lymphatic drainage to rare *lingual lymph nodes* associated with the sublingual gland between the mucosa of the floor of the mouth and the mylohyoid muscle can result in regional metastatic failure above the mylohyoid muscle.[28,29] The buccal mucosa contains a dense lymphatic system that drains via eight to 10 collecting vessels that traverse the buccinator muscle primarily into the *submandibular space*. These lymph vessels interconnect with the lymphatics of the maxillary and mandibular gingiva overlying the alveolar ridges. The mucosa of the hard and soft palate have a dense superficial lymphatic system. Lymphatic vessels occasionally cross the midline of the hard palate, whereas crossover is more frequent in the soft palate.[26] These lymphatic vessels provide the pathways for metastatic tumor deposition into the cervical lymphatics that are discussed in Chapter 14.

◆ The Mandible

The bony *mandible* is composed of a horseshoe-shaped horizontally positioned body whose anteriormost apex forms the *mandibular symphysis* (symphysis menti) and two flattened *rami* jutting vertically from the two ends of the body in a posterosuperior direction. The posteriormost extent of the body of the mandible joins the posterior border of the ramus at the angle of the mandible. Just anterior to the angle, the *groove for the facial artery* creates a slight concavity along the inferior border of the mandible.

The external surface of the body of the mandible is distinguished by the presence of the *mental foramen,* located inferior to the first and second premolars. This foramen has a beveled opening that faces in a posterior direction and transmits the mental nerve, artery, and vein. Also on this surface the oblique line is evident as it progresses from the anterior edge of the ramus to the mental tubercle, located at the inferolateral border of the mandibular symphysis. Posteriorly, just distolateral to the third molar, the oblique line forms the lateral boundary of the *retromolar fossa*, medial to which is the *retromolar triangle,* a depression between the fused buccal and lingual alveolar crests just behind the third molar.

Anteriorly, the internal surface of the body of the mandible is marked by the presence of the two (or occasionally four) spine-like protuberances, the superiorly positioned *genial tubercles* that form the site of attachment of the *genioglossus muscles,* and the two inferiorly positioned *inferior mandibular spines* that act as the attachment sites of the *geniohyoid muscles.* A linear protuberance, the *mylohyoid line,* extends from the mandibular symphysis as far posteriorly as the third molar, and serves as the origin of the *mylohyoid muscle.* This line also separates the superiorly positioned *sublingual fossa* from the inferiorly situated *submandibular fossa,* depressions housing the major salivary glands of those names. The soft tissue anatomy of the floor of the mouth and submandibular space is detailed in Chapter 11.

The *ramus of the mandible* is a flattened structure whose superiormost extent sports the anteriorly positioned, flat, triangular extension, the *coronoid process* and the posteriorly situated extension, the *condyloid process*. The coronoid process functions as the site of insertion of the temporalis muscle. It is important to note that the temporalis muscle continues to insert along the anterior border of the ramus, and its tendinous sheath frequently conceals the *buccal nerve* as well as the *buccal artery and vein*. The condylar process has a slender region, the *neck of the mandible,* and ends in an articular surface, the *condyle* that, at rest, occupies the mandibular fossa of the temporal bone. The *lateral pterygoid muscle* inserts in a small depression, the *pterygoid fovea,* on the medial surface of the neck of the mandible. The concave depression between the coronoid and condylar processes, the *mandibular notch,* is traversed by the *masseteric nerve* and *vessels* to pierce the posterior aspect of the masseter and provide that muscle with nerve and vascular supply. The lateral surface of the ramus has a roughened texture attesting to the attachment of the *masseter muscle.* The central region of the medial surface of the ramus displays the *mandibular foramen,* the opening of the mandibular canal, which houses the *inferior alveolar nerve, artery,* and *vein.* The *lingula,* a small, sharp, triangular projection of bone is located anterior to the foramen, and is the site of attachment of the *sphenomandibular ligament.* A thin but well-defined *mylohyoid groove,* housing the *mylohyoid nerve* and *vessels,* extends inferiorly from the lingula toward the base of the mandible. The rough appearance of the medial surface of the ramus and of the angle of the mandible indicates the insertion of the *medial pterygoid muscle.*

The temporomandibular joint (TMJ) receives its blood supply via the *maxillary* and *superficial temporal arteries.* The *mandibular portion of the maxillary artery* supplies the TMJ via its *middle meningeal, deep auricular,* and *anterior tympanic* branches. The condyle is perfused by perforating branches of these arteries that enter through the retained periosteum, lateral pterygoid insertion, and TMJ capsule, and also receives vascular supply through its marrow spaces from the inferior alveolar artery.[30] Because the condyle is supplied by numerous sources and is not reliant on the inferior alveolar artery, segmental mandibulectomy with preservation of the condyle to facilitate reconstruction and improve postoperative function can usually be performed without the risk of avascular necrosis. In fact, mandibulectomy with condylar head preservation via performance of an osteotomy at the junction of the condylar head and neck has been performed in children with condylar growth documented postoperatively.[31]

Surgeons must have a thorough understanding of mandibular anatomy and the variability of the course of the inferior alveolar nerve (IAN) within the mandible to preserve the IAN during mandibular resective surgery (**Fig. 5–7**). A summary of the course of the IAN in the average adult dentate mandible has been compiled from numerous disparate published descriptions of its course. The *mandibular foramen* is located below the plane of the *occlusal surface* of the mandibular teeth in 75% of individuals. The foramen is located 12 to 16 mm posterior to the anterior edge of the ramus and 17 to

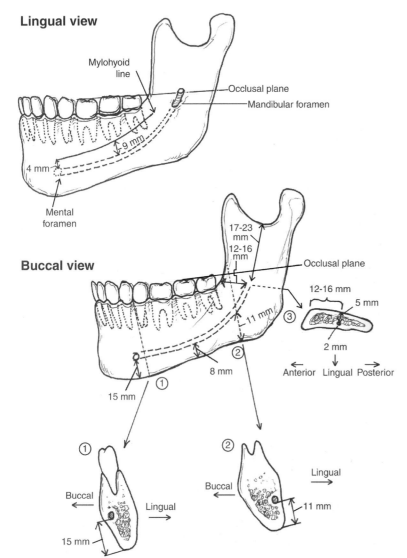

Figure 5–7 The intramandibular course of the inferior alveolar nerve (IAN): buccal and lingual views. Cross-sectional views of the mandible (*insets*) are provided at locations 1, 2, and 3 to illustrate how the location of the IAN changes within the mandible.

23 mm inferior to the mandibular notch.[32,33] Within the ramus, the *mandibular canal* is generally midway between the anterior and posterior borders of the ramus, approximately 2 mm from the medial or lingual surface and 5 mm from the lateral surface. As the nerve courses mesially (anteriorly) within the mandibular canal, it travels close to the lingual cortical plate in a bone-encased tunnel within a noncompartmentalized medullary core.[34] The medullary core is relatively large with a thin cortical rim ranging from 2 to 4 mm. Although the IAN may be encased within a bony mandibular canal, this is not a constant feature and the canal frequently lacks definite walls.[35] Distally (posteriorly), the nerve courses within 3 to 6 mm of the apex of the third molar, approximately 11 mm above the inferior mandibular border. The mandibular canal courses further inferiorly from the root apices and more mesially until the mandibular canal reaches its lowest point at the distal half of the first molar, where the canal courses within 8 mm of the inferior border of the mandible.[34,35] Similarly, the mandibular canal is located approximately 9 mm below the mylohyoid line in the second molar region but only 4 mm below the mylohyoid line in the premolar region.[36] The relationship between the IAN and the inferior mandibular border is less variable than its relationship with the crest of the alveolus, because alveolar bone height can vary in dentate patients with periodontal bone loss as well as in edentulous patients who may experience progressive superior alveolar ridge resorption with dehiscence of the mandibular canal along the occlusal surface.

The nerve continues to travel close to the lingual cortex within the medullary cavity until it reaches the mental foramen, which is consistently located higher then the nerve.[33,34] In the dentate mandible, the foramen is typically 15 to 19 mm above the mandible's inferior border. The location of the mental foramen has been evaluated in a large series of cadaveric mandibles.[37] The mental foramen was located below the apex of the second premolar in 60% of the mandibles, between the apices of the first and second premolars in 20%, and posterior to the second premolar in 20%. Anterior, or mesial to the mental foramen, a well-defined incisive nerve is inconsistently present, and marked variability in the innervation of the anterior teeth exists.

Evaluation of the course of the IAN using CT with a standard axial acquisition protocol provides limited information about its location in the ramus. Kane et al[33] were able to visualize reliably the bony canal only over an average distance 12.7 mm within the ascending ramus. Stein et al[38] have shown that the canal can be visualized with CT when the slices intersect the nerve perpendicularly, and have developed a protocol to allow visualization of the nerve through its entire course by optimal patient positioning and gantry tilt of the scanner.

◆ Dentoalveolar Anatomy

The periodontal tissues that support and invest the tooth are composed of the *gingiva, periodontal ligament (PDL), cementum,* and *alveolar bone* (**Fig. 5–8**).[39] The root of the tooth is housed within the bony *alveolus,* or tooth socket. Periodontal ligament fibers, which are bundles of collagen fibers, are

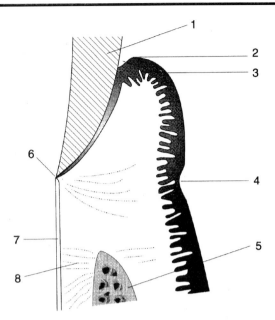

Figure 5–8   1, enamel; 2, gingival margin; 3, small gingival sulcus; 4, free gingival groove; 5, alveolar bone; 6, cementoenamel junction; 7, cementum; 8, periodontal ligament. Between 2 and 4 is free gingiva. (From Holmstrup P. The macroanatomy of the periodontium. In: Wilson TG, Kornman KS, eds. Fundamentals of Periodontics. Carol Stream, IL: Quintessence, 1996:19, with permission.)

embedded in cementum at one end and in bone at the other end, anchoring the tooth to the surrounding alveolar bone. The embedded portions of the fiber bundles at either end are termed *Sharpey's fibers* and are named for Scottish anatomist William Sharpey.[40] The *alveolar processes* are covered by compact bone, and the compact bone that lines the socket is termed the *alveolar bone proper* (**Fig. 5–9**).

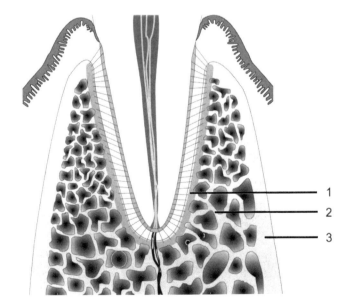

Figure 5–9   Alveolar bone structure: 1, alveolar bone proper (lamina dura in radiograph); 2, trabecular bone; 3, compact bone (cortical plate). (From Holmstrup P. The macroanatomy of the periodontium. In: Wilson TG, Kornman KS, eds. Fundamentals of Periodontics. Carol Stream, IL: Quintessence, 1996:21, with permission.)

The radiographic appearance of the alveolar bone proper is termed the *lamina dura*, and its appearance can be altered by periapical or periodontal pathology. The supporting *cancellous bone* (spongiosa) which is housed between the compact bone that forms the alveolar bone proper and the cortical plates of the mandible and maxilla, contains trabecular struts that strengthen the compact bone and the marrow-containing medullary cavities.[41]

The gingiva, whose mucosa is masticatory mucosa that covers the alveolar process, joins with the lining alveolar mucosa at the *mucogingival junction* (**Fig. 5–2**). The attached gingiva overlying the alveolar bone is "attached" to the cortical bone via collagen bundles that are embedded into the lamina propria of the masticatory mucosa, creating a mucoperiosteum. Once again, these fibers embedded in bone are Sharpey fibers. The attached gingiva continues coronal to the alveolar bone, where dentogingival fibers attach the cementum to the subepithelial lamina propria of the gingiva.[42] Fibers from the PDL do not insert into the gingiva. The gingiva coronal to the floor of the *gingival sulcus* is termed the *free gingiva* because it is no longer attached. In health, a shallow epithelial-lined gingival sulcus is present between the free gingiva and the tooth. Gingivitis injures the sulcular epithelium and can ultimately progress to periodontitis, which is characterized by the loss of periodontal connective tissue attachment and destruction of the alveolar bone proper.[42]

◆ Conclusion

Symptoms such as pain and paresthesia frequently result from invasion of soft tissue, bone, and nerve by oral cancer that correlate with anatomically based clinical and radiographic findings. Such anatomic considerations can in turn be exploited to guide the performance of surgical resection and radiation therapy that improves disease control and minimizes morbidity. This topical overview illustrates how anatomic knowledge can directly impact clinical care and patient outcomes, and establishes the undeniable linkage between anatomy and oral oncology that will be reinforced throughout the remainder of this book.

References

1. Lip and oral cavity. In: Greene FL, Page DL, Fleming ID, eds. AJCC Cancer Staging Manual, 6th ed. New York: Springer-Verlag, 2002: 23–32

2. Funk GF, Karnell LH, Robinson RA, Zhen WK, Trask DK, Hoffman HT. Presentation, treatment, and outcome of oral cavity cancer: a National Cancer Data Base report. Head Neck 2002;24:165–180

3. Hoffman HT, Karnell LH, Funk GF, Robinson RA, Menck HR. The National Cancer Data Base report on cancer of the head and neck. Arch Otolaryngol Head Neck Surg 1998;124:951–962

4. Canto MT, Devesa SS. Oral cavity and pharynx cancer incidence rates in the United States, 1975–1998. Oral Oncol 2002;38: 610–617

5. Squier CA, Hill MW. Oral Mucosa. In: Ten Cate AR, ed. Oral Histology: Development, Structure, and Function, 4th ed. St. Louis: Mosby-Year Book, 1994:389–431

6. Whitson SW. Bone. In: Ten Cate AR, ed. Oral Histology: Development, Structure, and Function, 4th ed. St. Louis: Mosby-Year Book, 1994: 120–146

7. Dale AC. Salivary Glands. In: Ten Cate AR, ed. Oral Histology: Development, Structure, and Function, 4th ed. St. Louis: Mosby-Year Book, 1994:356–388

8. Klein RM. Development, Structure, and Function of Salivary Glands. In: Avery JK, ed. Oral Development and Histology, 2nd ed. New York: Thieme, 1994:352–381

9. Thilander B. Innervation of the temporomandibular joint disc in man. Acta Odontol Scand 1964;22:151–156

10. Davidson JA, Metzinger SE, Tufaro AP, Dellon AL. Clinical implications of the innervation of the temporomandibular joint. J Craniofac Surg 2003;14:235–239

11. Zur KB, Genden EM, Urken ML. Sensory topography of the oral cavity and the impact of free flap reconstruction: a preliminary study. Head Neck 2004;26:884–889

12. Bodin I, Jaghagen EL, Isberg A. Intraoral sensation before and after radiotherapy and surgery for oral and pharyngeal cancer. Head Neck 2004;26:923–929

13. Pinar YA, Bilge O, Govsa F. Anatomic study of the blood supply of the perioral region. Clin Anat 2005;18:330–339

14. Magden O, Edizer M, Atabey A, Tayfur V, Ergur I. Cadaveric study of the arterial anatomy of the upper lip. Plast Reconstr Surg 2004;114: 355–359

15. Zhao Z, Li S, Yan Y, et al. New buccinator myomucosal island flap: anatomic study and clinical application. Plast Reconstr Surg 1999;104:55–64

16. Whetzel TP, Saunders CJ. Arterial anatomy of the oral cavity. Plast Reconstr Surg 1997;100:582–587

17. Houseman ND, Taylor GI, Pan WR. The angiosomes of the head and neck: anatomic study and clinical applications. Plast Reconstr Surg 2000;105:2287–2313

18. Muraki AS, Mancuso AA, Harnsberger HR, Johnson LP, Meads GB. CT of the oropharynx, tongue base, and floor of the mouth: normal anatomy and range of variations, and applications in staging of carcinoma. Radiology 1983;148:725–731

19. Foster PK, Weed DT. Tongue viability after bilateral lingual artery ligation and surgery for recurrent tongue-base cancer. Ear Nose Throat J 2003;82:720–722, 724

20. Bell WH. Revascularization and bone healing after anterior maxillary osteotomy: a study using adult rhesus monkeys. J Oral Surg 1969;27:249–255

21. Bell WH, Levy BM. Revascularization and bone healing after posterior maxillary osteotomy. J Oral Surg 1971;29:313–320

22. Bell WH, Fonseca RJ, Kennedy JW, Levy BM. Bone healing and revascularization after total maxillary osteotomy. J Oral Surg 1975;33: 253–260

23. Dodson TB, Bays RA, Neuenschwander MC. Maxillary perfusion during Le Fort I osteotomy after ligation of the descending palatine artery. J Oral Maxillofac Surg 1997;55:51–55

24. Taylor GI, Palmer JH. The vascular territories (angiosomes) of the body: experimental study and clinical applications. Br J Plast Surg 1987;40:113–141

25. Callegari PR, Taylor GI, Caddy CM, Minabe T. An anatomic review of the delay phenomenon. I. Experimental studies. Plast Reconstr Surg 1992;89:397–407

26. Werner JA, Dunne AA, Myers JN. Functional anatomy of the lymphatic drainage system of the upper aerodigestive tract and its role in metastasis of squamous cell carcinoma. Head Neck 2003;25: 322–332

27. Abe M, Murakami G, Noguchi M, Yajima T, Kohama GI. Afferent and efferent lymph-collecting vessels of the submandibular nodes with special reference to the lymphatic route passing through the mylohyoid muscle. Head Neck 2003;25:59–66

28. Dutton JM, Graham SM, Hoffman HT. Metastatic cancer to the floor of mouth: the lingual lymph nodes. Head Neck 2002;24:401–405

29. Ozeki S, Tashiro H, Okamoto M, Matsushima T. Metastasis to the lingual lymph node in carcinoma of the tongue. J Maxillofac Surg 1985;13:277–281

30. Ash MM, Nelson SJ, eds. Dental Anatomy, Physiology, and Occlusion, 8th ed. Philadelphia: WB Saunders, 2003

31. Nahabedian MY, Tufaro A, Manson PN. Improved mandible function after hemimandibulectomy, condylar head preservation, and vascularized fibular reconstruction. Ann Plast Surg 2001;46:506–510

32. Nicholson ML. A study of the position of the mandibular foramen in the adult human mandible. Anat Rec 1985;212:110–112

33. Kane AA, Lo LJ, Chen YR, Hsu KH, Noordhoff MS. The course of the inferior alveolar nerve in the normal human mandibular ramus and in patients presenting for cosmetic reduction of the mandibular angles. Plast Reconstr Surg 2000;106:1162–1174

34. Haribhakti VV. The dentate adult human mandible: an anatomic basis for surgical decision making. Plast Reconstr Surg 1996;97:536–541 discussion 542–533

35. Anderson LC, Kosinski TF, Mentag PJ. A review of the intraosseous course of the nerves of the mandible. J Oral Implantol 1991;17:394–403

36. Gowgiel JM. The position and course of the mandibular canal. J Oral Implantol 1992;18:383–385

37. Wang TM, Shih C, Liu JC, Kuo KJ. A clinical and anatomical study of the location of the mental foramen in adult Chinese mandibles. Acta Anat (Basel) 1986;126:29–33

38. Stein W, Hassfeld S, Muhling J. Tracing of thin tubular structures in computer tomographic data. Comput Aided Surg 1998;3:83–88

39. Holmstrup P. The macroanatomy of the periodontium. In: Wilson TG, Kornman KS, eds. Fundamentals of periodontics. Chicago: Quintessence, 1996:17–25

40. Freeman E. Periodontium. In: Ten Cate AR, ed. Oral Histology: Development, Structure, and Function, 4th ed. St. Louis: Mosby-Year Book, 1994:276–312

41. Avery JK. Histology of the periodontium: alveolar bone, cementum, and periodontal ligament. In: Avery JK, ed. Oral Development and Histology, 2nd ed. New York: Thieme, 1994:144–163

42. Holmstrup P. The microanatomy of the periodontium. In: Wilson TG, Kornman KS, eds. Fundamentals of Periodontics. Chicago: Quintessence, 1996:27–45

6

Imaging of Patients with Oral Cancer

Jeffrey A. Bennett,
Parminder Deol, and
James J. Abrahams

Diagnostic imaging has an essential role in the evaluation and management of patients with oral cancer. Radiographic findings complement the clinical examination and pathologic data as part of the original staging process. Computed tomography (CT) and magnetic resonance imaging (MRI) are routinely used during the initial pretreatment evaluation for this purpose, providing additional prognostic information such as perineural invasion and lymph node extracapsular spread that is not included in the tumor, node, and metastasis (TNM) classification scheme. Radiographic investigation has refined the diagnostic criteria for metastatic nodal disease and early mandibular invasion, and has characterized patterns of tumor spread from different sites within the oral cavity. Significant advances continue to be made in posttreatment surveillance for persistent or recurrent cancer. The interdependence between radiographic assessment and health care delivery requires clinicians who evaluate and manage patients with oral cancer to have a working knowledge of diagnostic imaging of the head and neck.

◆ General Considerations

The imaging assessment of the oral cancer patient is focused on answering the following questions that directly affect prognosis and treatment decisions:

1. What is the full local extent of the primary lesion?
2. Is there bony invasion?
3. Is there evidence of perivascular or perineural spread?
4. Is there evidence of regional metastatic lymphadenopathy?
5. Is there distant metastatic spread?

Because the clinician can directly visualize the mucosal extent of the primary lesion, imaging is performed to determine the extent of tumor invasion into the submucosal tissues and deep spaces of the neck, which cannot be assessed by clinical examination. Radiographically, invasive carcinoma appears as a mass that infiltrates, replaces, and displaces normal tissue. The site of origin of the cancer is often suggested by the center of the tumor mass, but this determination may not be possible if the tumor is large and occupies multiple anatomic spaces. Thorough knowledge of normal anatomy, the imaging appearance of normal and abnormal tissues, and characteristic tumor spread patterns is necessary to understand and describe the full extent of the primary tumor.

A critical feature of the radiologic analysis is the presence of fat, which is normally seen throughout the various anatomic spaces of the head and neck, separates individual muscle bundles, and is present in small fat pads at neural foramina. Fat is easily seen on CT as low-density, nonenhancing tissue. On MRI, fat is seen as high signal intensity on pre- and postcontrast T1-weighted images, and on fast spin echo T2-weighted images. Therefore, fat provides a natural contrast to tumor on both CT and MRI, and its replacement is suggestive of tumor involvement (**Fig. 6–1**).

On noncontrast CT, carcinoma has a similar density to muscle and lymphoid tissue, which obscures visualization of the tumor. Fortunately, tumor enhances following the intravenous administration of iodinated contrast, and appears as a bright mass compared with fat and muscle (**Fig. 6–2**). On MRI, carcinoma typically appears as an intermediate signal intensity mass on noncontrast T1-weighted images, similar to the signal intensity of muscle. However, tumor has higher signal intensity than muscle on T2-weighted images and enhances following the intravenous

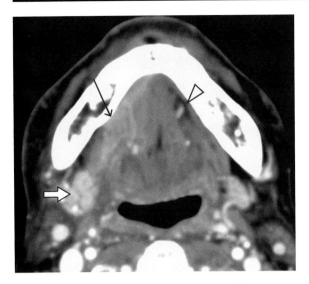

Figure 6–1 Axial contrast enhanced CT scan demonstrates squamous cell carcinoma of the floor of the mouth on the right (*arrow*). Note the replacement of low-density fat, which is seen in the sublingual space on the normal side (*arrowhead*). The right submandibular gland is enlarged and contains dilated ducts secondary to obstructive sialadenitis (*open arrow*).

administration of gadolinium diethylenetriamine pentaacetic acid (Gd-DTPA) (**Fig. 6–3**). Careful attention to the CT density of a lesion, or its MRI signal intensity on different sequences, aids in the differential diagnosis of lesions, and can help to avoid pitfalls, such as mistaking muscle denervation, which in its later stages consists of fatty infiltration, for tumor (see Fig. 28–6 in Chapter 28).

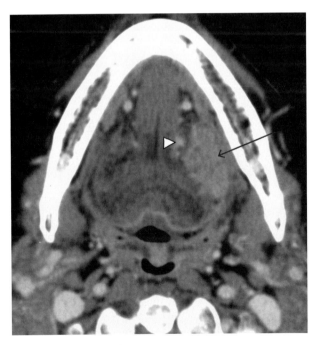

Figure 6–2 Axial contrast-enhanced CT scan demonstrates an infiltrating squamous cell carcinoma of the lateral surface of the tongue (*arrow*). There is no extension to bone and no involvement of the neurovascular bundle (*arrowhead*).

◆ Selection of an Appropriate Imaging Modality

Accurate radiographic assessment is dependent on excellent-quality images, which are essential to confidently answer the relevant clinical questions that guide patient care. Of the major diagnostic imaging modalities, CT and MRI provide the most complete evaluation. Debate continues as to whether CT or MRI is better as the initial diagnostic modality.[1] The bottom line is that either modality can produce a diagnostic-quality study, if performed with an appropriate dedicated protocol on a cooperative patient. Often, the information obtained from both studies is complementary. Other modalities such as DentaScan (GE Medical Systems, Global Center, Milwaukee, WI), plain film panoramic imaging, ultrasound, and positron emission tomography (PET), can be used to answer more specific diagnostic questions, as discussed below.

Computed Tomography

Advantages of multidetector CT include its wide availability and decreased cost relative to MRI. Image acquisition is extremely fast, making it well tolerated by patients, and nearly eliminating image distortion caused by patient motion. Very thin sections can be obtained that permit the reformation of data in multiple planes without compromising image quality. Software is available that allows data to be reformatted at the workstation by the radiologist in any plane. Three-dimensional reconstructions can be obtained, which may aid surgical planning, especially with respect to bony landmarks. Thin-section CT is superior to MRI for the evaluation of the cortical margins of bone. Axial images give good resolution of the lingual and buccal surfaces of the mandible and maxilla, whereas reformatted images, especially in the coronal plane, are best for assessing bony invasion of the alveolar ridges and the hard palate (**Fig. 6–4**). CT is slightly superior to MRI for the detection of metastatic deposits within lymph nodes.[2] CT-guided biopsy is also commonly performed to obtain a tissue diagnosis.

Disadvantages of CT include radiation exposure, poorer soft tissue contrast than MRI, and the need to administer iodinated intravenous contrast that carries the risks of contrast reactions and adverse effects on renal function. Dental amalgam and dental hardware also produce beam-hardening artifact, which can severely limit the evaluation of soft tissues within the oral cavity.

Magnetic Resonance Imaging

Compared with CT, MRI produces excellent soft tissue contrast. More specific tissue characterization can be made by comparing the signal intensity of a lesion on different imaging sequences. This is particularly useful when attempting to differentiate residual or recurrent tumor from posttreatment changes. MRI may provide a more accurate representation of the full extent and borders of the primary lesion.[3] Acquisitions can be obtained in any plane to aid in this analysis. The use of fat saturation, which causes fat to be low signal intensity, further increases contrast between tumor and normal tissue. Bone marrow infiltration is better visualized with MRI; on T1-weighted images, intermediate signal intensity tumor

A

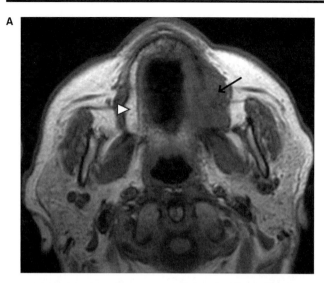

B

C

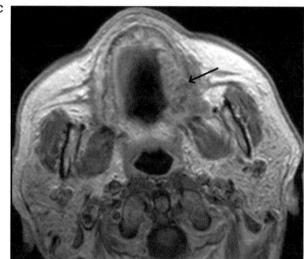

Figure 6–3 Axial T1-weighted **(A)**, axial T2-weighted **(B)**, and axial postgadolinium T1-weighted **(C)** images demonstrate a mass (*arrow*) involving the left maxillary alveolar ridge, confirmed to be squamous cell carcinoma. The mass is isointense to muscle on the T1-weighted image, hyperintense to muscle on the T2-weighted image, and enhances following intravenous gadolinium diethylenetriamine pentaacetic acid (Gd-DTPA). Note the normal high signal intensity of the bone marrow on the T1-weighted image (*arrowhead* in **A**) that is replaced by tumor on the involved side.

replaces the normally bright fatty marrow. MRI is superior to CT for evaluation of perineural tumor spread in the region of the skull base and cavernous sinus, as well as tumor spread to the cranial nerve root entry zones at the brainstem.

However, MRI also has a few important limitations. Some patients with pacemakers or other metal in their bodies are unable to undergo MRI. Because the study takes much longer than CT, the images are prone to motion artifact, such as those that occur with swallowing or tongue movement. Dental hardware, as with CT, can significantly degrade the images, and fat suppression techniques are particularly prone to artifacts. Intravenous gadolinium administration is necessary when evaluating oral cavity cancer, although this has significantly fewer risks than iodinated contrast material. Clinicians also tend to be less familiar with MR images and find the CT images easier to interpret.

At the University of Florida, CT is usually the preferred initial imaging modality for the assessment of oral cavity cancer. MRI is used as a complementary study when the primary lesion cannot be fully assessed with CT. For example, MRI provides additional information when there is excessive dental amalgam artifact, or when the presence of retrograde perineural spread toward the skull base must be evaluated.

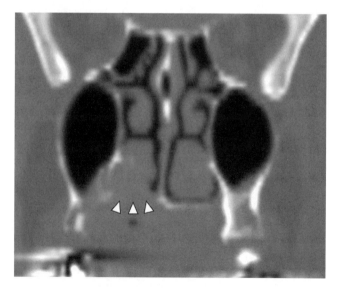

Figure 6–4 Coronal reformatted CT scan with bone algorithm demonstrates an aggressive pattern of bony destruction from adenocarcinoma involving the hard palate on the right (*arrowheads*), extending into the nasal cavity and maxillary tuberosity.

Plain Films and DentaScan

Plain films such as panoramic radiography or occlusal radiographs can be used to evaluate the alveolar ridge for the presence of bone invasion by malignant neoplasms. CT image reformatting software such as DentaScan, which was developed as an imaging tool for the precise placement of dental implants, has also been used to detect early cortical bone invasion (see Table 12–2 in Chapter 12; see also Chapter 23). Neurovascular foramina, nutrient foramina, and muscular insertions into bone are other sites of tumor invasion that can be evaluated with these techniques, although conventional CT usually provides comparable diagnostic information.

Ultrasound

Sonography is relatively inexpensive and is well tolerated by patients, but it provides a limited field of view and less anatomic detail than CT or MRI. A highly skilled operator is required to obtain diagnostic images, and artifact frequently limits the evaluation of pathology that abuts an air column or bone. Although the popularity of sonography as a diagnostic tool for the assessment of pathology in the head and neck region is dwindling, it remains extremely useful as a tool to guide fine-needle aspirations and core biopsies of soft tissue lesions and lymph nodes.

Positron Emission Tomography

At the present time, PET is primarily used to locate an unknown primary site of squamous cell carcinoma and in selective situations where tumor recurrence following treatment is a concern.[4] The co-registration of PET and CT data increases the accuracy of anatomic localization of the metabolic uptake of 2-[^{18}F]fluoro-2-deoxy-D-glucose (^{18}F-FDG).[5] Newer radiotracers continue to be developed that may have greater specificity for tumors, including tracers that image sites of cellular proliferation and tumor hypoxia.[6,7]

◆ Technique

Computed Tomography

Computed tomography data should be obtained following intravenous contrast with the gantry angled to avoid dental amalgam artifact, as well as with the gantry parallel to the body of the mandible. The collimator should be chosen to allow 1-mm-thick or thinner slices to optimally evaluate bone and to facilitate multiplanar reformations of diagnostic quality. The smallest possible field of view should be chosen to maximize resolution. Imaging should include the skull base and cavernous sinuses and the neck to the thoracic inlet. Three-millimeter-thick axial reconstructed slices with soft tissue algorithm are routinely used to evaluate the soft tissues.

Magnetic Resonance Imaging

Magnetic resonance imaging should also be performed to evaluate the skull base to the thoracic inlet. Axial, sagittal, and coronal images using a combination of T1-weighted, T2-weighted, and post–Gd-DTPA T1-weighted images should be obtained. Fat saturation can be applied to at least one of the postgadolinium T1-weighted images to enhance the delineation between tumor and normal tissue. The field of view, matrix size, slice thickness, and number of signal averages are chosen to maximize spatial resolution and signal-to-noise ratio, while maintaining a manageable imaging time.[8]

Positron Emission Tomography

Positron emission tomography is a functional study that relies on the use of radiotracers to measure metabolic activity in tissues. Because increased glycolysis is characteristic of tumors, the use of ^{18}F-FDG, which is incorporated into the cell by the glycolytic pathway, has become one of the most common tracers for head and neck cancer imaging.[9] However, ^{18}F-FDG is not a specific marker for cancer, and some tissues in the head and neck region normally demonstrate increased uptake, including salivary tissue, skeletal muscle, and macrophages.

Image quality in FDG-PET relies on proper patient preparation as well as proper technique of image acquisition.[10] Elevated circulating blood glucose levels reduce FDG tumor uptake because of potential competition at the tumor level, so FDG-PET may be less accurate if the blood glucose exceeds 200 mg/dL at the time of the scan. During the 1 hour uptake period after the initial ^{18}F-FDG injection, the patient should rest quietly with no talking and minimal movement to minimize extraneous muscular uptake.[9] Physiologic accumulation of FDG in the lymphatic tissue of Waldeyer's ring results in low-to-moderate uptake in the tonsils and base of tongue, and moderately increased uptake may be seen in the anterior floor of mouth from the genioglossus muscle, which prevents the tongue from relaxing posteriorly in the oropharynx when the patient is supine. Patients who speak or are anxious may have increased uptake in the masticatory musculature, tongue, face, neck, and larynx.[9]

A PET scan has two phases: emission and transmission. Emission scans are produced from the patient and must be adjusted for the attenuation that is caused by the varying thickness of patient tissues. The transmission phase results in attenuation-corrected images, which represent a quantitative distribution of the FDG. The resolution of current FDG-PET scans with attenuation correction is 3 to 4 mm.[9]

There are several ways in which FDG tracer uptake can be quantified, and the best method remains unproved. For attenuation-corrected PET images, the standardized uptake value (SUV) is a differential uptake ratio that describes tissue and tumor uptake. Several factors can affect the SUV level and complicate its interpretation, and no threshold level has been established that distinguishes benign from malignant processes.

◆ Radiographic Evaluation of Tumor Spread Patterns

Low-volume, superficial mucosal lesions are not well visualized on radiological studies, as they are difficult to distinguish from normal enhancing mucosa. Therefore, evaluation is made by clinical exam. Radiology becomes essential to evaluate the submucosal extent of disease and invasion into the deep spaces of the neck. This assessment is aided by an understanding of the characteristic patterns of invasion of malignant neoplasms that arise from specific locations within the oral cavity.

Cancer of the Lip

Lip cancers typically do not require imaging unless they are locally advanced or recurrent lesions, in which case imaging is performed primarily to look for bone invasion. Squamous cell carcinoma involves the lower lip much more frequently than the upper lip, and typically starts on the vermilion.[11] Invasion of the skin and the orbicularis muscle can occur. More advanced lesions can invade the adjacent buccal mucosa and bone of the mandible or maxilla. Perineural spread from lower lip cancer that involves the mental nerve can travel in a retrograde fashion along the inferior alveolar nerve in the absence of obvious mandibular marrow infiltration. Perineural spread from upper lip cancer usually involves the infraorbital branch of V2. Therefore, radiographic assessment should image the entire course of V2 and V3, including careful evaluation of the infraorbital, mandibular, mental foramina, pterygopalatine fossa, and cavernous sinuses (**Fig. 6–5**).

Cancer of the Floor of the Mouth

The majority of floor of mouth cancers arise within 2 cm of the midline anteriorly.[11] Early spread is to the sublingual gland, the genioglossus and geniohyoid muscles, and the periosteum of the lingual surface of the mandible. The periosteum acts as a barrier to tumor spread, with tumor preferentially extending along it, rather than through it. Bone invasion is a late finding, and tumor often extends along or over the alveolar ridge prior to bone invasion. Slow-growing lesions, which tend to remodel bone, causing a smooth

indentation on the cortex, invade the mandible in an *erosive* pattern (**Fig. 6–6**).[12] In contrast, aggressive lesions that demineralize and destroy bone cortex, typically with an ill-defined margin, invade the mandible in an *infiltrative* pattern (**Fig. 6–7**). Additional discussion of these patterns of mandibular invasion is provided in Chapter 12.

Posterior and inferior spread begins in the sublingual space, defined by the genioglossus and geniohyoid muscles medially, and the mylohyoid muscle laterally. The sublingual space contains fatty and glandular tissues, which provide good contrast to muscle on both CT and MRI. Replacement of sublingual space fat is one of the radiographic signs of tumor involvement. Tumor can spread along the mylohyoid muscle and hyoglossus muscle to the hyoid bone and suprahyoid neck. Spread can also occur through these muscles, although the mylohyoid muscle acts as a relatively effective barrier to lateral spread. Invasion posteriorly to the tongue base and superiorly to the oral tongue also occurs.

The submandibular duct and lingual nerve run in the sublingual space lateral to the hyoglossus muscle. Periductal spread may cause ductal obstruction, leading to enlargement and inflammation of the submandibular gland. Differentiation of tumor invasion of the submandibular gland from inflammatory change can be difficult radiographically, as both cause enlargement, increased density, and enhancement.

It is important to evaluate spread across the midline. The lingual septum mostly contains fat, which is not an effective barrier to tumor spread. Medial spread can also occur through the potential space between the genioglossus and geniohyoid muscle, or directly through the genioglossus muscle. The lingual artery and vein, as well as the hypoglossal nerve, lie medial to the hyoglossus muscle. Involvement of this neurovascular bundle must be assessed (**Fig. 6–8**). Tumor spread across the midline and involvement of the contralateral neurovascular bundle requires either total glossectomy or nonsurgical therapy.[13]

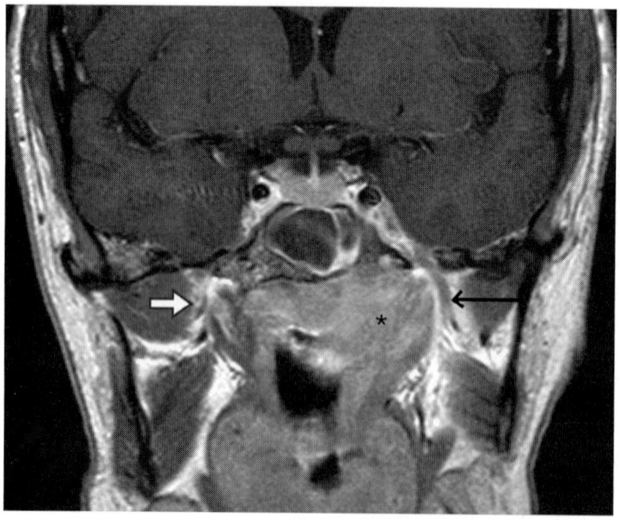

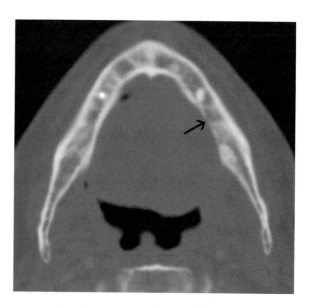

Figure 6–5 Coronal contrast enhanced T1-weighted image demonstrates perineural spread of a nasopharyngeal carcinoma (*asterisk*) along the mandibular division of the trigeminal nerve into the cavernous sinus. Notice the thickened V3 branch (*arrow*) medial to the lateral pterygoid muscle ascending to the foramen ovale. Compare the normal mandibular nerve on the right (*open arrow*).

Figure 6–6 Axial CT scan at bone window setting in a patient with squamous cell carcinoma of the left floor of the mouth demonstrates demineralization and thinning of the lingual cortex of the mandible (*arrow*), indicating bony invasion.

A

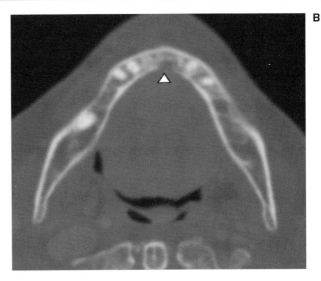

B

Figure 6–7 Axial contrast-enhanced CT scan at soft tissue window **(A)** and bone window **(B)** demonstrates a floor of mouth squamous cell carcinoma anteriorly (*arrow*), which has crossed the midline. Bony invasion through the lingual cortex of the mandible is also present (*arrowhead*).

Cancer of the Oral Tongue

Two thirds of oral tongue cancers arise from the lateral surface of the middle third of the tongue, and one third originate from the ventrolateral or anterior undersurface (**Fig. 6–2**).[11] On CT, normal tongue has a fairly homogeneous appearance, whereas carcinoma is seen as an enhancing mass. On MRI, the intrinsic muscle bundles of the tongue are usually visualized as intermediate T1-weighted signal intensity, separated by strands of high T1-weighted signal intensity fat. Carcinoma typically appears as an intermediate T1-weighted signal intensity and slightly high T2-weighted signal intensity mass, which disrupts the normal intrinsic muscle bundles. The tumor enhances following gadolinium administration. Although it may be difficult to determine the junction between the oral tongue and the floor of the mouth on axial images, this distinction can usually be made on coronal views that are either directly obtained or reformatted from axial data.

Carcinoma can invade the intrinsic muscles of the tongue and spread inferiorly along the hyoglossus muscle to the floor of the mouth, medially across the midline, or posteriorly to the anterior tonsillar pillar, glossotonsillar sulcus, and tongue base. Mandibular invasion is a late finding that usually occurs after the tumor has invaded the floor of the mouth adjacent to the bone.[11] Occasionally, tumors can spread along the styloglossus muscle to its attachment on the styloid process. Encasement of the lingual artery, as it courses medial to the hyoglossus muscle, can also be determined by imaging.

Cancer of the Buccal Mucosa

The buccal mucosa covers the inner lips and cheeks, which are composed primarily of the orbicularis oris muscle anteriorly and the buccinator muscles posterolaterally. It extends superoinferiorly to the gingivobuccal sulcus (the mucogingival junction) and posteriorly to the retromolar trigone. The buccal space is largely composed of the buccal fat pad, which is lateral to the buccinator muscle. The parotid duct courses through the buccal space to open into the buccal mucosa at the level of the second maxillary molar.

Early lesions of the buccal mucosa, which are not routinely imaged, can occasionally be seen on radiologic studies, particularly with a "puffed cheek" CT scan. Advanced lesions are imaged primarily to evaluate deep extension and bone invasion, which usually occurs at the maxillary or mandibular alveolar ridges. Lateral soft tissue invasion into the buccal fat pad can occur (**Fig. 6–9**). Because the buccal fat pad is contiguous with the retroantral fat of the masticator space,

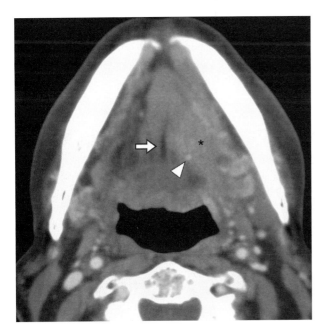

Figure 6–8 Axial contrast-enhanced CT scan demonstrates squamous cell carcinoma of the floor of the mouth (*asterisk*). The infiltrating mass extends to the fatty lingual septum (*open arrow*), but does not cross the midline. The contrast enhancing lingual artery is seen encased by tumor (*arrowhead*), indicating involvement of the neurovascular bundle.

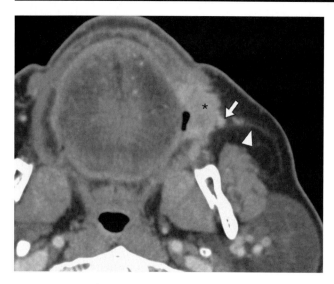

Figure 6-9 Axial contrast-enhanced CT scan demonstrates squamous cell carcinoma of the left buccal mucosa (*asterisk*). The parotid duct is seen entering into the mass (*arrowhead*). The facial vein (*open arrow*) is in close proximity to the tumor.

involvement of the bone of the maxillary antrum can occur. This is best imaged by coronal CT. Stensen's duct may become obstructed, leading to parotid gland enlargement. Periductal tumor spread as well as perineural spread along the facial nerve just deep to the superficial musculoaponeurotic system can also occur. Patients with trismus may have tumor spread along the masseter and pterygoid muscles to the coronoid process and ascending ramus of the mandible.[11] Tumor can involve the pterygomandibular raphe, from which spread can take place in the same manner as retromolar trigone tumors.

Cancer of the Upper and Lower Alveolar Ridge and Hard Palate

The upper alveolar ridge is covered by gingiva, or attached mucosa, that extends from the buccal mucogingival junction to the hard palate. The lower alveolar ridge is similarly covered by gingiva that extends from the buccal mucogingival junction to the lining mucosa of the floor of the mouth. Most gingival neoplasms are squamous cell carcinomas, whereas hard palate neoplasms are most frequently minor salivary gland tumors.

Carcinoma of the lower alveolar ridge spreads to the buccal mucosa and floor of the mouth, and can invade the periosteum of the mandible. Bone invasion occurs mainly at the occlusal surface, as the lingual and buccal plates have a thicker cortical margin, providing some resistance to tumor spread (Chapter 12). Spread within medullary bone is best seen on MRI, where intermediate signal intensity on T1-weighted images is seen replacing the normal high T1-weighted signal intensity fatty marrow. Perineural spread can also occur within the mandible along the inferior alveolar nerve. There is a small amount of fat at the mandibular foramen where the mandibular nerve enters the canal. This fat pad is normally seen on both CT and MRI, and its replacement by soft tissue is highly suggestive of perineural spread (**Fig. 6-10**). Involvement of tumor at the foramen ovale is evaluated in similar fashion.

Upper alveolar ridge cancer also tends to invade bone through the occlusal surface of the alveolar ridge (**Fig. 6-11**). Contiguous spread to the buccal mucosa, mucosa of the hard and soft palate, and underlying bone of the hard palate can occur. Invasion into the maxillary sinus or nose can also develop. Bony involvement of the hard palate is best evaluated with thin-section coronal CT. Perineural spread through the incisive canal and the greater and lesser palatine foramina to

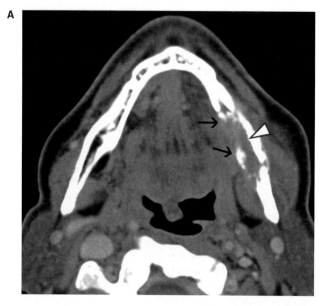

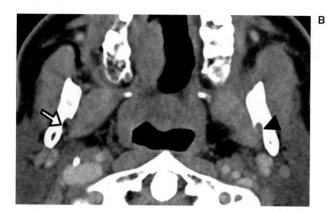

Figure 6-10 (**A**) Axial contrast-enhanced CT scan at the level of the body of the mandible demonstrates an enhancing squamous cell carcinoma of the mandibular alveolar ridge (*arrows*). There is destruction of both the lingual and buccal surfaces of the mandible, and tumor is seen replacing the bone marrow (*open arrowhead*). This finding is concerning for involvement of the inferior alveolar nerve. (**B**) Axial contrast-enhanced CT scan through the mandibular ramus demonstrates obliteration of the fat pad at the mandibular foramen by a soft tissue mass (*solid arrowhead*). Compare the normal fat density at the right mandibular foramen (*open arrow*). This finding is highly suggestive of perineural tumor spread.

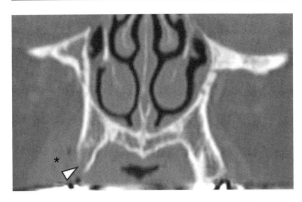

Figure 6–11 Coronal reformatted CT scan with bone algorithm demonstrating an infiltrating squamous cell carcinoma of the right maxillary alveolar ridge (*asterisk*). The tumor extends to both the lingual and buccal surfaces of the maxilla, and erosive changes extend from the occlusal surface (*arrowhead*).

the pterygopalatine fossa must also be excluded (**Fig. 6–12**). Both CT and MRI can be used to evaluate for obliteration of fat within the pterygopalatine fossa, indicating tumor involvement (**Fig. 6–13**). MRI, however, is the preferred imaging modality to evaluate for perineural spread into the cavernous sinus.

Cancer of the Retromolar Trigone

The retromolar trigone is a small triangular area posterior to the third mandibular molar extending along the anterior surface of the ascending ramus of the mandible to the maxillary tuberosity. Deep to the mucosa of the retromolar trigone is the pterygomandibular raphe. This is a band of connective tissue that serves as the insertion site for the buccinator, orbicularis oris, and superior constrictor muscles. It attaches inferiorly to the mylohyoid ridge of the mandible, and superiorly to the hamulus of the medial pterygoid plate. The pterygomandibular space, containing the lingual nerve, lies posterior to the raphe, between the ascending ramus of the mandible and the medial pterygoid muscle.

The spread of carcinoma from the retromolar trigone is to some extent guided by the pterygomandibular raphe. The adjacent buccal mucosa, lower gingiva, and anterior tonsillar pillar may become involved through contiguous spread (**Fig. 6–14**). Inferior spread to the floor of the mouth and lingual surface of the mandible may also occur. Tumor can extend posteriorly to invade the medial pterygoid muscle, or posterolaterally to invade the masseter muscle and ascending ramus of the mandible. Invasion through the buccinator muscle results in buccal space involvement. Superior spread to the maxillary tuberosity tends to continue along the posterior wall of the maxillary antrum, and irregularities within the bone of the posterior wall of the maxillary sinus or replacement of the retroantral fat pad may be seen on CT and MRI. The tumor can also course along the posteroinferior alveolar neurovascular bundle to the pterygopalatine fossa and cavernous sinus, to the root entry zone of the trigeminal nerve in the brainstem.

◆ Radiographic Evaluation of the Cervical Lymph Nodes

Computed tomography and MRI provide valuable information regarding the presence of metastatic tumor deposits within cervical lymph nodes that cannot be obtained via clinical examination, which has a relatively high false-negative rate. Characteristics used to determine metastatic lymph node involvement include size, shape, rim enhancement, foci of parenchymal necrosis, and extranodal spread.

When determining the size of a lymph node, the diameter is measured in the axial plane. The axial diameter that is most suggestive of metastatic involvement, however, has not been established. The specificity increases as a larger diameter is chosen, but the sensitivity is diminished.[2] Many clinicians use a cutoff of 15 mm in levels I and II, and 10 mm elsewhere, except for the retropharyngeal nodes, where 8 mm is suspicious. However, many radiologists

A

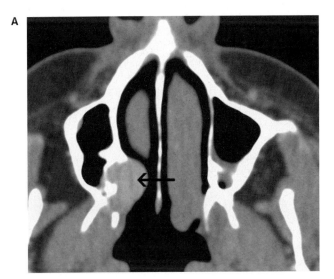

B

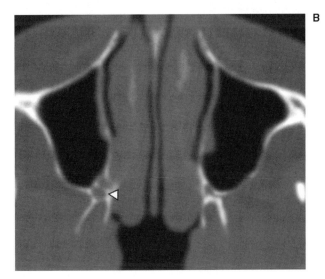

Figure 6–12 **(A)** Axial contrast-enhanced CT scan demonstrates squamous cell carcinoma of the right maxillary alveolar ridge (*arrow*) with bony invasion into the base of the pterygoid plates.

(B) Axial CT image at bone window slightly superior to **A** demonstrates enlargement of the greater and lesser palatine foramina (*arrowhead*) secondary to perineural spread.

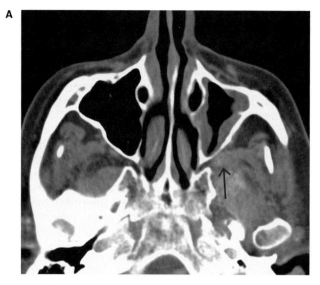

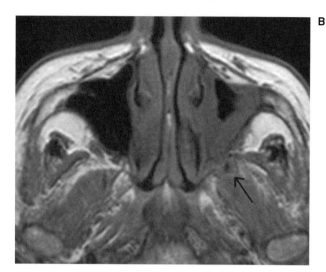

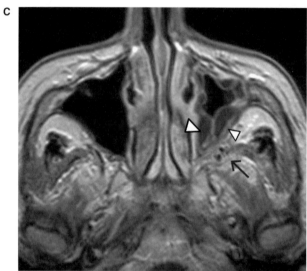

Figure 6–13 **(A)** Axial contrast-enhanced CT scan in a patient with maxillary alveolar ridge squamous cell carcinoma demonstrates replacement of retroantral fat with an enhancing soft tissue mass (*arrow*). Axial T1-weighted image **(B)** and axial T1-weighted post gadolinium image **(C)** in the same patient also show replacement of retroantral fat by enhancing soft tissue (*arrow*), secondary to perineurovascular spread of carcinoma to the pterygopalatine fossa. Note enhancing mucosal disease in the maxillary sinus (*arrowheads*).

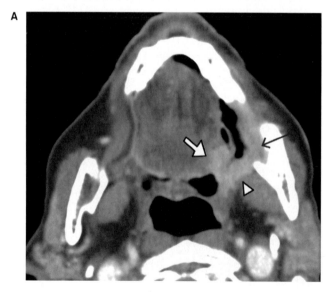

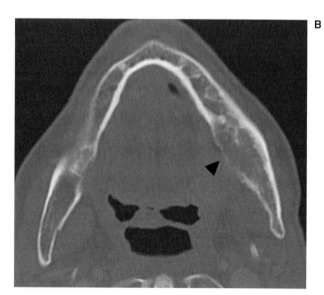

Figure 6–14 **(A)** Axial contrast-enhanced CT scan demonstrates a retromolar trigone squamous cell carcinoma (*arrow*) extending posteromedially along the anterior tonsillar pillar (*arrowhead*) to the tongue base (*open arrow*). **(B)** Axial CT scan at bone window demonstrates aggressive invasion of the lingual cortex of the mandible (*solid arrowhead*).

would minimize the importance of a 15-mm level II lymph node that has no other features of metastatic disease. Clustering and conglomeration of lymph nodes is a suspicious feature. Calcification within a node also increases the likelihood of malignancy. Rim enhancement is a suspicious but nonspecific finding seen on CT and MRI, especially with fat suppression. Reactive or infected nodes as well as malignant lymph nodes may demonstrate this feature.

Squamous cell carcinoma within lymph nodes tends to undergo necrosis, leading to filling defects within an otherwise enhancing lymph node. Necrosis is more optimally evaluated with CT than MRI and should be considered a suspicious finding, even when the node is smaller than 10 mm (**Fig. 6–15**). The presence of necrosis is often referred to as *central necrosis*, but this term is somewhat misleading because early necrosis typically occurs in the periphery of the node. This is logical given the anatomy of afferent lymphatics entering the node at multiple sites in the periphery, and efferent lymphatics exiting the node at the hilum. A focal filling defect is not a specific finding for carcinoma because it is also seen in suppurative nodes, granulomatous disease, and other neoplasms.

Curtin et al[2] studied CT and MRI for detection of lymph node metastases, using a size of greater than 10 mm or an internal abnormality to define a metastatic node. CT performed slightly better, with a negative predictive value of 84% for CT and 79% for MRI, and a positive predictive value of 50% for CT and 52% for MRI.

Extracapsular spread is best seen on CT as an indistinct margin of the lymph node. Infiltration of the surrounding fat may also be seen. This may have implications for treatment if the extranodal spread extends to encase the carotid artery (**Fig. 6–16**).

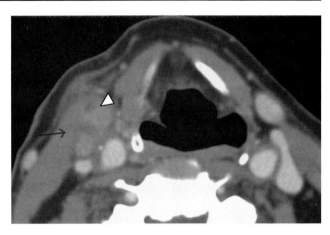

Figure 6–16 Axial contrast-enhanced CT scan demonstrates a conglomerate of sublevel IIA lymph nodes harboring metastatic squamous cell carcinoma. Note the presence of internal filling defects (*arrowhead*). The indistinct margin of the lymph nodes (*arrow*) is indicative of extracapsular spread.

These imaging features have also been used to evaluate cervical metastases following radiation therapy, in an attempt to minimize the performance of unnecessary neck dissections.[14] In a recent study, a contrast-enhanced CT scan was obtained about 4 weeks following the completion of radiation therapy for head and neck cancer with positive lymph nodes. When all of the lymph nodes in the irradiated neck measured less than 15 mm and did not contain a focal abnormality, the negative predictive value for the absence of disease in the neck specimen was 94%. The authors concluded that a neck dissection is indicated if a lymph node measures greater than 15 mm in axial diameter, or if a node contains a focal lucency, enhancement, or calcification.[15]

FDG-PET has been evaluated for the pretreatment evaluation of cervical lymphadenopathy in patients with head and neck cancer, but the criteria for the detection of metastatic nodes have not been established. In one investigation where clinically negative necks were evaluated with PET and correlated with pathologic findings of lymph nodes that were evaluated with 2-mm sections, sensitivity and specificity was 25% and 88%, respectively. Although micrometastases ranging from 1.2 mm to 3.4 mm were present in the specimens, FDG-PET was able to detect only a 3.4-mm metastasis, which correlates with the 3- to 4-mm limit of resolution of these scanners.[9] FDG-PET also has been utilized to evaluate active disease in residual neck nodes following therapy. One study found a negative predictive value of 97% for detecting viable tumor in a residual neck abnormality 12 weeks following treatment.[16]

◆ Radiological Criteria for the Classification of Cervical Lymph Node Disease

The American Head and Neck Society and the American Academy of Otolaryngology–Head and Neck Surgery have developed a classification scheme that divides each side of the neck into several anatomically defined levels and sublevels (see Table 14–2 in Chapter 14).[17] This classification

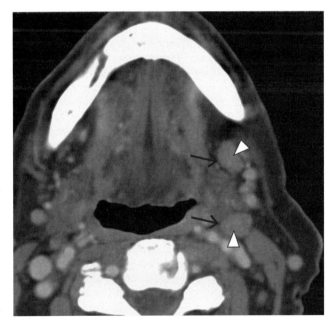

Figure 6–15 Axial contrast-enhanced CT scan of a patient with maxillary alveolar ridge squamous cell carcinoma demonstrates positive lymph nodes in sublevels IB and IIA (*arrows*). Despite measuring less than 1 cm in diameter, the internal filling defects are highly suspicious for tumor involvement (*arrowheads*).

Table 6–1   Summary of the Imaging-Based Nodal Classification*

Level	Definition
Level I	The submental and submandibular nodes. They lie above the hyoid bone, below the mylohyoid muscle, and anterior to the back of the submandibular gland.
Sublevel IA	The submental nodes. They lie between the medial margins of the anterior bellies of the digastric muscles.
Sublevel IB	The submandibular nodes. On each side, they lie lateral to the level IA nodes and anterior to the back of each submandibular gland.
Level II	The upper internal jugular nodes. They extend from the skull base to the level of the bottom of the body of the hyoid bone.
Sublevel IIA	A level II node that lies anterior, medial, lateral, or posterior to the internal jugular vein. If posterior to the vein, the node is inseparable from the vein.
Sublevel IIB	A level II node that lies posterior to the internal jugular vein and has a fat plane separating it and the vein.
Level III	The middle jugular nodes. They extend from the level of the bottom of the body of the hyoid bone to the level of the bottom of the cricoid arch. They lie anterior to the back of the sternocleidomastoid muscle.
Level IV	The low jugular nodes. They extend from the level of the bottom of the cricoid arch to the level of the clavicle. They lie anterior to a line connecting the back of the sternocleidomastoid muscle and the posterolateral margin of the anterior scalene muscle. They are also lateral to the carotid arteries.
Level V	The nodes in the posterior triangle. They lie posterior to the back of the sternocleidomastoid muscle from the skull base to the level of the bottom of the cricoid arch posterior to a line connecting the back of the sternocleidomastoid muscle and the posterolateral margin of the anterior scalene muscle from the level of the bottom of the cricoid arch to the level of the clavicle. They also lie anterior to the anterior edge of the trapezius muscle.
Sublevel VA	Upper level V nodes extend from the skull base to the level of the bottom of the cricoid arch.
Sublevel VB	Lower level V nodes extend from the level of the bottom of the cricoid arch to the level of the clavicle, as seen on each axial scan.
Level VI	The upper visceral nodes. They lie between the carotid arteries from the level of the bottom of the body of the hyoid bone to the level of the top of the manubrium.
Level VII	The superior mediastinal nodes. They lie between the carotid arteries below the level of the top of the manubrium and above the level of the innominate vein.
Supraclavicular nodes	They lie at or caudal to the level of the clavicle and lateral to the carotid artery on each side of the neck, as seen on each axial scan.
Retropharyngeal nodes	Within 2 cm of the skull base, they lie medial to the internal carotid arteries.

*The parotid nodes and other superficial nodes are referred to by their anatomical names.
From Som PM, Curtin HD, Mancuso AA. An imaging-based classification for the cervical nodes designed as an adjunct to recent clinically based nodal classifications. Arch Otolaryngol Head Neck Surg 1999;125:388–396, with permission. Copyright © 1999, American Medical Association. All rights reserved.

scheme has also been used to divide the cervical lymph nodes into several groups (see Table 14–1 in Chapter 14). Division of the neck into levels and sublevels allows clinicians to describe the location of lymph node metastases, and facilitates surgical or radiotherapeutic treatment to selected regions of the neck. Radiologic criteria have also been integrated into the classification of cervical lymph node disease, which correlate with the anatomic boundaries that have been established for each level and sublevel (**Table 6–1**).[18] Because radiographic assessment is routinely performed as a component of the pretreatment evaluation for most patients who are diagnosed with head and neck cancer, the imaging-based classification is used to evaluate and manage patients who have cervical metastases. Furthermore, the precise pretreatment localization of lymph node metastasis facilitates the evaluation of response to treatment and posttreatment surveillance. The patterns of lymph node metastasis associated with cancer arising from different sites within the oral cavity is discussed in Chapter 14.

◆ Radiographic Evaluation of Persistent or Recurrent Cancer

Widely accepted guidelines for cancer surveillance imaging after the completion of treatment have not been established. Although the use of CT has been advocated by some investigators, others continue to rely on clinical assessment to guide decision making. This controversy has been heightened by the introduction of functional imaging modalities such as PET/CT, which are now the subject of extensive investigative effort.

Posttreatment changes at the primary site and in the neck differ according to the treatment modality. Following surgical therapy, the initial tissue inflammatory response appears similar to tumor on imaging. This granulation tissue is isointense to slightly hypointense to muscle on T1-weighted images and hyperintense to muscle on T2-weighted images, and it enhances. Over a 3- to 4-month period, this usually resolves, leaving residual fibrosis that appears hypointense to muscle on both T1-weighted and T2-weighted images, and that does not enhance.[11]

Imaging during radiation therapy is not typically performed, but usually demonstrates necrosis and edema within the primary site, and surrounding edema. Following radiation therapy, the primary lesion usually decreases in size, leaving some residual fibrosis or no mass after 3 to 4 months. Postradiation mucosal and salivary gland enhancement and edema within the radiation portal usually persist longer. Given the above changes, some investigators have proposed performing a pretreatment PET scan followed by a posttreatment scan 2 to 4 months following treatment to evaluate for persistent or recurrent tumor.[19]

The approach to interpretation of posttreatment imaging is slightly different from pretreatment radiographic assessment because evaluation must include an analysis of the primary site for evidence of posttreatment complications such as osteoradionecrosis, a search for perineural tumor spread and second primary tumors, as well as an assessment for residual lymphadenopathy. An enlarging mass on follow-up scans should raise suspicion for residual tumor. The appearance of the primary site may be complicated by posttreatment hemorrhage or seroma. If a residual or recurrent mass is suspected, its local extent and any bony invasion should be assessed. In addition, perineural spread is a more frequent finding in the setting of recurrent squamous cell carcinoma. Osteoradionecrosis typically has the appearance of bone demineralization and fragmentation on CT that may or may not be associated with an inflammatory mass.

◆ Conclusion

The role of diagnostic imaging in the evaluation and management of oral cancer continues to rapidly evolve. As the role for CT and MRI in the pretreatment assessment and post-treatment surveillance has become better defined, the desire for new technology has led to applications for FDG-PET and PET/CT to fill the voids that have not been addressed by more conventional imaging modalities. Despite refinements in imaging protocols and techniques, controversy about several treatment-related issues in head and neck cancer persist, including the best modality for the detection of early bone invasion or lymph node metastases, and the best modality for early detection of persistent nodal disease following radiation therapy. The role of emerging diagnostic technology such as FDG-PET and PET/CT in a variety of clinical situations requires clarification. For example, several potential aspects of PET technology must be investigated, including the establishment of criteria for detecting metastatic lymphadenopathy, the evaluation of new tracers that may provide more information regarding tumor proliferation than FDG, and the development of radiopharmaceuticals with labeled antibodies that can image growth factor receptors such as the epidermal growth factor receptor, which could allow for targeted molecular therapy for the treatment of squamous cell carcinoma.

References

1. Som PM. The present controversy over the imaging method of choice for evaluating the soft tissues of the neck. AJNR Am J Neuroradiol 1997;18:1869–1872

2. Curtin HD, Ishwaran H, Dalley RW, Caudry DJ, McNeil BJ. Comparison of CT and MR imaging in staging of neck metastases. Radiology 1998;207:123–130

3. Crecco M, Vidiri A, Palma O, et al. T stages of tumors of the tongue and floor of the mouth: correlation between MR with gadopentetate dimeglumine and pathologic data. AJNR Am J Neuroradiol 1994;15:1695–1702

4. Goerres GW, Schmid DT, Bandhauer F, et al. Positron emission tomography in the early follow-up of advanced head and neck cancer. Arch Otolaryngol Head Neck Surg 2004;130:105–109

5. Kapoor V, Fukui MB, McCook BM. Role of ^{18}FDG PET/CT in the treatment of head and neck cancers: principles, technique, normal distribution, and initial staging. AJR Am J Roentgenol 2005;184:579–587

6. Mankoff DA, Shields AF, Krohn KA. PET imaging of cellular proliferation. Radiol Clin North Am 2005;43:153–167

7. Rajendran JG, Krohn KA. Imaging hypoxia and angiogenesis in tumors. Radiol Clin North Am 2005;43:169–187

8. Sigal R, Zagdanski AM, Schwaab G, et al. CT and MR imaging of squamous cell carcinoma of the tongue and floor of the mouth. Radiographics 1996;16:787–810

9. Greven KM. Positron-emission tomography for head and neck cancer. Semin Radiat Oncol 2004;14:121–129

10. Goerres GW, Von Schulthess GK, Hany TF. Positron emission tomography and PET CT of the head and neck: FDG uptake in normal anatomy, in benign lesions, and in changes resulting from treatment. AJR Am J Roentgenol 2002;179:1337–1343

11. Million RR, Cassisi NJ, Mancuso AA. Oral cavity. In: Million RR, Cassisi NJ, eds. Management of Head and Neck Cancer: A Multidisciplinary Approach, 2nd ed. Philadelphia: JB Lippincott, 1994:321–400

12. Mukherji SK, Isaacs DL, Creager A, Shockley W, Weissler M, Armao D. CT detection of mandibular invasion by squamous cell carcinoma of the oral cavity. AJR Am J Roentgenol 2001;177:237–243

13. Mukherji SK, Pillsbury HR, Castillo M. Imaging squamous cell carcinomas of the upper aerodigestive tract: what clinicians need to know. Radiology 1997;205:629–646

14. Ojiri H, Mendenhall WM, Stringer SP, Johnson PL, Mancuso AA. Post-RT CT results as a predictive model for the necessity of planned post-RT neck dissection in patients with cervical metastatic disease from squamous cell carcinoma. Int J Radiat Oncol Biol Phys 2002;52:420–428

15. Liauw SL, Mancuso AA, Amdur RJ, et al. Post-radiotherapy neck dissection for lymph node positive head and neck cancer: the use of computed tomography to manage the neck. J Clin Oncol 2006;24:1421–1427

16. Porceddu SV, Jarmolowski E, Hicks RJ, et al. Utility of positron emission tomography for the detection of disease in residual neck nodes after (chemo)radiotherapy in head and neck cancer. Head Neck 2005;27:175–181

17. Robbins KT, Clayman G, Levine PA, et al. Neck dissection classification update: revisions proposed by the American Head and Neck Society and the American Academy of Otolaryngology–Head and Neck Surgery. Arch Otolaryngol Head Neck Surg 2002;128:751–758

18. Som PM, Curtin HD, Mancuso AA. An imaging-based classification for the cervical nodes designed as an adjunct to recent clinically based nodal classifications. Arch Otolaryngol Head Neck Surg 1999;125:388–396

19. Kubota K, Yokoyama J, Yamaguchi K, et al. FDG-PET delayed imaging for the detection of head and neck cancer recureence after radiochemotherapy: comparison with MRI/CT. Eur J Nucl Med Mol Imaging 2004;31:590–595

7

Staging of Oral Cancer

William M. Lydiatt

A clinically useful classification scheme for cancer should embody the features of a malignant neoplasm that describe its behavior.[1] The staging of cancer defines the extent of disease in terms of anatomic spread and is vital to the development of evidence-based approaches to therapy. Staging also provides a framework that enables the scientific community to characterize and study factors that impact prognosis, facilitates the comparison of treatment strategies, and allows different investigators to compare the outcomes of treatment.[2] Defining prognosis and comparing different treatment strategies are essential aspects of the current staging system advocated by the American Joint Committee on Cancer (AJCC) and the International Union Against Cancer (*Union Internationale Contre le Cancer*, UICC). This chapter details the staging of oral cancer and the inherent strengths and weaknesses of the present classification scheme.

The staging system proposed by the AJCC and the UICC is the product of an evolutionary process that has spanned more than 45 years.[3] This process began in 1959 with the efforts of the American Joint Committee for Cancer Staging and End-Results Reporting and culminated in 1977 with publication of the *Manual for Staging of Cancer*.[4] Using the principle that anatomic extension (T) and spread to lymph nodes (N) and elsewhere (M) best defined the life history of cancer, the tumor, node, and metastasis (TNM) classification system was developed, and a single TNM classification has been used worldwide since 1987. This shorthand method of indicating disease extent was also used to form stage groupings, with the assumption that more advanced stages would manifest progressively worse behavior.[4] Since its initial inception, the TNM system has undergone several revisions to account for new developments in diagnostic assessment and recently published therapeutic outcomes. The most recent update, the *AJCC Cancer Staging Manual*, 6th edition, was published in 2002.[1]

The principal advantages of this internationally accepted staging system are its longevity and ease of use. Clinicians throughout the world are familiar with the AJCC staging system, and historical comparisons are possible because the classification scheme has remained relatively uniform over time. The methods of clinical and pathologic staging are standardized and are accessible to most clinicians who treat patients with cancer, and the staging system can be used to estimate prognosis.

◆ Staging of Oral Cancer

Clinical stage is determined by physical examination supplemented by computed tomography (CT), magnetic resonance imaging (MRI), ultrasound (US), or plain radiographs (panoramic radiographs, occlusal films, etc.). Size can often be determined by inspection, although deep extension is usually more completely characterized with radiographic imaging. The role of positron emission tomography (PET) to determine nodal and distant metastasis is currently evolving. The ability to detect lymph node metastasis utilizing PET has been found to range from 70 to 100%.[5,6] This modality may be used in certain situations as an adjunct to standard imaging but is not routinely employed or recommended. PET may improve the detection of distant metastasis in advanced disease.[7,8]

Table 7–1   Definition of TNM: Oral Cavity

Stage	Definition
Primary tumor (T)	
TX	Primary tumor cannot be assessed
T0	No evidence of primary tumor
Tis	Carcinoma in situ
T1	Tumor 2 cm or less in greatest dimension
T2	Tumor more than 2 cm but not more than 4 cm in greatest dimension
T3	Tumor more than 4 cm in greatest dimension
T4 (lip)	Tumor invades through cortical bone,* inferior alveolar nerve, floor of mouth, or skin of face, i.e., chin or nose
T4a	Oral cavity: Tumor invades adjacent structures (e.g., through cortical bone,* into deep [extrinsic] muscle of tongue [genioglossus, hyoglossus, palatoglossus, and styloglossus], maxillary sinus, skin of face)
T4b	Tumor invades masticator space, pterygoid plates, or skull base and/or encases internal carotid artery
Regional lymph nodes (N)	
NX	Regional lymph nodes cannot be assessed
N0	No regional lymph node metastasis
N1	Metastasis in a single ipsilateral lymph node, 3 cm or less in greatest dimension
N2	Metastasis in a single ipsilateral lymph node, more than 3 cm but not more than 6 cm in greatest dimension; or in multiple ipsilateral lymph nodes, none more than 6 cm in greatest dimension; or in bilateral or contralateral lymph nodes, none more than 6 cm in greatest dimension
N2a	Metastasis in a single ipsilateral lymph node, more than 3 cm but not more than 6 cm in greatest dimension
N2b	Metastasis in multiple ipsilateral lymph nodes, none more than 6 cm in greatest dimension
N2c	Metastasis in bilateral or contralateral lymph nodes, none more than 6 cm in greatest dimension
N3	Metastasis in a lymph node more than 6 cm in greatest dimension
Distant metastasis (M)	
MX	Distant metastasis cannot be assessed
M0	No distant metastasis
M1	Distant metastasis

*Superficial erosion alone of bone/tooth socket by gingival primary is not sufficient to classify a tumor as T4.
Adapted from Greene FL, Page DL, Fleming ID, et al, eds. AJCC Cancer Staging Manual, 6th ed. New York: Springer-Verlag, 2002, with permission.

Two-centimeter increments in size of the primary tumor are used to differentiate between T1, T2, or T3 lesions of the oral cavity (**Table 7–1**).[1] Patterns of tumor invasion, on the other hand, are used to designate an oral cavity tumor as a T4a lesion. Tumors that invade through cortical bone into the deep (extrinsic) musculature of the tongue, the maxillary sinus, or the skin of the face are T4a lesions. Superficial cortical bone erosion is not sufficient to classify a tumor as T4. The criteria that result in a T4a designation for lip cancer differ somewhat from the criteria used to assign T4a tumors arising from other sites within the oral cavity. The sixth edition of the *AJCC Cancer Staging Manual* has modified the staging of oral cavity cancer by the addition of T4b, which denotes the presence of unresectable disease.[1] Tumor invasion of the masticator space, the pterygoid plates, or skull base and tumor encasement of the internal carotid artery are considered unresectable.

The criteria used to assign a value to N for the extent of regional lymph node metastasis from oral cancer is identical to the criteria used for the larynx and the pharynx, with the exception of the nasopharynx (**Table 7–1**).[1] A single ipsilateral lymph node 3 cm or less in greatest dimension is classified as N1, whereas a single ipsilateral lymph node greater than 3 cm in size or the presence of multiple lymph node metastases results in an N2 designation. A lymph node greater than 6 cm in size is assigned N3 status.

The absence of metastatic disease is classified as M0, whereas the presence of distant metastasis is assigned M1 status.[1] The resultant values for T, N, and M are combined to classify the tumor. The notation for clinical staging is cTNM, or simply TNM.

The AJCC classification scheme assigns each possible combination of the values for T, N, and M into one of several TNM stage groupings (**Table 7–2**).[1] The stage groupings are intended to make each stage group "relatively homogeneous with respect to survival" so "that the survival rates of these stage groupings for each cancer site are distinct," and are ultimately intended to provide a mechanism for comparing similar groups of patients who may be candidates for

Table 7–2   Stage Grouping: Oral Cavity

Stage	Grouping
0	Tis*N0M0
I	T1N0M0
II	T2N0M0
III	T3N0M0
	T1N1M0
	T2N1M0
	T3N1M0
IVA	T4aN0M0
	T4aN1M0
	T1N2M0
	T2N2M0
	T3N2M0
	T4aN2M0
IVB	Any T N3M0
	T4b Any N M0
IVC	Any T Any N M1

*In situ.
Adapted from Greene FL, Page DL, Fleming ID, et al, eds. AJCC Cancer Staging Manual, 6th ed. New York: Springer-Verlag, 2002, with permission.

particular therapeutic options.[1] Early primary tumors that have a single lymph node metastasis (N1) and cT3N0M0 tumors are assigned to the stage III group. The division of T4 lesions into T4a (resectable) and T4b (unresectable) has led to the division of stage IV into stages IVA, IVB, and IVC. The stage IVA group includes patients with T4a primary tumors or N2 regional nodal disease, whereas stage IVB includes patients who have been assigned either T4b or N3 status. The stage IVC grouping denotes the presence of distant metastasis (M1).[1]

Prefixes or suffixes are added to TNM to provide additional descriptive information so that these cases are analyzed separately. Pathologic staging, which should be performed whenever possible, is denoted by a lower case p that precedes the TNM classification (pTNM). The pathologic classification provides additional data that can be used to estimate prognosis and calculate end results.[1] It is important to appreciate that because mucosal margins can shrink by as much as 30% following resection, pathologic T categorization may be an underestimation of actual tumor size.[9] Retreatment classification (rTNM) is assigned when further treatment is planned for recurrent cancer following a disease-free interval. If stage is determined at autopsy for cancer that was not evident prior to death, the prefix "a" is used (aTNM). The m suffix denotes multiple primary tumors in a single site and is recorded parenthetically following the T characterization [pT(m)NM]. The y prefix denotes staging during or following multimodality therapy and should precede either the c or p (ycTNM or ypTNM). This prefix should only be used in the period *following* completion of multimodality therapy when a decision regarding further surgical therapy is being contemplated. Typically this decision is made within 2 months following completion of multimodality therapy.

These staging guidelines apply to all forms of carcinoma. Sarcomas, lymphomas, and melanomas should be staged via their respective guidelines. Histologic grade, which is a qualitative assessment that is not used to stage oral cancer, is included on the tumor staging form in the sixth edition of the *AJCC Cancer Staging Manual*.[1] For squamous cell carcinoma, histologic grade is subjectively categorized as either well, moderately, or poorly differentiated carcinoma in relation to its similarity to normal mucosa. Histologic grading is also performed for most minor salivary gland cancers. Mucoepidermoid carcinoma is classified as low, intermediate, or high grade, whereas adenocarcinoma is classified as low or high grade.

Following resection, the presence of residual tumor should be noted by using the following designations: presence of residual tumor cannot be assessed (RX), no residual tumor (R0), microscopic residual tumor (R1), and macroscopic residual tumor (R2). The staging form also allows for the addition of descriptors that denote the presence of lymphatic and venous invasion. The presence of perineural invasion should also be recorded. These have prognostic import even though they are not used to determine actual stage, and should be noted in the box for prognostic indicators provided on the second page of the staging form.[10] Similarly, characteristics of the tumor can be noted as exophytic, ulcerated, or endophytic. Tumor thickness or depth of invasion should be determined and included as an important

adjunct to the stage.[1] Two additional important descriptors that pertain to nodal disease are extranodal extension and nodal metastasis to the upper or lower neck, and should also be noted in the box labeled "Prognostic Indicators."

◆ Prognostic Indicators

Tumor Stage

Numerous investigations have shown that stage is an important predictor of prognosis. In a recent multivariate analysis of numerous biomarkers in squamous cell carcinoma of the tongue, for example, stage emerged as the most significant prognostic indicator.[11] Lo et al[12] documented 5-year survival of 75%, 65.5%, 49%, and 30% for stage I, II, III, and IV cancers of the oral cavity, respectively. According to the AJCC, the 5-year relative survival for squamous cell carcinoma of the oral cavity by stage is as follows: stage I, 65 to 70%; stage II, 50 to 55%; stage III, 38 to 44%; and stage IV, 25 to 29%.[1] Sessions et al[13] reported the 5-year disease-specific survival (DSS) for 227 patients with floor of mouth cancer by stage: stage I, 72.4%; stage II, 62.8%; stage III, 44.4%; and stage IV, 46.9%. The same investigators also reported the 5-year DSS in a retrospective case series of 279 patients with oral tongue cancer by stage: stage I, 75.8%; stage II, 63.5%; stage III, 38.5%; and stage IV, 26.5%.[14] These findings validate the utility of the AJCC staging system as a predictor of prognosis and survival.

Bone Invasion

Bone invasion has remained as one of the criteria for assigning the T4 designation since the first edition of the *Manual for Staging of Cancer* was published in 1977. This designation was based on the consensus opinion of the committee members that bone invasion portended a worse clinical course.[4] The sixth edition of the *AJCC Cancer Staging Manual* has clarified the relationship between bone invasion and regional metastasis.[1] Minimal cortical invasion is insufficient to classify a tumor as a T4 lesion.

Some authors report that frank bone invasion is prognostically important, and univariate analysis has demonstrated an adverse impact on survival.[15,16] However, bone invasion has not been a consistent independent predictor of survival on multivariate analysis.[15,17,18] Although bone invasion may have prognostic import, this association remains ill-defined.

Depth of Invasion

Tumor thickness and depth of invasion are important prognostic factors in oral cancer that are not utilized for T staging in the present AJCC classification scheme.[1] Tumor thickness and depth of invasion are predictive of occult nodal metastasis in the clinically negative neck of patients with oral cavity cancer.[19–23] The critical thickness that is associated with an increased risk of metastasis, however, remains ill-defined, and may not be uniform throughout the oral cavity (see Table 14–5 in Chapter 14). Future

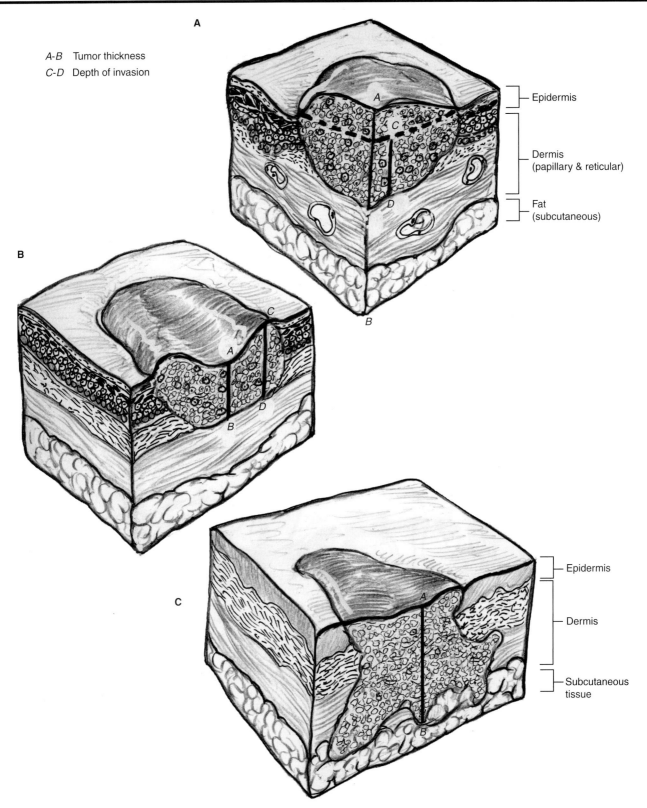

A-B Tumor thickness
C-D Depth of invasion

Figure 7–1 Characteristics of lip and oral cavity tumors. Measurements are performed with an ocular micrometer and recorded in millimeters. **(A)** Exophytic: The *tumor thickness* is measured perpendicular from *A*, the surface of the tumor, to *B*, the deepest area of involvement. The *depth of invasion* is measured perpendicular from *C*, the surface of the adjacent normal mucosa to *D*, the deepest portion of the tumor. **(B)** Ulcerated: The *tumor thickness* is measured perpendicular from *A*, the surface of the tumor, to *B*, the deepest area of involvement. The *depth of invasion* is measured perpendicular from *C*, the surface of the adjacent normal mucosa, to *D*, the deepest portion of the tumor. **(C)** Endophytic: The *tumor thickness* is measured perpendicular from *A*, the surface of the tumor, to *B*, the deepest area of involvement. In this situation, *tumor thickness* and *depth of invasion* are the same. (Adapted from Lip and oral cavity. In: Greene FL, Page DL, Fleming ID, et al, eds. AJCC Cancer Staging Manual, 6th ed. New York: Springer-Verlag, 2002:25–26, with permission.)

investigative efforts to characterize the relationship between depth of invasion and occult metastatic disease could be facilitated by routinely measuring depth of invasion in a prospective manner and recording these findings on the tumor staging form (**Fig. 7–1**).[1] This topic is reviewed in greater detail in Chapter 14.

◆ Limitations of TNM Staging in Predicting Prognosis

A staging system must establish a delicate balance between competing needs. Groome et al[24] defined four attributes of an effective staging system:

1. Hazard consistency: There should be homogeneity within each stage grouping so that survival rates are similar between members of the stage group. For example, T3N0M0 and T1N1M0, members of TNM stage group III, should exhibit similar survival rates.
2. Hazard discrimination: There should be heterogeneity between each stage grouping so that survival rates differ. In other words, the survival rate of patients in TNM stage group III should be worse than that for those in stage group II.
3. Predictive power: The prediction of cure for a particular stage grouping should be high. For instance, a group of stage I patients should manifest similar prognoses over time.
4. Balance: A balanced distribution of patients into each stage grouping permits meaningful statistical comparisons between groups.

One shortcoming of the present AJCC/UICC scheme is the relatively poor hazard consistency between different TNM members in stage IV, particularly if distant metastatic disease is present.[3] This lack of homogeneity has been partially addressed by subdividing the various TNM classifications into subgroups IVA, IVB, and IVC. Although hazard discrimination in the current AJCC/UICC system is relatively good, different groupings can be made that result in a wider distribution of prognosis between stages. For example, statistical analysis can be used to create a different breakdown of the TNM components that should be used to determine each stage.[25–27] These TNM components may differ for each subsite of the head and neck and may increase the complexity of the system, which could result in loss of the uniformity and ease of use that now exists in the present TNM classification system. Alternatively, a less complex system such as the integer system proposed by Jones et al[28] could be employed to determine stage. In this system, the values for T and N are added together to arrive at a score between 1 and 7. The score is known as TANIS (tumor and nodal integer score). For example, a T1N0 would be a TANIS 1, a T2N0 a TANIS 2, up to a T4M3, which is a TANIS 7. M1 disease is automatically assigned a score of TANIS 7. Jones and others have found that using all seven categories creates some categories with little difference in prognosis

between scores.[28–30] To remedy this, several authors have proposed combining certain TANIS scores together to arrive at either three or four different stages.[28,29] This naturally increases the complexity, and it is not clear exactly which combination is better. This scheme also lacks internal consistency because a T2N0 lesion does not have the same prognosis or behavior as a T1N1 lesion, even though both lesions are TANIS 2 tumors. These controversies illustrate some of the difficulties in developing a balanced staging system.

Lydiatt and Schantz[31] proposed a staging system that is more heavily based on the biology of the disease, incorporating factors such as tumor thickness and molecular markers. This temporally structured system attempts to incorporate all phases of the natural history of head and neck cancer, and broadly categorizes patients into four groups: stage I, intraepithelial neoplasia (precancer); stage II, early invasion in the absence of metastasis; stage III, extensive local invasion and metastasis that is potentially curable (most patients with head and neck cancer); stage IV, incurable or recurrent (therapeutically refractory) disease. The authors have proposed this staging system to address the shortcomings of the existing AJCC/UICC system, but further investigation is necessary to validate its usefulness for the staging of head and neck cancer.

Prior to making any changes in the present staging system, the ramifications of such a change must be predicted and balanced. For example, the impact of *stage migration* must be considered, since artifactual changes in prognosis will complicate comparisons between new treatment modalities and historic controls, and could accentuate or obliterate true differences in survival outcomes. It is important to note, however, that stage migration already occurs with the presently used TNM classification system for oral cancer. For instance, a comparison between the third and sixth editions of the *AJCC Cancer Staging Manual*, published in 1988 and 2002, respectively, demonstrates that the criteria for defining N stage remain identical.[1,32] Advances in diagnostic imaging that improve the detection of early nodal metastatic deposits, such as CT, shift patients with early regional metastatic disease into a higher stage grouping and out of the lower stage grouping. This shift, or stage migration, creates a statistical artifact whereby stage-specific survival improves for both stage groupings even though no overall improvement in survival may have actually occurred.[33]

◆ Conclusion

Staging of oral cancer is an important step in defining the natural history and prognosis of the disease. The AJCC system displays acceptable hazard discrimination and consistency, is well known by clinicians, and is easy to use. Continual critical assessment of the strengths and shortcomings of this staging system is essential to ensure that relevant prognostic parameters are incorporated into future staging classifications so that the features that define the behavior of malignant neoplasms are more completely encompassed.

References

1. Greene FL, Page DL, Fleming ID, et al, eds. AJCC Cancer Staging Manual, 6th ed. New York: Springer-Verlag, 2002

2. Piccirillo JF. Purposes, problems, and proposals for progress in cancer staging. Arch Otolaryngol Head Neck Surg 1995;121: 145–149

3. Lydiatt WM, Shah JP, Hoffman HT. AJCC stage groupings for head and neck cancer: should we look at alternatives? A report of the Head and Neck Sites Task Force. Head Neck 2001;23:607–612

4. American Joint Committee on Cancer Staging. Manual for Staging of Cancer. Philadelphia: JB Lippincott, 1977

5. Stuckensen T, Kovacs AF, Adams S, Baum RP. Staging of the neck in patients with oral cavity squamous cell carcinomas: a prospective comparison of PET, ultrasound, CT and MRI. J Craniomaxillofac Surg 2000;28:319–324

6. Myers LL, Wax MK. Positron emission tomography in the evaluation of the negative neck in patients with oral cavity cancer. J Otolaryngol 1998;27:342–347

7. Betka J. Distant metastases from lip and oral cavity cancer. ORL J Otorhinolaryngol Relat Spec 2001;63:217–221

8. Wax MK, Myers LL, Gabalski EC, Husain S, Gona JM, Nabi H. Positron emission tomography in the evaluation of synchronous lung lesions in patients with untreated head and neck cancer. Arch Otolaryngol Head Neck Surg 2002;128:703–707

9. Johnson RE, Sigman JD, Funk GF, Robinson RA, Hoffman HT. Quantification of surgical margin shrinkage in the oral cavity. Head Neck 1997;19:281–286

10. Lydiatt DD, Robbins KT, Byers RM, Wolf PF. Treatment of stage I and II oral tongue cancer. Head Neck 1993;15:308–312

11. Vora HH, Shah NG, Patel DD, Trivedi TI, Chikhlikar PR. Prognostic significance of biomarkers in squamous cell carcinoma of the tongue: multivariate analysis. J Surg Oncol 2003;82:34–50

12. Lo WL, Kao SY, Chi LY, Wong YK, Chang RC. Outcomes of oral squamous cell carcinoma in Taiwan after surgical therapy: factors affecting survival. J Oral Maxillofac Surg 2003;61:751–758

13. Sessions DG, Spector GJ, Lenox J, et al. Analysis of treatment results for floor-of-mouth cancer. Laryngoscope 2000;110(10 pt 1):1764–1772

14. Sessions DG, Spector GJ, Lenox J, Haughey B, Chao C, Marks J. Analysis of treatment results for oral tongue cancer. Laryngoscope 2002;112: 616–625

15. Soo KC, Spiro RH, King W, Harvey W, Strong EW. Squamous carcinoma of the gums. Am J Surg 1988;156:281–285

16. Jones AS, England J, Hamilton J, et al. Mandibular invasion in patients with oral and oropharyngeal squamous carcinoma. Clin Otolaryngol Allied Sci 1997;22:239–245

17. O'Brien CJ, Carter RL, Soo KC, Barr LC, Hamlyn PJ, Shaw HJ. Invasion of the mandible by squamous carcinomas of the oral cavity and oropharynx. Head Neck Surg 1986;8:247–256

18. Ash CS, Nason RW, Abdoh AA, Cohen MA. Prognostic implications of mandibular invasion in oral cancer. Head Neck 2000;22: 794–798

19. Spiro RH, Huvos AG, Wong GY, Spiro JD, Gnecco CA, Strong EW. Predictive value of tumor thickness in squamous carcinoma confined to the tongue and floor of the mouth. Am J Surg 1986;152:345–350

20. O-charoenrat P, Pillai G, Patel S, et al. Tumour thickness predicts cervical nodal metastases and survival in early oral tongue cancer. Oral Oncol 2003;39:386–390

21. Gonzalez-Moles MA, Esteban F, Rodriguez-Archilla A, Ruiz-Avila I, Gonzalez-Moles S. Importance of tumour thickness measurement in prognosis of tongue cancer. Oral Oncol 2002;38:394–397

22. Mishra RC, Parida G, Mishra TK, Mohanty S. Tumour thickness and relationship to locoregional failure in cancer of the buccal mucosa. Eur J Surg Oncol 1999;25:186–189

23. Yuen AP, Lam KY, Wei WI, Ho CM, Chow TL, Yuen WF. A comparison of the prognostic significance of tumor diameter, length, width, thickness, area, volume, and clinicopathological features of oral tongue carcinoma. Am J Surg 2000;180:139–143

24. Groome PA, Schulze K, Boysen M, Hall SF, Mackillop WJ. A comparison of published head and neck stage groupings in carcinomas of the oral cavity. Head Neck 2001;23:613–624

25. Hall SF, Groome PA, Rothwell D, Dixon PF. Using TNM staging to predict survival in patients with squamous cell carcinoma of head and neck. Head Neck 1999;21:30–38

26. Hart AA, Mak-Kregar S, Hilgers FJ, et al. The importance of correct stage grouping in oncology. Results of a nationwide study of oropharyngeal carcinoma in The Netherlands. Cancer 1995;75:2656–2662

27. Berg H. Die prognostische relevanz des TNM-systems fur oropharynzkarzinome. Tumor Diagn Ther 1992;13:171–177

28. Jones GW, Browman G, Goodyear M, Marcellus D, Hodson DI. Comparison of the addition of T and N integer scores with TNM stage groups in head and neck cancer. Head Neck 1993;15:497–503

29. Snyderman CH, Wagner RL. Superiority of the T and N integer score (TANIS) staging system for squamous cell carcinoma of the oral cavity. Otolaryngol Head Neck Surg 1995;112:691–694

30. Carinci F, Pelucchi S, Farina A, Calearo C. A comparison between TNM and TANIS stage grouping for predicting prognosis of oral and oropharyngeal cancer. J Oral Maxillofac Surg 1998;56:832–836 discussion 836–837

31. Lydiatt WM, Schantz SP. Biological staging of head and neck cancer and its role in developing effective treatment strategies. Cancer Metastasis Rev 1996;15:11–25

32. American Joint Committee on Cancer Staging. Manual for Staging of Cancer, 3rd ed. Philadelphia: JB Lippincott, 1988.

33. Feinstein AR, Sosin DM, Wells CK. The Will Rogers Phenomenon: stage migration and new diagnostic techniques as a source of misleading statistics for survival in cancer. N Engl J Med 1985;312: 1604–1608

8

Pretreatment Dental Evaluation and Management of the Oral Cancer Patient

Pamela L. Sandow

Multidisciplinary collaboration between health care providers is critical to minimize treatment delays and facilitate appropriate oral care before, during, and after cancer therapy. Increased life expectancy and improvements in dental health care have resulted in longer retention of teeth and a greater need for dentists to become an integral part of the cancer care team. It is incumbent upon the oncologist to refer each patient to a dentist for a pretreatment oral evaluation when the anticipated cancer therapy has the potential to affect the quality and quantity of saliva, alter the normal morphology of the oral cavity, or reduce the healing capacity of the oral hard and soft tissues. This chapter discusses the pretreatment dental evaluation for patients with head and neck cancer who will require radiation therapy or chemotherapy.

◆ Background

Dental disease is common in patients who have been diagnosed with oral cancer. Lockhart and Clark[1] reported that 97% of 131 dentate patients examined prior to radiation therapy (RT) required dental care for caries, poor oral hygiene, inadequate restorations, or periodontal disease. They also found that at follow-up visits, 81% of these patients failed to complete the recommended pretreatment dental procedures. In a separate investigation, 68% of dentate patients examined prior to RT required immediate dental treatment, and 21% of edentulous patients required treatment for ill-fitting dentures. Interestingly, only 11% of patients who reported previous regular dental visits had no dental needs that required attention before RT.[2] These

findings emphasize the importance of the pretreatment dental evaluation in all head and neck RT patients, dentate or edentulous, to identify and reduce dental disease that could increase the risk of post-RT sequelae.

◆ Radiation Therapy and Dental Disease

Dental Caries

Radiation-induced hyposalivation can result in rampant dental caries despite the complete absence of carious lesions prior to RT (**Fig. 8–1**). Radiation caries that results from quantitative and qualitative changes in saliva can develop within weeks to months after xerostomia develops. Radiation-induced salivary hypofunction often leads to rapidly developing caries in atypical locations such as the incisal, cuspal, and cervical areas of the teeth. The buffering capacity of saliva is reduced by hyposalivation because HCO_3^- concentration is directly related to the salivary secretion rate. A low salivary pH favors the survival of cariogenic bacteria such as lactobacilli and *Streptococcus mutans*. Although most oral bacteria are unable to tolerate acidic conditions for long periods, lactobacilli and *S. mutans* are both aciduric (acid loving) and acidogenic, which further propagates the demineralization of enamel. Low salivary pH may also be undersaturated with hydroxyapatite that is necessary for continuous remineralization of tooth enamel. Impaired salivary flow also decreases the mechanical cleansing ability of the saliva, which leads to inefficient clearance of sugar that in turn is fermented into acid by acidogenic bacteria.[3,4]

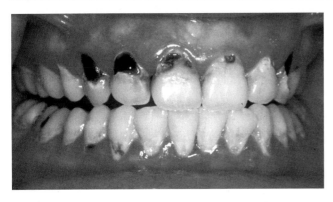

Figure 8–1 Numerous class V (cervical) carious lesions in a 21-year-old woman 3 years after the delivery of 37.5 Gy to the mantle field for lymphoma. There is extensive plaque accumulation along the gingival margin in the cervical region of the crowns.

Periodontal Disease

In the absence of periodontal bone loss, the depth of the periodontal sulcus typically measures 3 mm or less. A periodontal sulcular depth of greater than 3 mm predisposes this region to oral microbial colonization that cannot be effectively addressed with standard dental hygiene measures such as tooth-brushing and dental flossing. In this situation, periodontitis is likely to occur if aggressive periodontal therapy is not instituted. Because periodontal disease typically develops and progresses over a period of several years, the effect of RT on the periodontium has been more difficult to establish and is less predictable than the development of radiation caries. A decrease in salivary flow can contribute to a general loss of epithelial attachment and alveolar bone loss.[5,6] Furthermore, the irradiated periodontal ligament may become ischemic, leading to decreased cellularity and healing capacity. These changes, in combination with the presence of bacterial colonization in the periodontal sulcus, increase the likelihood of and sequelae from periodontitis. An ischemic or unhealthy periodontal ligament equates to the loss of insertion of Sharpey's fibers (collagen bundles) from the alveolar bone proper into the cementum, leading to apical migration of the epithelial attachment (see Chapter 5). A widened periodontal ligament space may become apparent on dental radiographs (**Fig. 8–2**). It is important to appreciate that preexisting periodontal disease, although stable prior to RT, may progress despite appropriate posttherapy dental care. Areas of chronic periodontal inflammation have also been reported to result in the development of osteoradionecrosis years after RT is completed.[7,8]

Osteoradionecrosis

Osteoradionecrosis (ORN) is a serious complication that can occur after high-dose RT to the oral cavity. Marx[9] described ORN as a radiation-induced, nonhealing defect, usually initiated by trauma to hypocellular-hypovascular-hypoxic irradiated tissue. The nonhealing wound, with associated necrotic bone, may require costly and extended treatment with hyperbaric oxygen therapy or debilitating surgery (see Chapter 26).[10] The risk of ORN increases with increasing radiation dose, with the greatest risk occurring in bone that has received in excess of 60 Gy.[11] Furthermore, the decrease in

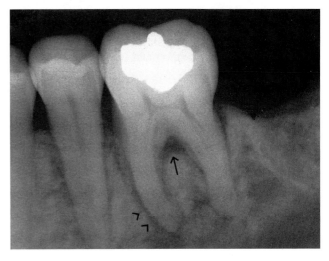

Figure 8–2 Periapical radiograph demonstrating a widened periodontal ligament space (*arrowhead*) in a 46-year-old woman 2 years after the delivery of 64 Gy for oral tongue cancer. There is also radiographic evidence of bone loss in the furcation region (*arrow*).

vascularity in irradiated bone and the risk of ORN has been shown to increase over the life of the patient. Extraction of teeth from irradiated bone can initiate osteoradionecrosis, and although the incidence is greater in the mandible, there have been numerous cases reported in the maxilla.[12] The incidence of post-RT bone necrosis ranges from 14 to 22%. There are reports that the incidence of ORN is reduced in patients who undergo pre-RT extractions.[13–16] However, a retrospective study of more than 400 patients who received RT at the University of Florida contradicted this finding. The time period that is required for healing prior to the initiation of RT and the risk factors (other than RT dose) associated with the development of ORN remain ill-defined. A retrospective evaluation of more than 400 patients who received RT is underway at the University of Florida to clarify the relationship between RT and the subsequent development of ORN in patients with or without preexisting dental disease.

◆ The Pretreatment Dental Evaluation

Communication between the oncologist and dentist prior to the initiation of cancer therapy is imperative. The treating dentist's knowledge of cancer treatment–related side effects and complications should be verified, particularly when there has been no previously established professional relationship between the oncologist and the dentist. The oncologist should apprise the dentist of the proposed treatment modalities, tumor location, size and pattern of spread, pertinent medical issues, and the overall prognosis of the patient. When head and neck RT is planned, the dentist should be informed of the proposed dose, fractionation, radiation treatment fields, and the impact that these factors will have on the future healing potential of the oral tissues. Furthermore, the timing of necessary dental procedures should be carefully coordinated with the oncologist so that adequate healing has occurred prior to the initiation of cancer therapy. Three to four weeks are typically required to schedule the pretreatment dental evaluation, perform any necessary extractions, and allow for adequate healing. During this period, preparation and planning for head and neck RT can be accomplished so that any pretreatment delay is minimized.

Subsequent to the initial consultation with the oncologist, the general dentist's primary objectives during the pretreatment oral evaluation should be to establish a baseline of oral health findings, identify dental problems, reduce potential post-RT complications, and initiate a protocol for caries and oral disease prevention.[17,18] In addition to instruction in proper oral hygiene procedures and caries prevention, both the dentist and the radiation oncologist should educate the patient about possible oral complications that could develop during and after head and neck RT. Through this dialogue, the health care provider can establish a clear relationship, in the mind of the patient, between compliance with the recommended oral health care regimen and reduction in the overall incidence of RT-induced complications. Consultation with other dental specialists, such as an oral and maxillofacial surgeon and a maxillofacial prosthodontist, may also be advisable during pretreatment planning to address surgical considerations and future prosthetic rehabilitation.

An essential part of the pretreatment oral assessment is a thorough medical and dental history. Of particular importance are habits and systemic diseases that have an impact on the healing potential of the oral cavity and affect the overall prognosis of the dentition, including tobacco use and alcohol abuse. There is a strong correlation between tobacco use and periodontal disease, ORN, and impaired oral healing. Tobacco use and alcohol abuse have also been associated with decreased compliance with health care.[1] The dentist must consider the patient's level of motivation to comply with a stringent daily oral hygiene and fluoride regimen if tooth preservation is planned.

A competent immune system and excellent oral hygiene are critical to the maintenance of dental and oral health during and after RT. Therefore, systemic diseases such as diabetes mellitus and AIDS should also be documented at the pretreatment oral evaluation because of their association with impaired healing and periodontal disease.[19] Furthermore, physical impairments that may affect the patient's ability to perform routine dental hygiene procedures should also be considered, because the inability to achieve excellent plaque control will increase the likelihood of future dental problems.

Once a comprehensive medical history has been obtained, a dental history should be performed that includes the frequency of past dental visits, a history of dental sensitivity, pain, infection, soft tissue lesions, bleeding, swelling, age and condition of existing dental prostheses, and a history of oral and periodontal surgery.[17] Obtaining past dental records, including radiographs, and consultation with other dentists involved in the patient's care should be considered, especially if the dentist performing the pretreatment dental evaluation is not the patient's usual dental provider. The dental history can also give insight into the patient's level of dental awareness and motivation to maintain optimum oral health. Inquiry into the patient's perceived reasons for lack of dental care may be predictive of future compliance.

For example, patients who have not received dental care because of limited financial resources or dental phobia will likely have similar issues after cancer therapy.

A radiographic evaluation is performed to evaluate the status of each tooth and its supporting periodontium. A panoramic radiograph (orthopantomograph, OPG) is a useful screening film for dental disease such as advanced caries and periodontal disease, and aids in the identification of impacted teeth, root tips, foreign bodies, and bony pathology. An OPG is easy to obtain and causes the patient minimal discomfort when compared with intraoral radiographs. However, panoramic radiography is very technique sensitive: (1) distortion of up to 25% can occur; (2) some structures can be outside of the focal trough (blurred) if the patient is improperly positioned; and (3) midline structures may appear flattened and spread out or can project as a double image, despite proper patient positioning.[20] Bite-wing, periapical, and occlusal radiographic studies can be used to supplement the information obtained from the panoramic radiograph. Periapical radiographs have the least distortion and provide excellent spatial resolution and superior detail, so they are useful in the detection of early dental caries, subtle periodontal bone loss, and early periapical pathology. Bite-wing radiographs provide similar levels of spatial resolution, and are used to screen for interproximal (mesial or distal) caries and periodontal defects. Occlusal radiographs can be used to evaluate the buccolingual position of impacted teeth, retained root tips, or intrabony pathology that requires treatment.

The findings from the radiographic evaluation are combined with the clinical examination to document abnormal tooth eruption, dental caries, defective dental restorations, previous root canal therapy, tooth vitality (pulpal viability), periapical pathology, root or crown fractures, and residual root tips. Dental restorations must demonstrate excellent marginal integrity (intimate adaptation of the edges of the restoration with the tooth surface) to minimize plaque accumulation. Dental restorations that are fractured or demonstrate poor marginal integrity predispose the tooth to dental caries. Sensitivity to percussion and periapical radiolucency are consistent with periapical pathology and loss of pulp viability. These findings usually require endodontic therapy (root canal) or extraction to eliminate a source of chronic infection that could lead to ORN. Residual root tips and tooth fractures that extend through the pulp canal also require endodontic therapy or extraction. In addition, the periodontal health of each tooth should be evaluated for mobility, gingivitis, gingival recession, abnormal periodontal sulcular depths (>3 mm), alveolar bone loss, and furcation involvement, which can occur in the presence of moderately advanced periodontal disease (**Fig. 8–2**). These findings are used to determine the long-term prognosis of each tooth so that treatment recommendations can be provided to the patient (**Table 8–1**).

◆ Dental Management

Prior to Radiation Therapy

The dentist should evaluate the teeth in the proposed high-dose field of radiation to determine whether they can be maintained relatively disease-free for the remainder of the

Table 8–1 Conditions Associated with Poor Dental Health and Tooth Loss Following Radiation Therapy

Medical history
  Diabetes
  HIV
  Diseases or medications that compromise immune system
  Tobacco and alcohol abuse
  Radiation dose >60 Gy to the oral cavity
Dental history
  General conditions
    Poor compliance with past medical/dental care
    Dental phobia
    Lack of financial resources for dental treatment
    Poor oral hygiene
  Periodontal conditions
    Pericoronitis
    Gingivitis
    Periodontal bone loss
      Tooth mobility
      Sulcular depths >5 mm
      Furcation involvement
      Poor crown to root ratio*
      History of periodontal surgery
  Endodontic conditions
    Internal or external root resorption
    Silver point root canal therapy
    Sensitivity to percussion
    Poorly obturated root canals
  Tooth-related conditions
    Bruxism
    Tooth pain and/or swelling
    Generalized high caries rate
    Deep carious lesions
    Nonvital teeth
    Fractured teeth
    Deep cervical/occlusal attrition or wear
    Numerous missing teeth
    Nonfunctional teeth
    Unopposed teeth
    Third molars
    Partially impacted teeth
    Root tips
  Pathology
    Periapical cysts/granulomas
    Dentigerous cysts
    Follicular cysts
Conditions resulting from cancer treatment
  Hyposalivation/xerostomia (Chapter 25)
  Trismus (Chapter 28)

*Crown to root ratio = (clinical crown in mm)/(clinical root in mm), where the clinical crown is measured from the cusp apex to the top of the alveolar bone proper and the clinical root is measured from the top of the alveolar bone proper to the root apex. In teeth with periodontal bone loss, the clinical crown (crown + root) is longer than the anatomic crown, and the clinical root is shorter than the anatomic root. Thus, periodontal bone loss results in a higher crown to root ratio, which is prognostically unfavorable.

patient's life. Once the prognosis of each tooth has been determined from the pretreatment evaluation, the patient should be informed of the risks and benefits of retaining teeth in the proposed high-dose radiation treatment field. This discussion should review the possible increased incidence of periodontal disease, xerostomia-induced caries, and the risk of ORN.

An appreciation for the likelihood and potential severity of radiation-induced adverse events is imperative before appropriate pretreatment recommendations can be made. The age of the patient and anticipated outcome of cancer therapy are important factors to consider when identifying teeth for extraction, because younger patients with a favorable chance of cure will likely need to maintain their teeth for a longer period of time. A patient's history of dental compliance with oral hygiene procedures and professional dental care are also major factors in the recommendation of retention or extraction of teeth before RT.

Teeth that are expected to receive more than 60 Gy should be evaluated for dental disease and possible extraction before RT is initiated to minimize the patient's lifelong risk of ORN. Grossly carious, symptomatic, unopposed, nonfunctional, or fractured teeth should be considered for removal if they will be located within the irradiated area. Teeth with periapical pathology and root canals that were filled with silver points should be evaluated for pretherapy extraction because of the potential for failed endodontic treatment.[21] Endodontic therapy prior to RT is frequently impractical, because inadequate time exists for complete resolution of the infection and for the final restoration of the tooth. If there are numerous carious, fractured, or poorly restored teeth, the dentist should carefully consider the patient's lack of previous motivation and susceptibility to dental disease. Numerous missing teeth may also indicate a vulnerability to dental disease. With these patients, poor oral health may persist after RT, so it may be prudent to remove all teeth within the proposed radiation treatment field to reduce the risk of post-RT complications.

The identification of teeth with a questionable long-term prognosis designates them as potential future sources of periodontal or endodontic infection, and their candidacy for extraction should be evaluated during the pretreatment phase. This can be a difficult decision-making process for the dentist and patient, and it is important for the dentist to discuss the potential adverse effects of RT so that the patient can make an informed decision. Generally, teeth within the proposed radiation treatment field that have periodontal sulcular depths greater than 5 mm, furcation involvement, mobility, or significant recession, should be extracted prior to RT.[2,7] Patients should be cautioned that the retention of irradiated teeth exhibiting early periodontal disease may present an increased lifelong risk of ORN. In a position paper, the Research, Science, and Therapy Committee of the American Academy of Periodontology recommended that invasive periodontal surgery and other surgical procedures in irradiated areas be avoided whenever possible.[22] With close follow-up and careful patient selection, however, it may be possible to safely perform conservative periodontal surgical procedures in patients receiving less than 65 Gy.[11] Because the incidence of ORN is extremely low in nonirradiated bone, teeth with a questionable long-term prognosis that will not be irradiated may be retained if they will improve masticatory function.

Additional areas of potential infection that should be eliminated prior to RT include retained root tips, failed dental implants, and partially impacted teeth. Full bony impacted teeth with pathology should be considered for extraction. However, the traumatic nature of the surgery may require additional healing time before the onset of RT, since ORN can develop in areas where surgery was performed 2 to 3 weeks prior to RT.[23] The oncologist should be advised of the risk of protracted healing prior to performing dental surgery so that the initiation of RT can be optimally timed. The decreased osteoblastic activity of irradiated bone presents another concern because the deposition of bone in an irradiated extraction site may be impaired. This can result in large bony defects several years after RT. With these potential complications in mind, the potential risks and benefits associated with the extraction of full bony impacted teeth prior to RT should be carefully considered prior to their removal.

Routine oral hygiene and restorative dental care may be difficult to perform if significant trismus develops from postsurgical or radiation-induced fibrosis of the muscles of mastication. Soft tissue fibrosis and trismus can occur months after RT is completed. Other postsurgical factors that may compromise the ability to perform adequate oral hygiene include paresthesia, loss of tongue mobility, and loss of oral soft and hard tissue structures. Teeth may become a chronic source of irritation after RT when adjacent tissues become indurated and lack salivary lubrication. Thus, it may be advisable to extract teeth that could irritate irradiated tissues or become difficult to clean due to limited interocclusal opening.

Stable, successfully osseointegrated implants can be retained in the proposed irradiated treatment field as long as impeccable oral hygiene is maintained.[24] Removal of healthy implants prior to RT, as with full bony impacted teeth, can increase the risk of ORN due to the traumatic nature of their removal. In contrast, patients who undergo implant placement at the time of surgical resection with subsequent postoperative RT may have compromised implant longevity. Some studies have demonstrated an increased failure rate in implants placed in these clinical situations.[25] Variables in implant retention include the interval between implant placement and irradiation, and the radiation dose that is delivered. The role for hyperbaric oxygen therapy prior to implant placement in irradiated bone has not been established, and additional well-designed prospective research is necessary to determine its potential benefit in this scenario. The lack of conclusive research pertaining to successful osseointegration in previously irradiated bone requires the dentist to consider dental implantation in carefully selected patients who will comply with the recommended maintenance regimen and required follow-up.

Discussions with the patient, rationale for the pretreatment dental recommendations, and ultimate treatment performed should be thoroughly documented in the patient's record. The oncologist should be informed of the need for pretreatment extractions to appropriately schedule other necessary cancer-related diagnostic and therapeutic procedures. Every attempt should be made to reduce the incidence of delayed healing when extracting teeth prior to RT. Postextraction alveoloplasty is recommended to achieve smooth bony contours and reduce the incidence of postsurgical bony dehiscence. Primary closure of the wound may improve healing as long as the gingival tissues are not stretched beyond their physiologic capacity. Gentle manipulation of tissue is desirable, and approximately 2 to 3 weeks of healing time is recommended prior to the initiation of RT. A greater interval between extraction and the onset of RT has been shown to decrease the incidence of ORN.[26]

Oral hygiene measures should also be reviewed with the patient in detail. Sharp teeth, overhanging restorations, and irregular prosthetic surfaces should be smoothed to

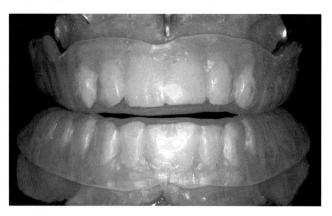

Figure 8–3   Vinyl custom fluoride trays.

eliminate potential sites of inflammation or irritation in preparation for RT. Products that facilitate cleansing of the teeth, soft tissues, and prostheses should be introduced. Pilocarpine, low-abrasion toothpastes, and super-soft toothbrushes may be instituted as part of the oral care regimen and to promote patient comfort during and after RT.[27,28] The most important caries preventive measure for the head and neck RT patient is the use of daily topical fluoride. Topical fluoride should be applied in custom vinyl trays as long as the natural dentition is retained (**Fig. 8–3**). The dentist should examine the fluoride trays to ensure proper coverage of all enamel and cementum surfaces. Either 1.1% sodium fluoride or 0.4% stannous fluoride gel may be used in the custom trays for 5 to 10 minutes daily, preferably at bedtime. Subsequent to fluoride use, the patient should not rinse, eat, or drink for at least 30 minutes. Other products that may assist the patient in the prevention of radiation-induced caries include a 2-week course of chlorhexidine rinse, fluoride varnish, and remineralizing dentrifices that contain sodium phosphate and calcium carbonate.[28] All health care providers involved in the patient's cancer therapy should provide lifelong reinforcement of compliance with the home fluoride regimen, oral hygiene procedures, and routine professional dental care.

Following Radiation Therapy

It is imperative that head and neck RT patients visit a dentist every 3 to 6 months for the remainder of their lives. Patients should be periodically counseled on the significant benefits of daily fluoride use and routine dental care to maintain a high level of oral hygiene and disease prevention. Radiographs, crowns, nonsurgical endodontic therapy, scaling and root planing, and restorative dentistry can be performed safely in irradiated patients, with careful tissue management. Amalgam is the recommended restorative material for class V carious lesions (cervical caries) in xerostomic patients who demonstrate compliance with daily topical fluoride application. For patients who are not compliant with daily fluoride application, resin-modified glass ionomers should be used for cervical restorations located at the gingival margin to take advantage of the fluoride-releasing capability of this material at a site that is predisposed to plaque accumulation.[28]

Following Chemotherapy

Patients who are scheduled to receive chemotherapy for the treatment of oral cancer should undergo the same pretreatment evaluation that is performed prior to RT. In most cases, chemotherapy is administered concomitantly with RT, which tends to exacerbate the severity of immediate adverse effects such as mucositis. Oral complications following chemotherapy vary depending on the type and dose of cytotoxic agents that are administered, the use of RT, and the patient's pretreatment dental status. Consultation with the oncologist is essential to optimize the timing of the patient's dental care with the administration of chemotherapy, and to determine whether prophylactic antibiotics are indicated for patients with central venous catheters. If myelosuppression is expected, interaction with the oncologist enables the dentist to appropriately modify dental therapy to avoid treatment-associated complications. Dentoalveolar surgery should be completed at least 2 weeks prior to the initiation of chemotherapy to maximize healing. Regularly scheduled follow-up evaluations are necessary to ensure the maintenance of dental health.

◆ Conclusion

Proper dental evaluation and management prior to the initiation of RT or chemotherapy is a critical component of every oral cancer patient's comprehensive cancer care. The pretreatment evaluation permits comprehensive dental evaluation and an opportunity to educate the patient about oral hygiene maintenance and dental care in the altered oral environment that results from cancer therapy. The sequelae of xerostomia and impaired tissue vascularization can have a significant impact on the cancer patient's quality of life. It is essential that every oral cancer patient has access to a dentist who is familiar with the evaluation process for patients who require radiation or chemotherapy, as well as the preventive measures that can be implemented to minimize the potential consequences of treatment for oral cavity cancer. Additional information pertaining to the maintenance of oral health in cancer patients is provided by the National Institute of Dental and Craniofacial Research at http://www.nidcr.nih.gov/HealthInformation/DiseasesAndConditions/CancerTreatmentAndOralHealth/.

References

1. Lockhart PB, Clark J. Pretherapy dental status of patients with malignant conditions of the head and neck. Oral Surg Oral Med Oral Pathol 1994;77:236–241
2. Epstein JB, Emerton S, Lunn R, Le N, Wong FL. Pretreatment assessment and dental management of patients with nasopharyngeal carcinoma. Oral Oncol 1999;35:33–39
3. Nauntofte B, Tenovuo JO, Lagerlof F. Secretion and composition of saliva. In: Fejerskov O, Kidd EAM, eds. Dental Caries: The Disease and Its Clinical Management. Malden, MA: Blackwell Munksgaard, 2003:7–27
4. van Houte J. Role of micro-organisms in caries etiology. J Dent Res 1994;73:672–681
5. Najera MP, al-Hashimi I, Plemons JM, et al. Prevalence of periodontal disease in patients with Sjogren's syndrome. Oral Surg Oral Med Pathol Oral Radiol Endod 1997;83:453–457
6. Epstein JB, Lunn R, Le N, Stevenson-Moore P. Periodontal attachment loss in patients after head and neck radiation therapy. Oral Surg Oral Med Oral Pathol Oral Radiol Endod 1998;86:673–677
7. Schiodt M, Hermund NU. Management of oral disease prior to radiation therapy. Support Care Cancer 2002;10:40–43
8. Epstein JB, Stevenson-Moore P. Periodontal disease and periodontal management in patients with cancer. Oral Oncol 2001;37:613–619
9. Marx RE. Osteoradionecrosis: a new concept of its pathophysiology. J Oral Maxillofac Surg 1983;41:283–288
10. Feldmeier JJ, Hampson NB. A systematic review of the literature reporting the application of hyperbaric oxygen prevention and treatment of delayed radiation injuries: an evidence based approach. Undersea Hyperb Med 2002;29:4–30
11. Epstein JB, Corbett T, Galler C, Stevenson-Moore P. Surgical periodontal treatment in the radiotherapy-treated head and neck cancer patient. Spec Care Dentist 1994;14:182–187
12. Tong AC, Leung AC, Cheng JC, Sham J. Incidence of complicated healing and osteoradionecrosis following tooth extraction in patients receiving radiotherapy for treatment of nasopharyngeal carcinoma. Aust Dent J 1999;44:187–194
13. Dreizen S. Oral complications of cancer therapies: description and incidence of oral complications. NCI Monogr 1990;9:11–15
14. Larson DL, Lindberg RD, Lane E, Goepfert H. Major complications of radiotherapy in cancer of the oral cavity and oropharynx: a 10 year retrospective study. Am J Surg 1983;146:531–536
15. Epstein JB, Rea G, Wong FL, Spinelli J, Stevenson-Moore P. Osteonecrosis: study of the relationship of dental extractions in patients receiving radiotherapy. Head Neck Surg 1987;10:48–54
16. Beumer J III, Harrison R, Sanders B, Kurrasch M. Preradiation dental extractions and the incidence of bone necrosis. Head Neck Surg 1983;5:514–521
17. Sonis ST, Woods PD, White BA. Oral complications of cancer therapies. Pretreatment oral assessment. NCI Monogr 1990;9:29–32
18. Stevenson-Moore P. Oral complications of cancer therapies: essential aspects of a pretreatment oral examination. NCI Monogr 1990;9:33–36
19. Neville BW, Damm DD, Allen CM, Bouquot JE. Periodontal Diseases. Oral and Maxillofacial Pathology, 2nd ed. Philadelphia: WB Saunders, 2002:137–161
20. Abrahams JJ, Hayt MW, Rock R. Dental CT reformatting programs and dental imaging. In: Som PM, Curtin HD, eds. Head and Neck Imaging. St. Louis: Mosby, 2003:907–918
21. Cohen S, Burns R. Retreatment: Pathways of the Pulp, 7th ed. St. Louis: Mosby, 1998:791–834
22. Periodontal considerations in the management of the cancer patient. Committee on Research, Science and Therapy of the American Academy of Periodontology. J Periodontol 1997;68:791–801
23. Jereczek-Fossa BA, Orecchia R. Radiotherapy-induced mandibular bone complications. Cancer Treat Rev 2002;28:65–74
24. Meraw SJ, Reeve CM. Dental considerations and treatment of the oncology patient receiving radiation therapy. J Am Dent Assoc 1998;129:201–205
25. Coulthard P, Esposito M, Worthington HV, Jokstad A. Therapeutic use of hyperbaric oxygen for irradiated dental implant patients: a systematic review. J Dent Educ 2003;67:64–68
26. Marx RE, Johnson RP. Studies in the radiobiology of osteoradionecrosis and their clinical significance. Oral Surg Oral Med Oral Pathol 1987;64:379–390
27. Warde P, Kroll B, O'Sullivan B, et al. A phase II study of Biotene in the treatment of postradiation xerostomia in patients with head and neck cancer. Support Care Cancer 2000;8:203–208
28. Rankin KV, Jones DL. Oral Health in Cancer Therapy. Texas Cancer Council, 1999

9

Cancer of the Lip

John W. Werning and
William M. Mendenhall

The upper and lower lips are important aesthetic features of the lower face that also serve a critical functional role in facial expression, speech articulation, and oral competence. As the site of transition between the skin of the face and the oral vestibule, the lips have anatomic and functional features that overlap with the face and the digestive system. Similarly, the epidemiology, etiology, and management of lip cancer share features with both oral cancer and skin cancer. The American Joint Committee on Cancer (AJCC) has addressed the unique characteristics associated with lip cancer by providing a staging classification for the lip and oral cavity that, at the same time, also acknowledges the mucosal lip as one of the eight oral cavity subsites.[1] This distinction facilitates our discussion of lip cancer as a distinct disease entity with unique management considerations.

The oral cavity begins at the skin-vermilion junction of the lips, or the vermilion line. The mucosal lip, according to the most recent edition of the AJCC, begins at the junction of the vermilion border with the skin and "includes only the vermilion surface or that portion of the lip that comes into contact with the opposing lip."[1] A translucent orthokeratinized stratified squamous epithelium overlies a profuse capillary bed that imparts its vermilion color. Predominantly mucous minor salivary glands are embedded in the tunica propria.

◆ Incidence and Epidemiology

Cancer of the lip consitutes 19.8% of all oral cavity cancers registered in the National Cancer Data Base (NCDB) and 24.5% of the oral cancers in the U.S. Surveillance, Epidemiology, and End Results (SEER) program registry (see Table 5–1 in Chapter 5).[2,3] Epidemiologic data pertaining to lip cancer are frequently published separately, because the etiology of lip cancer differs from cancers arising from other mucosal regions of the oral cavity. Lip cancer was the second most common site of oral cancer after tongue cancer in the SEER database and ranks third behind oral tongue and floor of mouth cancer in the NCDB registry.[2–4] Lip cancer is predominantly diagnosed in white individuals, comprising 99.4% of the cancerous lesions entered into the SEER registry between 1975 and 1998.[3] Although the incidence of lip and tongue cancer is similar among white males, lip cancer is less common than cancer of the tongue and floor of mouth in white females.[3] The median age at the time of diagnosis is 68 years for males and 73 years for females.[5] More than 95% of the diagnosed cases of lip cancer arise from the lower lip, and less than 1% of lip cancers exclusively involve the labial commissure.[5–7] This predilection for the lower lip is directly related to the etiology of lip cancer, which is discussed in the next section of this chapter.

According to data from the NCDB, squamous cell carcinoma (SCC) is the histologic diagnosis in 87.4% of lip cancers, followed by adenocarcinoma (2.6%) of the minor salivary glands and verrucous carcinoma (0.7%), with several other histologic types making up nearly 10% of the remaining histologies.[2] In a series of 1036 lip cancers reviewed by Zitsch et al,[6] however, SCC made up 96% of all diagnosed lip cancers. Basal cell carcinoma (BCC) frequently arises from the skin of the upper lip adjacent to the mucocutaneous junction and is therefore not typically considered to arise from the mucosal lip of the oral cavity. Some published reports have documented the occurrence of BCC on the vermilion border, but these malignancies most likely originated from the cutaneous side of the vermilion border.[8] Since SCC and BCC demonstrate differing rates of local-regional control and survival following treatment, this chapter focuses on the outcomes of therapy for SCC.

◆ Etiology

The potential etiologic agents responsible for SCC of the lips have been the subject of numerous epidemiologic investigations.[5,7,9–12] Individuals with outdoor occupations and chronic sun exposure have a significantly higher rate of SCC of the lip than the general population. A case-control study of fishermen documented a statistically significant age-adjusted relative risk for lip cancer of 1.65.[7] Several other investigations have bolstered these findings, including a meta-analysis of the literature that evaluated cancer rates in farmers.[10] In this meta-analysis, lip cancer was the only malignancy that occurred with greater frequency among farmers, with a relative risk of 1.95 [95% confidence interval (CI) 1.82–2.09].[10] A Finnish study also showed that individuals who worked as farmers, foresters, or fishermen were five times more likely to develop lip cancer than individuals employed as administrators or who performed clerical work.[11] The association between chronic sun exposure and SCC of the lip provides the most plausible explanation for its relatively high incidence in fair-skinned individuals. The overwhelming tendency for cancer to develop in the lower lip has also been attributed to chronic sun exposure, because the lower lip receives more sunlight than the upper lip.[12] Others have suggested that the lower incidence of lip cancer in women may be a consequence of less frequent outdoor employment and the use of lipstick, which inadvertently acts as a protective agent against ultraviolet light.[13]

The association between tobacco use and lip cancer continues to be controversial. In 1996, Doll[14] stated that "there can be no doubt that the disease is caused by pipe smoking," a contention that was based on the results of six retrospective series published between 1920 and 1970. Broders[15] reported that individuals diagnosed with lip cancer were twice as likely to be pipe smokers than cigarette smokers, but these findings were confounded by the unmeasured impact of chronic sun exposure, since 57% of the individuals were also farmers. A 1971 case-control study of fishermen by Spitzer et al[7] similarly showed a statistically significant relative risk of 1.5 for pipe smokers. However, the same study failed to detect a distinct association between lip cancer and tobacco use in general. In 2000, a prospective cohort study of more than 33,000 Swedish concrete workers followed for more than 19 years was unable to prove an increased risk of lip cancer among cigarette smokers and pipe smokers.[16] The combination of smoking and outdoor occupation has also been purported to carry a markedly increased risk for lip cancer in an investigation that extracted data from the Finnish Cancer Registry, but the study findings did not support these conclusions.[11] Thus, the role of tobacco in the causation of lip cancer has not been clearly elucidated, and additional prospective epidemiologic research is necessary to minimize the impact that confounders such as sun exposure may have on the results.

Other potential etiologic factors that have been associated with lip cancer include herpes simplex virus and human papilloma virus, familial and genetic predisposition, poor oral hygiene, and immunosuppression.[17,18] Unlike other sites within the oral cavity, an association between alcohol use and lip cancer has not been established.

◆ Prevention

Tobacco cessation, sunlight avoidance, and protective lip balms are effective preventive measures. The sunscreen selected should provide maximal protection against ultraviolet B (UVB) radiation (wavelength, 290 to 320 nm), a property that several commercial products fail to provide (**Table 9–1**).[19] Protection against UVA II (320 to 340 nm) and UVA I (340 to 400 nm) is also beneficial, although the degree of sun-induced damage sustained from this region of the UV spectrum is significantly less.[19] Sunscreens should be recommended with the understanding that there is limited evidence to support their use as protective agents against the development of BCC and melanoma.[20]

◆ Actinic Cheilitis

Chronic sun exposure results in ultraviolet light-induced, actinic changes to the lip, commonly known as actinic cheilitis. Clinically, the lips become dry, scaly, and fissured. The microscopic features of actinic cheilitis are similar to

Table 9–1   Common Sunscreen Ingredients*

Ingredient	Maximum Amount (%)	UVB Protection	UVA Protection
Chemical absorbers			
Avobenzone (Parsol 1789)	3	No	Yes
Cinnamates	7.5	Yes	No
Octocrylene	10	Yes	No
Oxybenzone (benzophenones)	6	No	Yes
PABA (para-aminobenzoic acid)	15	Yes	No
Padimate-O (octyl dimethyl PABA)	8	Yes	No
Salicylates	5	Yes	No
Physical blockers			
Titanium dioxide	25	Yes	Yes
Zinc oxide (including transparent)	25	Yes	Yes

*Among the less commonly used Food and Drug Administration–approved ingredients are dioxybenzone, menthyl anthranilate, phenylbenzinidazole, sulisobenzone, cinoxate, homosalate, and trolamine salicylate.
From Gasparro FP, Brown D, Diffey BL, Knowland JS, Reeve V. Sun protective agents: formulations, effects, and side effects. In: Freedberg IM, Eisen AZ, Wolff K, Austen KF, Goldsmith LA, Katz SI, eds. Fitzpatrick's Dermatology in General Medicine, 6th ed. New York: McGraw-Hill, 2003:2345, with permission of the McGraw-Hill Companies.

actinic keratosis, and include keratinocyte atypia, irregular acanthosis, hyperkeratosis, and parakeratosis. Actinic cheilitis is a premalignant condition of the lips, but the frequency with which actinic cheilitis evolves into SCC is not known. Topical therapy for actinic cheilitis includes the cytotoxic agent fluorouracil and imiquimod, an immunomodulator.[21] Chemical peels and carbon dioxide laser removal have also been effectively used.[22] The end point of treatment during laser resurfacing is complete epidermal ablation with superficial submucosal coagulation, because ablation of only the epidermis frequently results in recurrent actinic cheilitis.[23] One study that evaluated the outcomes of patients treated with topical 5-fluorouracil, medium-depth chemical peel, carbon dioxide laser resurfacing that extended to the papillary dermis, or surgical vermilionectomy showed persistent atypia on punch biopsy 1 year following treatment with fluorouracil or chemical peel, whereas no atypia was seen with use of the other two modalities.[24] One drawback of nonsurgical management, however, is that it precludes the identification of focal areas of invasive carcinoma that should be treated more aggressively. Consequently, posttreatment surveillance should be routinely recommended for patients with actinic cheilitis who undergo nonsurgical management.

Vermilionectomy is the surgical procedure of choice for diffuse actinic cheilitis.[25-27] This procedure requires an incision at the mucocutaneous junction that extends to the commissures followed by excision of the mucosa of the entire lower lip and advancement of a mucosal flap from the inside of the lip to re-create the vermilion (**Fig. 9–1**). If necessary, vermilionectomy can be combined with wedge resection when actinic cheilitis and focal carcinoma coexist (see Chapter 15). Modifications of this procedure to improve the cosmetic result have also been advocated, including the use of an adjacent buccal musculomucosal flap to improve lip fullness, or placement of a mucosal graft borrowed from the upper lip to minimize decreased lip fullness and to make the upper and lower lips appear similar.[28-30] Although vermilionectomy has been used to treat lip cancers as thick as 3 mm, this application is discouraged because the plane of dissection would likely result in an inadequate margin of resection.[31] Vermilionectomy should not be used in situations where invasion is suspected.

◆ Natural History and Clinical Presentation

Lip cancers are typically diagnosed earlier than other cancers of the oral cavity because of their conspicuous location. Lip cancer typically develops in areas of preexisting actinic cheilitis as an indolent, slowly growing lesion that enlarges over the course of months. Atrophy of the vermilion border and a mottled, patternless appearance of the lip mucosa may be seen, consisting of fissures, crusts, scales, and erythema. Erosion and ulceration of the lip eventually occurs, with partial healing followed by recurrence. An evolving cancer appears as an indurated, nonhealing ulcer, or less commonly, an exophytic mass.

Clinical evaluation should include careful inspection of the lips and the perioral region for actinic changes, and the patient's face and scalp similarly requires scrutiny for other suspicious skin lesions. A bimanual examination of the lips should be performed to determine the extent of subcutaneous and submucosal involvement. The presence of cutaneous sensory deficits should be noted. The horizontal length of affected mucosal and submucosal lip and the presence of labial commissure invasion should be carefully assessed preoperatively to estimate the size and nature of the surgical defect that will require reconstruction.

The tumor, node, and metastasis (TNM) staging criteria that are used for lip cancer correspond to the criteria used throughout the oral cavity with the exception of T4 lesions (see Chapter 7).[1] Primary tumors are staged by the following criteria: T1, ≤ 2 cm; T2, >2 and ≤ 4 cm; T3, >4 cm. Tumors of the lip are designated as T4a lesions when there is invasion through cortical bone or the tumor invades the inferior alveolar nerve, floor of mouth, or the skin of the face (i.e., chin or nose).[1] Superficial cortical bone erosion of the maxilla or mandible is not sufficient to apply the T4 designation. Invasion of the masticator space, pterygoid plates, or skull base, and/or internal carotid artery encasement is assigned T4b status.[1]

Several investigators have shown that 75 to 80% of lip cancers are T1 lesions at the time of diagnosis, which contributes to the improved survival rates seen in patients with lip cancer.[6,13,32] Radiographic evaluation should be considered for T2 lesions, palpable submucosal invasion of more than 3 to 4 mm, advanced histologic grade, and involvement of the labial commissure. Computed tomography (CT) can be performed to determine the extent of soft tissue invasion and to evaluate for mandibular or maxillary bone destruction as well as cervical adenopathy. Magnetic resonance imaging (MRI) can provide a more detailed assessment of soft tissue involvement, and is the preferred imaging modality to evaluate for perineural involvement.[33] A normal radiographic appearance of the nerve on MRI, however, does not exclude the presence of tumor involvement. Clinical suspicion of perineural invasion should be supplemented by imaging the retrograde course of any implicated nerve to the skull base and the cavernous sinus. Coronal sections optimize the evaluation of infraorbital nerve spread from the upper lip, and coronal images of the cavernous sinus and the trigeminal cistern should also be performed. Axial images are necessary to evaluate the pterygopalatine fossa, where fat obliteration raises concern for proximal perineural spread along the maxillary nerve.[33]

◆ Prognostic Factors

Regional nodal metastasis is the most important prognostic factor in patients diagnosed with lip cancer, and several parameters are predictive of regional metastatic disease and survival.[6] The most important prognostic factors are tumor thickness, tumor size, perineural invasion, and histologic grade.

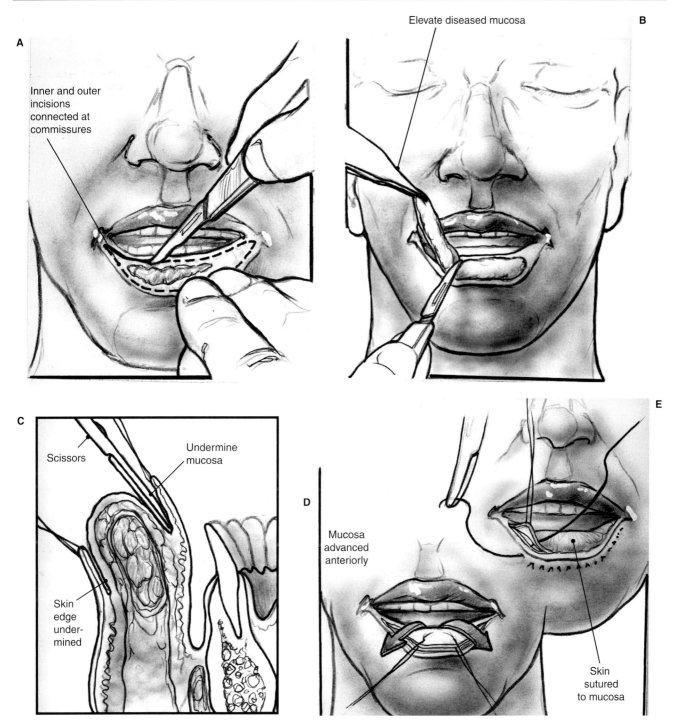

Figure 9–1 Vermilionectomy followed by reconstruction with a labial mucosal advancement flap. **(A)** Inner and outer incisions are performed that encompass the actinically altered mucosa. These incisions are connected laterally at the labial commissures. The outer incision can be extended beyond the vermilion border to include actinic changes involving this region. **(B)** Diseased mucosa is elevated with a scalpel in a submucosal plane deep to the minor salivary glands and immediately superficial to the orbicularis oris muscle. The resected tissue is oriented and submitted for pathologic evaluation. **(C)** A labial mucosal advancement flap is developed by undermining the mucosa into the apex of the vestibule, preserving the labial artery and its attachments to the underlying orbicularis oris. **(D)** The labial mucosal advancement flap is advanced to meet the outer incision line so that a tension-free closure is possible. **(E)** The flap is sutured to the cutaneous edge, re-creating the vermilion line.

Tumor thickness has been associated with regional metastasis in several studies. In one review of 187 SCC lesions of the lower lip, the mean thickness of cancers with a clinically node-negative neck was 2.5 mm, whereas those with cervical nodal metastases had a mean thickness of 7.5 mm.[34] Seventy-seven percent of the metastasizing carcinomas were at least 6 mm thick. Onerci et al[35] demonstrated a mean tumor thickness of 3.8 mm in patients without metastasis and 5.6 mm in those with neck metastasis ($p < .05$), and Rodolico and colleagues[36] documented a statistically significant association between tumor thickness and nodal metastatic disease. De Visscher et al[37] found that a tumor thickness of 5 mm or less was associated with a 5% rate of metastasis versus a metastatic rate of 26% for lesions $\geq$6 mm in thickness ($p < .01$).

Primary tumor size is predictive of regional metastatic disease. Zitsch et al[6] found cervical nodal metastasis in 7% of T1 lesions and 16% of T2–T4 lesions. Lip cancers greater than 4 cm in size demonstrated an 8% incidence of occult nodal metastases while cancers $\leq$1 cm demonstrated a 2% rate of occult metastasis. Another series documented that 84% of lip cancers without metastasis had T1 lesions and only 19% of patients with metastases had T1 lesions ($p < .01$).[37]

In one retrospective case series, perineural invasion was associated with a 30% rate of regional metastasis, and a statistically significant relationship between perineural invasion and regional metastases has been noted by other investigators.[34,37] Other investigators, however, were unable to document a statistically significant association.[36]

Some published data suggest that tumor grade impacts the rate of cervical nodal metastasis. Frierson and Cooper[34] showed that 37% of the metastasizing tumors were poorly differentiated, whereas only 0.6% of the nonmetastasizing tumors were poorly differentiated. Advanced histologic grade also correlated with the presence of nodal metastases in Rodolico et al's[36] series ($p < .01$) and with the risk of occult nodal metastasis (ONM) in the study by Zitsch et al[38] ($p < .01$).

Location of the primary tumor on the lips may have an impact on prognosis. In Zitsch et al's[6] review of 1036 patients diagnosed with lip cancer, there were 39 upper lip cancers. The labial commissure was involved in 2.2% of the cancers, but only seven patients (0.06%) had cancers that exclusively involved the labial commissure. The difference in the frequency of cervical nodal metastasis between the upper and lower lip was not statistically significant when basal cell carcinomas were excluded from the analysis. Labial commissure involvement, however, was associated with a higher frequency of metastasis ($p < .01$). In a follow-up study, however, location of the primary tumor on the upper lip, lower lip, or labial commissure was not associated with an increased rate of ONM.[38]

Several investigators have noted the risk of ONM for cancer of the lip. In the largest available retrospective series of 1001 patients, the rate of ONM was 4%.[38] Two other large retrospective reviews of lower lip cancer documented ONM in 6% and 7% of the patients, respectively.[37,39] McGregor et al[40] documented a 15% rate of ONM in a series of 118 patients with SCC of the lip. Investigators from the University of Palermo reported an unusually high 30% rate of regional metastasis and a 17% rate of ONM in a series of 54 cancers of the lower lip.[36] With the exception of these two studies, however, the published rates of ONM are considerably lower, and most clinicians observe the clinically negative neck in patients with early stage lesions.

The site of cervical nodal metastasis depends on the location of the primary tumor. Zitsch et al[38] found that lower lip cancers originating in the lateral third of the lip metastasize exclusively to the ipsilateral cervical nodes in 84% of cases, whereas contralateral-only and bilateral metastases were found in 10% and 6% of the patients, respectively. Most of the patients with contralateral metastases had large lesions that also involved the middle third of the lip. Regionally metastasizing lower lip cancers that primarily involve the middle third of the lip metastasize bilaterally in 23% of the patients.[38] In 85 patients with lower lip cancer who had regional metastases, lymph node level I was involved in 95%, level II was involved in 9%, and level V in 1% of the patients. In 33 patients with upper lip cancer, metastasis only occurred ipsilaterally: level I was involved in five patients, level II in two patients, and level III in one patient. Metastasis to the intraparotid lymph nodes did not occur.[38]

◆ Treatment

Surgical Considerations

Surgical resection of lip cancer typically necessitates a full-thickness resection that attends to both the surface lesion as well as the palpable subcutaneous and submucosal aspects of the lesion. In general, resection should be performed with margins of at least 0.5 to 1 cm. De Visscher et al[41] reported that margins of as little as 3 mm may be appropriate with frozen section verification. Surgical margins of greater than 1 cm can complicate reconstruction of the resultant defect, because the lip measures only 7 to 8 cm in length. For example, resection of a 3-cm tumor of the lower lip with 1-cm margins would result in resection of more than 60% of the lower lip. Such issues should be considered preoperatively in preparation for the possible reconstructive needs of the patient, because resection margins must not be compromised to provide for a more optimal reconstructive choice. Incisions should exploit existing facial contours such as the nasolabial crease and the mental crease to facilitate cosmetic closure. The intraoral mucosal incisions should mirror the external incisions to ensure that inadvertent beveling of the incision toward the tumor does not occur. Frozen section examination of the margins and the mental nerve may be necessary to verify complete resection prior to reconstruction. A multilayered primary closure of the mucosa, submucosa, orbicularis oris muscle, subcutaneous tissues, and skin should be carefully performed, reapproximating the vermilion and the orbicularis oris to optimize postoperative cosmesis and function (**Fig. 9–2**). Chapter 15 provides a comprehensive overview of lip reconstruction.

Radiation Therapy Technique

Radiotherapy to the lip can utilize either external beam radiation or interstitial therapy.

T1–T2 Lesions

Radiotherapy (RT) for early-stage cancers is usually directed to the primary site alone because the risk of occult neck disease is less than 15 to 20%. Exceptions would be patients with recurrent, poorly differentiated lesions, or those who exhibit perineural invasion.

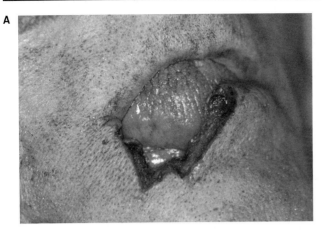

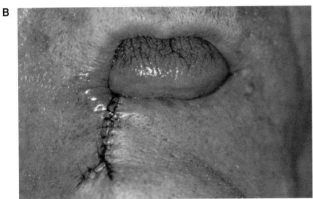

Figure 9–2 **(A)** A W-shaped full-thickness lip resection was performed to excise a squamous cell carcinoma. The W-shaped resection allows for more substantial tissue resection than a V-shaped wedge resection because the lines of resection do not need to completely converge at the apex. The lateral apex of the W is wider and terminates more inferiorly than the medial apex to be more congruent with the relaxed skin tension lines. **(B)** Closure of the defect with careful reapproximation of the vermilion border. The closure of the lateral apex lies in the mental crease.

Treatment may be administered with either brachytherapy or external beam RT. Lesions suitable for brachytherapy alone must be 1 cm or less in thickness so the cancer will be adequately irradiated with a single-plane implant. The implant may be performed with rigid cesium needles mounted in a bar with the needles organized vertically 1 cm apart and one or two horizontal crossing needles mounted on the bar to ensure an adequate dose on the surface of the lip (**Fig. 9–3**).[42] An alternative method is to use iridium 192 (^{192}Ir) via the plastic tube technique. The sources are arranged horizontally 10 to 12 mm apart with crossing sources on the lateral aspects of the implant. Three to five horizontal sources are used depending on the size of the lesion. The advantage of the plastic tube technique is the volume of the implant is more easily adapted to the extent of the tumor and the lateral commissure is readily included, if necessary.

Tumors more than 1 cm thick are initially treated with external beam RT using either orthovoltage x-rays or electrons. A lead shield is used to collimate the beam on the skin surface, and lead is also placed behind the lip to reduce the dose to the oral cavity. Because of beam

constriction, electron beam fields must be approximately 1 cm larger than orthovoltage x-ray fields. Lesions not suitable for brachytherapy may be treated alone with external beam RT. The total dose delivered to the primary tumor varies from 65 to 70 Gy, depending on the overall time. Brachytherapy is administered at approximately 10 to 12 Gy per day. External beam RT is administered at approximately 2 Gy per day, 5 days a week in a continuous course. It is desirable to shorten the overall treatment time so that, if external beam RT is combined with brachytherapy, a short course of RT administered at 1.6 Gy per fraction twice daily to 32 to 38.4 Gy may be used.

T3–T4 Lesions

Low-volume T3 cancers may be treated with primary RT, preferably combining external beam RT to the primary lesion and neck followed by a brachytherapy boost. External beam RT is administered with parallel-opposed fields, including the lip lesion and the level I and II lymph nodes (see **Fig. 9–4** on p. 86). A cork is placed in the mouth to displace the maxilla and upper lip and reduce the volume of normal tissues included in the fields. A separate anterior field is used to treat the level III and IV lymph nodes with a tapered midline block over the larynx (see **Fig. 9–5** on p. 86).[43] The supraclavicular lymph nodes are at low risk and are not included in the fields. Both sides of the neck are treated with RT because it is unlikely that T3–T4 primary lesions would be well lateralized.

The junction between the parallel-opposed fields and the low neck field is at the thyroid notch. The dose fractionation schedule used varies from 38.4 Gy at 1.6 Gy twice daily to 50 Gy at 2 Gy per fraction once daily, followed by a brachytherapy boost. Low-energy photons such as 4 MeV or 6 MV beams are recommended.

High-volume T3 and T4 cancers are unlikely to be cured with RT alone and are better treated with surgery and postoperative RT. Radiotherapy fields are similar to those used to treat patients with RT alone. A Vaseline gauze bolus is placed over incisions to ensure the surface dose is adequate. The fields are extended to the skull base along the course of the third division of the fifth cranial nerve if perineural invasion is present. The dose depends on the surgical margins: negative (R0), 60 Gy; microscopically positive (R1), 66 Gy; and gross residual disease (R2) 70 Gy. Patients are treated once daily at 2 Gy per fraction, 5 days a week, in a continuous course. Consideration should be given to using an altered fractionation schedule to reduce the overall treatment time for patients with positive margins or extensive perineural invasion.

◆ Outcomes

In general, patients with stage I or II lip cancer have an excellent prognosis following treatment. De Visscher et al[37] documented a 4.9% local recurrence rate for 171 T1 lower lip cancers, using surgery as the primary treatment modality. The 5-year disease-free survival for all 184 patients in this

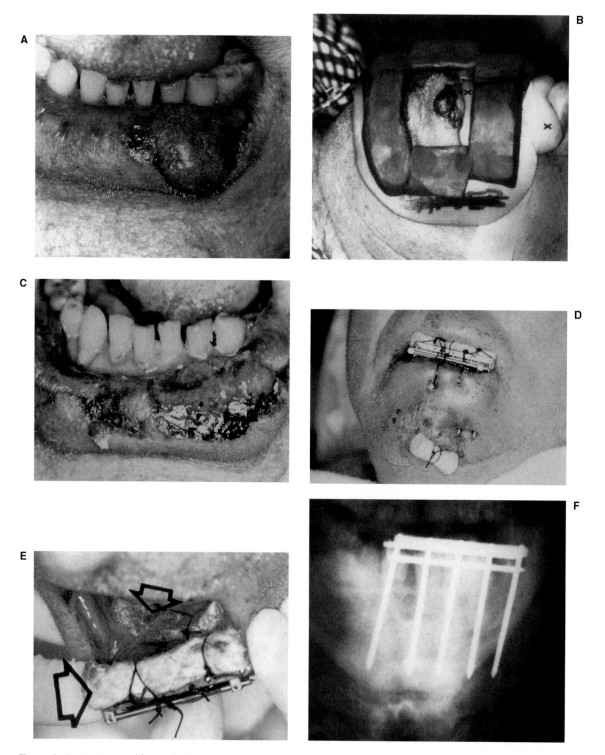

Figure 9–3 A 67-year-old man had a T2N0 squamous cell carcinoma of the lower lip. **(A)** The lesion measured 3.0 × 2.0 × 1.5 cm. Radiotherapy was elected because of the functional deficit likely to result from excision of the large lesion. **(B)** A 2-mm-thick lead mask was designed to outline the portal. A separate lead shield covered with beeswax was inserted behind the lower lip (X). He received 30 Gy over 2 weeks, 3 Gy per fraction, 250 kV (0.5 mm Cu). Lead putty was added to the shield to reduce transit radiotherapy to less than 1%. **(C)** By the completion of 30 Gy, he had a brisk mucositis of the lip and 60 to 70% regression of the obvious tumor. **(D)** A single-plane radium needle implant with double crossing. A gingivolabial pack was tied to the top of the bar to displace the upper lip. A chin pack was used to anchor the gingivolabial pack in place (see **E**). **(E)** A gauze pack was sewn into the gingivolabial gutter to displace the radium from the mandible and upper lip. **(F,G)** Roentgenograms of implant. The implant added 35 Gy specified at 0.5 cm from the plane of the needles. (*Continued*)

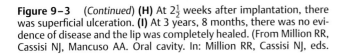

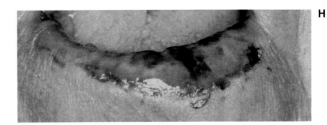

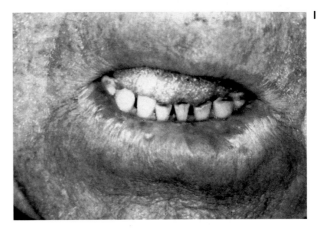

Figure 9–3 (*Continued*) (H) At $2\frac{1}{2}$ weeks after implantation, there was superficial ulceration. (I) At 3 years, 8 months, there was no evidence of disease and the lip was completely healed. (From Million RR, Cassisi NJ, Mancuso AA. Oral cavity. In: Million RR, Cassisi NJ, eds.

Management of Head and Neck Cancer: A Multidisciplinary Approach, vol 1, 2nd ed. Philadelphia: JB Lippincott, 1994;330, with permission from Lippincott Williams & Wilkins.)

investigation was 86%. De Visscher et al[32] also demonstrated local control rates of greater than 95% with either radiotherapy or surgery as the primary treatment modality for stage I lower lip cancer. Investigators from Vancouver, British Columbia, demonstrated a 98% 2-year local control rate following treatment with surgery or radiotherapy or both.[40] The Princess Margaret Hospital in Toronto documented a 5-year local control rate and 5-year disease-specific survival of 96% and 99%, respectively, following treatment with surgery, radiation, or surgery followed by radiation for 117 lip cancers, 86% of which were T1 lesions.[44] Gooris and colleagues[45] from the Netherlands documented local control rates of 100% for T1 lesions versus 80% for T2 lesions treated with external beam radiotherapy. Brachytherapy doses of 6000 to 7000 cGy were used in 12 additional patients, resulting in 100% local control; 42% of the tumors were T2 or T3 lesions. The efficacy of brachytherapy for 237 patients with lower lip cancer has been reported by French investigators from the Centre Alexis Vautrin: 67% were T1 lesions, 25% were T2 lesions, and 8% were T3–T4 lesions.[39] Treatment doses of 65 to 68 Gy using ^{192}Ir wires achieved a 5-year local control rate of 95%. The University of Turin published a 94% 5-year local control rate utilizing ^{192}Ir interstitial brachytherapy.[46]

Five-year determinate survival in the University of Missouri series was associated with tumor size: tumors less than 1 cm in diameter demonstrated 94% survival, whereas tumors greater than 4 cm demonstrated 62% survival ($p < .01$).[6] Cancer of the upper lip or commissure fared worse than lower lip cancers, although only 26 cancers of the upper lip and commissure were included in the analysis ($p = .04$). Treatment modality made no impact on survival:

determinate survival with radiotherapy alone was 87%, and survival following surgery with negative margins was 94%. Patients with positive margins, however, were less likely to survive than patients with negative margins or those treated by radiotherapy. Regional metastasis and advanced histopathologic grade were associated with worse survival.

Cancers of the upper lip and commissure have typically been considered to carry a poorer prognosis. However, there is a paucity of data to characterize the behavior of these tumors, and patterns of nodal metastasis, treatment, and outcomes are similarly limited by scant data. No definite conclusions about the prognosis of cancers of the upper lip and commissure can be derived from the limited number of patients in the studies that have been published.

Several clinicians have advocated Mohs micrographic surgery for the surgical management of lip cancer. Indeed, Frederic Mohs reviewed his personal experience with 1119 SCCs of the lower lip in 1985.[47] A 5-year cure rate of 96.6% was reported for T1 lesions versus only 59.6% for patients with T2 lesions or greater. Cure was obtained in 99.6% of the patients without regional metastasis versus 27.3% for those with regional metastatic disease, substantiating the adverse impact of cervical nodal disease. The neck was not treated unless clinically evident nodal metastases developed. Subsequent series by other investigators have documented local control rates of 92 to 100% in patients with T1-T2N0 lesions.[48,49]

Radiotherapy is associated with early complications such as acute mucositis, and late complications, including persistent ulceration, osteoradionecrosis, fibrosis, and skin changes such as pallor, atrophy, and telangiectasia.[39,44,45] Delayed healing and late complications following brachytherapy are more likely to occur with a treated tissue volume of

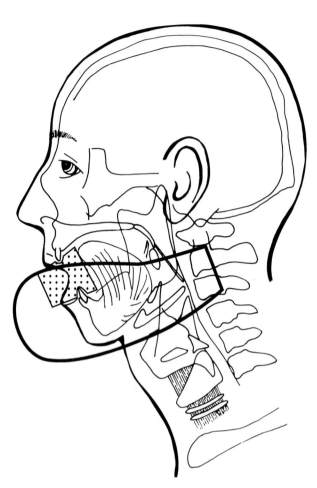

Figure 9–4 Parallel-opposed fields used to treat a carcinoma of the lower lip in conjunction with the level I and level II lymph nodes.

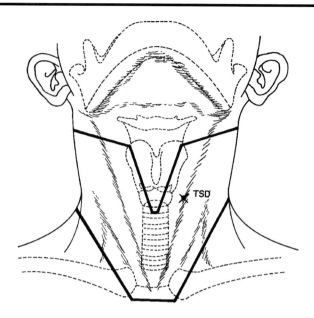

Figure 9–5 Fields for bilateral lower neck radiotherapy for the N0 neck. The larynx shield should be carefully designed. Because the internal jugular vein lymph nodes lie adjacent to the posterolateral margin of the thyroid cartilage, the shield cannot cover the entire thyroid cartilage without producing a low-dose area in these nodes. A common error in the treatment of the lower neck is to extend the low neck portal laterally out to the shoulders, encompassing lateral supraclavicular lymph nodes that are at negligible risk, while partially shielding the high-risk midjugular lymph nodes with a large rectangular laryngeal block. The inferior extent of the shield is at the cricoid cartilage or first or second tracheal ring; the shield must be tapered because the nodes tend to lie closer to the midline as the lower neck is approached. TSD, target-to-skin distance. (From Parsons JT, Mendenhall WM, Moore GJ, Million RR. Radiotherapy of tumors of the oropharynx. In: Thawley SE, Panje WR, Batsakis JG, Lindberg RD, eds. Comprehensive Management of Head and Neck Tumors, 2nd ed. Philadelphia: WB Saunders, 1999;861–875, with permission.)

$\geq 8 \, \text{cm}^3$ ($p = .03$).[39] Brachytherapy by itself results in minimal reduction of salivary flow rates, whereas external beam RT leads to clinically significant xerostomia in approximately one third of treated patients if the dose to the parotid glands is limited.

◆ Minor Salivary Gland Malignancies

Minor salivary gland malignancies make up 80% of the salivary gland tumors of the lips and buccal mucosa. Mucoepidermoid carcinoma and adenocarcinoma together made up more than 70% of the minor salivary gland malignancies of the lips and buccal mucosa in the series by Memorial Sloan Kettering Cancer Center (MSKCC), whereas the M. D. Anderson Cancer Center (MDACC) documented adenoid cystic carcinoma in 47% of 19 minor salivary malignancies of the lips.[50,51] The MSKCC experience documented a 5-year determinate cure rate of 48%, which decreased to 37% at 10 years. Sixteen percent of the patients in the MDACC series died of adenoid cystic carcinoma of the lip.

Treatment of the primary lesion is similar to the management of SCC of the lip. Surgery and radiotherapy for adenoid cystic carcinoma must account for the neurotropic

behavior of this malignancy. Occult nodal metastases are present in less than 10% of patients diagnosed with minor salivary gland malignancies, so treatment of the clinically negative neck is generally not necessary. In a series of 378 minor salivary gland malignancies treated at MSKCC, 14% presented with cervical nodal metastases and 7% more developed delayed regional metastatic disease.[52] The MDACC experience with 160 tumors of the minor salivary glands documented an 8% rate of regional metastasis.[53] More recently, Lopes et al[54] documented clinical evidence of regional metastatic disease in 16.4% of patients prior to treatment, but 45% of the patients in this series from Brazil had T3-T4 lesions. Tumors at high risk for local failure should receive postoperative radiotherapy. These features include locally advanced disease; recurrent disease; high-grade lesions; perineural spread; close, uncertain, or positive surgical margins; and cervical nodal disease. Perineural invasion of the mental nerve, especially in patients with adenoid cystic carcinoma, requires radiotherapy along the neural pathway to the skull base. The evaluation and management of minor salivary gland malignancies is discussed in greater detail in Chapter 13.

◆ Conclusion

The epidemiology and etiology of squamous carcinoma of the mucosal lip differs from the other mucosal regions of the oral cavity, and patients must be counseled to minimize their exposure to ultraviolet radiation and tobacco products. Stage I or II lesions can be treated with either radiotherapy or surgery with similar efficacy, whereas surgery combined with radiotherapy should be considered for stage III or IV disease. Well-designed prospective studies must be conducted to clarify the role of nonsurgical treatment modalities for actinic cheilitis and the application of micrographic surgery for early invasive cancers of the lip.

References

1. Lip and oral cavity. In: Greene FL, Page DL, Fleming ID, eds. AJCC Cancer Staging Manual, 6th ed. New York: Springer-Verlag, 2002:23–32
2. Hoffman HT, Karnell LH, Funk GF, Robinson RA, Menck HR. The National Cancer Data Base report on cancer of the head and neck. Arch Otolaryngol Head Neck Surg 1998;124:951–962
3. Canto MT, Devesa SS. Oral cavity and pharynx cancer incidence rates in the United States, 1975–1998. Oral Oncol 2002;38:610–617
4. Funk GF, Karnell LH, Robinson RA, Zhen WK, Trask DK, Hoffman HT. Presentation, treatment, and outcome of oral cavity cancer: a National Cancer Data Base report. Head Neck 2002;24:165–180
5. de Visscher JG, Schaapveld M, Otter R, Visser O, van der Waal I. Epidemiology of cancer of the lip in The Netherlands. Oral Oncol 1998;34:421–426
6. Zitsch RP III, Park CW, Renner GJ, Rea JL. Outcome analysis for lip carcinoma. Otolaryngol Head Neck Surg 1995;113:589–596
7. Spitzer WO, Hill GB, Chambers LW, Helliwell BE, Murphy HB. The occupation of fishing as a risk factor in cancer of the lip. N Engl J Med 1975;293:419–424
8. de Sousa J, Sanchez Yus E, Rueda M, Rojo S. Basal cell carcinoma on the vermilion border of the lip: a study of six cases. Dermatology 2001; 203:131–134
9. Hakansson N, Floderus B, Gustavsson P, Feychting M, Hallin N. Occupational sunlight exposure and cancer incidence among Swedish construction workers. Epidemiology 2001;12:552–557
10. Acquavella J, Olsen G, Cole P, et al. Cancer among farmers: a meta-analysis. Ann Epidemiol 1998;8:64–74
11. Pukkala E, Soderholm AL, Lindqvist C. Cancers of the lip and oropharynx in different social and occupational groups in Finland. Eur J Cancer B Oral Oncol 1994;30B:209–215
12. Ju DM. On the etiology of cancer of the lower lip. Plast Reconstr Surg 1973;52:151–154
13. Wurman LH, Adams GL, Meyerhoff WL. Carcinoma of the lip. Am J Surg 1975;130:470–474
14. Doll R. Cancers weakly related to smoking. Br Med Bull 1996;52:35–49
15. Broders AC. Squamous cell epithelioma of the lip. JAMA 1920;74:656–664
16. Knutsson A, Damber L, Jarvholm B. Cancers in concrete workers: results of a cohort study of 33,668 workers. Occup Environ Med 2000;57:264–267
17. de Visscher JG, van der Waal I. Etiology of cancer of the lip: a review. Int J Oral Maxillofac Surg 1998;27:199–203
18. King GN, Healy CM, Glover MT, et al. Increased prevalence of dysplastic and malignant lip lesions in renal-transplant recipients. N Engl J Med 1995;332:1052–1057
19. Gasparro FP, Brown D, Diffey BL, Knowland JS, Reeve V. Sun protective agents: formulations, effects, and side effects. In: Freedberg IM, Eisen AZ, Wolff K, Austen KF, Goldsmith LA, Katz SI, eds. Fitzpatrick's Dermatology in General Medicine, 6th ed. New York: McGraw-Hill, 2003: 2344–2351
20. Vainio H, Bianchini F, eds. Sunscreens. In: International Agency for Research on Cancer, ed. IARC Handbooks of Cancer, No. 5. Lyon: World Health Organization, 2001
21. Smith KJ, Germain M, Yeager J, Skelton H. Topical 5% imiquimod for the therapy of actinic cheilitis. J Am Acad Dermatol 2002;47:497–501
22. Zelickson BD, Roenigk RK. Actinic cheilitis: treatment with the carbon dioxide laser. Cancer 1990;65:1307–1311
23. Hruza G, Dover JS, Arndt KA. Skin resurfacing: laser. In: Freedberg IM, Eisen AZ, Wolff K, Austen KF, Goldsmith LA, Katz SI, eds. Fitzpatrick's Dermatology in General Medicine, 6th ed. New York: McGraw-Hill, 2003:2538–2544
24. Robinson JK. Actinic cheilitis. A prospective study comparing four treatment methods. Arch Otolaryngol Head Neck Surg 1989;115:848–852
25. Birt BD. The "lip shave" operation for pre-malignant conditions and micro-invasive carcinoma of the lower lip. J Otolaryngol 1977;6:407–411
26. Kolhe PS, Leonard AG. Reconstruction of the vermilion after "lip-shave." Br J Plast Surg 1988;41:68–73
27. Kurul S, Uzunismail A, Kizir A. Total vermilionectomy; indications and technique. Eur J Surg Oncol 1995;21:201–203
28. Field LM. An improved design for vermilionectomy with a mucous-membrane advancement flap. J Dermatol Surg Oncol 1991;17:833–834
29. Ono I, Gunji H, Tateshita T, Sanbe N. Reconstruction of defects of the entire vermilion with a buccal musculomucosal flap following resection of malignant tumors of the lower lip. Plast Reconstr Surg 1997;100:422–430
30. Kroll SS, Weber RS, Goldberg DP, Pisano S. The vermilion-sharing graft for repairing a vermilionectomy defect. Plast Reconstr Surg 1996;98:876–879
31. van der Wal JE, de Visscher JG, Baart JA, van der Waal I. Oncologic aspects of vermilionectomy in microinvasive squamous cell carcinoma of the lower lip. Int J Oral Maxillofac Surg 1996;25:446–448
32. de Visscher JG, Botke G, Schakenraad JA, van der Waal I. A comparison of results after radiotherapy and surgery for stage I squamous cell carcinoma of the lower lip. Head Neck 1999;21:526–530
33. Mancuso AA. Diagnostic Imaging. In: Weber RS, Miller MJ, Goepfert H, eds. Basal and Squamous Cell Skin Cancers of the Head and Neck. Baltimore: Williams & Wilkins, 1996:79–113
34. Frierson HF Jr, Cooper PH. Prognostic factors in squamous cell carcinoma of the lower lip. Hum Pathol 1986;17:346–354
35. Onerci M, Yilmaz T, Gedikoglu G. Tumor thickness as a predictor of cervical lymph node metastasis in squamous cell carcinoma of the lower lip. Otolaryngol Head Neck Surg 2000;122:139–142
36. Rodolico V, Daniele E, Leonardi V, et al. Node status in lower lip squamous cell carcinoma in relation to tumor size, histological variables and DNA ploidy. Anticancer Res 1998;18:911–914
37. de Visscher JG, van den Elsaker K, Grond AJ, van der Wal JE, van der Waal I. Surgical treatment of squamous cell carcinoma of the lower lip: evaluation of long-term results and prognostic factors—a retrospective analysis of 184 patients. J Oral Maxillofac Surg 1998;56: 814–820 discussion 820–811
38. Zitsch RP III, Lee BW, Smith RB. Cervical lymph node metastases and squamous cell carcinoma of the lip. Head Neck 1999;21:447–453
39. Beauvois S, Hoffstetter S, Peiffert D, et al. Brachytherapy for lower lip epidermoid cancer: tumoral and treatment factors influencing recurrences and complications. Radiother Oncol 1994;33:195–203
40. McGregor GI, Davis NL, Hay JH. Impact of cervical lymph node metastases from squamous cell cancer of the lip. Am J Surg 1992;163: 469–471
41. de Visscher JG, Gooris PJ, Vermey A, Roodenburg JL. Surgical margins for resection of squamous cell carcinoma of the lower lip. Int J Oral Maxillofac Surg 2002;31:154–157
42. Million RR, Cassisi NJ, Mancuso AA. Oral cavity. In: Million RR, Cassisi NJ, eds. Management of Head and Neck Cancer: A Multidisciplinary Approach, 2nd ed. Philadelphia: JB Lippincott, 1994: 321–400
43. Parsons JT, Mendenhall WM, Moore GJ, Million RR. Radiotherapy of tumors of the oral cavity. In: Thawley SE, Panje WR, Batsakis JG, Lindberg RD, eds. Comprehensive Management of Head and Neck Tumors, vol 1, 2nd ed. Philadelphia: WB Saunders, 1999:695–719
44. Cerezo L, Liu FF, Tsang R, Payne D. Squamous cell carcinoma of the lip: analysis of the Princess Margaret Hospital experience. Radiother Oncol 1993;28:142–147
45. Gooris PJ, Maat B, Vermey A, Roukema JA, Roodenburg JL. Radiotherapy for cancer of the lip. A long-term evaluation of 85

treated cases. Oral Surg Oral Med Oral Pathol Oral Radiol Endod 1998;86:325–330

46. Orecchia R, Rampino M, Gribaudo S, Negri GL. Interstitial brachytherapy for carcinomas of the lower lip: results of treatment. Tumori 1991;77:336–338

47. Mohs FE, Snow SN. Microscopically controlled surgical treatment for squamous cell carcinoma of the lower lip. Surg Gynecol Obstet 1985;160:37–41

48. Holmkvist KA, Roenigk RK. Squamous cell carcinoma of the lip treated with Mohs micrographic surgery: outcome at 5 years. J Am Acad Dermatol 1998;38(6 pt 1):960–966

49. Mehregan DA, Roenigk RK. Management of superficial squamous cell carcinoma of the lip with Mohs micrographic surgery. Cancer 1990; 66:463–468

50. Spiro RH. Salivary neoplasms: overview of a 35-year experience with 2,807 patients. Head Neck Surg 1986;8:177–184

51. Weber RS, Palmer JM, el-Naggar A, McNeese MD, Guillamondegui OM, Byers RM. Minor salivary gland tumors of the lip and buccal mucosa. Laryngoscope 1989;99:6–9

52. Spiro RH, Thaler HT, Hicks WF, Kher UA, Huvos AH, Strong EW. The importance of clinical staging of minor salivary gland carcinoma. Am J Surg 1991;162:330–336

53. Garden AS, Weber RS, Ang KK, Morrison WH, Matre J, Peters LJ. Postoperative radiation therapy for malignant tumors of minor salivary glands. Outcome and patterns of failure. Cancer 1994;73:2563–2569

54. Lopes MA, Santos GC, Kowalski LP. Multivariate survival analysis of 128 cases of oral cavity minor salivary gland carcinomas. Head Neck 1998;20:699–706

10

Cancer of the Buccal Mucosa

John W. Werning and
William M. Mendenhall

The buccal mucosa, as defined by the American Joint Committee on Cancer (AJCC), "includes all the membrane lining of the inner surface of the cheeks and lips from the line of contact of the opposing lips to the line of attachment of mucosa of the alveolar ridge (upper and lower) and pterygomandibular raphe."[1] Using this definition, the lining mucosa of the labial vestibule, or labial mucosa, is considered a part of the buccal mucosa. The lining mucosa of the labial vestibule extends from the internal aspect of the mucosal lip to the mucogingival junction. Cancers arising from the labial vestibule tend to invade the adjacent perioral musculature and mandible, and the pattern of invasion dictates management. Consequently, the treatment of cancer involving the upper and lower labial vestibular regions is largely contingent on the patterns of invasion that are present, and is reviewed in Chapters 9, 12, and 13, which detail the management of cancers of the lip and alveolar ridges. This chapter focuses on the management of buccal mucosal cancers that arise from the cheek posterior to the labial commissure.

The cheek is a complex anatomic region that serves an important functional and aesthetic role. Contraction of the buccinator muscles improves masticatory efficiency by compressing the cheeks and positioning food over the occlusal surfaces of the teeth, and assists the lips with sucking, as well as air expulsion. Normal cheek appearance and contour rely on the fullness provided by the buccal fat pad, the skeletal support of the zygoma and mandible, and the baseline tonicity provided by the confluence of several muscles innervated by the facial nerve. Treatments for cancer of the buccal mucosa such as full-thickness cheek resection often disrupts a delicate balance between function and aesthetics that cannot be restored through reconstruction and rehabilitation. This chapter reviews the evidence that provides the basis for the evaluation and management of buccal mucosal cancer and the indications for recommending treatment that results in "acceptable" morbidity in exchange for a chance at improved local-regional control.

The cheek is lined intraorally by the buccal mucosa and externally by the skin. As dissection is continued lateral to the buccal mucosa, the following loosely partitioned soft tissue layers are traversed: submucosa, buccinator, buccal space, muscles of facial expression (i.e., risorius, zygomaticus major), superficial fascia, and skin (**Fig. 10–1**). The submucosa contains multiple minor salivary glands. The buccal mucosa and submucosa have a dense lymphatic system that drains through 8 to 10 collecting vessels that extend through the buccinator primarily into the submandibular space.[2] Anterior to the masseter muscle and posterior to the orbicularis oris muscle, there is a potential fascial space termed the *buccal space*. The anatomic boundaries of the buccal space are as follows: posterior, masseter muscle; anterior, orbicularis oris muscle; medial, buccinator muscle; lateral, muscles of facial expression and superficial fascia; superior, zygomatic arch; inferior, mandible.[3] The buccal space includes portions of the parotid duct, the anterior facial vein and the facial artery, lymphatic vessels, branches of the facial nerve, and the buccal fat pad, which is interspersed between the muscles and acts to facilitate gliding of the muscles during mastication and mimetic function.[3,4] The parotid duct turns medially along the anterior edge of the masseter muscle and courses through the buccal fat pad and the buccinator muscle, draining through the parotid duct orifice in the buccal mucosa.[3] The anterior facial vein and facial artery pass through the

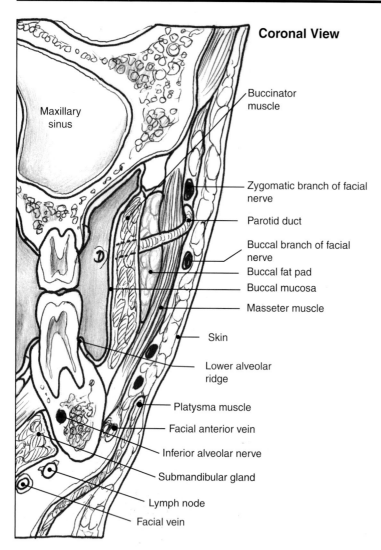

Coronal View

Buccinator muscle

Maxillary sinus

Zygomatic branch of facial nerve

Parotid duct

Buccal branch of facial nerve

Buccal fat pad

Buccal mucosa

Masseter muscle

Skin

Lower alveolar ridge

Platysma muscle

Facial anterior vein

Inferior alveolar nerve

Submandibular gland

Lymph node

Facial vein

Figure 10–1 Cross-sectional anatomy of the cheek in the coronal plane at the anterior aspect of the masseter muscle. The anatomic boundaries of the buccal space are as follows: posterior, masseter muscle; anterior, orbicularis oris muscle; medial, buccinator muscle; lateral, muscles of facial expression and superficial fascia; superior, zygomatic arch; inferior, mandible. The buccal space includes portions of the parotid duct, the anterior facial vein and the facial artery, lymphatic vessels, branches of the facial nerve, and the buccal fat pad, which is interspersed between the muscles.

buccal fat pad lateral to the parotid duct. The facial nerve, which is located lateral to these vessels on the outer surface of the capsule of the buccal fat pad, innervates the buccinator from its lateral surface and the risorius and zygomaticus major from their medial surface. The skin, subcutaneous tissues, and superficial musculoaponeurotic system (SMAS) are located immediately superficial to the facial nerve.

◆ Incidence, Epidemiology, and Etiology

Cancer of the buccal mucosa made up 5.8% of all cancers of the oral cavity compiled by the National Cancer Data Base (NCDB), ranking as the sixth most common mucosal region for oral cancer (see Table 5–1 in Chapter 5).[5] Only cancers of the upper and lower alveolar ridges are less common. In contrast, buccal carcinoma is one of the most common cancers in central Asia and Southeast Asia because of the frequent use of tobacco together with preparations that also contain derivatives of the areca nut. For example, carcinoma

of the buccal mucosa is the most frequent intraoral malignancy in India, and is the most common cancer in men and third most common cancer in women.[6] Data from the Tata Memorial Hospital in Bombay, India, report that 39% of the diagnosed oral cancers originate from the buccal mucosa.[7]

Several studies from the United States and Western Europe have shown that 50 to 91% percent of patients with carcinoma of the buccal mucosa were tobacco users and 17 to 82% used alcohol.[8-13] Sixty-nine percent of the 119 patients reviewed by Diaz et al[12] used tobacco products: 74% were cigarette users, 17% chewed tobacco, and 9% were cigar smokers. Extensive epidemiologic evidence supports the carcinogenic role of betel quid-chewing, which is a popular oral habit in South Africa, central Asia, and Southeast Asia, with 600 million quid-chewers worldwide.[14] Most tobacco consumed in India is in the form of unregulated tobacco products.[15] "Bidis" are hand-rolled filterless tobacco cigarettes largely produced at home by millions of poor women and children, and account for at least 40% of all tobacco consumed in India.[16] Betel quid is a combination of areca nut, tobacco, and lime. "Pano," which is commonly chewed in India, is composed of betel leaf, lime, catechu, and areca nut, and is also frequently mixed with tobacco. The use of tobacco-free pano and betel quid without tobacco are also strong risk factors for oral carcinoma.[14,17,18] The inclusion of tobacco in most of the betel quid that is chewed has often confounded investigations that attempted to evaluate the carcinogenic role of the other ingredients in betel quid. Recent case-control studies from regions such as Taiwan where betel quid does not contain tobacco, however, have established a strong association between betel quid without tobacco and precancer as well as oral cancer.[19,20] Another case-control study documented a relative risk for oral cancer of 14.6 in subjects that chewed betel quid with tobacco compared with controls.[21] Betel quid without tobacco has recently been classified as human carcinogen by the International Agency for Research on Cancer, and much of the evidence points to the areca nut as the most important carcinogen in these preparations.[14,18]

Of the cases compiled by the NCDB, squamous cell carcinoma (SCC) was diagnosed in 74.6% of the patients, followed by adenocarcinoma (11.8%) and verrucous carcinoma (6.0%).[5] The buccal mucosa was the most common location for verrucous carcinoma.[5]

Buccal carcinoma in the United States and Europe is most frequently diagnosed in individuals older than 60 years of age, whereas the average age is younger in Asia, with series from India and Taiwan documenting average ages of less than 50.[5,10,12,22–26] Buccal carcinoma is generally diagnosed 1.5 to 2 times more frequently in males, but retrospective data suggest that geographic differences in this ratio exist.[6,10,22,26,27] For example, females made up less than 5% of the diagnosed cases in one retrospective case series from Taiwan but more than 85% of the diagnosed cases in another series from Alabama.[23,25] Although the authors of the Alabama study provided no insights into the reasons for the disproportionately high number of females with cancer of the buccal mucosa, the use of snuff by elderly women in certain geographic regions may provide the explanation. A case-control study from North Carolina, for example, documented a nearly 50-fold risk of cancer of the buccal mucosa and alveolar ridge among women who dipped snuff for more than 50 years.[28]

◆ Natural History and Clinical Presentation

Most early carcinomas are asymptomatic and may begin as a region of leukoplakia or erythroplakia. The most common complaint on initial presentation is an intraoral mass (55%), a nonhealing oral ulcer (39%), or intractable pain (28%).[8,9] Patients with undiagnosed buccal carcinoma are also referred for evaluation of leukoplakia, lymphadenopathy, or trismus. Facial paralysis and skin ulceration are unusual findings on initial presentation.[8,9] The tumor is frequently exophytic in nature and may be morphologically verruciform.

Clinical evaluation of the patient with carcinoma of the buccal mucosa requires careful assessment of the buccal mucosa for surrounding mucosal changes (**Fig. 10–2**). Bimanual palpation helps to quantify the extent of tumor invasion. Impairment of facial nerve function is indicative of deep invasion through the buccinator muscle and the buccal space, which may necessitate full-thickness cheek resection. Soft tissue, bone invasion, and cervical adenopathy can be evaluated with computed tomography (CT). Magnetic resonance imaging (MRI) is capable of providing more detailed assessment of buccal space involvement and perineural or parotid gland invasion. Imaging can also evaluate the extent of submucosal travel beyond the surface lesion as well as extension along the buccinator muscle posteriorly to the pterygomandibular raphe, which is the anterior boundary of the parapharyngeal space and forms a portion of the enveloping fascia of the masticator space that contains the muscles of mastication.[29,30] MRI can also provide information regarding early invasion through buccinator muscle into the buccal fat pad with T2 sequences, a finding that may impact prognosis and surgical decision making.[31] Changes in the character of the buccal fat pad can be an early marker of tumor invasion that may be appreciated on either CT or MRI.[31]

Tumor staging for the buccal mucosa corresponds to the criteria utilized throughout the oral cavity (see Chapter 7).[1] Primary tumors are staged by the following criteria: T1, ≤2 cm; T2, >2 and ≤4 cm; T3, >4 cm. Invasion through cortical bone, into the deep (extrinsic) tongue musculature (genioglossus, hyoglossus, palatoglossus, and styloglossus), the maxillary sinus, or the skin of the face are designated T4a lesions.[1] Superficial cortical bone erosion of the maxilla or mandible is not sufficient to apply the T4 designation. Invasion of the masticator space, pterygoid plates, or skull base, and/or internal carotid artery encasement is assigned T4b status.[1]

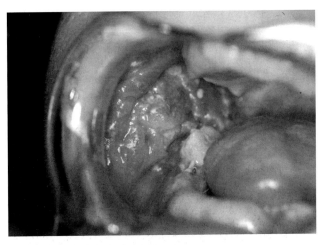

Figure 10–2 Locally advanced squamous cell carcinoma of the buccal mucosa with extension to the retromolar trigone region. There is no evidence of trismus on clinical examination. Radiographic evaluation provides important supplemental information pertaining to the extent of submucosal invasion, involvement of the buccal, masticator, and parapharyngeal spaces, and parotid gland involvement.

A compilation of 587 buccal mucosal cancers from seven published retrospective series provides the following T-stage distribution at the time of initial presentation: T1, 14.8%; T2, 38.5%; T3, 28.5%; T4, 18.2%.[6,8-10,12,23,25] The rate of clinically positive cervical adenopathy ranges from 10 to 45.6% and is directly related to T stage: T1, 11 to 12%; T2, 20 to 43%; and T3, 41 to 56%.[8,12,22,23,25] The frequency of occult nodal metastasis (ONM) in one retrospective case series of 147 patients was 14%, and by T stage, the rate of ONM was as follows: T1, 14%; T2, 14%; and T3, 17%.[13] Three additional retrospective cases series each documented a 26% rate of occult nodal metastases, which usually occurs in lymph node levels I and II.[8,10,12,32] In one retrospective review of radical neck dissections for 181 T3-T4 lesions of the alveolobuccal complex, which included lesions arising from the buccal mucosa, gingivobuccal sulcus, and lower alveolar ridge, 51% of the neck dissection specimens were pathologically positive and 67% of these patients had ONM.[33] Lymph node levels I and II harbored metastases in 85% and 51% of the pathologically positive necks, respectively. Isolated level I disease was present in 46% of the specimens, whereas 81% of the necks with level II disease also manifested level I metastases. Lymph node levels III, IV, and V contained metastatic nodal disease in 19%, 18%, and 5% of the specimens, respectively. Isolated involvement of level IV or V in the absence of nodal disease in other regions of the neck (skip metastases) was present in only 4% of the specimens. Metastases to the buccal nodes and retropharyngeal nodes have also been documented.[34]

◆ Treatment

Surgical Considerations

Because the cheek can measure less than 3 cm in thickness, surgeons are prone to compromise the deep margin of resection to avoid injury to the facial nerve and the need for reconstruction of a full-thickness defect. Buccinator muscle involvement has been documented in more than 60% of stage I or II tumors, so the buccinator muscle should be resected as the deep surgical margin for superficial lesions.[11] Extension into the buccal fat leads to unpredictable patterns of tumor invasion because there are no good anatomic barriers to spread. Furthermore, the adequacy of surgical margins cannot be assessed because of the inaccuracy of using fat as a frozen-section margin. In this situation, parotidectomy may be performed to preserve the branches of the facial nerve, because facial nerve preservation via the transbuccal approach is impractical.[11] Full-thickness cheek resection should be seriously considered when radiographic or clinical evidence of invasion through the lateral aspect of the fat pad or the buccal space is present. The SMAS, which is a thick structure in the parotid region, becomes thin and discontinuous in the cheek anterior to the parotid gland. Consequently, the SMAS is an unreliable barrier to tumor invasion and cannot be used as a deep margin so that the adjacent skin and subcutaneous tissue can be preserved.[35]

Deeply infiltrating tumors that extend close to the skin or manifest facial nerve weakness require full-thickness cheek resection without regard for the reconstructive implications.

The extent of tumor resection is dictated by combining clinical examination with radiologic assessment by MRI or CT, presenting clinicians with three different management scenarios: (1) superficial lesions of the buccal mucosa that are not fixed to the underlying musculature should undergo resection that includes the buccinator muscle as the deep margin; (2) lesions suspected of invading or extending through the buccinator muscle should be evaluated for resection of the buccal space, and parotidectomy may be performed to preserve the facial nerve; (3) tumors with extensive buccal space involvement or that invade the soft tissues lateral to the buccal space often require full-thickness cheek resection with wide margins and intentional sacrifice of the facial nerve branches in this region. Facial nerve preservation should not be attempted unless an oncologically sound en bloc resection can be successfully accomplished.

In a recent review of 119 buccal mucosal cancers, 73% of the lesions were resected transorally, whereas 27% required a cheek flap for exposure.[12] Resection of the mandible was required in 23% of the cases, and partial maxillectomy was performed in 16%. Reconstruction was achieved by primary closure and split-thickness skin graft in 26% and 55% of the patients, respectively. Ten percent of the resultant defects required free tissue transfer, and myocutaneous flaps were used in 6%, whereas regional skin flaps were utilized to close 3% of the defects. Another retrospective review by Bloom and Spiro[22] noted that 67% of T1 lesions and 31% of T2 lesions were amenable to transoral resection without performance of a cheek flap.

Early-stage lesions with a clinically negative neck may be managed expectantly, whereas T2 to T4 lesions mandate prophylactic surgical or radiation therapy (RT). Cervical lymphadenectomy for buccal mucosal cancer is covered in great detail in Chapter 14.

Radiation Therapy Technique

The preferred treatment for patients with carcinoma of the buccal mucosa is surgery. RT alone is used to treat patients by default in the uncommon situation where primary surgery is not feasible.

Patients with T1 to T2 cancers may be treated with a combination of external beam RT and an interstitial implant. External beam RT is administered with an ipsilateral field arrangement that includes the primary lesion and the level I and II lymph nodes. Patients may be treated with either a "wedge pair" of 6 MV x-ray beams or an en face "mixed beam" of 6 MV x-rays and electrons (**Fig. 10-3**). The electron energy used in the mixed beam technique varies depending on the depth of the target volume. Because of the steep falloff of the electron beam at depth, it is preferable to risk overshooting rather than underdosing the deep extent of the tumor, and to use higher electron beam energies such as 15 MeV or 20 MeV beams. The RT dose fractionation schedule is 38.4

chemotherapy regimen that is well tolerated with this dose fractionation schedule is once-weekly cisplatin, 30 mg/m². Well-lateralized tumors may be treated with the ipsilateral field arrangement as previously described. Patients with significant tumor extension toward the midline are treated with parallel-opposed fields weighted 3:2 toward the side of the lesion. Field reductions occur at 40.8 to 45.6 Gy and at 60 Gy. The low neck is treated with an anterior field with a 6 MV x-ray beam to 50 Gy in 25 fractions once daily. Thereafter, part or all of the low neck may be boosted depending on the presence and location of clinically positive neck nodes.

Patients with advanced cancers unsuitable for aggressive therapy are treated with palliative RT using either 20 Gy in two fractions with a 1-week interfraction interval, or 30 Gy in 10 fractions over 2 weeks.

◆ Outcomes

A few retrospective series have evaluated the role of definitive RT for the management of buccal mucosal cancer. Nair and colleagues[6] from Kerala, India, evaluated the role of external beam and interstitial RT in the management of 234 patients with carcinoma of the buccal mucosa. Forty-five patients with T1, T2, and early T3 lesions were treated with interstitial radium implants delivered to a tumor dose of 6500 cGy. Radium implantation resulted in the following 3-year disease-free survival (DFS) rates: T1, 75%; T2, 65%; and T3, 46%. External beam RT was administered using either 5000 to 5250 cGy in 15 fractions over 19 days or 6000 cGy in 25 fractions over 33 days. Small-volume external irradiation with wedge filters resulted in the following 3-year DFS rates: T1, 66%; T2, 75%; and T3, 50%. Treatment with an uninterrupted continuous course of external beam RT using a single lateral field resulted in the following 3-year DFS rates: T2, 36%; T3, 40%; and T4, 22%. The overall local failure rates in this retrospective series were T1, 0%; T2, 27%; T3, 31%; and T4, 50%. Tata Memorial Hospital in Mumbai, India, reported a 59% local-regional control rate for stage I to II disease and a 10% local-regional control rate for stage III to IV disease 2 years following treatment when patients lost to follow-up were excluded from the analysis.[24] The patients evaluated in this analysis were treated by a variety of regimens that utilized external beam and interstitial therapy alone or in combination, and patients with stages III and IV were treated with a palliative course of 5000 to 6000 cGy in 5 to 6 weeks. The Centre Alexis Vautrin in France reported its experience with interstitial brachytherapy, documenting a local control rate of 74% and 5-year disease-specific survival (DSS) of 73.6%.[10] Five-year DSS was 93% for T1 lesions and 67.5% for T2 lesions ($p = .09$).

Tata Memorial Hospital recently published its experience with wide local excision without RT for 147 patients with cT1-T3N0 squamous carcinoma of the buccal mucosa.[13] The neck was not electively treated. Nineteen percent developed local recurrence and 14% developed regional recurrence with a 77% 3-year disease-free survival (DFS) rate. Local recurrences were successfully salvaged in 83% of the cases.

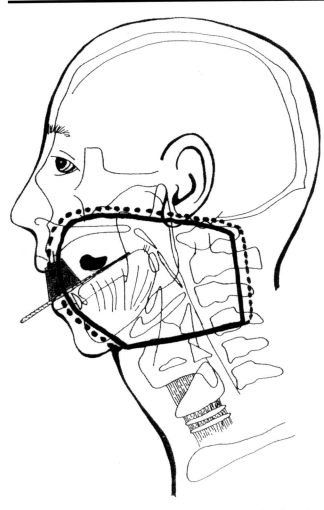

Figure 10–3 Radiation therapy: buccal mucosa. Mixed ipsilateral en face 6 MV x-rays (*solid line*) and electrons (*dotted line*). The electron field is 1 cm larger in all dimensions, due to beam constriction, except where it matches the anterior low neck field at the thyroid notch.

Gy at 1.6 Gy per fraction, twice daily. The ipsilateral low neck is treated with en face 6 MV x-ray field matched at the level of the thyroid notch. Interstitial implantation is accomplished using iridium 192 (¹⁹²Ir) via the plastic tube technique. The implant consists of a single plane of three to five horizontal tubes spaced 10 to 12 mm apart with crossing tubes at either end of the horizontal tubes. Ribbons containing ¹⁹²Ir seeds are afterloaded into the tubes to deliver approximately 30 to 35 Gy at 10 to 12 Gy per day specified at 5 mm from the plane of the sources.

The preferred treatment for patients with T3 to T4 cancers is resection of the primary tumor in conjunction with a neck dissection followed by postoperative RT. Patients who are not surgical candidates are treated with external beam RT and concomitant chemotherapy. Although it would be desirable to include brachytherapy as part of the treatment, the likelihood of adequately encompassing an advanced tumor with an interstitial implant is remote, and so these patients are treated with external beam RT to 76.8 Gy in 64 twice-daily fractions over 6.5 weeks. A

Subsequent development of regional metastatic disease occurred in 14% of the patients, and there was no difference in the regional recurrence rate between T stages.[13] The experience reported by other cancer centers, however, document dismal local control rates following surgical resection. Roswell Park Cancer Institute reported its outcomes following surgery without RT for 24 patients with buccal mucosal cancer, noting local recurrence rates of 40% and 80% for T1–2 and T3–4 lesions, respectively, when negative margins were attained.[8] The University of Michigan reported a 100% local recurrence rate for patients with stage I or II disease who were treated with surgical resection alone.[11]

There are a few large retrospective case series that report the efficacy of surgery in combination with postoperative RT. Fang et al[25] evaluated the role of surgery and postoperative RT for squamous carcinoma of the buccal mucosa in 57 patients from Taiwan with a median duration of follow-up of 42 months. All patients received postoperative RT, 1.8 Gy per fraction 5 days per week with a median dose of 61.2 Gy (range: 45 to 68.4 Gy) to the buccal region and 46.8 Gy to the neck. Three-year local and regional control rates were 68% and 86%, respectively, and the 3-year DFS rate was 62%. Multivariate analysis demonstrated that tumor invasion into the skin of the cheek was the only significant prognostic factor ($p < .01$), and 90% of the patients with cheek invasion failed locally within 1 year after completing RT. Tata Memorial Hospital recently reported its experience with composite resection and postoperative RT for 428 cancers of the lower gingivobuccal complex, which included lesions arising from the buccal mucosa and gingivobuccal sulcus (78%), lower alveolar ridge (17%), and retromolar trigone (5%).[36] Pathologic mandibular invasion was present in 40% of the resections evaluated. On multivariate analysis, skin infiltration and extracapsular spread were associated with poorer disease-free survival, whereas RT combined with surgery resulted in improved disease-free survival.

Diaz and colleagues[12] from M. D. Anderson Cancer Center reported the outcomes following the treatment of 119 patients with buccal mucosal cancers. Seventy-one percent of the patients were treated with surgery and 29% received surgery and RT. The reported 5-year survival rates by stage were as follows: I, 78%; II, 66%; III, 62%; and IV, 50%.[12] The 5-year survival rates by T stage were as follows: T1, 79%; T2, 65%; T3, 56%; and T4, 69%. Twenty-three percent developed local recurrence, 11% developed regional recurrence, and 9% developed local and regional recurrence. Tumor location relative to Stensen's duct and buccinator muscle invasion had no impact on local-regional recurrence. Five-year survival rates for patients with N0 and N+ neck disease were 70% and 49%, respectively ($p = .01$). The local-regional control rates accomplished with surgery and surgery in combination with postoperative therapy were not analyzed separately. Similar findings have been documented by smaller retrospective case series.[9,37]

Investigators from Orissa, India, conducted a nonrandomized prospective study comparing treatment outcomes following surgery ($n = 60$) and surgery plus postoperative RT ($n = 80$) for T3–4 buccal mucosal lesions.[26] Fifty-eight percent of the patients treated with definitive surgery were clinically node-negative, whereas 70% of the patients receiving postoperative RT were node-positive ($p < .05$). Three-year DFS was 38% in the surgery group and 47% in the postoperative RT group ($p < .005$).

Tumor-specific factors that have been shown to adversely affect prognosis include skin invasion, T stage, pN stage, extracapsular spread, and tumor thickness.[12,23,25,27,36] A tumor thickness of more than 4 mm was associated with higher rates of lymph node metastasis, and a tumor thickness of greater than 6 mm has been associated with worse survival.[23,27] Surprisingly, depth of tumor invasion was not associated with worse prognosis in an investigation conducted at the University of Alabama in Birmingham.[23]

◆ Verrucous Carcinoma

The buccal mucosa is the most frequent intraoral location for verrucous carcinoma, a variant of well-differentiated SCC, constituting 6% of the cancers diagnosed at this site.[5] Grossly, verrucous carcinoma demonstrates wart-like exophytic growth secondary to extensive surface keratinization (**Fig. 10–2**). Biopsy of suspected verrucous carcinoma is best performed by excision of the lesion to evaluate the interface between the tumor and the submucosa. Isolated biopsies of these exophytic lesions usually show thickened keratinized mature epithelium, preventing evaluation of the epithelial-submucosal interface.[38] Excision is typically necessary to differentiate verrucous carcinoma from proliferative verrucous hyperplasia or verrucous carcinoma with focal areas of typical squamous cell carcinoma.[38] Verrucous carcinoma is a well-differentiated malignancy that has low metastatic potential.

Verrucous carcinomas have traditionally been treated with surgical resection because of the fear that dedifferentiation can be induced by RT. This premise remains largely unfounded, and subsequent investigation has documented foci of less-differentiated squamous carcinoma within nearly 20% of untreated verrucous carcinomas as the most probable cause of treatment failures.[39] There are now several published series documenting the efficacy of RT for these tumors, with survival rates comparable to well-differentiated squamous carcinoma.[40–42] Surgery, however, remains the mainstay of therapy for most lesions, and complete excision provides additional prognostic information regarding foci of higher grade carcinoma that may suggest the need for postoperative RT. Medina et al[39] documented 82% local control following definitive surgery and 58% local control with RT. Local failures following treatment with RT, however, were documented exclusively with T4 lesions. The rate of local control correlated closely with the T stage in this retrospective case series. The NCDB compiled 2350 cases of verrucous carcinoma with an overall 5-year relative survival rate of 80%, and a 5-year survival rate of 74% for oral cancers.[43] Survival rates progressively worsen as disease stage advances, from 87% for stage I disease to 47% for stage IV lesions. In the series of 236 cases of verrucous carcinoma of the buccal mucosa compiled by the NCDB, 76% were treated with surgery, 9% received RT, and 6% were treated with surgery and radiation.[43] The 5-year relative survival rate in this series, which is the ratio of the observed survival rate to the expected rate for a similar group of people from the general population, was 76%.

◆ Minor Salivary Gland Malignancies

According to Spiro,[44] the cheek and lips composed 17% of the minor salivary gland malignancies diagnosed in the oral cavity (this series did not differentiate malignancies of the hard and soft palate). Mucoepidermoid carcinoma was diagnosed most frequently, followed by adenocarcinoma and adenoid cystic carcinoma. The buccal mucosa was more frequently involved than the lip in another retrospective case review, and adenoid cystic carcinoma was the most common histologic type, followed by mucoepidermoid carcinoma, adenocarcinoma, and acinic cell carcinoma.[45] Minor salivary gland malignancies of the buccal mucosa should undergo a management strategy similar to squamous cell carcinoma. Adenoid cystic carcinoma, perineural invasion, resection margin status, and stage have been associated with poor prognosis.[46,47] Advanced grade is also associated with poorer outcome with the exception of adenoid cystic carcinoma.[46,47] The site of origin was not a significant predictor of survival. Garden et al[48] found that adenoid cystic carcinoma histology, perineural invasion, nodal disease, and an increased time interval between surgery and radiation were associated with a greater risk of distant metastasis.

◆ Conclusion

Buccal carcinoma, like other cancers of the oral cavity, is most effectively managed via prevention and early detection. In India, where resources for health care are limited and much of the tobacco industry is unregulated, 5-year relative survival rates for oral cancer are in the range of 45% because only one third of patients present with localized disease.[49] Efforts to educate the public about the dangers of tobacco use and the importance of early detection have been effective in India, but need to be implemented nationwide and throughout the developing world.[15]

Preoperative clinical and radiographic evaluation of the depth of tumor invasion and its relationship to the buccinator, buccal space, and facial nerve are paramount considerations that can be used to estimate the extent of surgical resection, the probability that facial nerve function will be lost, and the likelihood that microvascular reconstruction will be necessary. In an attempt to avoid the cosmetic and functional sequelae associated with full-thickness cheek resection, surgeons may be tempted to compromise the width of the deep surgical margin. The high published local recurrence rates following resection of T1 and T2 lesions, however, emphasize the importance of achieving clean surgical margins and the need to maintain a low threshold for administering postoperative RT.[8,11,25]

References

1. Lip and oral cavity. In: Greene FL, Page DL, Fleming ID, eds. AJCC Cancer Staging Manual, 6th ed. New York: Springer-Verlag, 2002:23–32

2. Werner JA, Dunne AA, Myers JN. Functional anatomy of the lymphatic drainage system of the upper aerodigestive tract and its role in metastasis of squamous cell carcinoma. Head Neck 2003;25:322–332

3. Gallia L, Rood SR, Myers EN. Management of buccal space masses. Otolaryngol Head Neck Surg 1981;89:221–225

4. Zhang HM, Yan YP, Qi KM, Wang JQ, Liu ZF. Anatomical structure of the buccal fat pad and its clinical adaptations. Plast Reconstr Surg 2002;109:2509–2518, discussion 2519–2520

5. Funk GF, Karnell LH, Robinson RA, Zhen WK, Trask DK, Hoffman HT. Presentation, treatment, and outcome of oral cavity cancer: a National Cancer Data Base report. Head Neck 2002;24:165–180

6. Nair MK, Sankaranarayanan R, Padmanabhan TK. Evaluation of the role of radiotherapy in the management of carcinoma of the buccal mucosa. Cancer 1988;61:1326–1331

7. Paymaster JC. Some observations on oral and pharyngeal carcinomas in the state of Bombay. Cancer 1962;15:578–583

8. Sieczka E, Datta R, Singh A, et al. Cancer of the buccal mucosa: are margins and T-stage accurate predictors of local control? Am J Otolaryngol 2001;22:395–399

9. Chhetri DK, Rawnsley JD, Calcaterra TC. Carcinoma of the buccal mucosa. Otolaryngol Head Neck Surg 2000;123:566–571

10. Lapeyre M, Peiffert D, Malissard L, Hoffstetter S, Pernot M. An original technique of brachytherapy in the treatment of epidermoid carcinomas of the buccal mucosa. Int J Radiat Oncol Biol Phys 1995;33:447–454

11. Strome SE, To W, Strawderman M, et al. Squamous cell carcinoma of the buccal mucosa. Otolaryngol Head Neck Surg 1999;120:375–379

12. Diaz EM Jr, Holsinger FC, Zuniga ER, Roberts DB, Sorensen DM. Squamous cell carcinoma of the buccal mucosa: one institution's experience with 119 previously untreated patients. Head Neck 2003;25:267–273

13. Iyer SG, Pradhan SA, Pai PS, Patil S. Surgical treatment outcomes of localized squamous carcinoma of buccal mucosa. Head Neck 2004;26:897–902

14. Jeng JH, Chang MC, Hahn LJ. Role of areca nut in betel quid-associated chemical carcinogenesis: current awareness and future perspectives. Oral Oncol 2001;37:477–492

15. Sturgis EM. A review of social and behavioral efforts at oral cancer preventions in India. Head Neck 2004;26:937–944

16. Shimkhada R, Peabody JW. Tobacco control in India. Bull World Health Organ 2003;81:48–52

17. Merchant A, Husain SS, Hosain M, et al. Paan without tobacco: an independent risk factor for oral cancer. Int J Cancer 2000;86:128–131

18. International Agency for Research on Cancer. Betel-Quid and Areca-Nut Chewing and Some Areca-Nut-Derived Nitrosamines, vol 85. Lyon, France: IARC Press, 2004

19. Jacob BJ, Straif K, Thomas G, et al. Betel quid without tobacco as a risk factor for oral precancers. Oral Oncol 2004;40:697–704

20. Lu CT, Yen YY, Ho CS, et al. A case-control study of oral cancer in Changhua County, Taiwan. J Oral Pathol Med 1996;25:245–248

21. Nandakumar A, Thimmasetty KT, Sreeramareddy NM, et al. A population-based case-control investigation on cancers of the oral cavity in Bangalore, India. Br J Cancer 1990;62:847–851

22. Bloom ND, Spiro RH. Carcinoma of the cheek mucosa: a retrospective analysis. Am J Surg 1980;140:556–559

23. Urist MM, O'Brien CJ, Soong SJ, Visscher DW, Maddox WA. Squamous cell carcinoma of the buccal mucosa: analysis of prognostic factors. Am J Surg 1987;154:411–414

24. Chaudhary AJ, Pande SC, Sharma V, et al. Radiotherapy of carcinoma of the buccal mucosa. Semin Surg Oncol 1989;5:322–326

25. Fang FM, Leung SW, Huang CC, et al. Combined-modality therapy for squamous carcinoma of the buccal mucosa: treatment results and prognostic factors. Head Neck 1997;19:506–512

26. Mishra RC, Singh DN, Mishra TK. Post-operative radiotherapy in carcinoma of buccal mucosa: a prospective randomized trial. Eur J Surg Oncol 1996;22:502–504

27. Mishra RC, Parida G, Mishra TK, Mohanty S. Tumour thickness and relationship to locoregional failure in cancer of the buccal mucosa. Eur J Surg Oncol 1999;25:186–189

28. Winn DM, Blot WJ, Shy CM, Pickle LW, Toledo A, Fraumeni JF Jr. Snuff dipping and oral cancer among women in the southern United States. N Engl J Med 1981;304:745–749

29. Mukherji SK, Pillsbury HR, Castillo M. Imaging squamous cell carcinomas of the upper aerodigestive tract: what clinicians need to know. Radiology 1997;205:629–646

30. Som PM, Curtin HD. Fascia and spaces of the neck. In: Som P, Curtin HD, eds. Head and Neck Imaging, 4th ed. St. Louis: Mosby, 2003: 1805–1827

31. Kahn JL, Wolfram-Gabel R, Bourjat P. Anatomy and imaging of the deep fat of the face. Clin Anat 2000;13:373–382

32. Shah JP, Candela FC, Poddar AK. The patterns of cervical lymph node metastases from squamous carcinoma of the oral cavity. Cancer 1990;66:109–113

33. Rao RS, Deshmane VH, Parikh HK, Parikh DM, Sukthankar PS. Extent of lymph node dissection in T3/T4 cancer of the alveolo-buccal complex. Head Neck 1995;17:199–203

34. Tiwari R. Squamous cell carcinoma of the superior gingivolabial sulcus. Oral Oncol 2000;36:461–465

35. Gardetto A, Dabernig J, Rainer C, Piegger J, Piza-Katzer H, Fritsch H. Does a superficial musculoaponeurotic system exist in the face and neck? An anatomical study by the tissue plastination technique. Plast Reconstr Surg 2003;111:664–672, discussion 673–665

36. Pathak KA, Gupta S, Talole S, et al. Advanced squamous cell carcinoma of lower gingivobuccal complex: patterns of spread and failure. Head Neck 2005;27:597–602

37. Pop LA, Eijkenboom WM, de Boer MF, et al. Evaluation of treatment results of squamous cell carcinoma of the buccal mucosa. Int J Radiat Oncol Biol Phys 1989;16:483–487

38. Crissman JD, Gnepp DR, Goodman ML, Hellquist H, Johns ME. Preinvasive lesions of the upper aerodigestive tract: histologic definitions and clinical implications (a symposium). Pathol Annu 1987; 22:311–352

39. Medina JE, Dichtel W, Luna MA. Verrucous-squamous carcinomas of the oral cavity: a clinicopathologic study of 104 cases. Arch Otolaryngol 1984;110:437–440

40. Nair MK, Sankaranarayanan R, Padmanabhan TK, Madhu CS. Oral verrucous carcinoma: treatment with radiotherapy. Cancer 1988; 61:458–461

41. Jyothirmayi R, Sankaranarayanan R, Varghese C, Jacob R, Nair MK. Radiotherapy in the treatment of verrucous carcinoma of the oral cavity. Oral Oncol 1997;33:124–128

42. Vidyasagar MS, Fernandes DJ, Kasturi DP, et al. Radiotherapy and verrucous carcinoma of the oral cavity: a study of 107 cases. Acta Oncol 1992;31:43–47

43. Koch BB, Trask DK, Hoffman HT, et al. National survey of head and neck verrucous carcinoma: patterns of presentation, care, and outcome. Cancer 2001;92:110–120

44. Spiro RH. Salivary neoplasms: overview of a 35-year experience with 2,807 patients. Head Neck Surg 1986;8:177–184

45. Weber RS, Palmer JM, el-Naggar A, McNeese MD, Guillamondegui OM, Byers RM. Minor salivary gland tumors of the lip and buccal mucosa. Laryngoscope 1989;99:6–9

46. Spiro RH, Huvos AG. Stage means more than grade in adenoid cystic carcinoma. Am J Surg 1992;164:623–628

47. Spiro RH, Thaler HT, Hicks WF, Kher UA, Huvos AH, Strong EW. The importance of clinical staging of minor salivary gland carcinoma. Am J Surg 1991;162:330–336

48. Garden AS, Weber RS, Ang KK, Morrison WH, Matre J, Peters LJ. Postoperative radiation therapy for malignant tumors of minor salivary glands: outcome and patterns of failure. Cancer 1994;73: 2563–2569

49. Yeole BB, Sankaranarayanan R, Sunny MSL, Swaminathan R, Parkin DM. Survival from head and neck cancer in Mumbai (Bombay), India. Cancer 2000;89:437–444

11

Cancer of the Oral Tongue and Floor of Mouth

John W. Werning and
William M. Mendenhall

The tongue and floor of mouth are mucosally contiguous regions that play a vital role in speech, mastication, and deglutition. Oral tongue and floor of mouth (FOM) cancers together account for over 50% of the malignant lesions that develop in the oral cavity, so much of our knowledge regarding the natural history of, and treatment outcomes for, oral cancer has been culled from the peer-reviewed literature pertaining to cancer arising from these two mucosal regions. The treatment of these cancers frequently alters the balanced functional relationship that exists between the oral tongue and the FOM. As our ability to control cancer in these regions has plateaued, increasing attention has been directed toward the preservation of functional integrity and quality of life. Clinicians are confronted with the need to preserve function without compromising oncologic efficacy in nearly every patient who presents with cancer of the tongue and FOM.

The oral tongue is the freely mobile anterior two thirds of the tongue that extends from the circumvallate papillae anteriorly to the undersurface of the tongue at the junction of the FOM. The oral tongue is composed of the tip, the lateral borders, the dorsum, and the undersurface, or nonvillous ventral surface, of the tongue.[1] The ventral surface is considered a separate site by the World Health Organization.[1] The ventral surface of the tongue is covered by a thin lining of mucosa and submucosa, whereas the dorsum of the tongue is covered by a thicker, specialized mucosa. The specialized mucosa has a thick, intermittently keratinized stratified squamous epithelium that forms three different types of lingual papillae and overlies a prominent lamina propria that binds directly to connective tissue surrounding the intrinsic tongue musculature.[2] The intrinsic musculature can be divided into transverse, longitudinal, and vertical fiber

groups, which alter the shape of the tongue during speech and swallowing. There are also four paired extrinsic tongue muscles, which move the tongue as a unit: the styloglossus, hyoglossus, genioglossus, and palatoglossus muscles.

The FOM is a horseshoe-shaped region of lining mucosa overlying the mylohyoid and hyoglossus muscles that extends from the mucogingival junction of the lingual mandibular alveolar ridge to the undersurface of the tongue.[1] The FOM extends posteriorly to the base of the anterior tonsillar pillar. It contains the ostia of the submandibular and sublingual salivary glands and is divided at the midline by the lingual frenulum. The mylohyoid muscles, which extend from the mylohyoid ridge on the medial aspect of each side of the mandible to a median raphe that extends between the inner aspect of the mandibular symphysis to the hyoid bone, supports the anterior FOM posteriorly to the molar region. The hyoglossus, which arises from the superior border of the greater horns of the hyoid bone, supports the posterior FOM. Medially, the hyoglossus, genioglossus, and styloglossus muscles lie between the mylohyoid muscle and the FOM mucosa. The hyoglossus muscle separates the medially positioned lingual artery from the sublingual glands and the lingual and hypoglossal nerves, which are lateral to the hyoglossus (**Figs. 11–1** and **11–2**).[3]

◆ Incidence, Epidemiology, and Etiology

Oral tongue cancer is the most commonly reported site for oral cancer in the United States, constituting 36.2% of the oral cancers compiled in the U.S. Surveillance, Epidemiology, and End Results program (SEER) and 27.5% of the oral

Coronal View

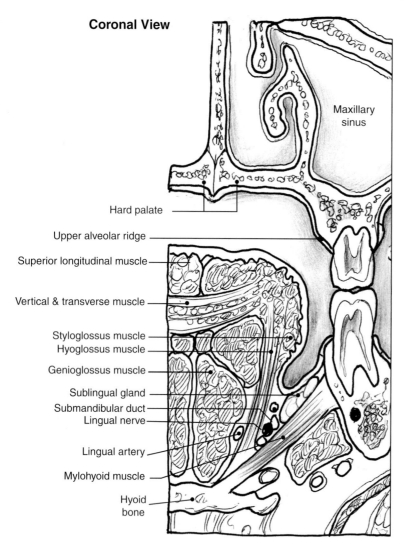

Maxillary sinus

Hard palate

Upper alveolar ridge

Superior longitudinal muscle

Vertical & transverse muscle

Styloglossus muscle
Hyoglossus muscle

Genioglossus muscle

Sublingual gland
Submandibular duct
Lingual nerve

Lingual artery

Mylohyoid muscle

Hyoid bone

Figure 11–1 Cross-sectional anatomy of the oral tongue and floor of mouth (FOM) in the region of the molar teeth (coronal plane). The hyoglossus muscle separates the lingual artery from the lingual nerve and submandibular duct.

cancers registered in the National Cancer Data Base (NCDB).[4–6] Cancer involving the FOM ranks third behind the oral tongue and the lip in the SEER database and second in the NCDB, constituting 19.8% and 24.5% of the oral cancers registered, respectively (see **Table 5–1** in Chapter 5 for the method of calculation).[4–6] The incidence of oral tongue and FOM cancer is more than 1.5 times greater in the male African-American population than in Caucasian males, whereas the incidence is similar in the female African-American and Caucasian populations.[4] The rates of oral tongue and FOM cancer in white males are 2.25 and 2.55 times greater, respectively, than in white females. This disparity is larger between black males and black females, with black males developing oral tongue and FOM cancer 3.4 and 4.2 times more frequently, respectively, than black females.[4]

Although the median age at the time of diagnosis for both oral tongue and FOM cancers is 62 years, 4.7% of oral tongue cancers registered in the NCDB were diagnosed in individuals 35 years of age or less, whereas less than 1% of FOM cancer occurred in this age group.[6] When SEER program data from 1973 to 1984 were compared with

data from 1985 to 1997, the incidence of oral tongue cancer in individuals younger than 40 years of age increased 60%, whereas the incidence of head and neck cancer remained stable.[7] Adults 40 years of age or younger also make up an increasing proportion of the individuals treated for oral tongue cancer at M. D. Anderson Cancer Center (MDACC) and the University of Madrid.[8,9] Interestingly, nearly half of the patients in both of these retrospective case series had no significant history of tobacco or alcohol use.

Greater than 94% of the diagnosed cancers of the oral tongue and FOM are squamous cell carcinomas (SCCs). Minor salivary gland malignancies constitute 1% and 2% of tongue and FOM cancers, respectively, and verrucous carcinoma accounts for 1% of the cancers at both sites.[6]

Most patients diagnosed with SCC of the oral tongue or FOM report a history of frequent alcohol or tobacco use.[10] Extensive epidemiologic evidence exists to substantiate the relationship between tobacco and alcohol use and the subsequent development of oral cancer (see Chapter 1). The combined use of alcohol and tobacco increases the risk of head and neck cancer in a multiplicative manner, and

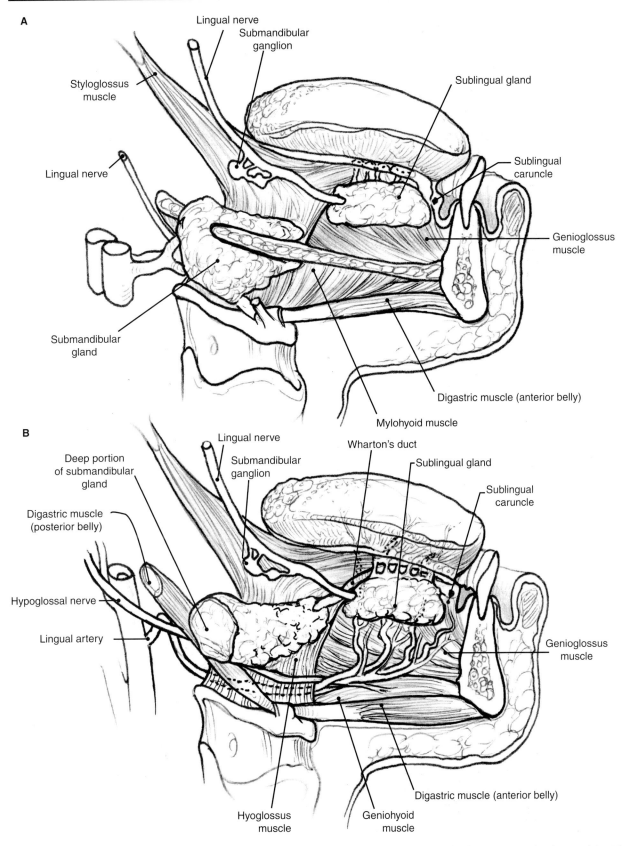

A

Lingual nerve

Submandibular ganglion

Styloglossus muscle

Sublingual gland

Lingual nerve

Sublingual caruncle

Genioglossus muscle

Submandibular gland

Digastric muscle (anterior belly)

Mylohyoid muscle

B

Deep portion of submandibular gland

Lingual nerve

Submandibular ganglion

Wharton's duct

Sublingual gland

Digastric muscle (posterior belly)

Sublingual caruncle

Hypoglossal nerve

Lingual artery

Genioglossus muscle

Digastric muscle (anterior belly)

Hyoglossus muscle

Geniohyoid muscle

Figure 11–2 **(A)** Lateral view of the FOM. The mylohyoid muscle, which lies deep to the genioglossus muscle, supports the FOM. The deep portion, or uncinate process, of the submandibular gland comes into close contact with the posterior sublingual glands on the superior surface of the mylohyoid muscle.

(B) Lateral view of the FOM with the mylohyoid muscle removed. The hyoglossus provides support for the posterior FOM. The lingual nerve, hypoglossal nerve, and Wharton's duct travel superficial to the hyoglossus, whereas the lingual artery lies deep to this muscle.

heavy smokers with high volumes of alcohol intake have a relative risk of more than 20 times that of individuals who do not use tobacco or alcohol.[11,12]

◆ Natural History and Clinical Presentation

Sixty to seventy percent of oral tongue cancers arise from the lateral surface of the middle third of the tongue (**Fig. 11–3**), and 30 to 40% originate from the ventrolateral or anterior undersurface.[13] Carcinoma arising from the dorsum of the tongue is an uncommon but real entity that accounts for 3 to 5% of oral tongue cancers, and carcinoma can rarely originate from the dorsal midline.[14,15]

Early oral tongue cancers typically arise within regions of leukoplakia or erythroplakia and are frequently asymptomatic. Progressive growth eventually results in surface ulceration and muscular invasion, which cause pain and limitation of motion. Tumor extension can proceed into the floor of the mouth and lingual alveolar lining mucosa and gingiva with underlying mandibular involvement. Growth can also occur posteriorly into the base of tongue, glossotonsillar sulcus, and anterior tonsillar pillar region. Extensive submucosal muscular invasion can occur in the absence of overlying mucosal abnormalities. Significant impairment of mobility may result from invasion of the deep or extrinsic tongue muscles, which include the genioglossus, hyoglossus, palatoglossus, and styloglossus. Physical examination should include close inspection of the surrounding mucosal surface and palpation to determine the extent of muscular involvement.

Similarly, FOM cancers are often asymptomatic until submucosal invasion or ulceration occurs. Approximately 80% of FOM cancers arise in the anterior FOM, and extension onto the lingual gingiva occurs in 15% of lesions less than 4 cm in size.[16,17] Contiguous involvement of the undersurface of the tongue progresses in an unhindered fashion, and involvement of the deep tongue musculature can develop with subsequent impairment in mobility. Once again,

careful inspection and palpation are necessary to quantify the extent of tumor involvement. The presence of periosteal or mandibular invasion can be assessed by using bimanual palpation to determine the mobility of the lingual alveolar mucosa, but this examination technique is frequently difficult to perform in the presence of painful, bulky tumors (**Fig. 11–4**). Radiographic evaluation must be combined with clinical examination to accurately detect the presence of mandibular invasion in most cases.[18] Mandibular invasion is reviewed in depth in Chapter 12.

Radiographic evaluation with computed tomography (CT) or magnetic resonance (MRI) provides important complementary information that impacts staging and therapy. Contrast-enhanced CT can be used to determine the extent of submucosal and muscular invasion, and bone algorithms are helpful in determining the presence of mandibular invasion. MRI detects perineural spread with greater sensitivity than CT, facilitates the detection of marrow replacement, and characterizes the extent and pattern of muscular invasion in greater detail than CT scan. The fibrous lingual septum, which vertically bisects the tongue, is seen as a hypodense midline structure on CT scan and has been referred to as the midline low-density plane.[3] The largely fat-filled sublingual compartment of the submandibular space, or sublingual space, is also hypodense on CT and is termed the *lateral low-density plane*.[3] Qualitative changes in these landmarks are useful for the assessment of tumor extension across the midline of the tongue and into the sublingual space, respectively. Radiographic imaging is also utilized to evaluate for regional nodal metastasis as an integral aspect of the staging workup.

Tumor staging for both sites corresponds to the criteria used for other oral cavity sites (see Chapter 7). Tongue and FOM lesions that invade through cortical bone, into the deep (extrinsic) tongue musculature (genioglossus, hyoglossus, palatoglossus, and styloglossus), or invade the skin of the face, are designated T4a lesions.[1] Superficial mandibular bone erosion is not sufficient to apply the T4 designation.[1] Internal carotid artery encasement resulting from contiguous tumor growth through the FOM into the neck is

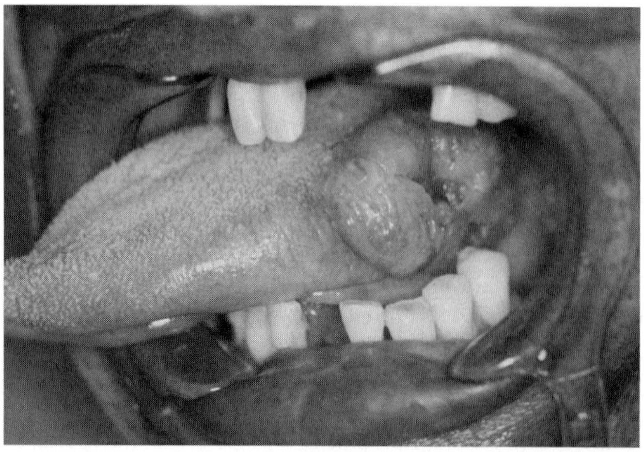

Figure 11–3 Squamous carcinoma arising from the posterolateral surface of the oral tongue.

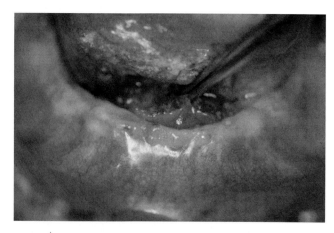

Figure 11–4 Anterior FOM tumor that extends up to the lingual mucogingival junction. The anterior portion of the tumor can be lifted away from the mandible with a forceps, and the lesion was not fixed to the mandible on bimanual palpation.

considered a T4b lesion. Invasion of the masticator space, pterygoid plates, and skull base are unusual manifestations of cancer arising from these areas that would result in the T4b designation.[1]

At the time of presentation, the T-stage distribution for oral tongue cancer is as follows: T1, 15 to 38%; T2, 36 to 53%; T3, 22 to 26%; T4, 4%.[19,20] The clinical N-stage distribution is as follows: N0, 75%; N1, 16%; N2, 6%; N3, 3%.[20] The clinical stage distribution is as follows: I, 37%; II, 28%; III, 24%; IV, 11%.[20] Overall, approximately 45% of patients with oral tongue cancer are pathologically node-positive, and 38% of these patients have extracapsular spread.[19]

The T-stage distribution of patients with FOM cancer at initial presentation is as follows: T1, 30 to 33%; T2, 32 to 37%; T3, 11 to 19%; T4, 14 to 23%. The N stage on presentation has been reported to be as follows: N0, 59 to 62%; N1, 23 to 24%; N2, 6 to 13%; N3, 2 to 11%. The stage distribution is as follows: I, 27 to 30%, II, 21 to 22%; III, 17 to 26%; IV, 25 to 31%.[21,22]

Occult nodal metastases (ONM) in patients with either oral tongue or FOM cancer most commonly occur in lymph node levels I and II. The rate of ONM in patients with oral tongue cancer by lymph node level is as follows: I, 14%; II, 19%; III, 16%; IV, 3%; V, 0%.[23] The frequency of ONM in patients with FOM cancer by lymph node level is as follows: I, 16%; II, 12%; III, 7%; IV, 2%; V, 0%.[23] Level IB metastases predominantly involve the prevascular or retrovascular nodes.[24,25] In clinically node-positive necks, the rate of nodal metastatic disease exceeds 30% in lymph node levels I through III for both oral tongue and FOM cancers.[23] Level IV contains metastatic disease in 21% and 12% of oral tongue and FOM cancers, respectively. Level V metastatic disease typically occurs only in the presence of nodal disease at other levels in less than 10% of clinically positive necks.[23] An increased risk of contralateral metastasis is associated with advanced T stage,

poorly differentiated lesions, multiple ipsilateral nodal metastases, FOM carcinoma, and tumors that extend to within 1 cm of the midline.[26,27]

"Skip metastases," which are metastases to levels IIB, III, or IV in the absence of level I or IIA metastases, were noted Byers and colleagues[28] in 16% of patients with oral tongue cancer. Other investigators have also documented the existence of skip metastases in patients with oral tongue cancer as well as oral cancer originating from other sites.[29,30] Although it is possible that skip metastases are due to histopathologic sampling error during evaluation of the neck dissection specimen, their existence should be acknowledged until more conclusive data from prospective sentinel lymphadenectomy research that evaluates the patterns of nodal metastasis from squamous cell carcinoma are available. The need for level IV dissection in patients with a clinically negative neck is controversial. Investigators who have found a 7% rate of skip metastases in level IV are strong advocates of level IV dissection, whereas others have documented a 4% rate of ONM in the clinically node-negative neck, leading them to conclude that removal of level IV is unnecessary.[28,31] Level IV dissection should be performed in the clinically positive neck, because the rate of level IV nodal disease in this case is 15%.[23]

Regional nodal metastases from oral tongue and FOM cancer have been associated with T stage, pattern of invasion, angiolymphatic invasion, perineural invasion, and degree of tumor differentiation.[25,32–37] Tumor thickness and depth of invasion, however, appear to be the best predictors of nodal metastatic disease (**Table 11–1**).[33,38–44] But attempts to define the tumor thickness or depth of invasion that requires treatment of the neck remain elusive. Two investigations documented regional metastatic rates of less than 20% when depth of tumor invasion was as great as 5 mm, whereas two other publications demonstrate metastatic rates of greater than 20%

Table 11–1   Relationship Between Tumor Thickness* (TT) or Depth of Invasion[†] (DI) and Occult Nodal Metastasis (ONM) in Patients with Cancer of the Oral Tongue or Floor of Mouth

First Author	Parameter Measured		Rate of ONM (%) when TT/DI is:	
	TT (mm)	DI (mm)	Shallower	Deeper
Oral tongue				
Spiro[38]	2		2[‡]	45[‡]
Yuen[39]	3		8	44
Byers[33]		4 (well)[§]	14	24
		4 (mod)[§]	29	43
		4 (poor)[§]	49	64
Kurokawa[40]		4	3	37
Fakih[43]		4	14	73
Fukano[41]		5	6	65
O-charoenrat[42]		5	16	64
Floor of mouth				
Mohit-Tabatabai[44]	1.5		2	33
Spiro[38]	2		2[‡]	45[‡]

*Tumor thickness is the measured thickness from the surface of the tumor using an optical micrometer.
[†]Depth of invasion is the measured thickness from the surface of the normal mucosa to the deepest portion of the tumor using an optical micrometer.
[‡]The results for oral tongue and floor of mouth were not analyzed separately.
[§]A logistic regression model was utilized to predict the risk of cervical metastases by accounting for clinical N stage, tumor differentiation (well = well differentiated; mod = moderately differentiated; poor = poorly differentiated) and depth of muscle invasion.

with a tumor thickness of only 2 mm.[38,41,42,44] Until further investigation clarifies this relationship, the risk of regional metastases should be considered significant for any lesion that exceeds 2 mm in thickness. The association between depth of invasion, tumor thickness, and regional metastatic disease is discussed at length in Chapter 14.

◆ Treatment

Surgical Approaches (That Improve Access)

Transoral resection of FOM and oral tongue cancer should be performed whenever circumferential tumor-free margins can be obtained with confidence. Frequently, however, transoral resection does not provide the access needed to resect bulky tumors of the oral tongue or tumors with significant extension into the posterior oral tongue or tongue base, FOM, or posterior mandibular alveolar ridge. A cheek flap that is elevated in the gingivobuccal sulcus can provide the access needed when posterior mandibular alveolar ridge or retromolar trigone resection is necessary. However, the mandible frequently precludes surgical access for the optimal resection of tumors of the oral tongue and FOM when the resection margin extends into the lingual alveolar sulcus or posterior oral tongue. Furthermore, performing a reconstruction of a large oral cavity defect that is housed within the confines of the oral cavity or oropharynx via a transoral approach can be inefficient and exasperating. In such cases, surgeons should consider performing either a mandibulotomy or a mandibular lingual releasing approach to improve their exposure. Both of these approaches provide excellent exposure and improve the surgeon's ability to resect malignancies in a three-dimensional fashion under direct visualization.

Mandibulotomy

In the past, resection of neoplasms of the posterior oral cavity and oropharynx was often achieved by resecting the mandible to give "adequate access."[45] The realization that mandibular resection was unnecessary in the absence of mandibular invasion led to the development of procedures that provided access without mandibular sacrifice. The mandibulotomy, popularized by Spiro and colleagues[46–48] at Memorial Sloan-Kettering Cancer Center (MSKCC), evolved into the procedure of choice to gain access whenever transoral resection was not feasible.

There are several considerations in the optimal performance of a mandibulotomy. Exposure for the mandibulotomy requires a lip-splitting incision. Originally, a straight midline incision was used that extended from the midline of the submental region through the soft tissues of the chin and through the midline of the lip. The straight midline chin-contour incision, a modification that was originally proposed by McGregor, courses around the chin pad and is now the most common incision used. This incision provides a superior aesthetic and functional result when compared with the straight midline incision.[49,50] Other modifications of this incision have been suggested to optimize the aesthetic outcome.[50]

Debate persists regarding the best location to perform the mandibular osteotomy. In situations where the mandible is going to be preserved, a lateral mandibulotomy posterior to the mental foramen is contraindicated, and the osteotomy should be performed anterior to the mental foramen so that lower lip sensation is preserved. However, the best location for a mandibular osteotomy placed anterior to the mental foramen remains unresolved. There are proponents of the midline mandibulotomy as well as of the paramedian or paramidline mandibulotomy. Those who advocate the paramedian mandibulotomy suggest that function is preserved because the procedure does not require division of the geniohyoid and genioglossus muscles.[51,52] Proponents of the midline mandibulotomy state that the paramedian osteotomy results in reliance on terminal branches of the contralateral inferior alveolar artery to vascularize the ipsilateral parasymphyseal mandibular segment.[53] The midline osteotomy also prevents irradiation of the osteotomy site, minimizing radiation-induced sequelae.[53] However, a comparison of midline and paramedian mandibulotomies demonstrated no difference in complication rates.[51]

Frequently, the extraction of a mandibular incisor facilitates the execution of an osteotomy, although a midline osteotomy can sometimes be performed without tooth extraction by using a thin osteotomy blade.[53] The unnecessary extraction of periodontally sound teeth should be avoided whenever feasible to optimize dental arch integrity and periodontal health. Some clinicians have converted from a midline osteotomy to a paramedian osteotomy between the lateral incisor and the canine because the roots of these two teeth diverge, facilitating mandibulotomy without dental extraction.[48] Plain film radiography has been used to quantify this relationship, confirming that the angle of divergence between the roots of the lateral incisor and canine was consistently greater than between the central incisors. Moreover, the horizontal distance between the canine and lateral incisor at the level of the alveolar crestal bone was greater than the horizontal distance between the central incisors.[52] Nevertheless, a tooth-sparing osteotomy should be cautiously considered, because the bony alveolar housing of two adjacent teeth can be mutilated by a poorly executed osteotomy.

The preferred type of osteotomy also remains a subject of debate. Osteotomies include the straight, stair-step, and notched osteotomies.[48,53,54] The stepped osteotomy was presumed to provide a broader surface for bony apposition and to minimize rotation at the osteotomy site.[54] Critics of this technique, however, point out that more bone is removed at the bone interface during the stair-step and notched osteotomies. Moreover, the use of rigid fixation with titanium plates affords greater stability than wire osteosynthesis, which was the primary method of fixation that was available when stair-stepped osteotomies were initially advocated. No comparative study exists to bolster the use of one osteotomy design over another.

Surgical Technique (Fig. 11–5). Typically, an apron incision that extends to the mid-submental region is performed that also provides exposure for performing an ipsilateral neck dissection. In situations where a neck dissection is not performed, the apron incision does not need to extend as

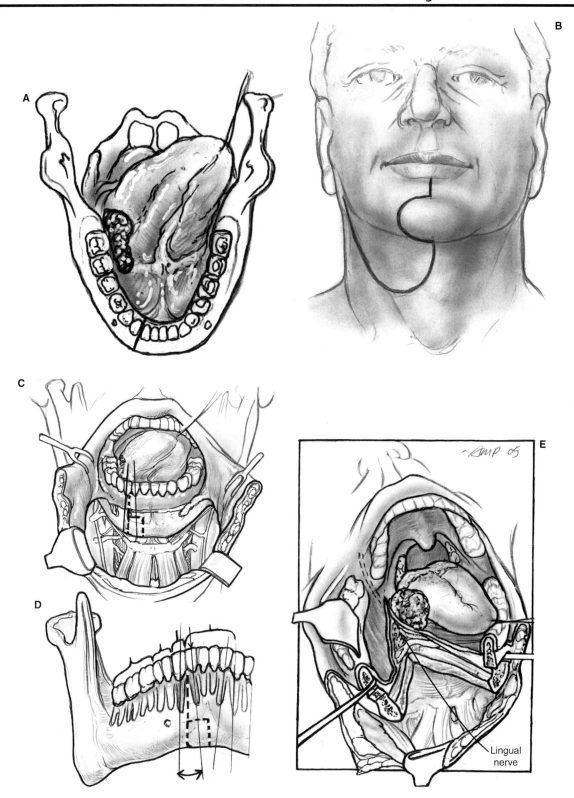

Figure 11–5 Mandibulotomy. **(A)** Tumor involving the lateral tongue and FOM that extends into the posterior oral cavity. A mandibulotomy will be performed to improve surgical access. **(B)** Apron incision extends to the submental crease and is connected to a straight midline chin-contour incision, which is used to split the lip at the midline. **(C)** The mucosal incision is extended into the labial vestibular sulcus, the mandibular periosteum is elevated, and a cheek flap is raised to the region of the planned osteotomy. The paramedian osteotomy is placed anterior to the mental foramen between the lateral incisor and the canine. The straight and stair-step osteotomies are depicted. **(D)** The angle of divergence between the mandibular lateral incisor and canine is greater than between the incisors. However, a tooth-sparing osteotomy should be considered only when adequate alveolar crestal bone exists to house both tooth roots following the osteotomy. **(E)** The mandible is lateralized and the soft tissues of the FOM are divided, preserving the lingual nerve whenever possible. Excellent access is gained by this approach to facilitate circumferential tumor resection and reconstruction.

far caudally unless the reconstructive phase requires such exposure. When bilateral neck dissections have been performed, a midline incision is created from the apron flap superiorly to the submental crease. The skin incision is continued superiorly from the mid-submental crease using a straight midline chin-contour incision that extends through the lip and into the depth of the labial alveolar sulcus, but an adequate cuff of alveolar mucosa should be left attached to the gingiva to facilitate incisional closure. The mucosal incision is then extended within the labial alveolar sulcus to the region of the mandible corresponding to the site of the mandibular osteotomy that is preferred by the surgeon. The periosteum is elevated in the region of the planned osteotomy in anticipation of placing the mandibular plate and performing the osteotomy. The cheek flap can be elevated by leaving a cuff of soft tissue over the mandible if tumor has invaded the labial cortical plate to ensure complete resection. Care is taken to preserve the mental nerve. The incision is then extended over the alveolar ridge into the lingual sulcus. If necessary, a tooth is extracted at the site of the planned osteotomy. A mandibular reconstruction plate is then fashioned to the shape of the mandible with at least three screw holes drilled on either side of the planned osteotomy. The osteotomy is then performed by using a sagittal saw. If a stair-step osteotomy is performed, the horizontal portion of the osteotomy must be at least 5 mm apical to the apices of the tooth roots to maintain pulpal viability.[55,56] An incision must be extended posteriorly within the lingual alveolar sulcus to allow for lateralization of the mandible to gain access for tumor resection. The lingual mucosal incision should be designed so that an adequate cuff of lining mucosa remains attached to the mandible to facilitate closure. Dissection is continued through the submucosal tissues, and the mylohyoid muscle must be divided to swing the mandible laterally so that tumor resection can be completed. The lingual nerve can frequently be preserved by dissecting the surrounding soft tissues away from the nerve so that the mandible can be swung laterally. The hypoglossal nerve is preserved unless its preservation would compromise the tumor resection. Preservation of the hypoglossal or lingual nerve may be facilitated by following the nerve from the submandibular triangle into the FOM and tongue.

Following tumor resection, the osteotomy is reapproximated by applying the previously contoured mandibular reconstruction plate. Although a single plate is typically adequate to reduce the osteotomy, a monocortical plate can be applied more superiorly to maximize immobilization and osteosynthesis. Closure of the lingual soft tissues is performed in multiple layers, and reapproximation of the suprahyoid musculature minimizes the risk of fistula formation. The cheek flap is closed in layers, carefully reconstructing the vermilion border and the patient's preoperative appearance.

Mandibular Lingual Releasing Approach

The mandibular lingual releasing approach is a technique that can be employed to improve surgical exposure without performing an osteotomy.[57,58] This approach is frequently less time-consuming than the mandibulotomy because a reconstruction plate is not required and there is no lip-splitting incision to close. The mandibular lingual releasing approach facilitates surgical resection and reconstruction by providing wide access to the posterior oral cavity and oropharynx.

Surgical Technique[57,58] **(Fig. 11–6).** A subplatysmal apron flap is elevated superiorly that extends to the inferior border of the mandible, exposing the soft tissues of the neck bilaterally. In most patients with large tumors of the oral tongue or FOM, the apron flap has already been performed to gain exposure so that bilateral neck dissections can be completed. After the submandibular and submental triangle contents have been removed, the suprahyoid musculature can be easily visualized. A mucosal incision is performed along the lingual vestibule of the FOM from first molar to first molar, ideally leaving a 1 cm cuff of lining mucosa attached to the lingual mucogingival junction to optimize closure of the FOM following tumor resection. Tumors that abut the mandible in the FOM may require extension of the incision onto the mucosa of the alveolar ridge to achieve an adequate tumor-free margin. If there are concerns about the relationship of the tumor to the mandible, these concerns may be more effectively addressed via performance of a mandibulotomy.

The mylohyoid, geniohyoid, and digastric muscles are divided bilaterally at their site of attachment to the mandible, and the tongue is freed from the lingual aspect of the mandible by division of the genioglossus muscle. The lingual and hypoglossal nerves, which were identified and preserved during the neck dissections, are preserved until their relationship to the tumor is clarified. The FOM incision is then connected to the dissection performed in the submental and submandibular regions, completely separating the tongue and involved FOM from the uninvolved mandible and lingual sulcular mucosa. A suture is passed through the body of the tongue, which is used to pull the tongue through the FOM into the submental region below the mandible. This approach usually provides transcervical access that extends posterior to the circumvallate papillae, facilitating extensive resections that extend into the base of the tongue (see **Fig. 11–7** on p. 107). Reconstruction of the resultant tongue and FOM defect typically requires the use of free tissue transfer, and this approach similarly simplifies transcervical reconstruction.

An incision through the lingual mucoperiosteum of the mandible in dentate patients and on the crest of the mandibular alveolar ridge in edentulous patients was previously advocated, but such an incision can increase the risk of mandibular exposure and devascularization.[58] A mucosal incision in the FOM is preferred unless attainment of an adequate mucosal margin requires extension onto the mucosa overlying the mandible. A mandibular lingual releasing incision in the lingual alveolar sulcus immediately adjacent to the mandible that leaves inadequate mucosa and submucosa for soft tissue reapproximation increases the risk of postoperative fistula formation and ablation of the lingual alveolar sulcus, which may consequently preclude functional rehabilitation with a removable denture.

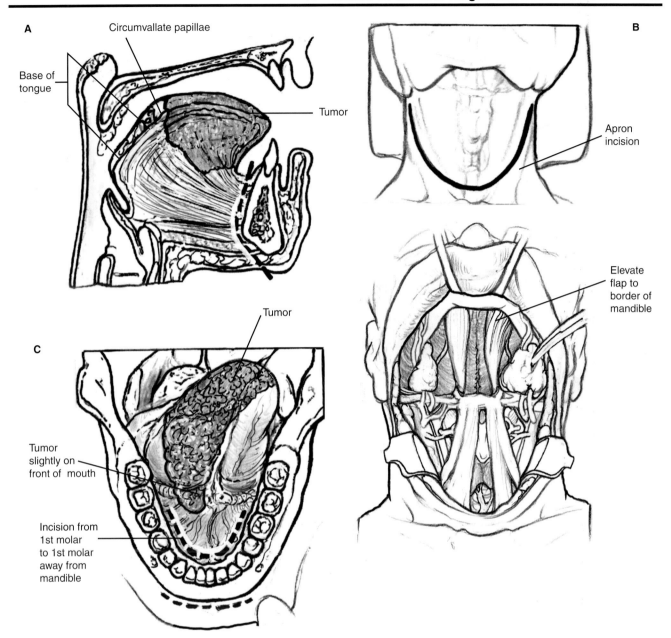

Figure 11–6 Mandibular lingual releasing approach (MLRA). **(A)** The transoral approach provides insufficient access to resect an extensive tumor that involves most of the oral tongue. The dashed line represents the planned path of entry into the FOM using the MLRA technique. **(B)** An apron flap is elevated to the inferior border of the mandible in a subplatysmal plane. **(C)** A mucosal incision is performed in the FOM from one first molar region to the other. Care must be taken to design an incision that widely resects the tumor. (*Continued*)

Surgical Considerations During Tumor Resection

The Management of Surgical Margins

Oral tongue and FOM cancers require careful resection, resulting in microscopically clear margins. Positive margins are associated with higher rates of local-regional recurrence and disease-specific mortality.[21,59–63] Frozen section analysis of surgical margins has an accuracy of 90% and can help to verify the adequacy of resection, particularly when the first set of margins are negative.[60,63] However, oral tongue cancer resections with initially positive frozen section margins that eventually become negative following additional tissue resection are associated with an increased rate of local recurrence and reduced survival.[64] Surgical resection through the oral tongue musculature is especially perilous, because cutting through regions of microscopic tumor foci can result in multifocal seeding as a result of muscle fiber retraction that is not amenable to re-resection that clears residual microscopic tumor foci with confidence. Mild to moderate epithelial dysplasia at the surgical margin has also been associated with an increased risk of local recurrence.[65] Consequently, concerted attempts to achieve negative surgical margins during the initial resection are paramount, and dysplasia-free margins should ideally be achieved, although field cancerization may thwart the attainment of dysplasia-free margins.

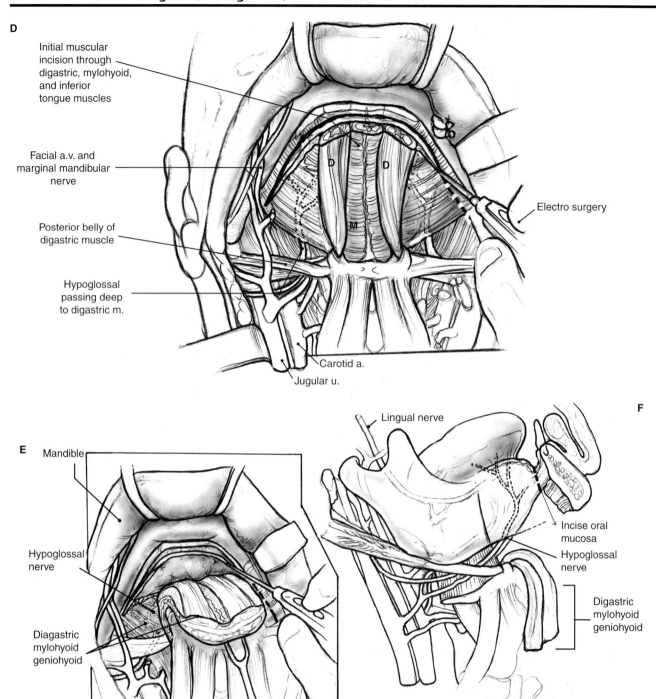

Figure 11–6 **(D)** The suprahyoid musculature is divided at the site of attachment to the mandible. The lingual and hypoglossal nerves on both sides are preserved until their relationship to the tumor can be evaluated. **(E)** Dissection is continued superiorly, connecting with the FOM mucosal incision. **(F)** Lateral view of the dissection following division of the suprahyoid musculature. A cuff of lining mucosa and soft tissue remains in the FOM to facilitate reconstruction following resection. Once access has been achieved into the FOM through the cervical region, the tongue and any attached FOM tissue can be pulled through this region so that tumor resection is possible (*arrow*). (*Continued*)

The attainment of initially negative margins, though, may not improve local-regional control or survival in the presence of close histologic margins. Looser and colleagues[66] from MSKCC observed that resection margins within 5 mm of the tumor were associated with a local recurrence rate of 73.7% and 5-year survival of 21%, figures that are comparable to those for patients with positive margins. Patients with marked atypia or carcinoma in situ at the margins also

G

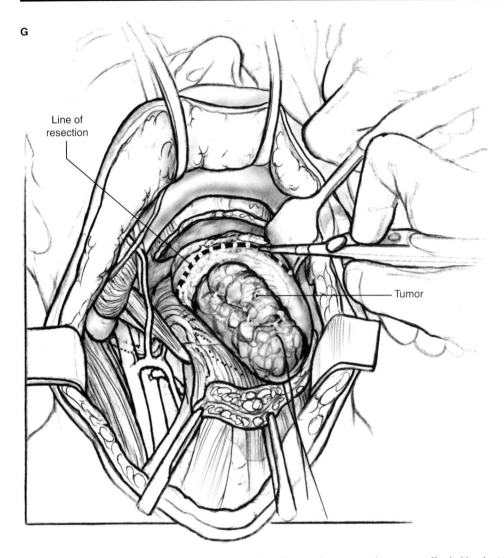

Line of resection

Tumor

Figure 11–6   (*Continued*) **(G)** The tumor is resected, exploiting the improved exposure afforded by the MLRA technique. Reconstruction is also facilitated by using this maneuver.

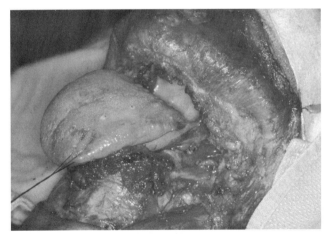

Figure 11–7   Surgical access that is achieved through the neck with the MLRA. The entire oral tongue is visualized, and resection can be extended into the base of tongue if indicated.

demonstrated higher rates of local recurrence than patients with negative margins of 5 mm or greater. This seminal work has shaped our present-day approach to head and neck cancer surgery, and several investigators have subsequently reconfirmed that margins of less than 5 mm have a worse prognosis.[59,67,68] If we assume that margin analysis was meticulously well-performed by both the surgeon and the pathologist, the explanation is most likely related to cellular abnormalities that are not appreciated on histologic examination. This assertion is supported by research performed at Johns Hopkins that found that if negative surgical margins contained p53 mutations specific for the primary tumor, the rate of local recurrence was significantly higher than negative surgical margins in which p53 mutations were not detected.[69]

Postoperative radiation therapy (RT), therefore, is indicated whenever resection margins of less than 5 mm are obtained.[61,68] Postoperative irradiation for oral cavity primary tumors results in local-regional control rates that are inferior to other head and neck primary sites, and the results of at least one investigation suggest that oral tongue cancers have worse outcomes than oral cancers arising from other sites.[70–73] Consequently, the importance of obtaining margins of at least 5 mm during oral cancer resection cannot be overemphasized. It is important to note that the width of the tumor-free margin frequently measures less during histopathologic assessment than the gross tumor-free margin that was obtained at the time of surgery. The adverse outcomes that are associated with close surgical margins have been largely derived from the evaluation of formalin-fixed, paraffin-embedded tissue. Johnson et al,[74] quantified the degree of shrinkage that occurs following the resection of oral cancers and found that the shrinkage resulting from electrosurgery, formalin fixation, and slide preparation is additive. Labiobuccal mucosal margins shrunk by more than 45% and tongue mucosal margins shrunk by an average of 30%. Deep tongue margins demonstrated a mean shrinkage of 35%, which means that a 7-mm pre-resection in-situ margin frequently results in a final margin of less than 5 mm, or a close surgical margin. Consequently, resection margins of at least 1 cm should be obtained to ensure that circumferentially negative final margins of greater than 5 mm are achieved to improve the rate of local-regional control.

In-Continuity and Discontinuous Neck Dissections

Historically, the principles of surgical resection for malignancies of the oral tongue and FOM evolved from Halsted's en bloc resective procedures for breast cancer. Ward and Robben[45] in 1951 advocated the performance of a composite operation that resected the mandible en bloc with the oral malignancy whenever the tumor extended "close to the lower jaw." Their rationale for this procedure derived from an anatomical study performed in 1902, which reported the presence of lymphatic vessels that traverse from the tongue and FOM through the mandibular periosteum and into the submandibular triangle.[75] This "anatomical fact" was challenged by researchers from Roswell Park Cancer Institute (Buffalo, NY) who found that no relationship existed between periosteal involvement and the development of cervical metastases.[76,77] The "pull-through" operation replaced the composite procedure as the preferred en bloc approach for tumors that were not fixed to the mandible. This technique, also referred to as an "in-continuity neck dissection," involves resection of the oral cancer primary, which is left attached to the neck dissection specimen and is subsequently "pulled through" the neck. The published outcomes of treatment for the pull-through operation have been mixed. Investigators from MSKCC failed to demonstrate a difference in local-regional control between in-continuity neck dissection and discontinuous primary tumor resection and cervical lymphadenectomy, whereas researchers from Amsterdam documented higher rates of regional recurrence and mortality following discontinuous resection.[78,79] Indeed, metastases to lingual lymph nodes in the superficial FOM have been demonstrated that may not be addressed by the discontinuous neck dissection.[80,81] In the absence of compelling evidence against discontinuous resection, however, the in-continuity neck dissection is infrequently performed in the United States.

Other Surgical Considerations

Marginal mandibulectomy is often necessary to ensure that a tumor-free margin is achieved when tumor extends onto the lingual alveolar ridge mucosa and whenever early mandibular cortical invasion is a possibility. The surgical techniques for marginal mandibulectomy are described in Chapter 12.

Resection of tumors involving the FOM that also require neck dissection frequently result in communication with the submandibular triangle despite mylohyoid muscle preservation. Following resection, the mylohyoid muscle should be retracted anteriorly to inspect for communications that must be properly addressed to prevent postoperative fistula formation. If a tension-free primary closure of the intraoral soft tissues is not feasible, a split-thickness skin graft may be used. For the skin graft to survive, however, a vascularized recipient bed must be constructed from the remaining soft tissues of the FOM and submandibular region by suturing the tissues together from the submandibular approach. An intraoral bolster dressing must be placed over the skin graft and a pressure dressing should be applied to the submandibular region following closure of the neck incision so that the skin graft is compressed between these two pressure dressings. Occasionally, inadequate lingual alveolar mucosa remains for suture placement. Spiro[82] has described a "transmandibular repair technique" for the closure of defects created by resection of sublingual gland cancers that can also be used in selected cases following resection FOM cancers in which inadequate lingual alveolar mucosa remains for suture placement. Horizontal mattress sutures are placed that pass through predrilled holes in the inferior mandibular body and through the remaining mucosa and soft tissues of the FOM and ventral tongue. These closure techniques, however, preclude the reestablishment of a new lingual vestibule, which is necessary if oral rehabilitation with a removable denture is desired. Tongue mobility can also become significantly impaired. Microvascular reconstruction should be considered in situations where appropriate closure of the FOM defect is not feasible.

Radiation Therapy Technique

Oral Tongue Cancer

T1–T2 Lesions. Comparison of overall treatment time is key to the successful treatment of oral tongue carcinomas with RT alone. Patients with well-differentiated carcinomas that are 4 mm or less in size are optimally treated with brachytherapy alone. Interstitial implantation may be accomplished using rigid cesium needles mounted in a bar or with iridium using the plastic tube technique. Rigid cesium needles mounted in a bar are difficult to position because of the length of the needles unless the lesion is relatively superficial. Therefore, the plastic tube technique is preferred. The total dose varies from 65 to 70 Gy over 5 to 7 days. Although intraoral cone RT has been used successfully to treat oral tongue cancers, it is often difficult to immobilize the lesion, so setup reproducibility may be problematic.

Patients who have poorly differentiated carcinomas, as well as those with 5 mm or more depth of invasion, should be treated with a combination of external beam RT (EBRT) and brachytherapy. Parallel-opposed fields include the primary tumor as well as the level I and II lymph nodes. A cork and tongue block displaces the tongue inferiorly and the maxilla superiorly to minimize the amount of normal tissue included in the portals (**Fig. 11–8**).[83] The fields are weighted 3:2 to the side of the tumor and either 30 Gy in 10 fractions once daily or 38.4 Gy at 1.6 Gy per fraction twice daily is delivered over 2 to 2.5 weeks with 4- or 6-MV x-rays. Although cobalt 60 (^{60}Co) is an ideal beam for treatment of patients with oral cavity cancers, it is not

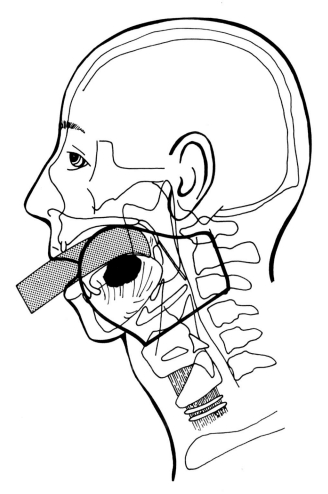

Figure 11–8 Example of portal for carcinoma of the oral tongue with an N0 neck. The field encompasses the submental, submandibular, and subdigastric lymph nodes; the sternocleidomastoid muscle plus 1 cm is included to ensure adequate posterior coverage of the subdigastric lymph nodes. The larynx is excluded from the radiation field. The anterior submental skin and subcutaneous tissues are shielded when possible to reduce submental edema and late fibrosis. The upper border is shaped to exclude part of the parotid gland. An intraoral lead block (*stippled area*) may be used in selected cases to shield the contralateral mucosa. The block is coated with beeswax to prevent a high-dose effect on the adjacent mucosa because of scattered low-energy electrons from the metal surface. An ipsilateral portal may be selected for superficial lesions; larger lesions are managed with parallel-opposed portals without an intraoral lead block. The lower neck is electively irradiated in all cases. (From Parsons JT, Mendenhall WM, Million RR. Radiotherapy of tumors of the oral cavity. In: Thawley SE, Panje WR, Batsakis JG, Lindberg RD, eds. Comprehensive Management of Head and Neck Tumors, 2nd ed, vol 1. Philadelphia: WB Saunders, 1999;695–719, with permission.)

available in most clinics. The level III and IV nodes are included in an anterior field as previously described. After EBRT, 35 to 40 Gy is added with an interstitial implant.

T3–T4 Lesions. Patients with T3–T4 oral tongue carcinomas are difficult to cure with RT alone. The ability to adequately encompass the primary tumor with an interstitial implant is difficult for all but the occasional patient with a favorable low volume T3 cancer. The risk of a major complication, such as a soft tissue or bone necrosis, is high after successful RT. Therefore, most patients are treated with surgery and postoperative RT. Dose depends on margin status: negative margins, 60 Gy in 30 fractions; microscopically positive margins, 66 Gy in 33 fractions; and gross residual disease, 70 Gy in 35 fractions. Patients with positive margins should be considered for treatment with an altered fractionation schedule, such as 74.4 Gy in 62 fractions over 6.5 weeks. RT portals are designed to include the primary tumor and both sides of the neck. The initial fields extend to the skull base to include the retropharyngeal nodes if the cervical nodes are involved. A Vaseline gauze bolus is placed on the incisions to ensure an adequate surface dose.

Patients with incompletely resected T3–T4 carcinomas have a poor prognosis and are treated with RT from 74.4 to 76.8 Gy at 1.2 Gy per fraction twice daily over 6.5 weeks with concomitant chemotherapy. Thereafter, patients are evaluated for resection of residual primary tumor (nidusectomy) versus an interstitial implant. Nidusectomy is preferred because of the high risk of necrosis associated with the addition of brachytherapy. Patients who have advanced, unfavorable oral tongue cancers and who are unsuitable for aggressive treatment are treated with palliative RT consisting of either 30 Gy in 10 fractions over 2 weeks or 20 Gy in two fractions with a 1-week interfraction interval.

Floor of Mouth Cancer

T1–T2 Lesions. Patients with superficial ($\leq$4 mm thick), well-differentiated squamous cell carcinoma of the FOM may be treated either with brachytherapy alone or intraoral cone RT. Brachytherapy is not feasible if the tumor abuts or extends onto the mandibular alveolar ridge because of the risk of bone exposure. Brachytherapy may be performed using either rigid cesium needles mounted in a customized template or iridium with the plastic tube technique. The rigid needles are preferable because, although the needles are active, the implant can be accomplished rapidly, as the needles are mounted in a rigid template (**Figs. 11–9 and 11–10**).[84,85] An additional advantage of this technique is that the geometry of the implant is optimal, and dosimetry can be obtained before the implant. The vertical needles are spaced approximately 1 cm apart with a crosser to ensure adequate surface dose. The implant is anchored in place by a suture placed through the submentum into the FOM.

Intraoral cone RT is administered with either orthovoltage x-rays or electrons. Orthovoltage x-rays are preferred because there is less beam constriction and the surface dose is higher. Before each treatment, it is necessary for the radiation oncologist to verify the position of the tumor

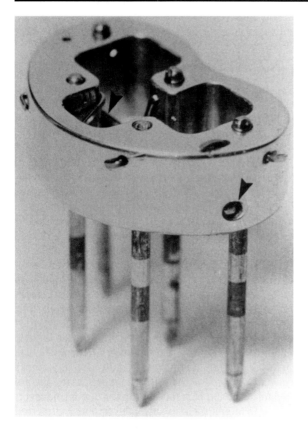

Figure 11–9   Custom-made implant device for stage T1–T2 cancers of FOM. Note single crossing needle through center of device (*arrowheads*). The device is now machined from nylon. Cesium needles have replaced the radium needles. (Modified from Marcus RB Jr, Million RR, Mitchell TA. A preloaded, custom-designed implantation device for stage T1–T2 carcinoma of the floor of mouth. Int J Radiat Oncol Biol Phys 1980;6:111, with permission.)

T3–T4 Lesions.   The likelihood of cure without a major complication after primary RT is low. Therefore, if patients are treated with curative intent, postoperative RT is combined with resection of the primary tumor and a neck dissection. The fields are similar to those described for patients treated with RT alone. The superior border of the field is extended to the skull base if there are multiple positive nodes or extracapsular extension. The portals are reduced off of the spinal cord at 44 to 46 Gy and, if necessary, the neck posterior to the reduced fields may be irradiated with 8 to 10 MeV electrons. A Vaseline gauze bolus is placed on the incision to ensure an adequate surface dose. The total dose depends on margin status: negative (R0), 60 Gy; microscopically positive (R1), 66 Gy; and gross residual disease (R2), 70 Gy. Patients were treated once daily at 2 Gy per fraction, 5 days a week, in a continuous course.

Altered fractionation should be considered for patients with positive margins and for those with a greater than 6-week interval between surgery and initiation of postoperative RT. The preferred schedule at the University of Florida is 74.4 Gy at 1.2 Gy per fraction administered twice daily in a continuous course over 6.5 weeks.

An occasional patient may present with an incompletely resectable tumor, usually because of fixed neck disease. In this event, RT precedes surgery in an effort to render the tumor resectable. Approximately 46 to 50 Gy is delivered to the primary tumor and both sides of the neck followed by a reduction and a boost to the area limiting resection to 60 to 70 Gy.

Patients with advanced disease and a remote chance of cure are treated with palliative intent. The dose fractionation schedules employed at the University of Florida are 20 Gy in two fractions with a 1-week interfraction interval or 30 Gy in 10 fractions over 2 weeks.

◆ Outcomes

Radiation Therapy

Low dose rate (LDR) interstitial brachytherapy has been assessed as the sole treatment to the primary site in oral tongue and FOM cancer. Lefebvre et al,[88] reported an 18% rate of local failure for 341 T1–T3 oral tongue cancers treated with 60 to 70 Gy of iridium 192 (^{192}Ir) brachytherapy administered over 4 to 8 days. Local control was 98% for T1 lesions and 89% for T2 lesions. The Curie Institute of Paris reported 5-year local control rates of 86%, 78%, and 71% for T1–T3 lesions, respectively, following the treatment of 602 oral tongue cancers with radium interstitial therapy alone or in combination with EBRT.[89] Comparable local control rates for FOM cancer have been reported with LDR ^{192}Ir interstitial brachytherapy as definitive therapy at the primary site. Piedbois and colleagues[90] documented an 87% 3-year local control rate for 233 T1–T2 lesions of the oral tongue and FOM using ^{192}Ir implants with doses ranging from 55 to 75 Gy. The Gustave-Roussy Institute reported 5-year local control rates of 93% and 88% for T1 and T2 FOM lesions, respectively, by delivering 58 to 80 Gy ^{192}Ir interstitial therapy at a mean dose rate of 0.5 Gy/h for a mean duration of 135 hours.[16] Mazeron et al,[91] documented 5-year local

relative to the intraoral cone (see **Fig. 11–11** on p. 112).[86] Because a small volume of tissue is included in the intraoral cone field, the dose per fraction may be increased from 2.5 to 3.0 Gy once daily.

Cancers thicker than 4 mm and those that are poorly differentiated have an increased risk of subclinical disease in the regional nodes. The first echelon nodes for the FOM are the level I and level II nodes. EBRT is delivered with either 6- or 4-MV x-rays to parallel-opposed fields that encompass the primary tumor as well as the first echelon nodes. A cork is placed in the mouth to displace the maxilla and upper lip out of the fields (see **Fig. 11–12** on p. 112).[83] The external beam fields are treated to 46 Gy in 23 fractions once daily or 38.4 Gy at 1.6 Gy per fraction twice daily. Brachytherapy follows the EBRT if that is the technique selected to boost the tumor. If intraoral cone RT is selected to boost the tumor, it precedes the EBRT so the extent of the tumor can be optimally defined and because it may be difficult to place the cone after EBRT because of patient discomfort. The total dose ranges from 65 to 70 Gy.

The low neck is irradiated with an anterior field, using 6- or 4-MV x-rays to 50 Gy in 25 fractions or 40.5 Gy in 15 fractions. A tapered midline block is used to shield the larynx. The junction between the parallel-opposed fields and the low neck field is at the thyroid notch (see **Fig. 11–13** on p. 113).[87]

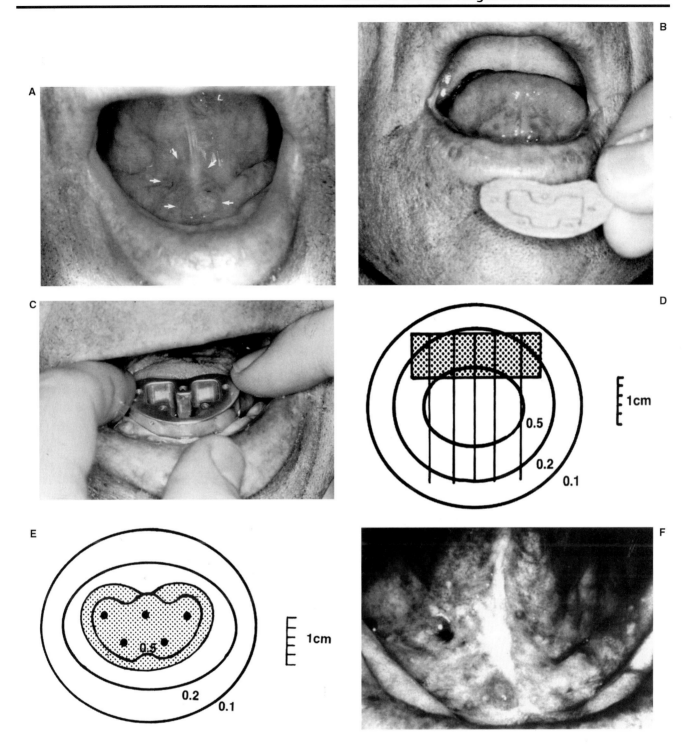

Figure 11–10 Squamous cell carcinoma of the FOM (T2N0). **(A)** The lesion (*arrows*) measured 2.5 × 2.5 cm, including the induration, and was tethered to the periosteum in the midline. The treatment plan was 50 Gy over 5 weeks with parallel-opposed portals that included the submaxillary and subdigastric lymph nodes. The midjugular lymph nodes were treated with an anterior portal. An implant was planned to add 15 Gy. **(B)** Cardboard template used for design of radium needle holder. **(C)** Implant in position. Device was secured with two sutures from the submental skin. There were five 2--cm-active-length, full-intensity needles without crossing. **(D)** Sagittal isodose distribution. The 0.5-Gy/h isodose line was selected for specification at dose, and the implant remained in place for hours. *Stippled area* represents the implant device. **(E)** Midplane isodose distribution. The 0.5-Gy/h isodose line is approximately 1 mm outside the needles. The highest dose rate to the anterior lingual gingiva would be about 0.30 to 0.35/h or at least 4.50 Gy lower than the minimum tumor dose. **(F)** Patient was free of disease at 4 years 8 months with no complications. (From Million RR, Cassisi NJ, Mancuso AA. Oral cavity. In: Million RR, Cassisi NJ, eds. Management of Head and Neck Cancer: A Multidisciplinary Approach, 2nd ed. Philadelphia: JB Lippincott, 1994:321–400, with permission.)

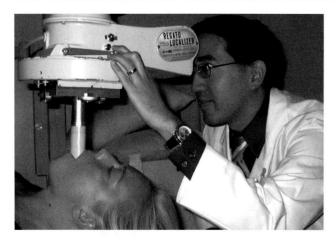

Figure 11–11 The position of the lead cone used for orthovoltage intraoral therapy is checked daily by physician. A good localizer, such as the one shown, is essential for final positioning.

control rates of 93.5% and 71% for T1 and T2 FOM lesions, respectively, with ^{192}Ir therapy. Extension onto the lingual gingiva resulted in a statistically significant reduction in local control, with a 50% local failure rate. Similar findings have been noted with gold 198 (^{198}Au) interstitial therapy, in which local control decreased from 82% to 55% for FOM lesions with gingival involvement.[92]

The local control rates achieved with brachytherapy have been evaluated against brachytherapy in combination with EBRT. Pernot and colleagues[93] reviewed the outcomes of 448 oral tongue cancers treated exclusively by irradiation with either ^{192}Ir or EBRT 2.0 Gy/fraction 5 days a week to a total dose of 40 to 50 Gy followed by interstitial brachytherapy, and found that brachytherapy resulted in a 5-year local control rate of 90% versus a local control rate of 50% with combination therapy for T2 lesions. These investigators also reported the outcomes of 207 FOM cancers with similar findings. Five-year local control was 97% and 72% for T1 and T2 lesions, respectively. Tumors with extension onto the lingual gingiva were not evaluated, eliminating its

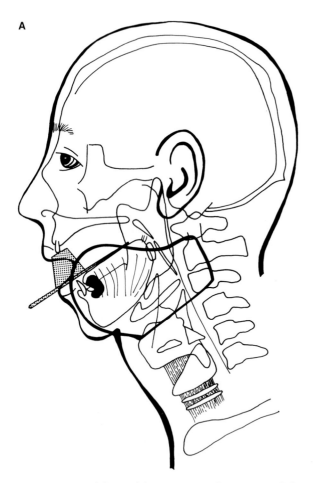

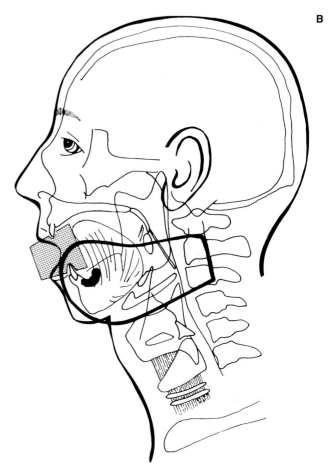

Figure 11–12 (A) Portal for treatment of carcinoma of the FOM with tongue invasion; the tongue is depressed into the FOM with a tongue blade and cork. **(B)** Portal for irradiation of limited anterior FOM carcinoma without tongue invasion. Two notches are cut on a cork so it can be held in the same position between the patient's upper and lower incisors during every treatment session; the tip of the tongue is displaced from the treatment field. The anterior border of the field covers the full thickness of the mandibular arch. The lower field edge is at the thyroid cartilage, ensuring adequate coverage of the submandibular lymph nodes. The superior border is shaped so that much of the oral cavity, oropharynx, and parotid glands are out of the portal. The minimum tumor dose is specified at the primary site (i.e., not along the central axis of the portal) with the aid of computer dosimetry. (From Parsons JT, Mendenhall EM, Moore GJ, Million RR. Radiotherapy of tumors of the oral cavity. In: Thawley SE, Panje WR, Batsakis JG, Lindberg RD, eds. Comprehensive Management of Head and Neck Tumors, 2nd ed. Philadelphia: WB Saunders, 1999:695–719, with permission.)

A   B

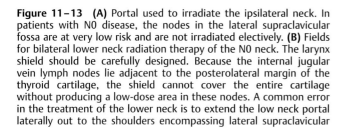

Figure 11–13 **(A)** Portal used to irradiate the ipsilateral neck. In patients with N0 disease, the nodes in the lateral supraclavicular fossa are at very low risk and are not irradiated electively. **(B)** Fields for bilateral lower neck radiation therapy of the N0 neck. The larynx shield should be carefully designed. Because the internal jugular vein lymph nodes lie adjacent to the posterolateral margin of the thyroid cartilage, the shield cannot cover the entire cartilage without producing a low-dose area in these nodes. A common error in the treatment of the lower neck is to extend the low neck portal laterally out to the shoulders encompassing lateral supraclavicular lymph nodes that are at negligible risk while partially shielding the high-risk midjugular lymph nodes with a large rectangular laryngeal block. The inferior extent of the shield is at the cricoid cartilage or first or second tracheal ring; the shield must be tapered because the nodes tend to lie closer to the midline as the lower neck is approached. TSD, target-to-skin distance. (From Parsons JT, Mendenhall WM, Million RR. Radiotherapy of tumors of the oropharynx. In: Thawley SE, Panje WR, Batsakis JG, Lindberg RD, eds. Comprehensive Management of Head and Neck Tumors, 2nd ed. Philadelphia: WB Saunders, 1999:861–875, with permission.)

role as a potential confounder.[17] Other retrospective investigations have documented similar treatment outcomes.[94,95] At the MDACC, the local control rate improved from 65 to 92% when higher interstitial doses and lower external doses were delivered.[96] Mendenhall et al,[95] found that local control of T2 lesions of the oral tongue and FOM was improved when a majority of the treatment dose was delivered by brachytherapy. Selection bias may have impacted the results of these retrospective studies, however. For example, Benk and co-investigators,[94] from Creteil, France, similarly found that brachytherapy was superior to external irradiation followed by brachytherapy in the management of T2 oral tongue cancers, but 74% of the tumors treated with interstitial therapy alone were less than 3 cm in size, whereas 68% of the lesions treated with EBRT and brachytherapy measured more than 3 cm. Moreover, treatment-selection bias was introduced into the University of Florida experience by inclusion of patients treated with a split-course technique.[95] A subsequent review of 42 T2 oral tongue cancers that excluded patients treated with the split-course technique, however, confirmed that local control was significantly better when ≥35 Gy was delivered via the implant.[97]

The efficacy of high dose rate (HDR) interstitial brachytherapy has also been assessed in the management of oral tongue cancer.[98,99] Investigators from Osaka University evaluated 51 patients with T1 or T2 oral tongue cancers that were randomized to treatment with either LDR using [192]Ir

implants to total doses of 65 to 75 Gy at a median dose rate of 0.60 Gy/h or HDR using ^{192}Ir with an after-loading system to a total dose of 60 Gy over 10 fractions at a median dose of 2.1 Gy/min.[98] Five-year local control rates for the LDR and HDR groups were 84% and 87%, respectively. The investigators subsequently evaluated T3 oral tongue cancers treated with either HDR or LDR, and demonstrated 3-year local control rates of 71% and 67%, respectively.[100] The HDR after-loading technique eliminates the risk of radiation exposure to medical staff and can result in a more homogeneous dose distribution by using computer optimization, but increasing dose rates have also been associated with higher rates of tissue necrosis.[99,101] Finally, Wang et al,[102] evaluated EBRT with intraoral cone RT as a boost to the primary site in place of interstitial brachytherapy in 66 patients with T1–T2 lesions of the oral tongue and FOM. Two-year local control for T1 and T2 oral tongue lesions was 77% and 82%, respectively, whereas local control for T1 and T2 FOM lesions was 92% and 95%, respectively.

The risk of soft tissue necrosis and osteoradionecrosis that can develop following definitive RT is not trivial. Mazeron et al[101] reported significant soft tissue necrosis and osteoradionecrosis in 24% and 14%, respectively, of the patients treated with RT. At the University of Florida, definitive RT for T2 oral tongue cancer resulted in a 33% complication rate, mostly soft tissue necrosis or bone exposure.[97] Similarly, management of FOM cancer by RT alone at the

University of Florida resulted in a 47% rate of complications, most of which were soft tissue necrosis or bone exposures.[103] Most of these complications were mild to moderate in nature, with severe soft tissue necrosis or bone exposure developing in only 9.5% and 6% of the patients treated for cancer of the oral tongue and FOM, respectively. This experience led to a shift in treatment philosophy at the University of Florida in 1985 from definitive RT alone to surgery alone or combined with RT based on clinical stage and pathologic findings.

Surgery

Surgical therapy for early-stage cancer achieves local control rates that are comparable to definitive RT. O'Brien and colleagues[104] in 1986 at the University of Alabama in Birmingham documented 2-year local control rates of 95% and 87% for T1 and T2 oral tongue lesions. Retrospective reviews of the MDACC experience with oral tongue and FOM cancer documented better local control with surgery than definitive RT, leading the authors to conclude that surgery was the best initial treatment.[105,106] Spiro et al,[107] reviewed the MSKCC experience with 105 cancers of the tongue and FOM in which surgery was the only treatment modality employed, noting a 12% local recurrence rate. The T-stage distribution of the cancers treated was as follows: T1, 46%; T2, 47%; T3, 7%. Each of these investigators concluded that surgery was the preferred treatment modality for early-stage cancer of the oral tongue or FOM.

Surgery and Radiation Therapy

Radiation therapy alone resulted in local control rates of 51 to 55% for T3 FOM cancers and 45% for T3 oral tongue cancers, leading radiation oncologists to advocate combined treatment with surgery and RT.[17,103,108] Surgical oncologists also realized that adjunctive RT was necessary to achieve superior rates of local control in cases with questionable margin status, and other pathologic findings from resection of the primary tumor that increased the risk of local-regional failure.[22,63,105] Furthermore, the growing body of evidence that demonstrated superior local-regional control and survival when postoperative radiation was employed led to a consensus that further solidified the role of surgery in combination with RT for stage III and IV disease.[68,109]

The use of postoperative ^{192}Ir brachytherapy for T1–T2 oral tongue and FOM cancers with close or positive margins has been investigated, achieving a 2-year local control rate of 89% and a disease-specific survival rate of 85%. Soft tissue necrosis or bone exposure developed in 28% of the treated cases that lasted a mean duration of 15 months.[110] Fein et al[108] compared RT alone with surgery alone or combined with RT for the treatment of oral tongue cancer. Although the 2-year local control rates were similar using either treatment modality for T1 or T2 lesions, 82% of T3 lesions treated with surgery alone or combined with RT were controlled, whereas only 45% of T3 lesions treated with RT alone were controlled at 2 years ($p = .03$). Surgery combined with RT also results in superior local control rates for T3–T4 FOM lesions.[103] Recently, the University of Florida updated its experience with external beam postoperative irradiation for 71 FOM tumors and 58 oral tongue cancers.[61] Indications for postoperative RT included T4 status, multiple positive nodes or extracapsular spread, perineural or vascular invasion, and margins that were positive, initially positive but negative after reexcision, close ($\leq$5 mm), or demonstrate dysplasia or carcinoma in situ. The 5-year local control rates were 84% and 85% for oral tongue and FOM cancer, respectively. This differs with the findings of Zelefsky et al,[73] from MSKCC, who noted 5-year local failure rates of 38% for oral tongue cancer versus 11% for FOM cancer treated with surgery and postoperative RT ($p = .02$). Altogether, these findings corroborate the conclusions of numerous other investigators that postoperative RT improves the rate of local-regional control and disease-specific survival for appropriately selected patients.[68,105,109,111]

Published Survival Rates

The published rates of 5-year disease-specific survival for patients with oral tongue cancer by stage are as follows: stage I, 63 to 90%; stage II, 72 to 82%; stage III, 54 to 74%; stage IV, 34 to 50%.[108,109] The published rates of 5-year disease-specific survival for patients with FOM cancer by stage are as follows: stage I, 88 to 95%; stage II, 80 to 86%; stage III, 66 to 82%; stage IV, 32 to 52%.[21,22]

Outcomes for Young Patients with Oral Tongue Cancer

The fate of younger patients with oral tongue cancer has been evaluated by several investigators. Clinicians from Tel Aviv University noted that oral tongue cancer was associated with worse 2-year disease-specific survival in patients younger than 45, leading them to conclude that oral tongue cancer appeared to follow a more aggressive course in younger individuals even though disease-specific survival at 5 years was similar.[112] Data from MDACC and the University of Madrid, however, showed that disease-specific survival following treatment was adversely impacted by advanced T stage, regional metastasis, surgical margins of less than 5 mm, and perineural invasion rather than the patient's age.[8,9] In fact, analysis of 749 oral tongue cancer patients from the SEER program tumor registry showed that the cohort of patients younger than 40 years old demonstrated the highest rate of disease-specific survival, and a 10-year increase in age was associated with an 18% increase in risk of death.[113] MSKCC data similarly failed to demonstrate a worse survival outcome for younger patients.[114]

◆ Verrucous Carcinoma

The NCDB reported the outcomes of 228 cases of verrucous carcinoma of the tongue and 60 additional cases involving the FOM.[115] Eleven percent of oral tongue lesions were stage III or IV at diagnosis, whereas 34% of FOM cancers were stage III or IV lesions. Surgical resection alone was used to treat 85% of the tongue lesions and 65% of the FOM cancers. Surgery in combination with RT was more frequently used for the treatment of FOM cancers because of the advanced stage of many of these cancers. The 5-year relative survival rate for oral tongue cancers was 75% and was similar to the survival rates for patients with alveolar ridge and buccal mucosal cancers. The outcomes of FOM cancers were not specifically addressed in this publication.

◆ Sublingual Gland Malignancies

The sublingual glands, which lie between the mucosa of the FOM and the mylohyoid muscle, are composed of a major sublingual gland and 8 to 30 minor sublingual glands. The deep portion of the submandibular gland, or the uncinate process, comes into close contact with the posterior sublingual glands on the superior surface of the mylohyoid muscle (**Fig. 11–2**). Malignant neoplasms of the sublingual glands make up 1.5% of all major salivary gland malignancies.[116] Between 80 and 90% of sublingual neoplasms are malignant.[117] The median age at the time of diagnosis is 59, and these neoplasms frequently present as an asymptomatic swelling in the FOM.[82] Adenoid cystic carcinoma is the most commonly diagnosed malignancy, followed by mucoepidermoid carcinoma.[82] The rate of regional metastasis has not been characterized because of their rarity, so management of the neck must be extrapolated from our experience with FOM squamous carcinoma and other salivary gland malignancies. Surgery is the treatment of choice, which should include wide local resection and neck dissection if deemed appropriate.[118] Postoperative RT similarly should be considered in cases with close margins, neural involvement, or nodal disease.

◆ Minor Salivary Gland Malignancies

Greater than 90% of the minor salivary gland neoplasms arising from these two oral cavity sites are malignant.[119–121] Cancers arising from the oral tongue and FOM make up 7 to 17% and 6 to 9%, respectively, of the minor salivary gland malignancies arising from the oral cavity.[119–121] The three most common histologic diagnoses at both anatomic sites are mucoepidermoid carcinoma, adenoid cystic carcinoma, and adenocarcinoma.[119–121] Survival data following treatment of oral tongue and FOM malignancies is scant and has been combined with the findings from other oral cavity sites. A detailed discussion of the management of these malignancies is presented in Chapter 13.

◆ Conclusion

Early-stage cancer of the oral tongue and FOM can be treated with either RT or surgery, whereas advanced malignant lesions are optimally treated by surgery and postoperative RT. Thorough preoperative clinical and radiographic evaluation is essential to evaluate the extent of soft tissue involvement and the presence of mandibular invasion, because these findings impact prognosis, surgical resection, surgical reconstruction, and the eventual functional outcome. Mandibulotomy or the mandibular lingual releasing approach should be considered whenever transoral access will compromise surgical resection or reconstruction. These diagnostic and treatment modalities should be exploited so that circumferential resection margins of greater than 5 mm are routinely achieved to minimize the need for postoperative RT and to maximize local-regional control and survival.

In most regions of the world, the oral tongue and FOM give rise to more than 50% of the cancerous lesions that are diagnosed in the oral cavity, providing us with the largest source of peer-reviewed literature pertaining to the natural history of oral cancer. Future prospective research that evaluates novel therapeutic strategies for the treatment of cancers involving these two regions will provide us with the best opportunity to improve treatment outcomes for malignant lesions originating from less common oral cavity locations.

References

1. Lip and oral cavity. In: Greene FL, Page DL, Fleming ID, eds. AJCC Cancer Staging Manual, 6th ed. New York: Springer-Verlag, 2002: 23–32
2. Squier CA, Hill MW. Oral mucosa. In: Ten Cate AR, ed. Oral Histology: Development, Structure, and Function, 4th ed. St. Louis: Mosby-Year Book, 1994:389–431
3. Smoker WRK. The oral cavity. In: Som PM, Curtin HD, eds. Head and Neck Imaging, 4th ed. St. Louis: Mosby, 2003:1377–1464
4. Canto MT, Devesa SS. Oral cavity and pharynx cancer incidence rates in the United States, 1975–1998. Oral Oncol 2002;38:610–617
5. Hoffman HT. The National Cancer Data Base Report on Cancer of the Head and Neck. Arch Otolaryngol Head Neck Surg 1998;124:951–962
6. Funk GF, Karnell LH, Robinson RA, Zhen WK, Trask DK, Hoffman HT. Presentation, treatment, and outcome of oral cavity cancer: a National Cancer Data Base report. Head Neck 2002;24:165–180
7. Schantz SP, Yu GP. Head and neck cancer incidence trends in young Americans, 1973–1997, with a special analysis for tongue cancer. Arch Otolaryngol Head Neck Surg 2002;128:268–274
8. Myers JN, Elkins T, Roberts D, Byers RM. Squamous cell carcinoma of the tongue in young adults: increasing incidence and factors that predict treatment outcomes. Otolaryngol Head Neck Surg 2000; 122:44–51
9. Martin-Granizo R, Rodriguez-Campo F, Naval L, Diaz Gonzalez FJ. Squamous cell carcinoma of the oral cavity in patients younger than 40 years. Otolaryngol Head Neck Surg 1997;117(3 pt 1): 268–275
10. Lewin F, Norell SE, Johansson H, et al. Smoking tobacco, oral snuff, and alcohol in the etiology of squamous cell carcinoma of the head and neck. Cancer 1998;82:1367–1375
11. Llewelyn J, Mitchell R. Smoking, alcohol and oral cancer in south east Scotland: a 10-year experience. Br J Oral Maxillofac Surg 1994;32: 146–152
12. Bundgaard T, Wildt J, Frydenberg M, Elbrond O, Nielsen JE. Case-control study of squamous cell cancer of the oral cavity in Denmark. Cancer Causes Control 1995;6:57–67
13. Mashberg A, Meyers H. Anatomical site and size of 222 early asymptomatic oral squamous cell carcinomas: a continuing prospective study of oral cancer. II. Cancer 1976;37:2149–2157
14. Goldenberg D, Ardekian L, Rachmiel A, Peled M, Joachims HZ, Laufer D. Carcinoma of the dorsum of the tongue. Head Neck 2000;22:190–194

15. Pogrel MA, Weldon LL. Carcinoma arising in erosive lichen planus in the midline of the dorsum of the tongue. Oral Surg Oral Med Oral Pathol 1983;55:62–66

16. Marsiglia H, Haie-Meder C, Sasso G, Mamelle G, Gerbaulet A. Brachytherapy for T1–T2 floor-of-the-mouth cancers: the Gustave-Roussy Institute experience. Int J Radiat Oncol Biol Phys 2002;52:1257–1263

17. Pernot M, Hoffstetter S, Peiffert D, et al. Epidermoid carcinomas of the floor of mouth treated by exclusive irradiation: statistical study of a series of 207 cases. Radiother Oncol 1995;35:177–185

18. Brown JS, Lewis-Jones H. Evidence for imaging the mandible in the management of oral squamous cell carcinoma: a review. Br J Oral Maxillofac Surg 2001;39:411–418

19. Myers JN, Greenberg JS, Mo V, Roberts D. Extracapsular spread: a significant predictor of treatment failure in patients with squamous cell carcinoma of the tongue. Cancer 2001;92:3030–3036

20. Callery CD, Spiro RH, Strong EW. Changing trends in the management of squamous carcinoma of the tongue. Am J Surg 1984;148:449–454

21. Hicks WL Jr, Loree TR, Garcia RI, et al. Squamous cell carcinoma of the floor of mouth: a 20-year review. Head Neck 1997;19:400–405

22. Shaha AR, Spiro RH, Shah JP, Strong EW. Squamous carcinoma of the floor of the mouth. Am J Surg 1984;148:455–459

23. Shah JP, Candela FC, Poddar AK. The patterns of cervical lymph node metastases from squamous carcinoma of the oral cavity. Cancer 1990;66:109–113

24. Lim YC, Kim JW, Koh YW, et al. Perivascular-submandibular lymph node metastasis in squamous cell carcinoma of the tongue and floor of mouth. Eur J Surg Oncol 2004;30:692–698

25. DiNardo LJ. Lymphatics of the submandibular space: an anatomic, clinical, and pathologic study with applications to floor-of-mouth carcinoma. Laryngoscope 1998;108:206–214

26. Kurita H, Koike T, Narikawa JN, et al. Clinical predictors for contralateral neck lymph node metastasis from unilateral squamous cell carcinoma in the oral cavity. Oral Oncol 2004;40:898–903

27. Kowalski LP, Bagietto R, Lara JR, Santos RL, Tagawa EK, Santos IR. Factors influencing contralateral lymph node metastasis from oral carcinoma. Head Neck 1999;21:104–110

28. Byers RM, Weber RS, Andrews T, McGill D, Kare R, Wolf P. Frequency and therapeutic implications of "skip metastases" in the neck from squamous carcinoma of the oral tongue. Head Neck 1997;19:14–19

29. Crean SJ, Hoffman A, Potts J, Fardy MJ. Reduction of occult metastatic disease by extension of the supraomohyoid neck dissection to include level IV. Head Neck 2003;25:758–762

30. Woolgar JA. Detailed topography of cervical lymph-note metastases from oral squamous cell carcinoma. Int J Oral Maxillofac Surg 1997;26:3–9

31. Khafif A, Lopez-Garza JR, Medina JE. Is dissection of level IV necessary in patients with T1–T3 N0 tongue cancer? Laryngoscope 2001;111:1088–1090

32. Sparano A, Weinstein G, Chalian A, Yodul M, Weber R. Multivariate predictors of occult neck metastasis in early oral tongue cancer. Otolaryngol Head Neck Surg 2004;131:472–476

33. Byers RM, El-Naggar AK, Lee YY, et al. Can we detect or predict the presence of occult nodal metastasis in patients with squamous carcinoma of the oral tongue? Head Neck 1998;20:138–144

34. Lindberg R. Distribution of cervical lymph node metastases from squamous cell carcinoma of the upper respiratory and digestive tracts. Cancer 1972;29:1446–1449

35. Hiratsuka H, Miyakawa A, Nakamori K, Kido Y, Sunakawa H, Kohama G. Multivariate analysis of occult lymph node metastasis as a prognostic indicator for patients with squamous cell carcinoma of the oral cavity. Cancer 1997;80:351–356

36. Bundgaard T, Rossen K, Henriksen SD, Charabi S, Sogaard H, Grau C. Histopathologic parameters in the evaluation of T1 squamous cell carcinomas of the oral cavity. Head Neck 2002;24:656–660

37. Umeda M, Yokoo S, Take Y, Omori A, Nakanishi K, Shimada K. Lymph node metastasis in squamous cell carcinoma of the oral cavity: correlation between histologic features and the prevalence of metastasis. Head Neck 1992;14:263–272

38. Spiro RH, Huvos AG, Wong GY, Spiro JD, Gnecco CA, Strong EW. Predictive value of tumor thickness in squamous carcinoma confined to the tongue and floor of the mouth. Am J Surg 1986;152:345–350

39. Yuen APW, Lam KY, Lam LK, et al. Prognostic factors of clinically stage I and II oral tongue carcinoma—a comparative study of stage, thickness, shape, growth pattern, invasive front malignancy grading, Martinez-Gimeno score, and pathologic features. Head Neck 2002;24:513–520

40. Kurokawa H, Yamashita Y, Takeda S, Zhang M, Fukuyama H, Takahashi T. Risk factors for late cervical lymph node metastases in patients with stage I or II carcinoma of the tongue. Head Neck 2002;24:731–736

41. Fukano H, Matsuura H, Hasegawa Y, Nakamura S. Depth of invasion as a predictive factor for cervical lymph node metastasis in tongue carcinoma. Head Neck 1997;19:205–210

42. O-charoenrat P, Pillai G, Patel S, et al. Tumour thickness predicts cervical nodal metastases and survival in early oral tongue cancer. Oral Oncol 2003;39:386–390

43. Fakih AR, Rao RS, Borges AM, Patel AR. Elective versus therapeutic neck dissection in early carcinoma of the oral tongue. Am J Surg 1989;158:309–313

44. Mohit-Tabatabai MA, Sobel HJ, Rush BF, Mashberg A. Relation of thickness of floor of mouth stage I and II cancers to regional metastasis. Am J Surg 1986;152:351–353

45. Ward GE, Robben JO. A composite operation for radical neck dissection and removal of cancer of the mouth. Cancer 1951;4:98–109

46. Spiro RH, Gerold FP, Shah JP, Sessions RB, Strong EW. Mandibulotomy approach to oropharyngeal tumors. Am J Surg 1985;150:466–469

47. Spiro RH, Gerold FP, Strong EW. Mandibular "swing" approach for oral and oropharyngeal tumors. Head Neck Surg 1981;3:371–378

48. Dubner S, Spiro RH. Median mandibulotomy: a critical assessment. Head Neck 1991;13:389–393

49. McGregor IA, MacDonald DG. Mandibular osteotomy in the surgical approach to the oral cavity. Head Neck Surg 1983;5:457–462

50. Rapidis AD, Valsamis S, Anterriotis DA, Skouteris CA. Functional and aesthetic results of various lip-splitting incisions: a clinical analysis of 60 cases. J Oral Maxillofac Surg 2001;59:1292–1296

51. Dai TS, Hao SP, Chang KP, Pan WL, Yeh HC, Tsang NM. Complications of mandibulotomy: midline versus paramidline. Otolaryngol Head Neck Surg 2003;128:137–141

52. Pan WL, Hao SP, Lin YS, Chang KP, Su JL. The anatomical basis for mandibulotomy: midline versus paramidline. Laryngoscope 2003;113:377–380

53. Amin MR, Deschler DG, Hayden RE. Straight midline mandibulotomy revisited. Laryngoscope 1999;109:1402–1405

54. Cohen JI, Marentette LJ, Maisel RH. The mandibular swing stabilization of the midline mandibular osteotomy. Laryngoscope 1988;98:1139–1142

55. Bell WH, Fonseca RJ, Kennedy JW, Levy BM. Bone healing and revascularization after total maxillary osteotomy. J Oral Surg 1975;33:253–260

56. Pepersack WJ. Tooth vitality after alveolar segmental osteotomy. J Maxillofac Surg 1973;1:85–91

57. Stanley RB. Mandibular lingual releasing approach to oral and oropharyngeal carcinomas. Laryngoscope 1984;94(5 pt 1):596–600

58. Stringer SP, Jordan JR, Mendenhall WM, Parsons JT, Cassisi NJ, Million RR. Mandibular lingual releasing approach. Otolaryngol Head Neck Surg 1992;107:395–398

59. Loree TR, Strong EW. Significance of positive margins in oral cavity squamous carcinoma. Am J Surg 1990;160:410–414

60. Byers RM, Bland KI, Borlase B, Luna M. The prognostic and therapeutic value of frozen section determinations in the surgical treatment of squamous carcinoma of the head and neck. Am J Surg 1978;136:525–528

61. Hinerman RW, Mendenhall WM, Morris CG, Amdur RJ, Werning JW, Villaret DB. Postoperative irradiation for squamous cell carcinoma of the oral cavity: 35-year experience. Head Neck 2004;26:984–994

62. Sessions DG, Spector GJ, Lenox J, Haughey B, Chao C, Marks J. Analysis of treatment results for oral tongue cancer. Laryngoscope 2002;112:616–625

63. Spiro RH, Guillamondegui O Jr, Paulino AF, Huvos AG. Pattern of invasion and margin assessment in patients with oral tongue cancer. Head Neck 1999;21:408–413

64. Scholl P, Byers RM, Batsakis JG, Wolf P, Santini H. Microscopic cut-through of cancer in the surgical treatment of squamous carcinoma of the tongue: prognostic and therapeutic implications. Am J Surg 1986;152:354–360

65. Weijers M, Snow GB, Bezemer PD, van der Wal JE, van der Waal I. The clinical relevance of epithelial dysplasia in the surgical margins of tongue and floor of mouth squamous cell carcinoma: an analysis of 37 patients. J Oral Pathol Med 2002;31:11–15

66. Looser KG, Shah JP, Strong EW. The significance of "positive" margins in surgically resected epidermoid carcinomas. Head Neck Surg 1978;1:107–111

67. Ravasz LA, Slootweg PJ, Hordijk GJ, Smit F, van der Tweel I. The status of the resection margin as a prognostic factor in the treatment of head and neck carcinoma. J Craniomaxillofac Surg 1991;19:314–318

68. Vikram B, Strong EW, Shah JP, Spiro R. Failure at distant sites following multimodality treatment for advanced head and neck cancer. Head Neck Surg 1984;6:730–733

69. Brennan JA, Mao L, Hruban RH, et al. Molecular assessment of histopathological staging in squamous-cell carcinoma of the head and neck. N Engl J Med 1995;332:429–435

70. Amdur RJ, Parsons JT, Mendenhall WM, Million RR, Stringer SP, Cassisi NJ. Postoperative irradiation for squamous cell carcinoma of the head and neck: an analysis of treatment results and complications. Int J Radiat Oncol Biol Phys 1989;16:25–36

71. Peters LJ, Goepfert H, Ang KK, et al. Evaluation of the dose for postoperative radiation therapy of head and neck cancer: first report of a prospective randomized trial. Int J Radiat Oncol Biol Phys 1993;26:3–11

72. Kramer S, Gelber RD, Snow JB, et al. Combined radiation therapy and surgery in the management of advanced head and neck cancer: final report of study 73–03 of the Radiation Therapy Oncology Group. Head Neck Surg 1987;10:19–30

73. Zelefsky MJ, Harrison LB, Fass DE, et al. Postoperative radiotherapy for oral cavity cancers: impact of anatomic subsite on treatment outcome. Head Neck 1990;12:470–475

74. Johnson RE, Sigman JD, Funk GF, Robinson RA, Hoffman HT. Quantification of surgical margin shrinkage in the oral cavity. Head Neck 1997;19:281–286

75. Polya AE, Navratil D. Unersuchungen uber die Lymphbahnen der Wangenschleimhaut. Dtsch Z Chir 1902;66:122–175

76. Marchetta FC, Sako K, Badillo J. Periosteal lymphatics of the mandible and intraoral carcinoma. Am J Surg 1964;108:505–507

77. Marchetta FC, Sako K, Murphy JB. The periosteum of the mandible and intraoral carcinoma. Am J Surg 1971;122:711–713

78. Spiro RH, Strong EW. Discontinuous partial glossectomy and radical neck dissection in selected patients with epidermoid carcinoma of the mobile tongue. Am J Surg 1973;126:544–546

79. Leemans CR, Tiwari R, Nauta JJ, Snow GB. Discontinuous vs in-continuity neck dissection in carcinoma of the oral cavity. Arch Otolaryngol Head Neck Surg 1991;117:1003–1006

80. Ozeki S, Tashiro H, Okamoto M, Matsushima T. Metastasis to the lingual lymph node in carcinoma of the tongue. J Maxillofac Surg 1985;13:277–281

81. Dutton JM, Graham SM, Hoffman HT. Metastatic cancer to the floor of mouth: the lingual lymph nodes. Head Neck 2002;24:401–405

82. Spiro RH. Treating tumors of the sublingual glands, including a useful technique for repair of the floor of the mouth after resection. Am J Surg 1995;170:457–460

83. Parsons JT, Mendenhall WM, Moore GJ, Million RR. Radiotherapy of tumors of the oral cavity. In: Thawley SE, Panje WR, Batsakis JG, Lindberg RD, eds. Comprehensive Management of Head and Neck Tumors, 2nd ed, vol 1. Philadelphia: WB Saunders, 1999:695–719

84. Marcus RB Jr, Million RR, Mitchell TP. A preloaded, custom-designed implantation device for stage T1–T2 carcinoma of the floor of mouth. Int J Radiat Oncol Biol Phys 1980;6:111–113

85. Million RR, Cassisi NJ, Mancuso AA. Oral cavity. In: Million RR, Cassisi NJ, eds. Management of Head and Neck Cancer: A Multidisciplinary Approach, 2nd ed. Philadelphia: JB Lippincott, 1994:321–400

86. Million RR, Cassisi NJ. General principles for treatment of cancers in the head and neck: radiation therapy. In: Million RR, Cassisi NJ, eds. Management of Head and Neck Cancer: A Multidisciplinary Approach. Philadelphia: Lippincott, 1984:77–90

87. Parsons JT, Mendenhall WM, Moore GJ, Million RR. Radiotherapy of tumors of the oropharynx. In: Thawley SE, Panje WR, Batsakis JG, Lindberg RD, eds. Comprehensive Management of Head and Neck Tumors, 2nd ed, vol 1. Philadelphia: WB Saunders, 1999:861–875

88. Lefebvre JL, Coche-Dequeant B, Castelain B, Prevost B, Buisset E, Ton Van J. Interstitial brachytherapy and early tongue squamous cell carcinoma management. Head Neck 1990;12:232–236

89. Decroix Y, Ghossein NA. Experience of the Curie Institute in treatment of cancer of the mobile tongue. II. Management of the neck nodes. Cancer 1981;47:503–508

90. Piedbois P, Mazeron JJ, Haddad E, et al. Stage I–II squamous cell carcinoma of the oral cavity treated by iridium-192: is elective neck dissection indicated? Radiother Oncol 1991;21:100–106

91. Mazeron JJ, Grimard L, Raynal M, et al. Iridium-192 curietherapy for T1 and T2 epidermoid carcinomas of the floor of mouth. Int J Radiat Oncol Biol Phys 1990;18:1299–1306

92. Matsumoto S, Takeda M, Shibuya H, Suzuki S. T1 and T2 squamous cell carcinomas of the floor of the mouth: results of brachytherapy mainly using 198Au grains. Int J Radiat Oncol Biol Phys 1996;34:833–841

93. Pernot M, Malissard L, Hoffstetter S, et al. The study of tumoral, radiobiological, and general health factors that influence results and complications in a series of 448 oral tongue carcinomas treated exclusively by irradiation. Int J Radiat Oncol Biol Phys 1994;29:673–679

94. Benk V, Mazeron JJ, Grimard L, et al. Comparison of curietherapy versus external irradiation combined with curietherapy in stage II squamous cell carcinomas of the mobile tongue. Radiother Oncol 1990;18:339–347

95. Mendenhall WM, Van Cise WS, Bova FJ, Million RR. Analysis of time-dose factors in squamous cell carcinoma of the oral tongue and floor of mouth treated with radiation therapy alone. Int J Radiat Oncol Biol Phys 1981;7:1005–1011

96. Ange DW, Lindberg RD, Guillamondegui OM. Management of squamous cell carcinoma of the oral tongue and floor of mouth after excisional biopsy. Radiology 1975;116:143–146

97. Mendenhall WM, Parsons JT, Stringer SP, Cassisi NJ, Million RR. T2 oral tongue carcinoma treated with radiotherapy: analysis of local control and complications. Radiother Oncol 1989;16:275–281

98. Inoue T, Yoshida K, Yoshioka Y, et al. Phase III trial of high- vs. low-dose-rate interstitial radiotherapy for early mobile tongue cancer. Int J Radiat Oncol Biol Phys 2001;51:171–175

99. Leung TW, Wong VY, Kwan KH, et al. High dose rate brachytherapy for early stage oral tongue cancer. Head Neck 2002;24:274–281

100. Kakimoto N, Inoue T, Murakami S, et al. Results of low- and high-dose-rate interstitial brachytherapy for T3 mobile tongue cancer. Radiother Oncol 2003;68:123–128

101. Mazeron JJ, Simon JM, Le Pechoux C, et al. Effect of dose rate on local control and complications in definitive irradiation of T1–2 squamous cell carcinomas of mobile tongue and floor of mouth with interstitial iridium-192. Radiother Oncol 1991;21:39–47

102. Wang CC, Doppke KP, Biggs PJ. Intra-oral cone radiation therapy for selected carcinomas of the oral cavity. Int J Radiat Oncol Biol Phys 1983;9:1185–1189

103. Rodgers LW Jr, Stringer SP, Mendenhall WM, Parsons JT, Cassisi NJ, Million RR. Management of squamous cell carcinoma of the floor of mouth. Head Neck 1993;15:16–19

104. O'Brien CJ, Lahr CJ, Soong SJ, et al. Surgical treatment of early-stage carcinoma of the oral tongue–wound adjuvant treatment be beneficial? Head Neck Surg 1986;8:401–408

105. White D, Byers RM. What is the preferred initial method of treatment for squamous carcinoma of the tongue? Am J Surg 1980;140:553–555

106. Guillamondegui OM, Oliver B, Hayden R. Cancer of the anterior floor of the mouth. Selective choice of treatment and analysis of failures. Am J Surg 1980;140:560–562

107. Spiro RH, Spiro JD, Strong EW. Surgical approach to squamous carcinoma confined to the tongue and the floor of the mouth. Head Neck Surg 1986;9:27–31

108. Fein DA, Mendenhall WM, Parsons JT, et al. Carcinoma of the oral tongue: a comparison of results and complications of treatment with radiotherapy and/or surgery. Head Neck 1994;16: 358–365

109. Franceschi D, Gupta R, Spiro RH, Shah JP. Improved survival in the treatment of squamous carcinoma of the oral tongue. Am J Surg 1993;166:360–365

110. Lapeyre M, Hoffstetter S, Peiffert D, et al. Postoperative brachytherapy alone for T1–2 N0 squamous cell carcinomas of the oral tongue and floor of mouth with close or positive margins. Int J Radiat Oncol Biol Phys 2000;48:37–42

111. Lydiatt DD, Robbins KT, Byers RM, Wolf PF. Treatment of stage I and II oral tongue cancer. Head Neck 1993;15:308–312

112. Popovtzer A, Shpitzer T, Bahar G, Marshak G, Ulanovski D, Feinmesser R. Squamous cell carcinoma of the oral tongue in young patients. Laryngoscope 2004;114:915–917

113. Davidson BJ, Root WA, Trock BJ. Age and survival from squamous cell carcinoma of the oral tongue. Head Neck 2001;23:273–279

114. Friedlander PL, Schantz SP, Shaha AR, Yu G, Shah JP. Squamous cell carcinoma of the tongue in young patients: a matched-pair analysis. Head Neck 1998;20:363–368

115. Koch BB, Trask DK, Hoffman HT, et al. National survey of head and neck verrucous carcinoma: patterns of presentation, care, and outcome. Cancer 2001;92:110–120

116. Spiro RH, Armstrong J, Harrison L, Geller NL, Lin SY, Strong EW. Carcinoma of major salivary glands. Recent trends. Arch Otolaryngol Head Neck Surg 1989;115:316–321

117. Eneroth CM. Salivary gland tumors in the parotid gland, submandibular gland, and the palate region. Cancer 1971;27:1415–1418

118. Rinaldo A, Shaha AR, Pellitteri PK, Bradley PJ, Ferlito A. Management of malignant sublingual salivary gland tumors. Oral Oncol 2004; 40:2–5

119. Spiro RH. Salivary neoplasms: overview of a 35-year experience with 2,807 patients. Head Neck Surg 1986;8:177–184

120. Waldron CA, el-Mofty SK, Gnepp DR. Tumors of the intraoral minor salivary glands: a demographic and histologic study of 426 cases. Oral Surg Oral Med Oral Pathol 1988;66:323–333

121. Eveson JW, Cawson RA. Tumours of the minor (oropharyngeal) salivary glands: a demographic study of 336 cases. J Oral Pathol 1985;14:500–509

12

Cancer of the Lower Alveolar Ridge and Retromolar Trigone

John W. Werning and
William M. Mendenhall

Malignant lesions that arise from the mucosa of the lower alveolar ridge and retromolar trigone often manifest aggressive patterns of tumor spread that lead to invasion of the underlying mandible and the surrounding soft tissues of the oral cavity and oropharynx. Failure to recognize transcortical bone invasion through the alveolar ridge or submucosal extension from the retromolar region into the masticatory musculature, cheek, or anterior tonsillar pillar can lead to suboptimal surgical resection and inferior rates of local-regional control and survival. These concerns have resulted in a plethora of investigative work that has critically evaluated our ability to clinically and radiographically discern various patterns of tumor invasion. Surgical approaches have also evolved to facilitate the resection of tumors that involve the posterior oral cavity and oropharynx, and the predictability of microvascular reconstruction allows surgeons to perform segmental mandibular resections without significantly impacting facial appearance and oromandibular function. Optimal management requires thoughtful pretreatment evaluation, aggressive surgical resection, careful surgical and prosthetic reconstruction, and judicious use of postoperative radiation therapy (RT). This chapter reviews the principles of, and rationale for, the evaluation and management of cancers originating from these two oral cavity sites.

The keratinized mucosa of the lower alveolar ridge (LAR) is intimately attached to the alveolar process of the mandible, giving rise to the term *attached mucosa*, or gingiva. This masticatory mucosa covers and protects the LAR and surrounds the mandibular teeth as a part of the periodontal apparatus. The junction between the epithelium and lamina propria is characterized by numerous deep papillary projections of connective tissue into the undersurface of the epithelium, contributing to the relative immobility of the masticatory mucosa. The lamina propria is firmly "attached" by bundles of collagen fibers to the underlying periosteum to form the mucoperiosteum. The embedded portions of these collagen fiber bundles, which extend from the lamina propria into the circumferential lamellae of the underlying bone, are termed *Sharpey's fibers*.[1] The gingiva of the LAR extends from the line of attachment at the mucogingival junction on the buccal surface of the alveolar ridge to the lingual mucogingival junction.[2] The mobile nonkeratinized lining mucosa continues from the buccal mucogingival junction into the mandibular buccal vestibule as the buccal mucosa, and from the lingual mucogingival junction into the lingual vestibule as mucosa of the floor of the mouth. Malignancies that arise from the attached masticatory mucosa of the LAR are LAR lesions, whereas cancers that originate buccal or lingual to the mucogingival junction should be considered lesions of the buccal mucosa or floor of mouth, respectively.

The retromolar trigone (RMT), as defined by the American Joint Committee on Cancer (AJCC), is the attached mucosa overlying the ascending ramus of the mandible from the level of the posterior surface of the last molar tooth to the apex superiorly adjacent to the tuberosity of the maxilla.[2] The retromolar gingiva is in continuity with the mucosa of the buccal region, the floor of mouth, the mandibular alveolar ridge, the maxilla, and the anterior tonsillar pillar and soft palate of the oropharynx.

◆ Incidence, Epidemiology, and Etiology

In the United States, cancer of the LAR makes up 5.2% of the oral cavity cancers registered in the National Cancer Data Base (NCDB) and is the second least common site for oral cancer, the upper alveolar ridge being the most infrequent location (see Table 5–1 in Chapter 5 for the method of calculation).[3] Cancer arising from the RMT constitutes 8% of the oral cavity cancers registered in the NCDB and is the fourth most frequent location for oral cancer after cancers of the oral tongue, floor of mouth, and lip (see Table 5–1 in Chapter 5 for the method of calculation).[3] However, cancer of the RMT and posterior LAR is more commonly diagnosed in South Africa, central Asia, and Southeast Asia, where betel quid chewing is commonly practiced (see Chapter 10).[4,5] The median age at the time of diagnosis was 69 years and 64 years for patients registered in the NCDB with cancer of the LAR and RMT, respectively.[3]

Squamous cell carcinoma (SCC) is the most common histologic type at both sites, making up 89% of LAR cancers and 92.5% of RMT malignancies. The second most frequent malignancy of the LAR was verrucous carcinoma followed by adenocarcinoma, at 4.2% and 2.4%, respectively. In contrast, adenocarcinoma (4.5%) is more frequently diagnosed than verrucous carcinoma (0.9%) in the RMT region.[3]

Tobacco and alcohol use are the primary etiologic agents associated with squamous carcinoma involving the LAR and RMT in North America and Europe. Betel quid with or without tobacco is an important etiologic agent in other regions of the world, including India and Taiwan.[6] Although chronic irritation from denture-wearing was purported to be a risk factor, no supporting epidemiologic evidence exists.[7,8]

◆ Natural History and Clinical Presentation

Cancerous lesions of the LAR frequently manifest a superficial spreading behavior, which may extend along a broad mucosal front with surrounding erythroleukoplakic changes. Tumors that arise in dentate regions frequently manifest an erythematous proliferation of abnormal tissue at the gingival margin with rolled borders. Dentists occasionally attribute this appearance to the presence of gingival inflammation, which may influence them to perform gingival curettage or periodontal surgery. Larger lesions may become ulcerated. Because inflammation of the periodontal apparatus is typically diffuse and nonulcerative, inflamed gingiva surrounding one or two teeth with or without ulceration suggests the need for a tissue biopsy. Lesions that have invaded the periodontal ligament space can lead to increased tooth mobility, and neoplastic replacement of the periodontal ligament in the apical region may lead to depressability of the tooth within the socket. Invasion of the underlying mandible of the underlying alveolar ridge is difficult to assess on clinical examination because the lamina propria is attached to the underlying bone. Anterior lesions can extend into the labial vestibule and the lip or lingually into the anterior floor of mouth. Posterior alveolar ridge lesions similarly can spread into the buccal vestibule and onto the buccal mucosa, into the lingual sulcus and floor of mouth, or posteriorly onto the RMT (**Fig. 12–1**). Computed tomography has limited ability to detect superficial mucosal involvement, but can be useful to ascertain the presence of mandibular invasion and soft tissue extension into adjacent anatomic regions.

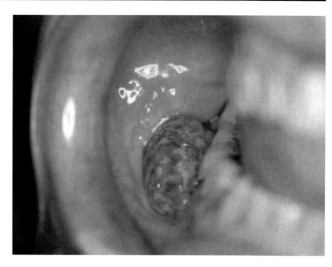

Figure 12–1 Squamous cell carcinoma of the posterior right lower alveolar ridge (LAR) and retromolar trigone that also invades the posterior buccal mucosa.

Tumor staging for both sites corresponds to the criteria used for other oral cavity sites (see Chapter 7).[2] Tumors that invade through cortical bone, into the deep (extrinsic) tongue musculature (genioglossus, hyoglossus, palatoglossus, and styloglossus), or invade the maxillary sinus or the skin of the face are designated T4a lesions.[2] Superficial mandibular bone erosion is not sufficient to apply the T4 designation. Invasion of the masticator space, pterygoid plates, skull base, and/or internal carotid artery encasement result in the T4b designation.[2]

The T-stage distribution of patients presenting with LAR lesions is as follows: T1, 23 to 31%; T2, 36 to 45%; T3, 13 to 21%; and T4, 11 to 20%.[7,9] The overall rate of clinically positive adenopathy is approximately 25% and is related to T-stage: T1 N+, 17%; T2 N+, 14%; T3 N+, 44%; and T4 N+, 44%.[9] Limited findings pertaining to the rate and pattern of occult nodal metastasis (ONM) in LAR cancer have been published. Eicher et al[9] demonstrated a 15% incidence of ONM in 127 patients staged T1 through T4 with a clinically negative neck. Ninety-three percent of the metastatic nodes were located in lymph node levels I or II, with the remaining 7% located in level III. In contrast, lymph node levels IV and V contained 10% and 11%, respectively, of the metastatic nodes that were identified in therapeutic neck dissections.

Tumors of the RMT can manifest aggressive patterns of local spread. The pterygomandibular raphe is a band of connective tissue situated beneath the mucosal surface of the RMT that attaches superiorly at the pterygoid hamulus of the medial pterygoid plate and inferiorly to the posterior aspect of the mylohyoid line of the mandible, and serves as a common insertion point for the buccinator muscle and the superior constrictor muscle. Superior spread along the pterygomandibular raphe provides access to the skull base and nasopharynx, whereas inferior growth facilitates floor of mouth invasion.[10] The pterygomandibular raphe lies between the anterior tonsillar pillar (ATP) and the RMT, helping to form the junction between the oropharynx and the oral cavity. The pterygomandibular raphe also forms the anterior border of the masticator space and the parapharyngeal space, which contains the lingual and the inferior alveolar nerves.[11] Consequently, RMT cancers can involve several adjacent regions, including the buccal space, the medial pterygoid muscle within the masticator space, the pterygopalatine fossa, the floor of the mouth and the mylohyoid muscle, and the tonsillar fossa and the superior constrictor muscle.

The most frequent presenting complaints of patients with cancer of the RMT include pain in the region of the primary, referred odynophagia, and trismus.[12] The anatomic location of the RMT over the alveolar ridge and ramus predisposes these lesions to early mandibular invasion, with a 14% rate of pathologically verified mandibular bone invasion documented in one series.[12] Retromolar trigone malignancies are also prone to extend onto the adjacent ATP (34–85%), soft palate (26–59%), buccal mucosa (43%), tongue base (19%), LAR (19–61%), and the maxillary tuberosity (**Fig. 12–2**).[12,13] These lesions can also invade the muscles of mastication, depending on the pattern of spread and infiltration.

Tumors involving the ATP-RMT region are often ill-defined lesions, which can demonstrate a superficial spreading behavior beyond the clinically evident lesion. Therefore, clinicians must closely evaluate the surrounding mucosa for subtle erythroleukoplakic changes that better define the actual extent of the lesion. Computed tomography (CT), with soft tissue and bone windows, and panoramic radiography are complementary diagnostic tools that can be used to ascertain the presence of bone invasion or extension into the pterygoid musculature or pterygopalatine fossa.

Computed tomography can identify perineural tumor involvement on thin-section coronal cuts and by the identification of widening of foramen ovale, whereas magnetic resonance imaging (MRI) is superior to CT in the evaluation of increased nerve diameter and intracranial neural involvement of the trigeminal cistern and the cavernous sinus.[11] Denervation muscle atrophy due to involvement of the mandibular division of the trigeminal nerve can be appreciated

on CT or MRI based on the presence of muscular atrophy and fatty replacement of the masticatory musculature (see Fig. 28–6 in Chapter 28).

The T-stage distribution of patients presenting with RMT lesions is as follows: T1, 10 to 22%; T2, 32 to 57%; T3, 15 to 20%; T4, 20 to 43%.[12–14] The overall rate of clinically positive adenopathy ranges from 18 to 33% and is directly rated to T stage: T1 N+, 7%; T2 N+, 21 to 32%; T3 N+, 40 to 50%; T4 N+, 50 to 56%.[12–14] The N-stage distribution at presentation is as follows: N0, 67 to 82%; N1, 11 to 19%; N2, 6 to 20%; N3, 0 to 5%.[12–14] Data pertaining to the rate and pattern of occult metastatic disease are scant. Byers et al[15] noted a 35% rate of ONM in 23 elective neck dissections, and Shah et al[16] observed a 44% rate of ONM in 16 dissected clinically negative necks. The distribution of ONM in Shah's series was as follows: level I, 19%; level II, 12%; level III, 6%; level IV, 6%; level V, 0%.

◆ Mandibular Invasion

Prior to 1964, the lymphatics of the tongue and the floor of the mouth were thought to pass through the mandibular periosteum on their way to the cervical lymph nodes. As a consequence, segmental resections were frequently performed in the absence of mandibular invasion to prevent the eventual development of cervical metastatic disease via the periosteal lymphatics. This belief, considered "anatomic fact" by Ward and Robben,[17] was challenged in 1964 and again in 1971 by Marchetta and his colleagues[18,19] at Roswell Park Cancer Institute (Buffalo, NY). Their important research showed that there was no association between mandibular periosteal involvement and the presence of cervical nodal metastases. They also demonstrated that periosteal involvement occurred solely when tumor directly abutted the mandible, and the mandible was involved only when there was direct extension through the periosteum. These findings provided the historical basis for periosteal stripping and mandibular conservation in situations where mandibular invasion is absent. Subsequent research by McGregor and MacDonald[20] that evaluated the location of invasion through the mandibular cortex found that the site of invasion was through the occlusal surface, or crest, of the alveolar ridge in nearly 90% of 46 nonirradiated mandibles and in almost 70% of 16 irradiated mandibles examined. However, 50% of the irradiated mandibles were invaded at multiple sites, with lingual cortical involvement in more than 60% and buccal cortical involvement in nearly 40% of the mandibles. In a retrospective series of 42 LAR cancers with histologically documented bone invasion, Totsuka et al[21] documented that invasion invariably occurred through the occlusal surface independent of the use of preoperative irradiation or the status of the dentition. In contrast, a prospective study of the histologic patterns of tumor invasion in nonirradiated mandibles demonstrated that tumor invasion occurs at the point of tumor abutment with the mandible rather than through the occlusal surface, neural foramina, or periodontal membrane.[22] The point of tumor abutment frequently occurred at the mucogingival junction in both dentate and edentulous mandibles.

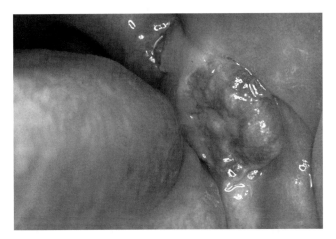

Figure 12–2 Left retromolar trigone tumor adjacent to the posterior oral tongue. The tumor involves the upper retromolar trigone region and extends toward the anterior tonsillar pillar.

Tumors of the tongue, floor of mouth, and buccal mucosa in this investigation were more likely to invade the buccal or lingual surface, whereas tumors of the LAR or RMT preferentially invaded through the occlusal surface.[22] These findings should be carefully considered prior to performing less than a segmental mandibulectomy.

Although tumor invasion can occur via named foramina (i.e., mental, mandibular foramen) or the periodontal ligament space, most invasion develops via defects, or "unnamed foramina," in the cortical bone.[20,21] Brown and Browne[23] from Liverpool surmise that the Sharpey's fibers, which are bundles of collagenous fibers that bind the attached mucosa to the alveolar ridge bone, are responsible for the primary cortical defects that predispose this region to transcortical invasion. The hard palate, another site of attached mucosa, has similar cortical defects that may explain the mechanism of bone invasion in this region.

Numerous authors have addressed the prognosis associated with mandibular invasion. In a retrospective series from M. D. Anderson Cancer Center (MDACC) of 155 previously untreated patients with carcinoma of the mandibular gingiva, mandibular involvement was not associated with local recurrence even though survival was adversely affected by cortical invasion ($p = .014$) as well as cancellous invasion ($p = .035$).[24] Local recurrence, however, was associated with tumor size larger than 3 cm. Other investigators have been unable to demonstrate a significant difference in recurrence or disease-free survival.[25–28] Another published analysis of the MDACC series that used multivariate analysis to evaluate the relationship between mandibular invasion and regional metastases found that advanced T stage and decreased tumor differentiation were the only factors that were predictive of regional metastases.[9] Most of the published evidence bolsters the assertion that tumor size is a more important prognostic factor than mandibular invasion.[25]

These investigations, however, did not address the possibility that prognosis may be affected by the pattern of mandibular invasion, an area of growing research interest. Mandibular invasion may occur via a predominantly erosive or infiltrative pattern, although these patterns likely represent the two ends of a spectrum of the patterns of invasion that can occur. The erosive or expansive pattern is characterized by a broad, pushing tumor front with a connective tissue layer and active osteoclasts at the interface between the bone and the tumor.[21,23,29] The infiltrative or invasive pattern exhibits nests and cords of tumor cells advancing independently along an irregular tumor front with no intervening layer of connective tissue and little osteoclastic activity.[23,29] Because either pattern causes bony destruction, "infiltrative" is more descriptive of this pattern than "invasive." Radiographically, the erosive pattern demonstrates loss of continuity of the cortex with a smooth, well-defined U-shaped or scalloped margin, whereas the infiltrative pattern has an irregular, poorly defined margin with either bony spicules or isolated fragments (see Figs. 6–6 and 6–7 in Chapter 6).[30] The pattern of invasion is more accurately characterized by CT than panoramic radiography.[31] CT findings suggest that an infiltrative pattern is associated with a poorer prognosis than CT findings consistent with an erosive pattern.[31] The width and depth of invasion is typically greater in tumors with an infiltrative pattern, so the erosive pattern may be an early manifestation of bone invasion that develops into an infiltrative pattern of invasion in some cases.[23] The infiltrative pattern is more likely to result in periodontal space and medullary space invasion, inferior alveolar nerve involvement, and a higher rate of positive bone margins. Infiltrative tumors also manifest higher rates of local recurrence and poorer disease-specific survival than malignancies with an erosive pattern of invasion.[29,32] Shaw et al[32] have found that a worse prognosis for infiltrative tumors persists after correcting for the soft tissue factors that affect prognosis, including tumor size and unfavorable patterns of soft tissue invasion. Moreover, they were unable to demonstrate any significant difference in prognosis between patients with the erosive pattern and patients without bone invasion. It appears that the T4 designation for bone invasion is an oversimplification because there is clearly a subset of individuals with a poorer prognosis.

Pretreatment Assessment of Mandibular Invasion

Investigative efforts aimed at elucidating the best modality to detect mandibular invasion have yielded widely disparate sensitivity and specificity values for each diagnostic test that has been evaluated (**Table 12–1**).[33–50] For instance, published values for the specificity of clinical examination,

Table 12–1   Detection of Mandibular Invasion: Range of Values for the Sensitivity and Specificity of Diagnostic Tests*

Diagnostic Test	Sensitivity (%)		Specificity (%)	
	Lowest Published Value	Highest Published Value	Lowest Published Value	Highest Published Value
Clinical examination	39[33]	87[34]	44[35]	100[33]
Plain radiography	40[36]	97[37]	65[37]	93[38]
Bone scintigraphy	80[36]	100[35,39–41]	47[42]	100[36]
SPECT	60[43]	100[44]	67[43]	100[44]
CT	50[45]	96[46]	80[42]	96[35]
DentaScan	—	95[47]	—	79[47]
MRI	92[38]	100[45,48]	40[48]	100[38]
Ultrasound	66[49]	93[50]	—	85[49]

*Published literature from 1990–2005.
SPECT, single photon emission computed tomography; CT, computed tomography; MRI, magnetic resonance imaging.

Table 12–2 Detection of Mandibular Invasion: Summary and Comparison of Imaging Techniques and Clinical Examination*

Imaging Technique	Number of Reports	Sensitivity (Mean %)	Specificity (Mean %)
Clinical examination	9	82	61
Plain radiography	18	76	81
Bone scintigraphy	15	93	74
SPECT	3	97	76
CT	7	75	86
DentaScan	3	—	—
MRI	4	85	72
Ultrasound	2	86	88

*Published literature from 1966–2000.
SPECT, single photon emission computed tomography; CT, computed tomography; MRI, magnetic resonance imaging. From Brown JS, Lewis-Jones HL. Evidence for imaging the mandible in the management of oral squamous cell carcinoma: a review. Br J Oral Maxillofac Surg 2001;39:411–418, with permission.

which is the ability to identify patients who do not have mandibular invasion, range from 44 to 100%.[33,35] Similarly, values for the sensitivity of CT, which is the ability to correctly identify patients who have mandibular invasion, range from 50 to 96%.[45,46] A systematic review of the peer-reviewed literature published from 1966 to 2000 was conducted to clarify the sensitivity and specificity obtained with each diagnostic modality (**Table 12–2**).[51] MRI demonstrated a higher sensitivity than CT, clinical examination, or plain film radiography, whereas CT demonstrated the highest specificity of these four treatment modalities. Thus, MRI resulted in the lowest false-negative rate, whereas CT provided the lowest false-positive rate. It is important to note, however, that the accuracy of diagnostic imaging can be adversely affected by suboptimal imaging technique. Mukherji et al[46] showed that the sensitivity and specificity of CT in detecting mandibular invasion is improved by customizing the CT protocol that is used. When the mandible was reconstructed by using a bone algorithm and a slice thickness of no more than 3 mm, a sensitivity of 96% and specificity of 87% were achieved. Moreover, the value of clinical examination may be affected by the diagnostic acumen of the examiner.[52] Therefore, the findings of the systematic review noted above should be applied to the clinical evaluation of mandibular bone invasion with caution.

Because there is no single investigation that can reliably predict the presence or absence of tumor invasion, accuracy may be improved by employing multiple diagnostic tests. Werning et al[26] documented greater diagnostic accuracy by combining clinical examination with radiography, exploiting the superior sensitivity and specificity, respectively, of these two modalities. Based on the findings of their systematic review, Brown and Lewis-Jones[51] similarly suggested that complementary sensitive and specific investigations should be combined, and that periosteal stripping also should be performed during surgery when the findings of these diagnostic studies are indeterminate.

Other investigators have combined radiographic studies to improve diagnostic accuracy. Clinicians from Brisbane, Australia, found that CT scan in combination with orthopantomograms (OPGs) resulted in a positive predictive value of 90%, which was superior to either CT (82%) or OPG (75%) alone.[43] In other words, 90% of the patients with abnormalities on both radiographic tests had pathologic mandibular invasion. The

negative predictive values were similar for all three diagnostic approaches. Dental radiologists have also suggested that panoramic radiography in combination with intraoral radiography provides comparable diagnostic accuracy to CT in the assessment of the superoinferior extent of mandibular invasion by gingival carcinoma.[31] This approach, however, does not address invasion of the lingual cortical plate that can be detected by using other available imaging modalities.

In general, high-quality radiographic studies should be combined with careful clinical examination by an experienced examiner to determine the likelihood of mandibular invasion. Intraoperative periosteal stripping should be employed whenever early cortical involvement could be present. Prospective investigations that correlate high- quality imaging using standardized imaging protocols with pathologic findings should provide the answers to this unresolved controversy.

The ability to predict *the extent of mandibular invasion* by using radiographic studies has also been studied. The degree of bone invasion that is seen on reformatted buccolingual cross-sectional CT images of the mandible has been associated with the presence of cervical metastasis and worse survival.[53] Panoramic radiography in another investigation correctly estimated the extent of histologic bone invasion in 67% of 24 patients.[54] Hong et al[55] correlated the histologic findings of 16 patients who had gingival carcinoma of the mandibular molar region with the extent of bone invasion that was demonstrated by intraoral periapical radiographs, panoramic radiography, bone scans, and CT scans. Radiologic assessment underestimated the histologic width of invasion to a greater degree than histologic depth of invasion. Histologic width of invasion was underestimated in 14 of 16 cases by an average distance of 8.5 mm, and histologic depth was underestimated in 10 of 16 cases by an average distance of 3.4 mm. In cases with an infiltrative pattern of invasion, the average difference between the radiologic and histologic width of tumor invasion was 10.9 mm. Brown et al[38] found that OPGs underpredicted the width and depth of invasion by an average 13 mm and 2 mm, respectively, whereas MRI overpredicted width of invasion by 19 mm and depth by 10 mm[38]; CT scans underpredicted width of invasion by 5 mm and overpredicted depth of invasion by 3 mm.

Once transcortical invasion has occurred, subcortical tumor spread within the medullary cavity typically extends no more than 1 cm from the region of overlying mucosal abnormality and the site of bony invasion.[54–56] Tumor can spread in a perineural or endoneural manner via the inferior alveolar nerve. Surrounding medullary space involvement is usually a precursor to nerve-related spread.[55,56] In their classic research, McGregor and McDonald[56] noted that nerve-related tumor spread occurred in more than 40% of edentulous nonirradiated mandibles invaded by squamous carcinoma, whereas nerve-related spread was less likely to occur if the mandible was dentate in the region of invasion. Prior radiation did not increase the rate of involvement. Skip lesions or extension of tumor from the perineural region into the surrounding medullary bone was not seen. Although there were no cases of perineural or endoneural extension from the intraosseous portion out of the inferior alveolar canal toward the skull base, others have documented proximal extension through the mandibular foramen.[54]

◆ Treatment

Surgical Considerations

The performance of mandibular resective surgery must account for particular patterns of tumor invasion and variations in mandibular bony anatomy that can impact the eventual oncologic and functional result. Segmental mandibulectomy should be considered the mandibular resective procedure of choice in patients with suspected mandibular bone invasion whenever less aggressive surgical resection could compromise local-regional control.

The performance of a conservation mandibulectomy procedure must preserve a biomechanically stable mandible that can withstand the load-bearing forces created by mastication and parafunctional habits such as bruxism. The changes in mandibular biomechanical stability that occur following marginal mandibulectomy were simulated in an investigation that subjected fresh cadaveric mandibles to strain analysis.[57] Five-millimeter increments of bone were removed from the crest of the anterior alveolar ridge posteriorly to the mental foramen region bilaterally. The mandibles were loaded after each incremental reduction to obtain strain curves. Strain significantly increased when the height of the residual mandible was reduced from 10 mm to 5 mm, suggesting that preservation of at least 1 cm of mandibular bone is necessary to prevent pathologic fracture.[57]

Surgical resection of advanced RMT lesions with transcortical invasion into the medullary cavity, or lesions that have failed RT, typically require an extensive resection of mandible, masticatory muscle, tonsillar fossa, and soft palate. Barbosa[58] in 1959 described the "retromolar operation," a procedure that consisted of a hemimandibulectomy with resection of the masseter and pterygoid muscles in continuity with an ipsilateral radical neck dissection. Kowalski et al[59] published their experience with the retromolar operation in 1993, describing the procedure as an extended "commando" operation that was a modification of the composite resection procedure described by Ward and Robben.[17] Kowalski et al reported the routine sacrifice of the condyle and 3 cm of bone anterior to the anteriormost region of gingival or mandibular involvement. The design of any composite resective procedure, however, should be dictated by the three-dimensional configuration of the tumor as determined by clinical exam and radiographic findings. Based on the evidence presented earlier in this chapter that spread within the medullary cavity typically extends no more than 1 cm from the region of overlying mucosal abnormality and the site of bony invasion, a safe tumor-free margin can usually be attained by resecting 2 to 2.5 cm of additional mandibular bone. Furthermore, our knowledge of the vascular supply to the condyle as well as the vast clinical experience we have gained from subcondylar trauma and vertical ramus osteotomies for orthognathic surgery suggests that condylar preservation is frequently possible as long as oncologic efficacy is not compromised.

Historically, RMT cancers were routinely treated by posterior segmental mandibulectomy or composite resection.[17,60] In 1984, Byers et al[12] described resection of "a margin of bone including the coronoid process resected with the retromolar trigone cancer" in five patients. The posterior marginal mandibulectomy with coronoid process resection can be a useful conservation mandibulectomy procedure in the carefully selected candidate with early cortical invasion of the RMT. Inclusion of the coronoid process is necessary to ensure that an adequate bone margin is obtained.

The periosteum can be elevated away from the mandible in situations where the tumor abuts the mandible but is not fixed to the periosteum so that the resection margin extends deep to the level of soft tissue invasion. Periosteal stripping is also an effective maneuver when the tumor appears to be fixed to the periosteum and the presence of mandibular invasion could not be excluded via preoperative diagnostic testing.[38] However, periosteal stripping must be judiciously used, because the risk of residual microscopic disease following resection may be increased if microperforations in the periosteum remain undetected. In situations where the tumor is fixed to the periosteum and early cortical invasion cannot be excluded, a marginal or sagittal mandibulectomy can achieve a resection that extends at least one anatomic plane deeper than the anticipated depth of tumor invasion. Segmental resection should be considered whenever there is any suspicion of more than early cortical invasion in the nonirradiated mandible, and whenever mandibular invasion of the irradiated mandible is suspected.

Severe alveolar resorption may necessitate segmental resection in some patients who would otherwise be candidates for mandibular conservation surgery. Investigators from Ohio State University found that frozen section analysis of cancellous bone can be used to verify the adequacy of mandibular resection prior to reconstruction, with a sensitivity of 89% and a specificity of 100%.[61] Employment of this technique, however, should only be considered as an adjunct to wide resection of the invaded mandibular bone so that grossly normal-appearing bony margins are achieved.

Surgical Approaches (That Improve Access)

The Visor Flap

When an anterior segmental mandibulectomy is required, the visor flap provides excellent access to the anterior mandible and oral cavity (**Fig. 12–3**). An apron incision that extends bilaterally to the inframastoid region is raised superiorly to the inferior mandibular border, preserving the marginal mandibular nerves. The apron flap is elevated above the mandible by performing a subperiosteal dissection along the buccolabial surface of the mandible. The dissection can be performed in the soft tissues superficial to the periosteum whenever tumor invasion has extended through the buccal cortical plate of the mandible. The tumor is inspected intraorally, and an incision is created in the labial vestibule that extends to the premolar region bilaterally (see **Fig. 12–5** on p. 127). The intraoral mucosal incision is connected with the subperiosteal dissection that was developed through the transcervical approach along the anterior face of the mandible, completing the development of the visor flap. The mental nerves can occasionally be preserved in situations where a limited anterior segmental mandibulectomy is planned, but frequently these nerves must be divided to perform the segmental mandibulectomy and to optimize surgical exposure. The

visor flap can be retracted superiorly by passing a Penrose drain around the flap at each labial commissure (see **Fig. 12–5** on p. 127). This maneuver provides visualization of the anterior mandible and oral cavity through the neck to facilitate segmental mandibular resection in continuity with contiguous oral cavity soft tissues involved by tumor (see **Fig. 12–6** on p. 127).

Mandibular Conservation Surgery

Anterior Marginal (Rim) Mandibulectomy

The marginal, or rim, mandibulectomy for the treatment of lesions that involve the floor of mouth or lingual mandibular gingiva requires circumferential mucosal incisions that are placed at least 1 cm from any evident mucosal abnormality (see **Fig. 12–7** on p. 128). These incisions extend through

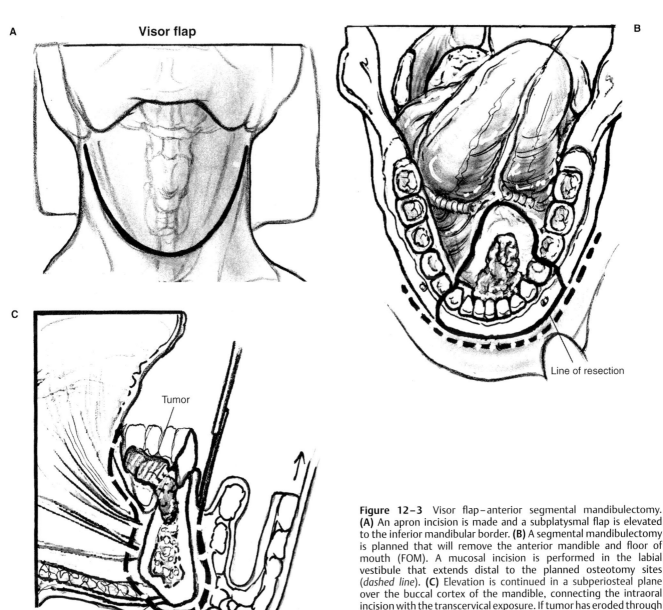

Figure 12–3 Visor flap–anterior segmental mandibulectomy. **(A)** An apron incision is made and a subplatysmal flap is elevated to the inferior mandibular border. **(B)** A segmental mandibulectomy is planned that will remove the anterior mandible and floor of mouth (FOM). A mucosal incision is performed in the labial vestibule that extends distal to the planned osteotomy sites (*dashed line*). **(C)** Elevation is continued in a subperiosteal plane over the buccal cortex of the mandible, connecting the intraoral incision with the transcervical exposure. If tumor has eroded through the buccal cortex, the dissection is performed through the soft tissues superficial to the mandible. (*Continued*)

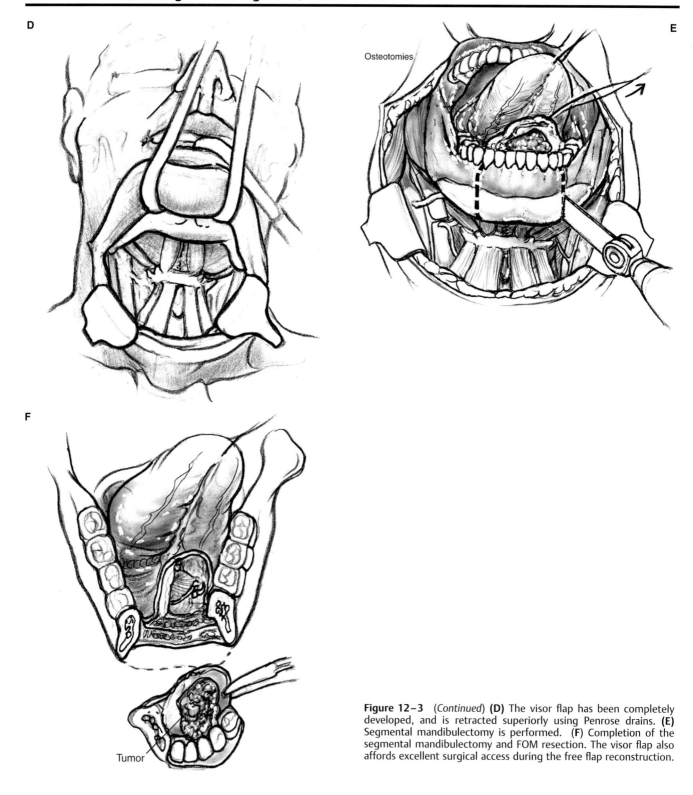

D

E

Osteotomies

F

Tumor

Figure 12–3 (*Continued*) **(D)** The visor flap has been completely developed, and is retracted superiorly using Penrose drains. **(E)** Segmental mandibulectomy is performed. **(F)** Completion of the segmental mandibulectomy and FOM resection. The visor flap also affords excellent surgical access during the free flap reconstruction.

the periosteum of the alveolar ridge mesial and distal to the tumor. Marginal mandibulectomy can be executed below the apices of the tooth roots, but dental extractions may be necessary at either end of the resection so that the osteotomies can traverse the dentate portion of the alveolar ridge. At least 1 cm of the mandible must be left intact to preserve mandibular stability. A subapical osteotomy is a more

difficult maneuver to perform in the molar region, where an osteotomy inferior to the molar root apices can damage the inferior alveolar nerve. If necessary, dental extractions can be performed prior to executing the osteotomies.

The osteotomy is performed by using an oscillating saw that is angled lingually toward the floor of the mouth, respecting the curvilinear contour of the mandibular arch.

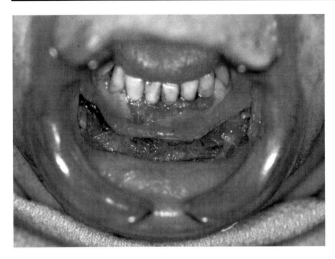

Figure 12–4   Visor flap. Labial vestibular incision used to elevate the soft tissues away from the mandible.

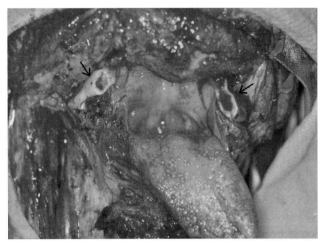

Figure 12–6   Surgical view from the neck following segmental mandibulectomy. The posterior mandibular remnants (*arrows*) are seen on either side of the tongue, which has been pulled forward. The entire oral cavity and oropharynx can be visualized through the neck, facilitating microvascular reconstruction.

The resection typically extends into the genioglossus muscle to ensure that a tumor-free deep soft tissue margin is achieved. Frequent palpation of the tumor and surrounding soft tissues facilitates soft tissue resection. If the mylohyoid muscle does not require resection, this muscle can be used to reconstruct the floor of the mouth. The resection must extend far enough beyond the area of tumor resection to avoid a steep bevel with the adjacent alveolar ridge, because abrupt transitions can give rise to a fracture-prone site. The resection edges should be rounded with a cutting bur to minimize the patient's postoperative bone exposure and to maximize the patient's comfort while wearing removable dental prostheses.

Following successful tumor resection, the floor of mouth should be carefully inspected for any communications with the submental or submandibular region. When the mylohyoid has been preserved, the surgeon should retract the posterior border of the mylohyoid anteriorly to inspect for communications because floor of mouth resection in combination with submandibular gland resection frequently

results in a communication (see **Fig. 12–8** on p. 129). The remaining soft tissues are closed using resorbable suture, and the posterior edge of the mylohyoid muscle, when present, is carefully sewn to the fascia overlying the hyoglossus muscle, taking care to avoid injury to the lingual and hypoglossal nerves and the lingual artery. Reconstruction is frequently performed using a split-thickness skin graft that is compressed with a pressure dressing to revascularize the graft. A customized acrylic stent may be used in lieu of a pressure dressing. The stent is lined by a moldable impression compound that closely conforms to the residual alveolar ridge, resulting in intimate adaptation of the skin graft to the residual alveolar ridge. Such a stent can re-create a new lingual and buccal alveolar sulcus to accommodate the flanges of a removable denture, and may circumvent the need for the tracheotomy that is frequently required when a bulky pressure dressing is applied that displaces the tongue base posteriorly into the oropharyngeal airway. An external pressure dressing can also be applied to facilitate revascularization of the skin graft and to optimize healing of the floor of mouth reconstruction to the soft tissues of the neck, thereby avoiding postoperative fistula formation. More extensive resections may necessitate pedicled or microvascular flap reconstruction to separate the oral cavity from the neck.

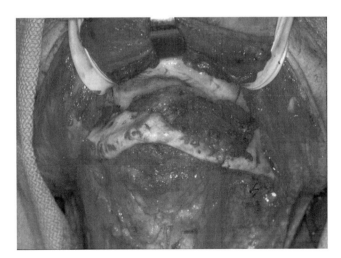

Figure 12–5   Visor flap retracted with Penrose drains, demonstrating the surgical access that is achieved in preparation for segmental mandibulectomy.

Posterior Marginal (Rim) Mandibulectomy

Marginal mandibulectomy of the posterior LAR or RMT usually requires resection of the posterior mandibular alveolar ridge as well as the coronoid process (see **Fig. 12–9** on p. 130). Resections of the posterior LAR that do not include the coronoid process may result in an inadequate bone margin posteriorly and may also result in an abrupt right angle at the posterior edge of the osteotomy. Although most marginal mandibulectomies that require resection of the coronoid process can be performed without performance of a cheek flap, a lip-splitting incision in combination with a

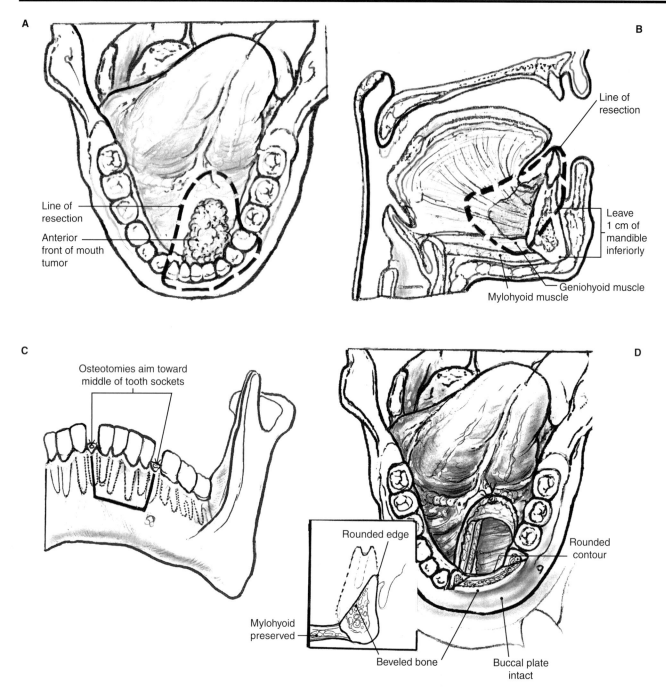

Figure 12–7 Anterior marginal mandibulectomy. **(A)** A tumor involves the anterior FOM and gingiva overlying the lingual cortex of the mandible to the gingival margin. Early mandibular cortical invasion is suspected. **(B)** Sagittal view. The tumor attaches to the mandible and invades the genioglossus muscle. The mylohyoid muscle is not involved. A marginal mandibulectomy is planned that preserves at least 1 cm of inferior mandible. **(C)** A tooth is extracted at either end of the planned resection so that osteotomies can be performed. The osteotomies should pass through the midportion of the tooth socket to ensure that adequate alveolar bone remains around the adjacent tooth. **(D)** The osteotomy is beveled toward the lingual cortex to preserve the inferior mandible. (*Inset*) The bone edges should be rounded with cutting bur prior to skin grafting. Preservation of the mylohyoid, when feasible, facilitates separation of the oral cavity from the dissected neck.

cheek flap may be necessary for more extensive resections that involve the buccal mucosa, maxilla, or soft palate, or in cases where trismus precludes adequate exposure. The presence of trismus secondary to significant masticatory muscle invasion, however, usually contraindicates conservative surgical resection.

When coronoidectomy is incorporated into the resection, an incision is extended posteriorly, immediately superficial to the underlying ramus. Dissection is continued through the soft tissues down to the ascending ramus, where subperiosteal dissection is performed up to the coronoid process and the attachments of the temporalis muscle are released.

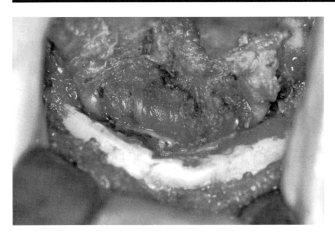

Figure 12–8   Appearance following marginal mandibulectomy prior to skin graft placement. The mandibular edges have been rounded off. The mylohyoid muscle remains intact.

Careful dissection along the lingual aspect of the ascending ramus must be performed to identify the mandibular foramen and to preserve the inferior alveolar and lingual nerves (see **Fig. 12–10** on p. 131). Once the coronoid process is isolated, an osteotomy is performed that extends from the sigmoid notch anteroinferiorly to the RMT region with an oscillating saw (see **Fig. 12–11** on p. 132). Alternatively, a reciprocating saw can be used to perform an osteotomy from the buccal aspect that extends from the RMT through the sigmoid notch. The marginal mandibulectomy is completed by using a sagittal saw to perform an osteotomy of the posterior alveolar ridge that meets the osteotomized bone from the ascending ramus (see **Figs. 12–12 and 12–13** on p. 133). Careful inspection of the radiographic inspection of the radiographic course of the inferior alveolar nerve (IAN) minimizes the risk of nerve transection during the mandibulectomy.

Sagittal (Coronal) Mandibulectomy

A sagittal mandibulectomy utilizes an osteotomy that resects the entire lingual cortical plate (see **Fig. 12–14** on p. 134). Anteriorly, the osteotomies are performed in the coronal plane, whereas osteotomies of the posterior mandible are performed in a sagittal plane. This technique does not completely resect the occlusal aspect of the alveolar ridge, although a marginal mandibulectomy can be performed in combination with a sagittal mandibulectomy using multiplanar osteotomies to preserve the inferior buccal mandibular plate.

The mucosal incisions required for a sagittal mandibulectomy are similar to those performed for a marginal mandibulectomy. In dentate patients, teeth must be extracted to remove the lingual plate, and the extraction sockets can be exploited to dictate the appropriate angulation of the osteotomy. The mandibular anterior teeth are axially inclined so that the incisal edges are labial to the root apices, and an osteotomy that extends from the alveolar crest through the apices of the alveolar sockets can be used to remove the entire lingual cortex. Extension of the osteotomy through the inferior border of the mandible also requires a deeper

dissection through the floor of the mouth than may be necessary for a marginal mandibulectomy. The height of the mandible may make completion of the osteotomy through the inferior border of the mandible difficult, so the osteotomy can also be approached inferiorly after exposing the mandible through an apron flap that was required during the neck dissections (see **Fig. 12–15** on p. 136). During posterior sagittal mandibulectomy, the relationship of the inferior alveolar nerve to the lingual plate of the mandible must be appreciated if preservation of the IAN is desired. Osteotomies that do not extend distal to the premolar region can safely resect the lingual plate with preservation of the IAN, whereas more posterior sagittal resections are more likely to result in neural injury.

Reconstruction following sagittal mandibulectomy may require reapproximation of the soft tissues of the floor of mouth to the mandible by passing nonresorbable suture through drilled holes in the residual mandible. Reconstruction may also be facilitated by using skin grafts, local intraoral flaps, or microvascular reconstructive surgery.

Radiation Therapy Technique

T1–T2 Lesions

The preferred treatment for patients with T1–T2 cancers of the LAR and RMT is surgery. Patients who are not deemed to be surgical candidates are treated with RT. Treatment may be administered with either an ipsilateral en face combination of 6-MV x-rays and electrons, or with two 6-MV x-ray beams arranged in a "wedge pair" (see **Fig. 12–16** on p. 136). The latter technique is preferred because it is possible to vary the depth of the target volume more precisely, and underdosing the medial extent of the tumor is less likely. Lesions that exhibit significant extension onto the soft palate or into the tongue (unusual for a T1 or T2 tumor) would be treated with parallel-opposed fields weighted 3:2 to the side of the tumor. Patients receive 74.4 Gy in 62 fractions over 6 weeks with a field reduction at 45.6 Gy. The low neck is treated with an anterior 6-MV x-ray field matched at the thyroid notch and receives 50 Gy in 25 fractions.

T3–T4 Lesions

Patients with T3–T4 carcinomas have a relatively low chance of cure with RT alone and are optimally treated with surgery and postoperative RT. The postoperative dose varies with the margins: negative (R0), 60 Gy; microscopically positive (R1), 66 Gy; and gross residual (R2), 70 Gy. Patients are treated once daily at 2 Gy/fraction, 5 days a week, in a continuous course. Patients with positive margins should be considered for treatment with an altered fractionation technique. Patients are treated with parallel-opposed portals that include the primary tumor and upper neck nodes (see **Fig. 12–17** on p. 136).[1] The fields are weighted 3:2 toward the side of the tumor. The anterior low neck is treated with an en face 6-MV x-ray field matched at the level of the thyroid notch. A Vaseline gauze bolus is placed on the incisions to ensure an adequate surface dose. Fields are reduced off of the spinal cord at approximately 45 Gy. An electron beam may be used to irradiate the posterior strips if

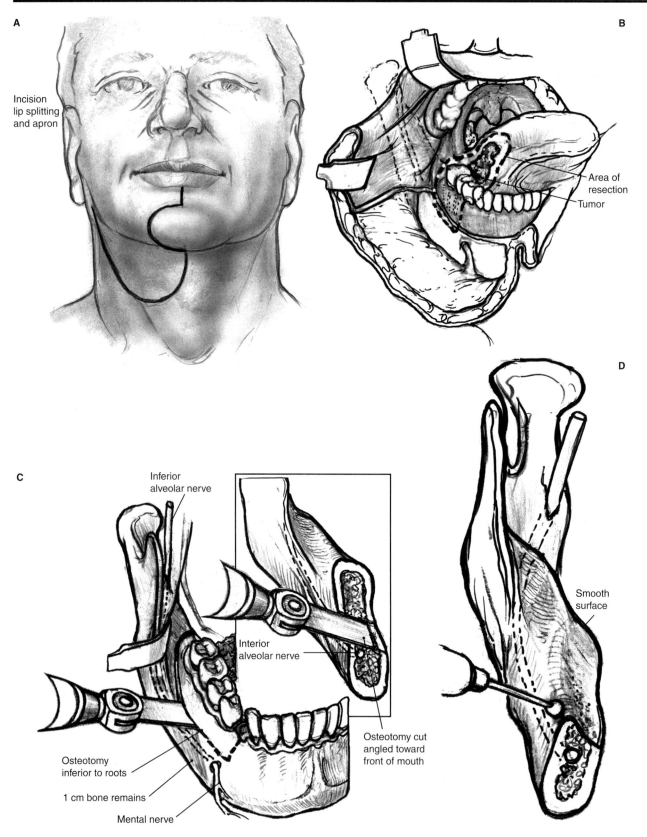

Figure 12–9 Marginal mandibulectomy of the posterior LAR. **(A)** A right-sided apron incision is performed that is combined with a straight midline chin-contour incision to split the lip so that a cheek flap can be elevated. **(B)** The cheek flap has been elevated, preserving the mental nerve. The tumor involves the LAR in the premolar-molar region and involves the FOM and lateral tongue. **(C)**

The intramandibular course of the inferior alveolar nerve (IAN) is radiographically evaluated. A sagittal saw is used to perform an osteotomy that is beveled to resect the lingual cortical plate and to preserve the inferior mandible. The IAN is preserved if this will not compromise the resection. **(D)** The edges of the residual mandible are rounded prior to skin graft placement and wound closure.

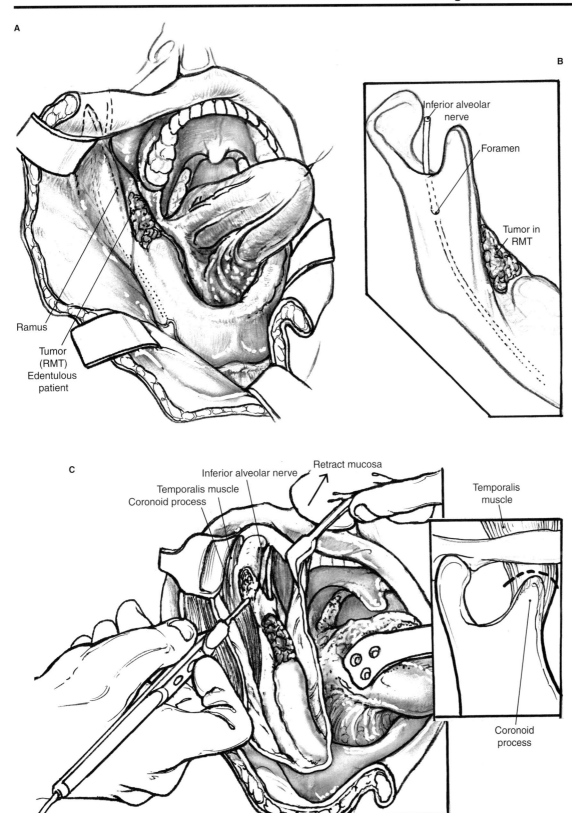

Figure 12–10 Marginal mandibulectomy for resection of a retromolar trigone (RMT) tumor: surgical access. **(A)** The tumor extends from the posterior alveolar ridge onto the RMT. **(B)** The course of the IAN is evaluated prior to resection to determine whether preservation is feasible. In this case, the course of the IAN prior to its entry into the inferior alveolar canal as well as the lingual nerve must be considered. **(C)** A circumferential mucosal incision has been performed around the tumor. Dissection is carried down to the anterior mandibular ramus. The IAN and lingual nerves are identified. (*Inset*) The insertion of the temporalis muscle onto the coronoid process is divided.

A

B

C

D

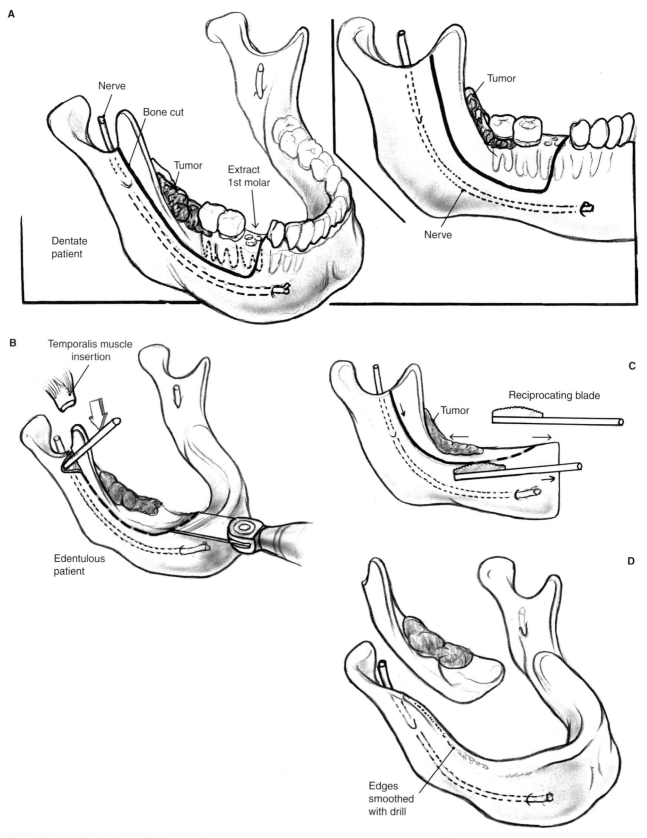

Figure 12–11 Marginal mandibulectomy for resection of a retromolar trigone tumor: mandibular resection. **(A)** The anterior osteotomy should be performed at least one tooth anterior to the extent of tumor involvement. The coronoid process is included in the resection. Once again, the osteotomy is beveled on the lingual aspect. The IAN and lingual nerves are protected during resection of the coronoid process. **(B)** A sagittal saw can be used to osteotomize the alveolar ridge, and an oscillating saw can be used to remove the coronoid process, or **(C)** a reciprocating blade may be used to develop the osteotomy. **(D)** The bone edges are smoothed off with a round cutting bur prior to closure.

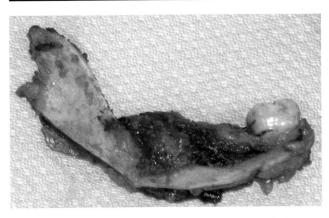

Figure 12–12 Posterior marginal mandibulectomy, including the coronoid process: en bloc specimen.

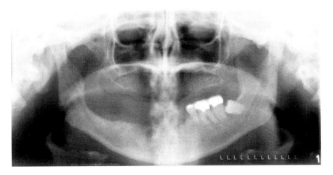

Figure 12–13 Panoramic radiograph demonstrating preservation of the inferior alveolar canal following posterior marginal mandibulectomy with resection of the coronoid process.

additional RT to these sites is indicated after off-cord reduction. Well-lateralized tumors may be treated with an ipsilateral wedge pair technique.

Patients who are not suitable for surgery are treated with twice-daily RT to 76.8 Gy in 64 fractions over 6.5 weeks combined with concomitant chemotherapy. The field arrangements are similar to those previously described. Patients who are unsuitable for aggressive treatment receive moderate dose palliative RT: 20 Gy in two fractions with a 1-week interfraction interval or 30 Gy in 10 fractions over 2 weeks.

◆ Outcomes

Mandibular Conservation versus Segmental Mandibulectomy

The local control rates achieved with conservation mandibulectomy procedures and segmental resection have not been rigorously evaluated in a prospective randomized trial (see **Table 12–3** on p. 137).[31,28,62–64] Furthermore, the available retrospective case series comparing these two approaches are impacted by selection bias, because larger tumors with bony invasion were more likely to undergo segmental resection. The unmeasured role of RT on tumor control also confounds the findings in many of these investigations because RT was used more frequently in patients treated by segmental mandibulectomy.

Only two of the publications that compare treatment outcomes following marginal mandibulectomy and segmental mandibulectomy document the presence of histologic bone invasion (see **Table 12–3** on p. 137).[28,34] Ord et al[34] documented bone invasion in 65% of the segmental group versus 7% of the marginal group, and Munoz Guerra and colleagues[28] from Madrid noted mandibular invasion twice as frequently in the segmental resection group, illustrating how preoperative evaluation for mandibular invasion results in selection bias. In the sole study that compared the impact of bone invasion on local control, marginal mandibulectomy resulted in a 75% local control rate versus a 66% rate of local control following segmental mandibulectomy.[28] In the absence of a

randomized clinical trial that contains treatment arms with subjects of similar stage and degree of mandibular invasion, marginal mandibulectomy appears to provide comparable rates of tumor control when compared with segmental resection in properly selected patients.

The local control rates that are attained with either marginal or sagittal mandibulectomy are summarized in **Table 12–4** on p. 137.[26,27,34,57,62–67] Marginal mandibulectomy results in 2-year local control rates that range from 75 to 100%. Two large retrospective case series have compared the outcomes of treatment following marginal and sagittal mandibulectomy.[26,27] Werning et al[26] documented a 2-year local control rate of 87% for marginal mandibulectomy versus 74% for sagittal mandibulectomy, a difference that was not statistically significant. Histologic bone invasion was present in 49% of the floor of mouth, 33% of the RMT, and 28% of the LAR cancers. Similarly, Guerra et al[27] published a 2-year local control rate of 82% for marginal mandibulectomy versus 76% for sagittal mandibulectomy, which was not statistically significant. Once again, 29% of the floor of mouth cancers demonstrated histologic bone invasion, the most common site of invasion. The presence of bone invasion did not increase the rate of local recurrence in either study. Because both techniques provided comparable local control in the presence of bone invasion, the outcome following different conservation mandibulectomy techniques is largely dependent on proper patient selection. For example, sagittal mandibulectomy would be contraindicated whenever tumor invasion through the occlusal surface of the mandible is suspected.

A few published retrospective case series have provided local control rates for RMT cancers that were treated with posterior marginal mandibulectomy. Petruzzelli et al[68] from Loyola University recently published a series of 16 patients using this procedure with a 94% local control rate. Neither of the two patients with mandibular invasion recurred locally. Werning et al[26] documented an 80% local control rate in 24 patients with RMT cancer treated by posterior marginal mandibulectomy with coronoid process resection. Of the 15 patients in whom bone histopathology was documented, 33% demonstrated bone invasion. The local control rate in these patients was 80%, and there were no local treatment failures in patients with bone invasion.

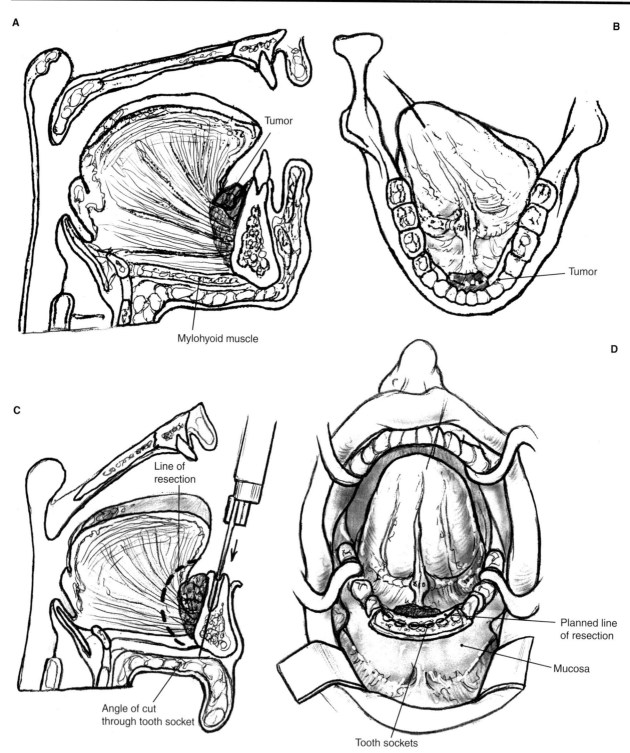

Figure 12–14 Sagittal mandibulectomy. **(A)** Sagittal view demonstrating a tumor involving the anterior FOM and lingual gingiva with suspected early lingual cortex invasion, and invasion through the FOM musculature to the mylohyoid muscle. In this case, a sagittal mandibulectomy that completely resects the lingual cortical plate would result in a wider margin of resection than a marginal mandibulectomy that passes through the lingual plate. **(B)** Intraoral view showing the extent of FOM involvement. **(C)** The anterior teeth have been extracted. A sagittal saw is used to perform the osteotomy, resecting the entire lingual plate. The tooth extraction sockets can be used to properly angle the saw so that the entire lingual plate is resected. **(D)** Intraoral view depicting the planned line of resection. At either end of the bony resection, the osteotomy gently curves lingually to provide a smooth contour to the bone edges. (*Continued*)

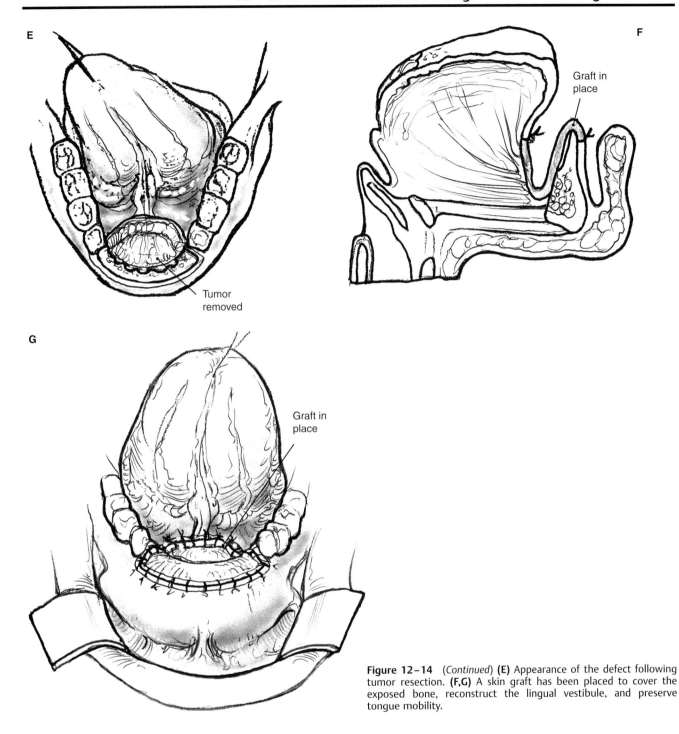

Figure 12–14 (*Continued*) **(E)** Appearance of the defect following tumor resection. **(F,G)** A skin graft has been placed to cover the exposed bone, reconstruct the lingual vestibule, and preserve tongue mobility.

Lower Alveolar Ridge

Only limited data are available pertaining to the outcomes of treatment for SCC of the LAR because most publications combined the treatment results of the upper and LARs.[69–71] For example, the most recent retrospective case series from Memorial Sloan-Kettering Cancer Center (MSKCC) documented a 5-year disease-specific survival rate of 54% following the treatment of 193 LAR lesions, 70 retromolar trigone lesions, and 83 upper alveolar ridge lesions that were analyzed

together.[70] Similarly, investigators from Massachusetts General Hospital noted a 49% 5-year overall survival rate for squamous carcinomas of the upper and LARs.[71]

In 1983, a retrospective case series from the University of California at Los Angeles (UCLA) documented the following 2-year disease-free survival rates for patients with LAR cancer who were treated with either marginal or segmental mandibulectomy with or without RT: stage I, 78%; stage II, 62%; stage III, 50%; stage IV, 25%.[62] Researchers

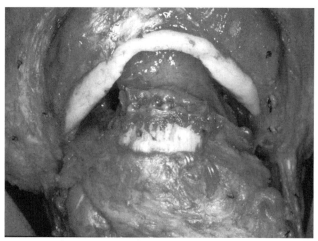

Figure 12–15 Sagittal mandibulectomy viewed from the neck. This view results from division of the suprahyoid musculature during the resection, so that the FOM contents collapse into the neck. The buccal cortical plate of the mandible has been preserved. The sagittal mandibulectomy specimen remains attached to the tissues of the FOM, and the anterior tongue can be seen above the resected bone specimen.

from Hokkaido University in Japan subsequently published a 2-year disease-free survival rate of 84% for 49 patients with LAR cancers treated by marginal or segmental mandibulectomy, many of whom were also treated with chemotherapy or RT prior to surgery.[63]

In 1981, Byers et al[7] documented a 5% rate of local-regional failure and a 2-year overall survival rate of 67% in 61 patients treated for LAR cancer at MDACC. Two subsequent retrospective case series from MDACC updated their treatment

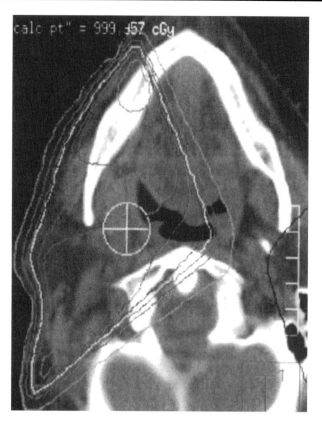

Figure 12–16 Patient with an early-stage carcinoma of the retromolar trigone. Radiation therapy is delivered with two 6 MV x-ray beams via a wedge-pair arrangement.

A

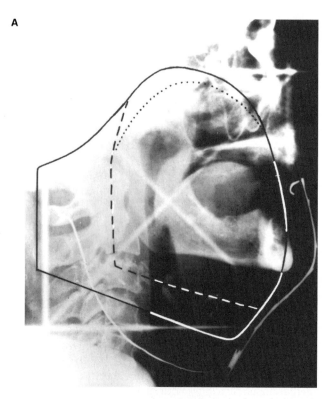

B

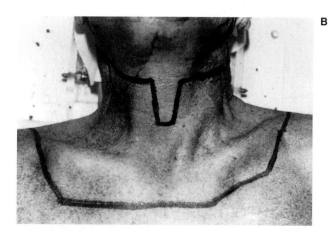

Figure 12–17 Typical portal for irradiation after hemimandibulectomy, partial maxillectomy, and radical neck dissection for pathologic T4N0 retromolar trigone lesion. **(A)** Field reductions made at 45 Gy (*dashed line*) and 60 Gy (*dotted line*). **(B)** Low neck received a 50-Gy dose (at D_{max}) given in 25 fractions. Larynx and a segment of spinal cord were shielded by tapered midline block. (From Amdur et al. Postoperative irradiation for squamous cell carcinoma of the head and neck: an analysis of treatment results and complications. Int J Radiat Oncol Biol Phys 1989; 16:25, with permission.)

Table 12–3 Studies Comparing Mandibular Conservation Surgery to Segmental Mandibulectomy

First Author	Year	Type of Resection	No. of Patients	2-Year Local Control (%)
Wald[62]	1983	Marginal	21	81
		Segmental	26	89
Totsuka[63]	1991	Marginal	21	86
		Segmental	28	75
Dubner[64]	1993	Marginal	79	19
		Segmental	51	94
Ord*[34]	1997	Marginal	26	92
		Segmental	20	100
Munoz Guerra†[28]	2003	Marginal	50	80
		Segmental	56	67

*Follow-up ranged from 1 to 60 months.

results for 155 patients treated for LAR carcinoma.[9,24] Surgical resection was the primary treatment modality, and postoperative RT was administered for positive margins, perineural invasion, multiple positive cervical lymph nodes, or extracapsular extension. Advanced T stage, decreased tumor differentiation, and mandibular invasion were predictive of regional metastasis, which adversely impacted survival.[9] Complete resection of the primary resulted in a 2-year local control rate of 87%. Tumor size larger than 3 cm strongly predicted local recurrence and worse survival. Persistently positive surgical margins were also associated with higher rates of local recurrence and worse disease-specific survival. Perineural invasion and histologic grade did not affect local control or survival even though advanced histologic grade correlated with the development of cervical metastases.[9] Mandibular invasion did not affect local control, but cortical invasion alone ($p = .014$), as well as cancellous involvement ($p = .035$), resulted in worse survival.[24] Five-year disease-specific survival by T stage was as follows: T1, 85%; T2, 84%; T3, 66%; T4, 64%.[24]

Retromolar Trigone

The outcomes of treatment for RMT cancer are provided by a limited number of retrospective case series. Moreover, the treatment-related outcomes for patients with cancer of the RMT have often been evaluated together with cancers of the LAR, soft palate, and ATP.

A few retrospective case series have been published that evaluate the local-regional control achieved with definitive external beam RT. Clinicians from Notre-Dame Hospital in Montreal recently reviewed the outcomes of 46 patients with SCC of the RMT that received once-daily fractions of 2 Gy/d to a median dose of 66 Gy (range, 60–70 Gy).[72] The 5-year local control rate achieved by RT was only 49%, with the following local control rates by T stage: T1, 25%; T2, 62%; T3, 59%; T4, 75%. However, the use of salvage surgery following RT failure resulted in 5-year ultimate local control, regional control, and disease-specific survival rates of 67%, 88%, and 78%, respectively. The authors concluded that RT with or without concurrent chemotherapy could be used with curative intent for RMT cancers, but lesions with bone invasion should receive surgery followed by RT. Another retrospective case series from MDACC reviewed 50 patients with RMT cancer and 87 patients with cancer of the ATP who were treated exclusively with RT.[73] Most of these lesions were treated to a total dose of 65 to 70 Gy at the primary site. The primary control rate was 66% for RMT cancers versus 77% for malignancies arising from the ATP ($p = .16$). Infiltrative or ulcerative tumors demonstrated a poorer prognosis than exophytic or superficial tumors ($p = .01$). There was no significant difference in control rates for T1, T2, or T3 tumors of the RMT.[73]

Most available retrospective series, however, report the results attained by the use of a variety of treatment modalities. In 1984, Byers and coauthors[12] published a review of

Table 12–4 Local Control Rates Following Mandibular Conservation Surgery

First Author	Year	Type of Resection	No. of Patients	2-Year Local Control (%)
Flynn[65]	1974	Marginal	23	83
Beecroft[66]	1982	Marginal	34	97
Wald[62]	1983	Marginal	21	81
Barttelbort[57]	1987	Marginal	16	75
Totsuka[63]	1991	Marginal	21	86
Shaha[67]	1992	Marginal	22	82
Dubner[64]	1993	Marginal	79	81
Ord*[34]	1997	Marginal	26	92
Werning[26]	2001	Marginal	182	87
		Sagittal	35	74
Guerra[27]	2003	Marginal	33	82
		Sagittal	17	76

*Follow-up ranged from 1 to 60 months.

110 patients treated at MDACC. Forty-two percent ($n = 46$) of the patients were treated by surgery alone at the primary site: 67% required segmental resection, 22% underwent transoral resection, and another 11% were treated with a marginal resection that included the coronoid process. Even though 42% of the lesions were classified as T3–T4 lesions, the local failure rate for patients treated with surgery alone was only 11%. The primary lesion was treated with RT in 45% ($n = 50$) of the patients, resulting in a local failure rate of 16%. There was a tendency to treat with RT when significant extension onto the ATP and soft palate was present. Fourteen patients (13%) received surgery in combination with either preoperative or postoperative RT. Primary control by T stage was as follows: T1, 92%; T2, 88%; T3, 90%; T4, 75%. The 2-year disease-specific survival rate was 85% and the 2-year disease-free survival rate was 46%, whereas the overall 5-year survival rate was only 26%. Osteoradionecrosis developed in 34% of the patients treated with RT; 41% of these patients subsequently required a partial mandibulectomy.

More recently, Washington University published a retrospective case series of 65 RMT cancers that were treated between 1971 and 1994.[13] Ten patients received preoperative RT and surgery, 39 received surgery and postoperative RT, and 16 received RT alone. The 5-year disease-free survival rates by treatment modality were as follows: preoperative RT and surgery, 90%; surgery and postoperative RT, 63%; and definitive RT, 31%. There was no difference in survival according to T stage. However, multivariate analysis showed that treatment modality had a significant impact on disease-free survival ($p < .01$) and local-regional control ($p = .05$). Advanced N stage was associated with worse disease-free survival ($p = .01$) and distant metastases ($p < .01$). Both forms of combined therapy were superior to RT alone; the local-regional recurrence rate was 11% for T1–T2N0 lesions that were treated with surgery and RT versus 54% for T1–T2N0 lesions that were treated with definitive RT. Furthermore, the overall local-regional control rate for patients treated with surgery and RT was 80% versus only 56% for definitive RT even though the frequency of nodal metastatic disease was much greater in the groups that were treated with RT and surgery (43% vs. 6%). Seven percent of these patients developed osteoradionecrosis from 6 months to 5.3 years after treatment, necessitating mandibulectomy in 40% of the cases.

Kowalski and colleagues[59] from São Paulo published their experience with the "retromolar operation" (discussed earlier; see Surgical Considerations) in 114 consecutive patients treated between 1960 and 1991. Fifty-eight percent of the patients received adjuvant postoperative RT (median dose, 50 Gy; range, 10–70 Gy) for positive margins or involved nodes. The median duration of follow-up was 25 months, and 19 patients who were lost to follow-up an average of 15 months after treatment were also included in their survival analysis. Five-year disease-free survival was 49%, and hard palate involvement and advanced stage were predictive of disease-free survival. Wound-related complications included wound dehiscence (20%), wound infection (18%), flap necrosis (12%), fistula (12%), seroma (7%), hematoma (4%), and carotid rupture in 2% of patients.

Investigators from the University of Florida recently reviewed their experience with RMT cancers treated by definitive RT or RT combined with surgery.[14] Cancers treated by surgery alone were not included in this retrospective case analysis. The 5-year local-regional control rates for patients treated with definitive RT versus surgery and RT were as follows: stage I to III, 51% and 87%; stage IV, 42% and 62%, respectively. The 5-year disease-specific survival rates after definitive RT compared with surgery and RT were as follows: stage I to III, 56% and 83%; stage IV, 50% and 61%, respectively. Multivariate analysis revealed that the likelihood of cure was better with surgery and RT compared with definitive RT. Twelve percent of the patients developed severe osteoradionecrosis following treatment.

◆ Verrucous Carcinoma

Two hundred seventy cases of verrucous carcinoma of the upper and lower alveolar ridges and 48 cases in the RMT region were compiled in the NCDB.[74] The alveolar ridges were the most frequent sites within the oral cavity, followed by the buccal mucosa. Thirty-five percent of alveolar ridge tumors and 30% of the RMT lesions were stage III or IV at the time of diagnosis. Surgery alone was the primary treatment modality in more than 70% of cases. Surgery in combination with RT was utilized in 21% of RMT lesions and was the most frequent site receiving this treatment approach. The 5-year relative survival rate for alveolar ridge cancers was 74%. Survival for RMT cancer was not reported, and disease-free survival statistics were not provided. No other series exists with an adequate number of cases to provide meaningful site-specific outcomes data for verrucous carcinoma.

◆ Minor Salivary Gland Malignancies

Malignancies arising from minor salivary glands of the LAR and RMT are uncommon, constituting less than 10% of the salivary gland malignancies arising in the oral cavity.[75–77] More than 90% of the neoplasms are malignant, with mucoepidermoid carcinoma and adenoid cystic carcinoma making up the majority.[75,77,78] Management of these malignancies is similar to the management of squamous cell carcinoma arising from this region, remaining cognizant of the additional treatment considerations that are required to address the neurotropism associated with adenoid cystic carcinoma. A full discussion of the management of these malignancies is offered in Chapter 13.

◆ Conclusion

The appropriate evaluation and management of malignant lesions that originate from the LAR and retromolar trigone frequently present clinicians with a variety of clinical dilemmas that can impact the ultimate outcome of therapy. Assessment for early mandibular invasion requires the employment of diagnostic tests that are both sensitive and specific so that the undertreatment of lesions that manifest mandibular invasion are eliminated and performing a segmental mandibulectomy for those lesions that do not invade the mandible is minimized. Candidates for mandibular conservation surgery should be carefully chosen to ensure that better postoperative function is not achieved at the expense of local-regional control. Postoperative RT, when indicated, must be administered to improve local-regional control and survival.

Prospective evaluation of high-quality imaging studies that are obtained by using standardized imaging protocols should help to determine whether a single diagnostic test can be reliably used to detect or exclude mandibular invasion. Future research endeavors should separately report the treatment outcomes that are achieved for cancers of the LAR and retromolar trigone, and a prospective randomized trial should be conducted to evaluate the outcomes following segmental mandibulectomy and mandibular conservation surgery.

References

1. Whitson SW. Bone. In: Ten Cate AR, ed. Oral Histology: Development, Structure and Function, 4th ed. St. Louis: Mosby-Year Book, 1994: 120–146

2. Lip and oral cavity. In: Greene FL, Page DL, Fleming ID, eds. AJCC Cancer Staging Manual, 6th ed. New York: Springer-Verlag, 2002:23–32

3. Funk GF, Karnell LH, Robinson RA, Zhen WK, Trask DK, Hoffman HT. Presentation, treatment, and outcome of oral cavity cancer: a National Cancer Data Base report. Head Neck 2002;24:165–180

4. Rao RS, Deshmane VH, Parikh HK, Parikh DM, Sukthankar PS. Extent of lymph node dissection in T3/T4 cancer of the alveolo-buccal complex. Head Neck 1995;17:199–203

5. Pathak KA, Gupta S, Talole S, et al. Advanced squamous cell carcinoma of lower gingivobuccal complex: patterns of spread and failure. Head Neck 2005;27:597–602

6. International Agency for Research on Cancer. Betel-Quid and Areca-Nut Chewing and Some Areca-Nut-Derived Nitrosamines, vol 85. Lyon, France: IARC Press, 2004

7. Byers RM, Newman R, Russell N, Yue A. Results of treatment for squamous carcinoma of the lower gum. Cancer 1981;47:2236–2238

8. Campbell BH, Mark DH, Soneson EA, Freije JE, Schultz CJ. The role of dental prostheses in alveolar ridge squamous carcinomas. Arch Otolaryngol Head Neck Surg 1997;123:1112–1115

9. Eicher SA, Overholt SM, el-Naggar AK, Byers RM, Weber RS. Lower gingival carcinoma. Clinical and pathologic determinants of regional metastases. Arch Otolaryngol Head Neck Surg 1996;122:634–638

10. Mukherji SK, Pillsbury HR, Castillo M. Imaging squamous cell carcinomas of the upper aerodigestive tract: what clinicians need to know. Radiology 1997;205:629–646

11. Smoker WRK. The oral cavity. In: Som PM, Curtin HD, eds. Head and Neck Imaging, 4th ed. St. Louis: Mosby, 2003:1377–1464

12. Byers RM, Anderson B, Schwarz EA, Fields RS, Meoz R. Treatment of squamous carcinoma of the retromolar trigone. Am J Clin Oncol 1984;7:647–652

13. Huang CJ, Chao KS, Tsai J, et al. Cancer of retromolar trigone: long-term radiation therapy outcome. Head Neck 2001;23:758–763

14. Mendenhall WM, Morris CG, Amdur RJ, Werning JW, Villaret DB. Retromolar trigone squamous cell carcinoma treated with radiotherapy alone or combined with surgery. Cancer 2005;103:2320–2325

15. Byers RM, Wolf PF, Ballantyne AJ. Rationale for elective modified neck dissection. Head Neck Surg 1988;10:160–167

16. Shah JP, Candela FC, Poddar AK. The patterns of cervical lymph node metastases from squamous carcinoma of the oral cavity. Cancer 1990;66:109–113

17. Ward GE, Robben JO. A composite operation for radical neck dissection and removal of cancer of the mouth. Cancer 1951;4:98–109

18. Marchetta FC, Sako K, Badillo J. Periosteal lymphatics of the mandible and intraoral carcinoma. Am J Surg 1964;108:505–507

19. Marchetta FC, Sako K, Murphy JB. The periosteum of the mandible and intraoral carcinoma. Am J Surg 1971;122:711–713

20. McGregor AD, MacDonald DG. Routes of entry of squamous cell carcinoma to the mandible. Head Neck Surg 1988;10:294–301

21. Totsuka Y, Usui Y, Tei K, et al. Mandibular involvement by squamous cell carcinoma of the lower alveolus: analysis and comparative study of histologic and radiologic features. Head Neck 1991;13:40–50

22. Brown JS, Lowe D, Kalavrezos N, D'Souza J, Magennis P, Woolgar J. Patterns of invasion and routes of tumor entry into the mandible by oral squamous cell carcinoma. Head Neck 2002;24:370–383

23. Brown JS, Browne RM. Factors influencing the patterns of invasion of the mandible by oral squamous cell carcinoma. Int J Oral Maxillofac Surg 1995;24:417–426

24. Overholt SM, Eicher SA, Wolf P, Weber RS. Prognostic factors affecting outcome in lower gingival carcinoma. Laryngoscope 1996;106:1335–1339

25. Ash CS, Nason RW, Abdoh AA, Cohen MA. Prognostic implications of mandibular invasion in oral cancer. Head Neck 2000;22:794–798

26. Werning JW, Byers RM, Novas MA, Roberts D. Preoperative assessment for and outcomes of mandibular conservation surgery. Head Neck 2001;23:1024–1030

27. Guerra MF, Campo FJ, Gias LN, Perez JS. Rim versus sagittal mandibulectomy for the treatment of squamous cell carcinoma: two types of mandibular preservation. Head Neck 2003;25:982–989

28. Munoz Guerra MF, Naval Gias L, Campo FR, Perez JS. Marginal and segmental mandibulectomies in patients with oral cancer: a statistical analysis of 106 cases. J Oral Maxillofac Surg 2003;61:1289–1296

29. Wong RJ, Keel SB, Glynn RJ, Varvares MA. Histological pattern of mandibular invasion by oral squamous cell carcinoma. Laryngoscope 2000;110:65–72

30. Nakayama E, Yoshiura K, Yuasa K, et al. A study of the association between the prognosis of carcinoma of the mandibular gingiva and the pattern of bone destruction on computed tomography. Dentomaxillofac Radiol 2000;29:163–169

31. Nakayama E, Yoshiura K, Yuasa K, et al. Detection of bone invasion by gingival carcinoma of the mandible: a comparison of intraoral and panoramic radiography and computed tomography. Dentomaxillofac Radiol 1999;28:351–356

32. Shaw RJ, Brown JS, Woolgar JA, Lowe D, Rogers SN, Vaughan ED. The influence of the pattern of mandibular invasion on recurrence and survival in oral squamous cell carcinoma. Head Neck 2004;26:861–869

33. Van den Brekel MW, Runne RW, Smeele LE, Tiwari R, Snow GB, Castelijns JA. Assessment of tumor invasion into the mandible: the value of different imaging techniques. Eur Radiol 1998;8:1552–1557

34. Ord RA, Sarmadi M, Papadimitrou J. A comparison of segmental and marginal bony resection for oral squamous cell carcinoma involving the mandible. J Oral Maxillofac Surg 1997;55:470–477

35. Zupi A, Califano L, Maremonti P, Longo F, Ciccarelli R, Soricelli A. Accuracy in the diagnosis of mandibular involvement by oral cancer. J Craniomaxillofac Surg 1996;24:281–284

36. Soderholm AL, Lindqvist C, Hietanen J, Lukinmaa PL. Bone scanning for evaluating mandibular bone extension of oral squamous cell carcinoma. J Oral Maxillofac Surg 1990;48:252–257

37. Muller H, Slootweg PJ. Mandibular invasion by oral squamous cell carcinoma: clinical aspects. J Craniomaxillofac Surg 1990;18:80–84

38. Brown JS, Griffith JF, Phelps PD, Browne RM. A comparison of different imaging modalities and direct inspection after periosteal stripping in predicting the invasion of the mandible by oral squamous cell carcinoma. Br J Oral Maxillofac Surg 1994;32:347–359

39. Bahadur S. Mandibular involvement in oral cancer. J Laryngol Otol 1990;104:968–971

40. Ahuja RB, Soutar DS, Moule B, Bessent RG, Gray HW. Comparative study of technetium-99 m bone scans and orthopantomography in determining mandible invasion in intraoral squamous cell carcinoma. Head Neck 1990;12:237–243

41. Higashi K, Wakao H, Ikuta H, Kashima I, Everhart FR. Bone scintigraphy in detection of bone invasion by oral carcinoma. Ann Nucl Med 1996;10:57–61

42. Kalavrezos ND, Gratz KW, Sailer HF, Stahel WA. Correlation of imaging and clinical features in the assessment of mandibular invasion of oral carcinoma. Int J Oral Maxillofac Surg 1996;25:439–445

43. Acton CH, Layt C, Gwynne R, Cooke R, Seaton D. Investigative modalities of mandibular invasion by squamous cell carcinoma. Laryngoscope 2000;110:2050–2055

44. Chan KW, Merrick MV, Mitchell R. Bone SPECT to assess mandibular invasion by intraoral squamous-cell carcinomas. J Nucl Med 1996; 37:42–45

45. Tsue TT, McCulloch TM, Girod DA, Couper DJ, Weymuller EA Jr, Glenn MG. Predictors of carcinomatous invasion of the mandible. Head Neck 1994;16:116–126

46. Mukherji SK, Isaacs DL, Creager A, Shockley W, Weissler M, Armao D. CT detection of mandibular invasion by squamous cell carcinoma of the oral cavity. AJR Am J Roentgenol 2001;177:237–243

47. Brockenbrough JM, Petruzzelli GJ, Lomasney L. DentaScan as an accurate method of predicting mandibular invasion in patients with squamous cell carcinoma of the oral cavity. Arch Otolaryngol Head Neck Surg 2003;129:113–117

48. Chung TS, Yousem DM, Seigerman HM, Schlakman BN, Weinstein GS, Hayden RE. MR of mandibular invasion in patients with oral and oropharyngeal malignant neoplasms. AJNR Am J Neuroradiol 1994;15: 1949–1955

49. Heppt WJ, Issing WJ. Assessment of tumorous mandibular involvement by transcutaneous ultrasound and flexible endosonography. J Craniomaxillofac Surg 1993;21:107–112

50. Millesi W, Prayer L, Helmer M, Gritzmann N. Diagnostic imaging of tumor invasion of the mandible. Int J Oral Maxillofac Surg 1990;19: 294–298

51. Brown JS, Lewis-Jones H. Evidence for imaging the mandible in the management of oral squamous cell carcinoma: a review. Br J Oral Maxillofac Surg 2001;39:411–418

52. Shaha AR. Preoperative evaluation of the mandible in patients with carcinoma of the floor of mouth. Head Neck 1991;13:398–402

53. Ogura I, Kurabayashi T, Amagasa T, Okada N, Sasaki T. Mandibular bone invasion by gingival carcinoma on dental CT images as an indicator of cervical lymph node metastasis. Dentomaxillofac Radiol 2002;31: 339–343

54. Lam KH, Lam LK, Ho CM, Wei WI. Mandibular invasion in carcinoma of the lower alveolus. Am J Otolaryngol 1999;20:267–272

55. Hong SX, Cha IH, Lee EW, Kim J. Mandibular invasion of lower gingival carcinoma in the molar region: its clinical implications on the surgical management. Int J Oral Maxillofac Surg 2001;30:130–138

56. McGregor AD, MacDonald DG. Patterns of spread of squamous cell carcinoma within the mandible. Head Neck 1989;11:457–461

57. Barttelbort SW, Bahn SL, Ariyan SA. Rim mandibulectomy for cancer of the oral cavity. Am J Surg 1987;154:423–428

58. Barbosa JF. Cancer of the retromolar area: a study of twenty-eight cases with the presentation of a new surgical technique for their treatment. AMA Arch Otolaryngol 1959;69:19–30

59. Kowalski LP, Hashimoto I, Magrin J. End results of 114 extended "commando" operations for retromolar trigone carcinoma. Am J Surg 1993; 166:374–379

60. Martin H. Cancer of the gum (gingivae). Am J Surg 1941;54:765–806

61. Forrest LA, Schuller DE, Karanfilov B, Lucas JG. Update on intraoperative analysis of mandibular margins. Am J Otolaryngol 1997;18:396–399

62. Wald RM Jr, Calcaterra TC. Lower alveolar carcinoma: segmental vs. marginal resection. Arch Otolaryngol 1983;109:578–582

63. Totsuka Y, Usui Y, Tei K, et al. Results of surgical treatment for squamous carcinoma of the lower alveolus: segmental vs. marginal resection. Head Neck 1991;13:114–120

64. Dubner S, Heller KS. Local control of squamous cell carcinoma following marginal and segmental mandibulectomy. Head Neck 1993;15: 29–32

65. Flynn MB, Moore C. Marginal resection of the mandible in the management of squamous cancer of the floor of the mouth. Am J Surg 1974; 128:490–493

66. Beecroft WA, Sako K, Razack MS, Shedd DP. Mandible preservation in the treatment of cancer of the floor of the mouth. J Surg Oncol 1982;19:171–175

67. Shaha AR. Marginal mandibulectomy for carcinoma of the floor of the mouth. J Surg Oncol 1992;49:116–119

68. Petruzzelli GJ, Knight FK, Vandevender D, Clark JI, Emami B. Posterior marginal mandibulectomy in the management of cancer of the oral cavity and oropharynx. Otolaryngol Head Neck Surg 2003;129: 713–719

69. Cady B, Catlin D. Epidermoid carcinoma of the gum: a 20-year survey. Cancer 1969;23:551–569

70. Soo KC, Spiro RH, King W, Harvey W, Strong EW. Squamous carcinoma of the gums. Am J Surg 1988;156:281–285

71. Ildstad ST, Bigelow ME, Remensnyder JP. Squamous cell carcinoma of the alveolar ridge and palate. A 15-year survey. Ann Surg 1984;199: 445–453

72. Ayad T, Gelinas M, Guertin L, et al. Retromolar trigone carcinoma treated by primary radiation therapy: an alternative to the primary surgical approach. Arch Otolaryngol Head Neck Surg 2005;131: 576–582

73. Lo K, Fletcher GH, Byers RM, Fields RS, Peters LJ, Oswald MJ. Results of irradiation in the squamous cell carcinomas of the anterior faucial pillar-retromolar trigone. Int J Radiat Oncol Biol Phys 1987;13: 969–974

74. Koch BB, Trask DK, Hoffman HT, et al. National survey of head and neck verrucous carcinoma: patterns of presentation, care, and outcome. Cancer 2001;92:110–120

75. Eveson JW, Cawson RA. Tumours of the minor (oropharyngeal) salivary glands: a demographic study of 336 cases. J Oral Pathol 1985;14: 500–509

76. Eveson JW, Cawson RA. Salivary gland tumours. A review of 2410 cases with particular reference to histological types, site, age and sex distribution. J Pathol 1985;146:51–58

77. Spiro RH, Koss LG, Hajdu SI, Strong EW. Tumors of minor salivary origin: a clinicopathologic study of 492 cases. Cancer 1973;31: 117–129

78. Waldron CA, el-Mofty SK, Gnepp DR. Tumors of the intraoral minor salivary glands: a demographic and histologic study of 426 cases. Oral Surg Oral Med Oral Pathol 1988;66:323–333

13

Cancer of the Hard Palate and Upper Alveolar Ridge

John W. Werning and
William M. Mendenhall

Cancers of the hard palate and upper alveolar ridge are relatively uncommon malignancies that manifest unique patterns of clinical behavior. The proximity of the maxilla to the nose, paranasal sinuses, orbit, and skull base must be considered during evaluation and management. Few well-performed retrospective reviews of treatment outcomes exist for either site, and no large prospective studies are available. Many larger retrospective studies of palate cancers combine malignancies of the hard and soft palate, and squamous carcinoma and minor salivary gland malignancies are evaluated together. Furthermore, most of the investigations reviewing alveolar ridge cancers do not differentiate between the upper and lower alveolar ridge. Collating data of different histologic types and sites would not be acceptable in more common sites such as the tongue or lip, and therefore we have made a concerted attempt to extract the relevant data from the existing literature for review in this chapter.

The hard palate is the semilunar area inside the upper alveolar ridge that is covered by keratinized masticatory mucosa that extends from the inner surface of the upper alveolar ridge to the posterior edge of the palatine bone at its junction with the soft palate.[1] The upper alveolar ridge refers to the keratinized mucosa overlying the alveolar process of the maxilla, which extends from the line of attachment of mucosa in the upper gingivobuccal sulcus to the junction of the hard palate.[1] Its posterior margin is the upper end of the pterygopalatine arch.[1]

Anteriorly, the lamina propria is attached to the underlying bone through collagenous bundles, or Sharpey's fibers, that form the mucoperiosteum. Posterolaterally, the connective tissue of the hard palate contains numerous purely mucous minor salivary glands, the palatine glands, which extend posteriorly onto the soft palate. At the midline of the hard palate,

or median raphe, there are dense fibrous attachments to the underlying bone and no submucosa is present, giving rise to the term *mucoperiosteum*. In contrast, the submucosa overlying the lateral hard palate contains fatty and glandular tissue (**Fig. 13–1**).[2] A dense superficial system of capillary-like lymph vessels exists within the mucosa of the hard palate, including a few lymph vessels that cross the midline of the hard palate. Lymph flows posteriorly from the hard palate into the collecting system of the soft palate, and laterally through the collecting system of the maxillary gingiva, which is continuous with the upper lymphatic drainage system of the buccal region.[3]

◆ Incidence, Epidemiology, and Etiology

In the United States, cancer of the hard palate makes up 6.7% of all oral cancer cases registered in the National Cancer Data Base (NCDB), whereas cancer of the upper alveolar ridge (UAR) made up only 2.5% of oral cancers (see Table 5–1 in Chapter 5 for the method of calculation).[4] UAR cancers make up less than one third of the cancers that arise from the upper and lower alveolar ridges. Squamous cell carcinoma (SCC) was the most common histologic type at both sites, making up 77% of cancers of the UAR and 43% of cancers of the palate. However, adenocarcinoma made up 31.6% of cancers of the palate, the most frequent site within the oral cavity, whereas adenocarcinoma was the diagnosis in only 3.2% of UAR cancers. Verrucous carcinoma made up 5.7% and 2.8% of UAR and palate cancers, respectively.[4]

The median age at the time of diagnosis was 68.8 years and 70.7 years for patients registered in the NCDB with cancer of the hard palate and UAR, respectively.[4] The etiologic agents

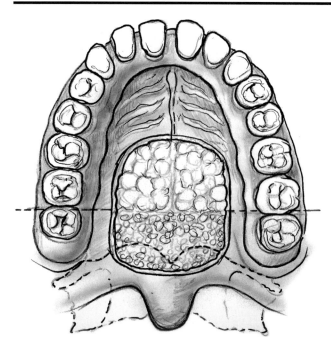

Figure 13–1 Mucosa and submucosa of the hard palate. The submucosa of the posterior hard palate and soft palate contains numerous minor salivary glands, whereas the submucosa anterior to this region contains fatty tissue.

most closely associated with cancer in these regions are similar to the causes at other sites within the oral cavity. In a series of 347 patients with squamous carcinoma of the upper or lower alveolar ridge, 71% regularly used tobacco products and 47% routinely consumed alcoholic beverages.[5] More than 90% of palatal squamous carcinomas have been associated with tobacco and alcohol use.[6] Although other factors such as poor oral hygiene and chronic irritation from denture use have been implicated, little evidence exists to substantiate any relationship.[7]

Chutta smoking is a habit that has been strongly associated with the development of cancer of the hard palate. Chutta is a coarsely prepared cheroot that is made by rolling a sun-dried tobacco leaf into a cylindrical shape that varies from 5 to 9 cm in length.[8,9] Chutta can be smoked conventionally or in reverse fashion, with the burning end inside the mouth. Inhalation and exhalation occur through the body of the cigar.[10] This peculiar habit is practiced in only a few areas of the world: the Philippines, Aruba, Venezuela, Colombia, Panama, Sardinia, and the states of Andhra Pradesh and Orissa along the east coast of India.[9,10] In India, women almost exclusively smoke chuttas in reverse fashion because this is considered a more feminine way to smoke.[8] A cross-sectional study performed in Andhra Pradesh found that 33% of the population practiced reverse chutta smoking, whereas only 12.5% of the population practiced conventional chutta smoking, mainly by men.[10] Palatal lesions were significantly more common in reverse chutta smokers than conventional chutta smokers, and all of the newly diagnosed palatal cancers were observed within the group of reverse smokers. More than 90% of the reverse chutta smokers had abnormal palatal mucosa, whereas approximately 55% of the conventional chutta smokers

demonstrated palatal mucosal abnormalities. Moreover, nearly 80% of all oral mucosal lesions were located solely on the hard palate.[10] Although cancer of the hard palate is rare in other areas of India and the world, it makes up 38% to 48% of the oral cancers in Andhra Pradesh.[11,12] The high levels of tobacco-specific *N*-nitrosamines contained in chutta as well as the production of intraoral temperatures as high as 58°C are thought to result in the elevated incidence of hard palatal cancer in reverse chutta.[9]

◆ Natural History and Clinical Presentation

Cancer of the hard palate frequently begins as a region of erythroplakia or leukoplakia that enlarges into a palatal swelling that can become ulcerated (**Fig. 13–2**). The most common complaints of patients diagnosed with cancer of the hard palate include the sensation of a lump or swelling in the roof of the mouth (34%), pain (27%), ulcer (12%), bleeding (12%), and poorly fitting dentures (8%).[13] The mean duration of symptoms is typically greater than 3 months prior to diagnosis.[6] Seventy percent of hard palate carcinomas extend beyond the hard or soft palate.[6] Carcinoma of the UAR similarly begins as a red or white patch that may appear as a thickened gingival margin adjacent to a tooth, and may be mistaken for gingivitis or periodontal disease. The lesion may extend over the gingiva into the interdental region, and tooth loosening may occur. Lesions are slightly more prone to develop in edentulous regions of the alveolar ridge rather than dentate areas, but this predilection may be related to the frequency of tooth loss in the elderly population at risk for oral cancer.[14] Soreness or gum pain is the most frequent complaint in 54% of patients. Other common symptoms include ulceration (16%) and toothache, as well as tooth-loosening or ill-fitting dentures (15%). Twelve percent were asymptomatic lesions that were incidentally found by their physician or dentist.[5] Determination of fixation to underlying bone is usually not feasible at either site due to the preexisting intimate relationship between the submucosa and the bone. The lesion may also extend

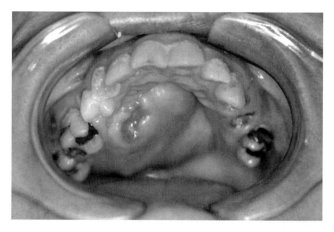

Figure 13–2 Carcinoma ex pleomorphic adenoma of the hard palate.

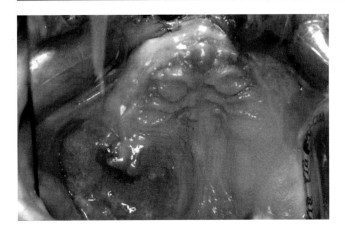

Figure 13–3 Squamous cell carcinoma of the posterior upper alveolar ridge (UAR) with involvement of the hard and soft palate and the gingivobuccal sulcus.

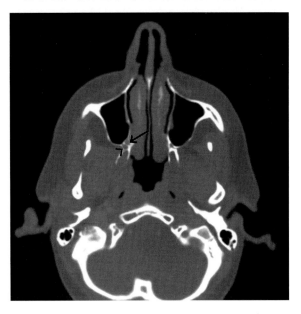

Figure 13–4 Computed tomography (CT) scan demonstrating retrograde perineural invasion from a polymorphous low-grade adenocarcinoma of the hard palate. There is widening of the greater (*arrow*) and lesser (*arrowhead*) palatine canals at the pterygomaxillary junction.

from the alveolar ridge onto the lining mucosa of the oral vestibule, or gingivobuccal sulcus (**Fig. 13–3**). Decreased mucosal sensation is suggestive of palatine nerve involvement, but intact sensation does not exclude nerve invasion. Perineural invasion may also result in facial pain and paresthesias related to branches of V_2, and involvement of the cavernous sinus can result in multiple cranial neuropathies. Posterior spread along the greater superficial petrosal nerve can extend to the geniculate ganglion. Tumors that erode bone may involve the nasal cavity floor or maxillary sinus.

Early lesions of the UAR and hard palate are frequently not easily appreciated on imaging studies, but may be appreciated as a subtle soft tissue thickening overlying the bone. Panoramic radiography may demonstrate obvious alveolar ridge resorption but is not useful in the assessment of the palate. Periapical radiographs may show alterations in the alveolar crestal bony margin and the trabecular bony pattern, but these changes must be differentiated from periodontal bone loss and the alveolar ridge resorption that occurs in the edentulous situation. Their diagnostic utility in the assessment of bone resorption of the maxilla from cancer has not been rigorously evaluated. Computed tomography (CT) provides invaluable information about bone destruction. Thin-section coronal CT is ideal for identifying palatal bone destruction and extension through the floor of the nasal cavity or maxillary sinus.[15] The site of origin in cases of advanced minor salivary gland malignancy is occasionally unclear because minor salivary glands are also present in the nose and maxillary sinus. Perineural spread via the anterior superior alveolar nerves and greater and lesser palatine nerves into the pterygopalatine fossa and foramen rotundum is best seen on coronal magnetic resonance imaging (MRI).[16] High-resolution CT scans with bone windows are invaluable in the assessment of palatine foraminal widening (**Fig. 13–4**).[17] Abnormal attenuation within the pterygopalatine fossa on soft tissue CT windows, or abnormal signal intensity on postcontrast T1-weighted fat-suppressed MRI is strongly suggestive of perineural spread.[17] High-resolution MRI can be used to examine foramen ovale and rotundum, the cavernous sinus, Meckel's cave, and the geniculate ganglion.[17]

Early lesions of the alveolar ridges are often initially evaluated during a visit to the dentist for gingival bleeding, pain, or tooth mobility. In one early review of 533 cancers of the upper and lower alveolar ridge, 62% were first evaluated by a dentist.[18] Fifty percent of them were not identified as cancerous lesions and the patients received other forms of treatment, 34% of whom received dental extractions. Such misdiagnosed gingival malignancies result in delays of diagnosis and could facilitate tumor growth into the extraction socket that could lead to invasion of the bone of the maxilla. The importance of the dental professional and the primary care physician in the early diagnosis of these lesions has been corroborated in subsequent investigations.[5]

Tumor staging for the hard palate and UAR corresponds to the criteria used for other oral cavity sites (see Chapter 7).[1] Tumors that invade through cortical bone, the maxillary sinus, or the skin of the face are designated T4a lesions.[1] Superficial cortical bone erosion of the maxilla is not sufficient to apply the T4 designation. Invasion of the masticator space, pterygoid plates, or skull base, and/or internal carotid artery encasement is assigned T4b status.[1]

Approximately 30% of UAR squamous carcinomas are T1 lesions and 50% are T2 lesions, whereas more than 50% of hard palate malignancies are T3 or T4 lesions.[5,13,19] Clinical evidence of bone invasion of the UAR using physical examination and panoramic radiography has been noted in 30% of UAR cancers.[5]

There are scant retrospective data pertaining to the rates of regional nodal metastasis from the hard palate and UAR. The rate of clinically evident regional metastasis at the time of presentation was 14% for cancer of the UAR in one series from Memorial Sloan-Kettering Cancer Center (MSKCC) and 17 to 29% for hard palate malignancies from a small group of retrospective case series.[5,6,13,19] One case series from the

University of Virginia noted a 14% rate of clinical metastasis for T1–T2 lesions and a 35% rate for T3–T4 lesions.[13] The frequency of occult nodal metastasis (ONM) associated with malignancies of the hard palate and UAR have not been documented, although the rate of ONM in two retrospective series that evaluated upper and lower alveolar ridge malignancies together was 13% and 38%, respectively.[5,20]

The patterns of regional metastasis for cancer arising from these two mucosal sites have not been rigorously evaluated. However, characterization of the lymph nodes at risk for metastatic disease arising from carcinoma of the adjacent buccal mucosa and soft palate suggests that lymph node levels I through IV would also be at risk for metastatic disease from the hard palate and UAR.[3] Metastases to the retropharyngeal nodes have been reported to occasionally develop from malignancies involving these two sites.[21]

Regional nodal metastases, advanced T stage, and positive surgical margins negatively impact disease-specific survival in patients with carcinoma of the UAR on multivariate analysis. The presence of bone invasion, however, has not been associated with worse survival.[5] Although Cady and Catlin[18] in 1969 documented worse survival in patients at MSKCC who underwent dental extractions prior to treatment, multivariate analysis of a subsequent series from MSKCC in 1981 was unable to confirm this association.[6] Regional metastasis is the most important prognostic factor for squamous carcinoma of the hard palate.[22]

◆ Treatment

Maxillectomy

Presurgical evaluation by a maxillofacial prosthodontist or microvascular reconstructive surgeon should be obtained whenever resection is expected to create a palatomaxillary defect that will require rehabilitation, because the functional and aesthetic outcome of surgery and rehabilitation is contingent upon close communication between surgeons and their colleagues. Careful consideration should be given to the preservation of the soft palate and critical abutment teeth that will optimize velopharyngeal function and improve the stability of the obturator, respectively. Scenarios of surgical outcomes that will not be optimally rehabilitated by the use of a prosthesis must be anticipated so that the patient and surgeon are prepared to proceed with microvascular reconstruction or osseointegrated implantation. Preoperative patient counseling should include a discussion of potential sequelae, including infraorbital anesthesia, epiphora and ectropion, velopharyngeal insufficiency, impairment of mastication and deglutition, and loss of vision or visual changes that could develop from orbital dystopia following loss of orbital floor support.

Bone resection is necessary to resect the majority of these malignancies to achieve tumor-free margins with confidence. According to Soo et al,[5] surgical resection of UAR cancers requires at least partial maxillectomy in 85% of the cases, whereas local excision without bony resection was successfully performed for 15% of the lesions. Only superficial mucosal lesions are amenable to wide local soft tissue resection with the underlying periosteum.

Many partial maxillectomy procedures can be performed transorally, although access to the posterior maxilla and the pterygomaxillary region frequently requires performance of a lip-splitting incision combined with a lateral rhinotomy incision and elevation of a cheek flap. The Weber-Fergusson extension of the incision along the lower eyelid frequently results in prolonged lower eyelid edema and ectropion, and can usually be avoided. If exposure is inadequate, an extended lateral rhinotomy incision can be employed to facilitate total maxillectomy with orbital preservation to avoid the subciliary extension (**Fig. 13–5**).[23] The intraoral gingivobuccal incision is performed through the lining mucosa of the buccal vestibule at least 5 mm away from the mucogingival junction. If pterygomaxillectomy dysjunction is planned, the mucosal incision must extend back to this region. Soft tissue elevation from the anterior face of the maxilla is usually performed in a subperiosteal plane unless there is radiographic evidence of tumor erosion through the anterior wall of the maxillary sinus. The zygomatic process of the maxilla is exposed in preparation for the lateral osteotomy. When palatal resection is planned, dissection through the soft tissues of the piriform aperture region into the nose permits retraction of the alar portion of the nose so that the resection can be extended through the palate into the nasal cavity.

The orbital floor can usually be preserved if there is no radiographic evidence of orbital floor destruction. This relationship can be directly inspected by entering the maxillary sinus superior to the anticipated intrasinus component of the tumor. A subperiorbital dissection can be performed if orbital preservation is a possibility in situations where preoperative clinical and radiographic assessment yield equivocal findings. Orbital preservation should be achieved whenever the orbital walls remain intact, and orbital preservation is usually possible if periorbital invasion has not developed in the presence of adjacent bone invasion. Resection of the periorbita to verify complete resection via frozen section examination is prudent. Periorbital tumor invasion must be evaluated on a case-by-case basis, but orbital exenteration must be seriously pondered, because orbital fat provides an ineffective barrier to tumor invasion.

The entire soft palate should be preserved whenever possible by extending the mucosal incision from the pterygomaxillary region over the pterygomaxillary junction to the soft palate–hard palate junction, where the remainder of the incision is dictated by the palatal extent of the tumor. If involvement is limited to the hard palate, a full-thickness incision is extended through the nasopharyngeal mucosa of the soft palate at the posterior aspect of the hard palate. If a significant anteroposterior portion of the soft palate must be resected, intraoperative discussion between the surgeon and prosthodontist may be necessary to determine whether a better functional result will be achieved by bisecting the remaining posterior soft palate so that a prosthesis with a palatal extension can be used. In these cases, the soft palate should be strategically divided and exploited as well-vascularized local rotational flaps to primarily close adjacent soft tissue defects of the lateral oropharyngeal walls.

Radiographic and clinical assessment of the patterns of tumor invasion should guide the placement of the osteotomies. For the purpose of this discussion, however, the

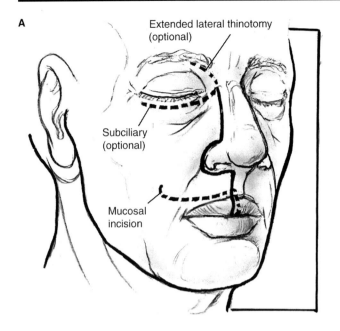

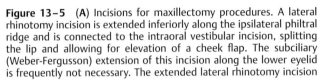

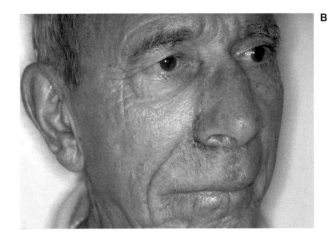

Figure 13–5 **(A)** Incisions for maxillectomy procedures. A lateral rhinotomy incision is extended inferiorly along the ipsilateral philtral ridge and is connected to the intraoral vestibular incision, splitting the lip and allowing for elevation of a cheek flap. The subciliary (Weber-Fergusson) extension of this incision along the lower eyelid is frequently not necessary. The extended lateral rhinotomy incision provides adequate exposure for performance of a total maxillectomy, eliminates lower eyelid complications, and results in a better cosmetic result. **(B)** Appearance of lateral rhinotomy incision in combination with lip-splitting incision 10 days following maxillectomy with orbital floor preservation. Cheek support has been reestablished by a maxillary obturator.

osteotomies that are performed for a "total" or "radical" hemimaxillectomy that resects the orbital floor but preserves the eye include the following (**Fig. 13–6**):

1. Division is performed through the nasal bone slightly above the nasomaxillary suture line, terminating the osteotomy inferior to the suture line at the junction of the frontal process of the maxilla and the frontal bone.
2. From the superior point of osteotomy No. 1, a horizontal osteotomy is performed inferior to the frontoethmoid suture line posteriorly through the lacrimal bone and orbital plate of the ethmoid bone to the inferolateral orbital wall at the inferior orbital fissure.
3. An angled osteotomy that passes from the pterygomaxillary junction through the anterior zygoma or zygomatic process of the maxilla and through the inferolateral orbital floor is connected to osteotomy No. 2 along the posterior orbital floor.
4. An osteotomy through the hard palate, or palatine process of the maxilla and the palatine bone, extends into the floor of the nose. If possible, the palatal bone supporting the anterior nasal septum should be preserved to maintain nasal tip support. Creation of an osteotomy that extends into the ipsilateral nasal cavity and avoids the nasal septum also facilitates prosthetic rehabilitation. This osteotomy is usually performed after the osteotomies Nos. 1 through 3 because more bleeding can be expected from this osteotomy.
5. The maxilla is usually somewhat mobile once the first four osteotomies have been completed. Pterygomaxillary dysjunction should be the last osteotomy that is performed because the potential for hemorrhage is most significant. Once the periosteum has been dissected away from the pterygomaxillary fissure, the region should be carefully palpated to identify the inferior aspect of the junction. A 15-mm curved osteotome should be positioned along the inferior portion of the fissure and directed anteriorly, inferiorly, and medially. The osteotomy can usually be performed without significant hemorrhage from the branches of the maxillary artery, but proper performance of each osteotomy with evidence of increasing maxillary mobility prior to pterygomaxillary dysjunction should allow for easy removal of the maxillectomy specimen and control of any bleeding via direct inspection. Tissue is sent for frozen section examination from all regions in proximity to the resected tumor prior to surgical reconstruction.

If the orbital floor has been resected, orbital floor reconstruction must be meticulously performed to precisely restore the position of the globe in all three planes to avoid postoperative diplopia and enophthalmos. A variety of modalities can be employed to reconstruct the floor, including temporalis muscle transposition and titanium mesh placement.

The soft tissue incisions and osteotomies for other maxillectomy procedures, once again, depend on the pattern of tumor invasion that is present (see **Figs. 13–7** to **13–10** on pp. 147 to 150). If an anterior maxillectomy must be performed that removes the anterior palatal support of the nasal septum, the surgeon must be prepared to reestablish nasal tip support by using a cantilevered cranial bone graft (see **Fig. 13–10** on p. 150). Maxillary resections that extend above the root apex of a tooth should be placed at least

A

Orbital plate of
ethmoid

Lacrimal
bone

Frontoethmoid
suture

#2

Nasomaxillary
suture

#1

#3

#4

Zygomaticomaxillary
suture

B

Pterygomaxillary fissure

Descending palatine
artery

Maxillary artery

Lateral
pterygoid plate

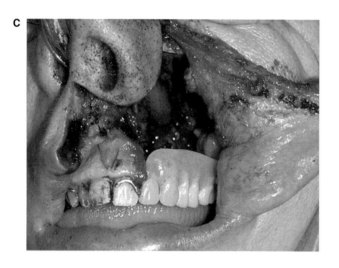

C

Figure 13–6 Total maxillectomy with orbital preservation. **(A)** Osteotomies: (1) through nasal bone, extending inferior to frontoethmoid suture line; (2) from 1 posterolaterally to inferior orbital fissure; (3) from pterygomaxillary junction to lateral portion of osteotomy 2 anterior to the inferior orbital fissure; (4) through palatine bone and palatine process of the maxilla into the floor of the nose. **(B)** Pterygomaxillary dysjunction. A 15-mm curved osteotome should be positioned at the inferior aspect of the suture, and the osteotomy should be directed anteriorly and inferiorly. **(C)** Appearance following maxillectomy with orbital floor preservation. An interim prosthesis has been placed, and a clasp engages the cervical region of the ipsilateral central incisor, which was preserved to optimize the cosmetic result. (Courtesy of Robin Windl, D.D.S., M.S.)

5 mm superior to the location of the root apex to maintain the viability of the tooth.[24,25] The inferior turbinate should be removed whenever the nasal floor has been resected, because contact of the obturator with the turbinate can complicate rehabilitation following surgery.

Vascular Considerations During Maxillectomy

Knowledge of vascular anatomy minimizes blood loss during maxillectomy and optimizes the vascular supply to the residual maxilla following surgical resection. The blood supply to the maxilla is derived from several branches of the external carotid artery, including the maxillary, facial,

and ascending pharyngeal artery. As the maxillary artery courses through the pterygopalatine fossa, it branches into its terminal vessels, including the sphenopalatine, descending palatine, and posterior superior alveolar arteries. The sphenopalatine artery gives rise to the nasopalatine artery, which travels through the incisive canal and exits through the incisive foramen behind the central incisors. The descending palatine artery passes through the greater palatine foramen at the junction between the maxillary alveolar ridge and the hard palate in the region of the maxillary second molar. The lesser palatine artery is formed by the confluence of the ascending palatine artery, a branch of the facial artery, and contributions from the ascending

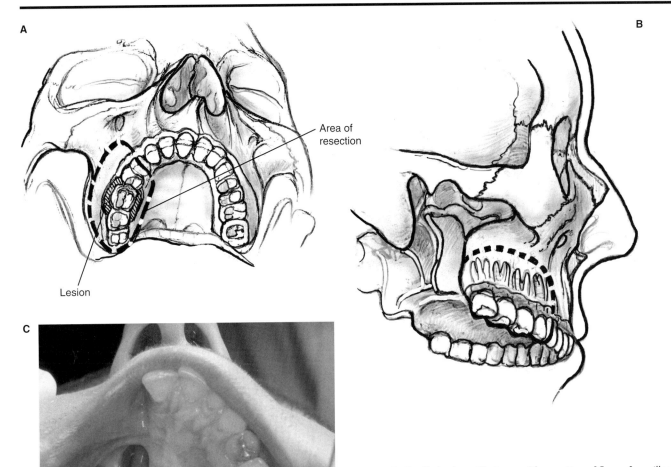

Figure 13–7 Limited maxillectomy with resection of floor of maxillary sinus. **(A)** Palatal view of planned resection. **(B)** Posterolateral view. **(C)** Appearance following resection, after mucosal healing. The mucosalized maxillary sinus is visualized laterally and the nasal cavity can be seen medially.

pharyngeal artery. The lesser palatine artery courses through the soft palate and anastomoses with the descending palatine artery to form the greater palatine artery.[26]

The LeFort I osteotomy, a frequently performed orthognathic surgical procedure, requires a circumvestibular incision that extends anteriorly from the first molar region bilaterally through the buccolabial periosteum with subperiosteal dissection over the anterior face of the maxilla followed by osteotomies that extend from the piriform aperture of the nose posteriorly and above the roots of the maxillary teeth to the pterygomaxillary junction. These osteotomies allow for down-fracture and mobilization of the maxilla, leaving the maxilla attached to a pedicle of soft tissue in the region of the soft palate and the posterior gingivobuccal sulcus. Bell[24,27,28] performed maxillary osteotomies on rhesus monkeys and found that the soft palate and gingivobuccal soft tissues provided adequate vascular supply to maintain viability of the osteotomized maxilla even if the descending palatine arteries were transected bilaterally. Subsequent research on human subjects who underwent Le Fort I osteotomy with bilateral descending palatine artery ligation demonstrated no significant decrease

in maxillary gingival blood flow when compared with patients who had both arteries preserved.[29] Perfusion following LeFort I osteotomy is maintained through the lesser palatine artery, which is formed by contributions of the facial and ascending pharyngeal arteries, as previously noted. When subapical osteotomies are performed, the bony cuts should be at least 5 mm above the apex of the tooth roots to preserve pulpal viability.[25,28]

Blood loss during maxillectomy can be minimized by carefully performing the osteotomy through the pterygomaxillary junction. The mean measured height of the pterygomaxillary junction (PMJ) is 14.6 mm in Americans and 19.5 mm in 100 Thai adult cadavers, suggesting that a racial disparity in the height of this suture line may exist. The maxillary artery has been shown to course through the pterygomaxillary fissure on its way into the pterygopalatine fossa 4 to 10 mm superior to the top of the pterygomaxillary suture line.[26,30,31] The mean distance from the inferior edge of the PMJ to the inferior aspect of the maxillary artery is 25.0 ± 1.5 mm in Americans according to Turvey and Fonseca,[31] and 23.5 ± 2.5 mm in Thai adults according to Apinhasmit and colleagues[30] from Bangkok. Using these measurements, an 8 to 10 mm margin

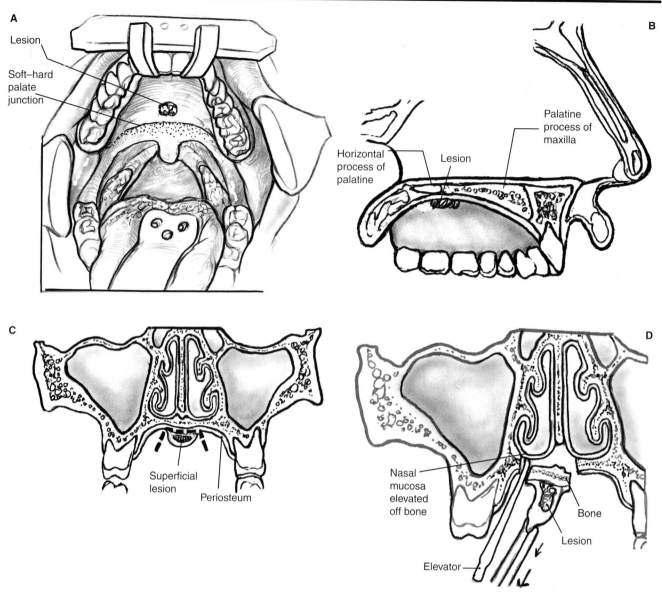

Figure 13–8   Resection of cancer involving the hard palate. **(A)** Cancerous lesion involving posterior hard palate, occlusal view. **(B)** Sagittal view. **(C)** Superficially invasive lesions can be resected in a submucoperiosteal plane. **(D)** Most malignant lesions require resection of palatal bone. Elevation of the nasal mucosa prior to performance of the osteotomy may avoid an oronasal communication in patients with early palatal bone invasion.

of safety exists between the superior aspect of a 15-mm osteotome that is placed so that the inferior aspect of the osteotome engages the inferior aspect of the PMJ.[30,31] Orienting the osteotome anteriorly and inferiorly further minimizes injury to the maxillary artery.

The descending palatine artery, which arises from the third portion of the maxillary artery, is also a vulnerable source of bleeding during maxillectomy due to its location in the posteromedial wall of the maxillary sinus.[26,30,31] This artery is a common source of significant bleeding during pterygomaxillary dysjunction, and transection is usually inevitable if the posterior wall of the maxillary sinus is resected. Once again, proper placement and orientation of the osteotome usually avoids injury during

separation of the PMJ so that significant hemorrhage is not experienced until the maxillectomy specimen has been mobilized, facilitating prompt visualization and hemostatic control.

In summary, the orthognathic surgical literature provides head and neck cancer surgeons with the following technical nuances that will improve the vascularity of the residual maxillary segment and minimize blood loss during maxillectomy:

1. Whenever possible, limit the posterior extent of the buccolabial circumvestibular incision to optimize ipsilateral blood supply to the residual maxilla and soft palate.

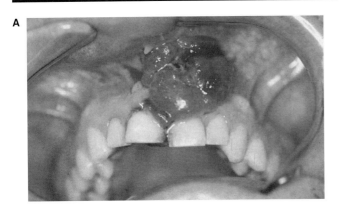

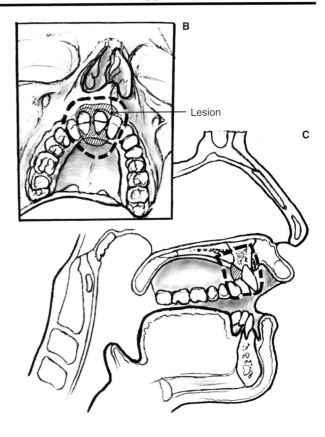

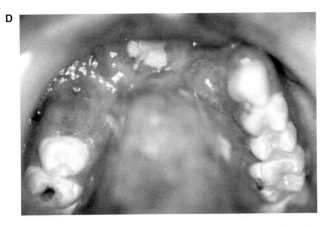

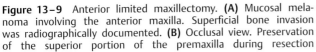

Figure 13-9 Anterior limited maxillectomy. **(A)** Mucosal melanoma involving the anterior maxilla. Superficial bone invasion was radiographically documented. **(B)** Occlusal view. Preservation of the superior portion of the premaxilla during resection preserves nasal tip support and avoids the creation of an oronasal fistula. **(C)** Sagittal view. **(D)** Appearance following resection. Residual bone separates the nose from the oral cavity. A skin graft was applied to the exposed bone.

2. If both greater palatine arteries require ligation, the residual soft tissue pedicle of the soft palate, the buccolabial gingiva, and the nasopalatine artery usually provide adequate vascular supply to the remaining maxilla. Atraumatic handling of these soft tissues is critical, and the surgeon should avoid extensive subperiosteal dissection to minimize devascularization of the residual bony maxillary segments.

3. Horizontal subapical osteotomies should be performed at least 5 mm above the tooth roots to preserve vascular supply to the dental pulp.

4. During pterygomaxillary dysjunction, the risk of arterial transection and clinically significant hemorrhage can be minimized by placing a curved osteotome along the inferior aspect of the pterygomaxillary fissure and angling the osteotome anteriorly and inferiorly (**Fig. 13-6B**).

Maxillectomy Classification

The term *total maxillectomy* usually refers to a total hemimaxillectomy that resects the maxilla as well as portions of the palatine, lacrimal, ethmoid, inferior concha, and the zygomatic contribution to the orbital floor. Resection of portions of the zygomatic bone that make up the zygomatic arch or the medial and lateral pterygoid plates may be required if dissection of the infratemporal fossa or pterygopalatine fossa region is indicated.

In broad terms, a partial maxillectomy includes any maxillectomy procedure that involves less than a total hemimaxillectomy, but the term *partial maxillectomy* encompasses a spectrum of surgical procedures, and the terminology used to describe these procedures is not standardized. Spiro and colleagues[32] from MSKCC recommend that terms such as *alveolectomy, medial maxillectomy*, and *infrastructure maxillectomy* should be discarded, and suggest a classification system that is based on the number of maxillary sinus walls that have been surgically removed:

1. Limited maxillectomy: resection of one wall of the maxillary sinus

2. Subtotal maxillectomy: resection of at least two walls of the maxillary sinus, not including the posterior wall (**Fig. 13-10**)

3. Total maxillectomy: complete resection of the maxilla with or without orbital exenteration (**Fig. 13-6**).

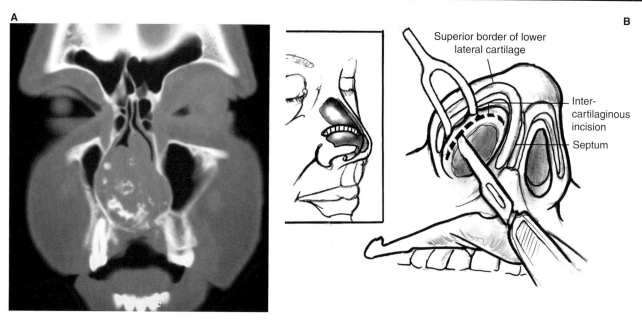

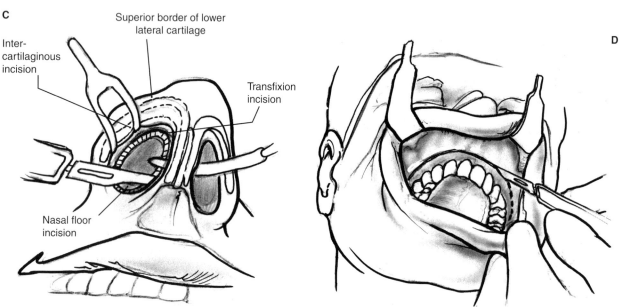

Figure 13–10   Subtotal maxillectomy for chondrosarcoma arising from the maxilla and nasal septum. This case is presented to illustrate resection of tumors that require full-thickness resection of the anterior maxilla. **(A)** Coronal CT scan demonstrating an expansile tumor with destruction of the anterior maxilla, nasal septum, and nasal bones. **(B–F)** Surgical access was achieved by using a midfacial degloving approach. **(B)** Bilateral intercartilaginous incisions between the upper and lower lateral cartilages were performed. The inset demonstrates the location of the incision. **(C)** A complete transfixion incision between the columella and nasal septum is performed, preserving the integrity of the medial crura of the lower lateral cartilages. An incision is then performed through the nasal floor immediately anterior to the face of the maxilla. These incisions are connected so that the nasal mucosa has been circumferentially incised on both sides of the nose. **(D)** A sublabial mucosal incision is created in the buccal vestibule to the first molar regions bilaterally. (*Continued*)

Using this classification, a palatectomy or an alveolectomy that resects the inferior wall of the maxillary sinus is termed a limited maxillectomy (**Fig. 13–7**). A medial maxillectomy is a limited maxillectomy that removes the medial wall of the maxillary sinus. Extensions of the procedure, such as the resection of skin, pterygoid plates, zygoma, or the contralateral maxilla, should also be documented to accurately depict the resection that was performed.

Although standardization of maxillectomy nomenclature is important, greater focus has also been placed on the significant rehabilitative issues that must be addressed following surgical resection. Although the maxillofacial prosthodontist and reconstructive surgeon can improve postsurgical outcomes, the resecting surgeon may be able to improve postoperative function by preservation of a critical abutment tooth or by increasing residual palatal or

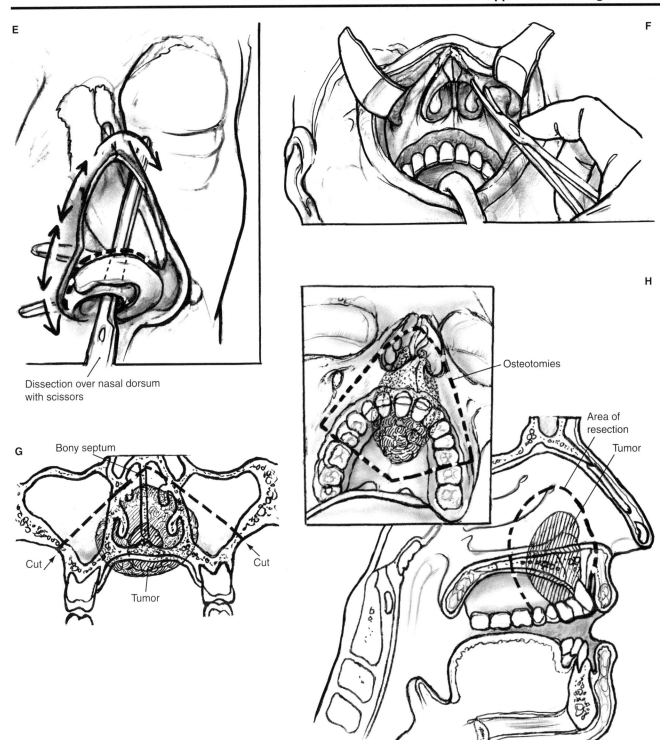

Dissection over nasal dorsum
with scissors

G

Bony septum

Cut

Tumor

Cut

Osteotomies

H

Area of
resection

Tumor

Figure 13–10 (*Continued*) **(E)** Using a scissors, dissection is performed through the intercartilaginous incisions superiorly over the nasal dorsum and laterally to the junction of the nasal bones with the maxilla. Dissection deep to the superficial musculoaponeurotic system (SMAS) of the nose minimizes bleeding. **(F)** Subperiosteal elevation of the soft tissues away from the anterior face of the maxilla is performed superiorly to the infraorbital foramen, preserving the infraorbital nerve. The midfacial degloving approach provides wide exposure of the maxilla and nose for subsequent tumor resection. **(G)** Planned lines of resection, coronal view. The inferior and medial walls of the maxillary sinus (two walls) will be resected bilaterally (a subtotal maxillectomy). **(H)** Sagittal view of planned resection lines. The inset illustrates the planned lines of resection through the UAR and hard palate anterior to the first molars. (*Continued*)

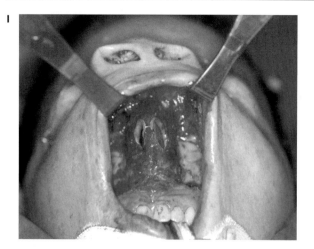

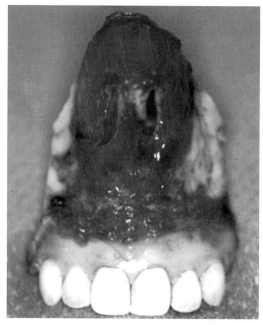

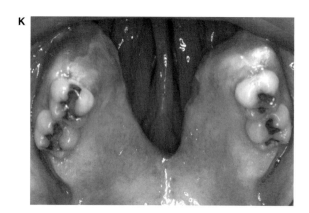

Figure 13–10 (*Continued*) **(I)** The osteotomies have been completed, and the anterior maxilla, nasal septum, and nasal bones have been resected en bloc. **(J)** Resected specimen. Nasal tip support was restored with a cranial bone graft. **(K)** Postresection defect. A maxillary obturator was used to effectively separate the nasal cavity from the oral cavity and restore upper lip support. The remaining molars and maxilla provided a stable base for the removable prosthesis.

alveolar ridge surface area without compromising the oncologic result. The execution of a maxillectomy, therefore, should be guided by the pattern of tumor invasion rather than by a predetermined formula provided by a how-to guide for maxillectomies. Preoperative communication between the surgeon and prosthodontist can circumvent the sacrifice of functionally and aesthetically critical soft tissue and bone.

Maxillectomy defects were traditionally managed by local flaps or the fabrication of a maxillary obturator, but the introduction of free tissue transfer has provided us with a greater spectrum of rehabilitative options that can be exploited to address particular functional and aesthetic needs.[33,34] Several classification systems for maxillectomy defects have consequently been developed so that clinicians are able to choose reconstructive and rehabilitative therapy that is defect-specific.[33,34] Brown and colleagues[33] from Liverpool note that the vertical component of the surgical defect primarily impacts the aesthetic outcome, whereas the horizontal component of the defect has greater functional implications, and propose a classification scheme that is intended to provide clinicians with rehabilitative options that correct the sequelae caused by the vertical and horizontal components (**Figs. 13–11**). The biomechanical principles that improve obturator stability are integrated into the palatomaxillary classification system proposed by clinicians from Mt. Sinai Medical Center (New York, NY),

which establishes a reconstructive algorithm that is intended to address midfacial deformities and restore optimal orodental function.[34] These classification schemes are reviewed in greater depth in Chapters 19 and 24.

Prosthetic Rehabilitation: Surgical Considerations

The surgeon may be able to preserve critical abutment teeth and portions of the alveolar ridge and hard palate that can simplify prosthetic rehabilitation and improve masticatory function. Mastication involves the subdivision of food by applied force, and can be quantified by measuring masticatory efficiency, which is the ability to reduce food to a certain size in a given time frame.[35] Masticatory efficiency and resistance to displacement of removable partial dentures, including obturators, depend on the support provided by the remaining teeth, bone, and soft tissues, and the stability and retention provided by the prosthesis. Stability is defined as the quality of a prosthesis to be firm and resist displacement by functional, horizontal, or rotational stresses. Retention is an inherent quality of the denture that resists vertical forces of dislodgment, including gravity and adhesive foods.[35] Retention of a removable prosthesis is provided by placing retaining elements such as carefully designed clasps that engage tooth surfaces and by the intimate relationship of denture bases and palatal connectors with underlying tissues.[36] A tooth-supported prosthesis

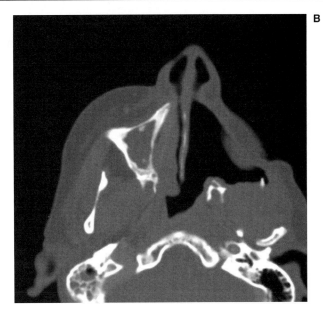

Figure 13–11 Total maxillectomy with orbital exenteration. The resection extends to the midline and to the skull base. Preservation of the anterior maxilla prevents collapse of the nasal tip. The vertical **(A)** and horizontal **(B)** components of the defect result in aesthetic and functional sequelae that must be restored. The pterygoid plates have been preserved **(B)**.

that restores a defect that has periodontally sound teeth on either side of the defect typically has the most support, stability, and retention. Such a prosthesis is fabricated for patients who undergo a limited anterior maxillectomy. A tooth- and tissue-supported prosthesis must rely on support that is provided by the teeth at one end of the prosthesis and the masticatory mucosa and surgical defect at the other end. Maxillectomies that extend through the pterygomaxillary fissure are restored with a distal tissue-supported prostheses that has less support, stability, and retention than a tooth-supported prosthesis. The acrylic denture base of such a prosthesis has a distal extension that is subject to significant movement as a consequence of the compressibility of the underlying soft tissues. Healthy masticatory mucosa overlying the alveolar ridge can be compressed as much as 3 mm, and the compressibility of tissues in a maxillectomy defect may be significantly greater.[37] These rotational forces result in denture instability and create pathologic lever forces that traumatize important abutment teeth by exacerbating periodontal bone loss.

Preservation of the residual UAR and hard palate improves support and retention by increasing the surface area for the denture base to rest upon, and also improves stability by minimizing the impact of rotational forces that result from an occlusal load that compresses an obturator into the maxillectomy defect. Careful surgical planning between the surgeon and the prosthodontist also provides an opportunity to exploit the biomechanical principles on which removable dental prostheses function by selecting potentially critical abutment teeth that can retain the prosthesis. The condition of the tooth that is located closest to the surgical defect is critical in predicting the resultant prosthetic result, so the root form and periodontal condition of this tooth as well as other potential abutment teeth must be evaluated.[34,38] For example, a healthy maxillary canine is usually preferred over the lateral incisor as an abutment

tooth for retention of a prosthesis because the canine has a superior root form and a greater root surface area.[34] Preservation of an important abutment tooth, when oncologically feasible, can markedly improve the prosthetic result that is achieved. Even if the canine cannot be preserved, a better cosmetic result can be achieved by preserving the ipsilateral central incisor and, if possible, the lateral incisor (**Fig. 13–6C**).

Preservation of the dentition and uninvolved maxilla can also create a favorable distribution of masticatory forces so that the "occlusal load" is evenly distributed, and an obturator bulb that intimately engages the structures within the defect helps to further diminish any counterproductive lever forces placed on the obturator, contributing to the support, stability, and retention of the prosthesis.[34] The two terminal abutment teeth and the canine furthest from the defect form a triangle that is directly associated with the stability of the obturator. As the maxillectomy defect increases in size, the area within the triangle diminishes, and the remaining palatal and dentoalveolar support becomes insufficient to prevent a cantilever effect around the fulcrum line, resulting in greater instability (**Fig. 13–12**). Thus, the nature and extent of surgical resection directly impacts the functional result that can be achieved following prosthetic restoration.

Radiation Therapy Technique

T1–T2 Lesions

The preferred initial treatment for patients with T1–T2 carcinomas of the UAR and hard palate is surgery. Radiation therapy (RT) is used by default to treat the occasional patient who is not a surgical candidate. Most of these lesions are not well lateralized; consequently, RT is administered with parallel-opposed fields encompassing the

A

B

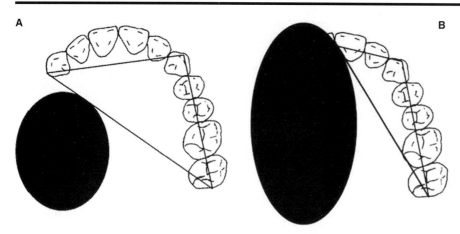

Figure 13–12 Relationship between maxillectomy defect size and stability of the obturator. **(A)** Triangle formed by fulcrum line of framework and tooth farthest from defect. Framework with complete palate major connector and direct retainers on teeth away from fulcrum line will resist destabilizing forces and contribute to stabilization of the obturator. **(B)** Supporting tissues diminish as defect enlarges, affecting prosthetic stability. Dental arch shortens, remaining palate decreases, and the superior root form of the canine as a terminal abutment is replaced with the less optimal root form of the incisor. All factors can contribute to instability of obturator (From Okay DJ, Genden E, Buchbinder D, Urken M. Prosthodontic guidelines for surgical reconstruction of the maxilla: a classification system of defects. J Prosthet Dent 2001;86:352–363, with permission from the Editorial Council of the *Journal of Prosthetic Dentistry.*)

primary tumor with a margin of 2 cm or less. A cork and tongue block is placed in the mouth to displace the tongue, mandible, and lower lip inferiorly and to reduce the amount of normal tissue included in the fields (**Fig. 13–13**). These lesions are not amenable to interstitial brachytherapy, and so patients are treated with external beam RT alone. The likelihood of cure with RT alone, even for early-stage lesions, is relatively low, so that an altered fractionation technique should be employed. We prefer hyperfractionated RT and we treat from 74.4 to 76.8 Gy at 1.2 Gy/fraction, twice daily, over 6 to 6.5 weeks. The fields are extended to include the regional lymph nodes (levels I and II) for patients with aggressive, poorly differentiated cancers (**Fig. 13–14**). The disadvantage of irradiating the regional lymph nodes is that the acute toxicity of the treatment is significantly increased. Fields are reduced at 45.6 Gy in 38 fractions to limited portals that adequately encompass the primary cancer. The low neck is irradiated with an interior field that abuts the primary fields at the level of the thyroid notch and receives 50 Gy in 25 fractions over 5 weeks.

T3–T4 Lesions

Patients with T3–T4 cancers are optimally treated with surgery and postoperative RT using fields encompassing the primary tumor and regional lymph nodes as previously described. Postoperative RT is initiated within 6 weeks of surgery. Patients are treated once daily at 2 Gy/fraction, 5 days a week in a continuous course: negative margins (R0), 60 Gy; microscopically positive margins (R1), 66 Gy; and gross residual disease (R2), 70 Gy. Reductions off of the spinal cord are performed at 44 to 46 Gy and the posterior strips are treated with 8- to 10-MeV electrons if it is necessary to irradiate these areas to a higher dose. An altered fractionation technique should be considered for those who have positive margins.

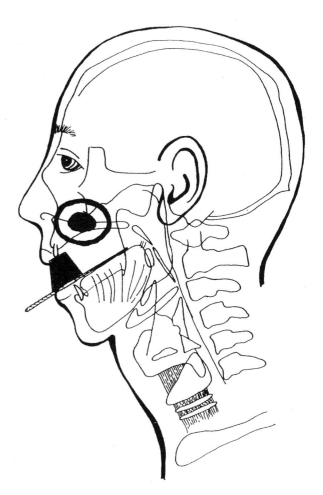

Figure 13–13 Early-stage hard palate carcinomas. Parallel-opposed 6 MV x-ray fields include the tumor with a 2-cm margin. Cork and tongue block displace the tongue and mandible inferiorly to minimize the amount of normal tissue included in the fields.

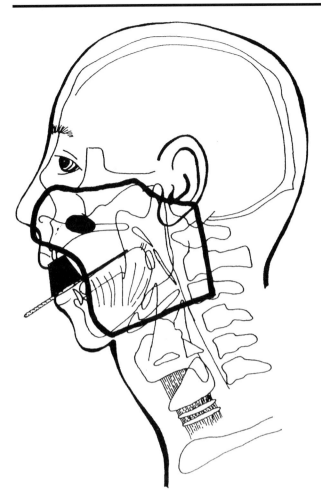

Figure 13–14 Advanced hard palate carcinoma. Portals include the primary tumor and upper neck nodes. The superior margin of the portals is extended to include V_2 to the skull base.

Patients with T3–T4 cancers who are not surgical candidates have a low chance of cure with RT. Patients are treated to 76.8 Gy at 1.2 Gy/fraction twice daily over 6.5 weeks combined with concomitant chemotherapy such as weekly cisplatin 30 mg/m^2. Patients who are not candidates for aggressive therapy are treated with moderate-dose palliative RT over 1 to 2 weeks.

◆ Outcomes

The peer-reviewed literature pertaining to the outcomes of therapy for squamous carcinoma of the hard palate and UAR is limited to a few retrospective case series. Meaningful interpretation of the findings from these investigations is limited by small sample size, failure to separately analyze outcomes by site and treatment modality, and treatment selection bias. Furthermore, tumor, node, and metastasis (TNM) distribution and the rates of local-regional recurrence, disease-free survival, and disease-specific survival are not consistently provided.

Treatment of squamous carcinomas of the hard palate and UAR range with RT alone achieves modest local control rates, ranging from 40 to 75%.[39,40] Chung and colleagues[40] from the

University of Virginia documented a 40% rate of local control with RT for cancers of the hard palate. In a series of 19 patients with cancer of the hard palate that received RT in Manchester, the 5-year local control rate and overall survival rate were 58% and 48%, respectively.[39]

The University of Virginia documented a 34% local recurrence rate and a 59% 5-year determinate survival rate for 32 patients with squamous carcinoma of the hard palate who were treated between 1932 and 1975.[13] Patients were treated with radiation therapy (RT), surgery, or surgery and RT. Fifty-five percent of the patients had T3–T4 lesions. The neck was clinically positive in 14% of the patients with T1–T2 lesions and 35% of those with T3–T4 lesions. Five-year determinate survival was 80% for stage I to II lesions versus 50% for stage III to IV lesions.

The outcomes of 62 patients that were treated at MSKCC for SCC of the hard palate were published in 1981.[6] Eighty-five percent of the patients were treated by surgery alone, whereas RT alone and surgery plus RT were employed for 10% and 5% of the patients, respectively. Determinate 5-year survival by stage was as follows: stage I, 75%; stage II, 46%; stage III, 36%; stage IV, 11%. The difference in survival between stages I to II and stage IV was statistically significant. There was no difference in survival between cancers of the soft or hard palate of the same stage.

In 1969, Cady and Catlin[18] reviewed the MSKCC experience with 95 patients treated for SCC of the UAR. The T stage distribution and the frequency of regional metastases were not provided. Sixty-six percent underwent surgical resection of the primary, 12% received local resection plus neck dissection, and 14% underwent RT. Local failure occurred in 17% of those patients who underwent local resection alone. Five-year determinate survival for all treated upper alveolar cancers was 47%. Cady and Catlin also noted that patients who underwent dental extractions prior to referral for cancer treatment demonstrated poorer 5-year survival.

In 1988, a follow-up study from MSKCC reviewed the outcomes of 83 patients with squamous carcinomas of the UAR.[5] Most patients underwent partial maxillectomy, and some of the patients received preoperative or postoperative RT. Determinate 5-year survival was 51% and multivariate analysis showed that survival was affected by T stage, regional nodal metastases, and positive surgical margins. The presence of bone invasion and the performance of dental extractions prior to treatment were not associated with worse survival in this series.

Investigators from the University of Cincinnati retrospectively reviewed their experience with 25 squamous carcinomas of the hard palate and UAR, 54% of which were T4 lesions.[19] Seventeen percent of the patients had clinically positive regional nodal metastatic disease.[19] All patients underwent surgical resection with or without postoperative RT. Patients with SCC had a local recurrence rate of 21%, and the overall 5-year survival rate was 76%.

Physicians from the Massachusetts General Hospital reviewed the treatment outcomes of 82 patients with SCC of the hard palate and upper and lower alveolar ridges.[22] Surgery was the primary treatment modality used for early carcinoma of the alveolar ridge or hard palate, whereas advanced disease was treated with surgery plus RT or RT alone. Overall 5-year survival rates for the hard palate and alveolar ridges were 57% and 49%, respectively. Stage I and II cancers of the hard palate demonstrated overall 5-year survival of 42% versus 20% for stage III to IV disease. There was, however, no significant difference in survival between patients with early-stage alveolar ridge cancer and those with more advanced disease. Patients with hard palate cancer that had clinically evident nodal metastases at the time of initial presentation demonstrated a 5-year survival of 0%. There was no statistically significant difference in survival between maxillary and mandibular alveolar ridge tumors, although disease-specific survival rates were not provided. Distant metastasis developed in 9% of patients diagnosed with alveolar ridge cancers and 14% of those with cancer of the hard palate.

Together, these retrospective case series document a significant risk of local recurrence following surgery or RT alone, reinforcing the need to perform aggressive surgical resection and to maintain a low threshold for postoperative RT. Larger case series that stratify treatment outcomes by T stage and primary tumor location so that cancers of the hard and soft palate and the upper and lower alveolar ridges are reported separately would improve the quality of the evidence pertaining to these uncommon sites.

◆ Verrucous Carcinoma

Verrucous carcinomas of the hard and soft palate have not been separately evaluated in the literature. Together, these two sites account for 7% of the verrucous carcinomas diagnosed in the head neck region.[41] More than 60% are diagnosed in stage I or II, and treatment is typically surgery alone (70%) or surgery and RT (12%).[41] Site-specific rates of local recurrence and survival for the hard and soft palate have not been individually reported. Similarly, the outcomes of therapy for verrucous carcinomas of the UAR are typically reported together with carcinomas of the lower alveolar ridge. Once again, greater than 60% of these lesions are stage I or II, and surgery is the most commonly used treatment modality (83%).[41] The 5-year relative survival rate for verrucous carcinoma of the alveolar ridges is 74%.[41] A detailed discussion of verrucous carcinoma is provided in Chapter 10.

◆ Minor Salivary Gland Malignancies

There are 450 to 750 minor salivary glands in the oral cavity and oropharynx.[42] After the parotid gland, the minor salivary glands are the second most common site of origin for benign and malignant salivary gland neoplasms. Approximately 14 to 22% of all diagnosed salivary gland neoplasms originate from these glands.[43–45] The hard palate is the location of more than 50% of the minor salivary gland neoplasms arising from the oral cavity and oropharynx because the posterior and lateral areas of the hard palate contain the greatest concentration of these glands (**Fig. 13–1** and **Table 13–1**).[43,45,46] Frequently, no differentiation is made between minor salivary gland cancers of the hard and soft palate in the literature, limiting our ability to separately assess the treatment outcomes

Table 13–1 Distribution of Minor Salivary Gland Malignancies within the Oral Cavity*

Region of Oral Cavity	Spiro[45] (n = 336)	Eveson and Cawson[43] (n = 150)	Waldron et al[46] (n = 181)
Palate	52%	57%	42%
Lips	17%[†]	13%	11%
Buccal mucosa	17%[†]	12%	17%
Tongue	14%	7%	ND
RMT	ND	2%	12%
FOM	5%	ND	9%
Alveolar ridge	8%	3%	1%
Others	4%	6%	8%
Total	100%	100%	100%

*Malignancies of the hard and soft palate were reported together in the retrospective case series published by Spiro[45] and Eveson and Cawson.[43] The data from Waldron et al[46] did not specify whether salivary gland malignancies of the soft palate were included.
[†]Minor salivary gland malignancies of the lips and buccal mucosa were accrued together.
ND, no data; RMT, retromolar trigone; FOM, floor of mouth.

of cancers involving the oral cavity and oropharynx. The precise origin of many of these lesions is difficult to pinpoint because they are typically found near the junction of the hard and soft palate, although investigators from São Paulo reported that 84% of palatal malignancies arose from the hard palate.[47] Most of these cancers present as painless swellings; only 15% of the patients complain of pain.[45] In a large series from Brazil, the most common complaint was the presence of a submucosal mass in the mouth for a median period of nearly 28 months.[47] The average age of patients diagnosed with minor salivary gland malignancies is 50.[43,45,46]

According to Spiro,[45] 82% of minor salivary gland neoplasms are malignant, but two other large retrospective series have documented malignancy rates of 42.5% and 46%, respectively.[43,46] Adenoid cystic carcinoma was the most common salivary gland malignancy of the oral cavity in two of these series, whereas mucoepidermoid carcinoma was the most common malignancy in the third series (**Table 13–2**).

Table 13–2 Minor Salivary Gland Malignancies of the Oral Cavity*

Type of Malignancy	Spiro[45] (n = 336)	Eveson and Cawson[43] (n = 150)	Waldron et al[46] (n = 181)
MEC	28%	20%	36%
ACC	38%	29%	22%
Adenocarcinoma	26%	26%	26%
MMT	7%	16%	3%
Others	1%	9%	13%
Total	100%	100%	100%

*Malignancies of the hard and soft palate were reported together in the retrospective case series published by Spiro[45] and Eveson and Cawson.[43] The data from Waldron et al[46] did not specify whether salivary gland malignancies of the soft palate were included.
MEC, mucoepidermoid carcinoma; ACC, adenoid cystic carcinoma; MMT, malignant mixed tumor (carcinoma ex pleomorphic adenoma).

At the time of diagnosis, more than 75% of the minor salivary gland malignancies of the palate and other sites within the oral cavity are stage I or II lesions.[48] There are a few retrospective case series that provide insight into the rates of clinically evident metastasis and ONM on initial presentation. In one large series of 434 patients with minor salivary gland malignancies from MSKCC, Spiro et al[49] noted a 22.8% overall rate of regional metastatic disease: 11.5% were clinically positive and 11.3% were ONM based on pathologic findings following elective radical neck dissection or the development of regional failure following initial treatment. Investigators from the University of Virginia documented a 5% rate of cervical nodal disease at presentation and a regional failure rate of 10%.[50] Thus, the rate of ONM and overall rate of regional metastatic disease in this series were 10% and 15%, respectively. The neck was clinically positive in 8% of the patients diagnosed with minor salivary gland malignancies in another series from M. D. Anderson Cancer Center (MDACC).[51] The rate of ONM in this series was difficult to assess because a significant number of patients with clinically negative necks were treated with postoperative RT, but only 5% of the untreated clinically node-negative necks developed regional failure. Based on these findings, the incidence of ONM in patients with minor salivary gland malignancies is less than 15%.

Radiographic imaging is recommended for all patients diagnosed with adenoid cystic carcinoma (ACC) of the hard palate because ACC is the most common histologic type to manifest perineural spread. Radiographic assessment can also be used to exclude the presence of bone invasion and to ascertain the extent of soft tissue spread.[17]

Treatment usually requires surgical excision followed by postoperative RT for high-risk situations, which include the presence of locally advanced disease, recurrence, high-grade histology, perineural spread, and regional metastases.[51] Aggressive surgical resection is indicated because of the propensity for perineural invasion and because the assessment of bony margins by frozen section is not possible. Physicians from the University of Cincinnati documented a 23% local recurrence rate following surgical resection and selective postoperative radiation in 21 salivary gland malignancies of the hard palate.[19] More extensive "radical surgery" demonstrated improved local control over wide local excision in a retrospective case series from the University of California at Los Angeles (UCLA).[52]

Published rates of local control following treatment for minor salivary gland malignancies range from 50 to 86% and survival rates following treatment vary from 57 to 91%.[19,40,47,48,50–53] At MSKCC, the 10-year disease-specific survival for all histologic subtypes was 93%, 68%, 32%, and 27% for patients with stages I through IV disease, respectively.[48] Patients with low-grade mucoepidermoid carcinoma, low-grade adenocarcinoma, or acinic cell carcinoma demonstrated significantly better overall 10-year survival rates

(93%) than patients with malignant mixed tumor, high-grade mucoepidermoid carcinoma, high-grade adenocarcinoma, ACC (42 to 58% at 10 years). At the University of Florida, adjuvant postoperative RT is delivered to all patients with ACC regardless of margin status, except for low-grade T1 lesions that are resected with widely negative margins.[54] Mendenhall et al[54] found that the 10-year local control rates achieved with surgery and postoperative RT were superior to RT alone ($p = .0008$).

Distant metastases are strongly associated with ACC histology, invasion of named nerves, and regional nodal disease.[51] Adenoid cystic carcinoma demonstrates a propensity for the eventual development of distant metastatic disease. In Spiro's[49] series, 40% of the patients with ACC developed distant metastases, and more than 60% of the cases of distant failure involved this histologic subtype. Two retrospective case series from MDACC similarly noted that distant metastasis was the most common failure pattern in patients diagnosed with ACC.[51,55] Several investigators have noted an overall 10-year disease-specific survival rate of approximately 70% for patients with ACC.[19,54,55] However, a decrease in disease-specific survival from 67.4% at 10 years to only 39.6% at 15 years has also been documented.[55]

Numerous investigators have shown that the treatment outcomes for minor salivary gland malignancies involving the oral cavity results in better rates of local control and survival than for malignancies arising from the paranasal sinuses.[48,50,51,53] At the University of Virginia, for example, the survival rate following treatment was 91% for malignancies of the hard palate versus 43% for malignancies of the maxillary sinus.[50] However, no such difference in local control or survival has been identified between the hard palate and other oral cavity sites. Stage, grade, and histologic classification appear to be more important prognostically than oral cavity site.

◆ Conclusion

Cancers arising from the hard palate and UAR present several diagnostic and therapeutic challenges that mandate the need for a multidisciplinary approach to management. Careful surgical, prosthetic, and radiotherapeutic planning can improve cure rates, minimize morbidity, and optimize functional outcomes. The reported rates of local-regional control and survival for these neoplasms have been derived from relatively small retrospective investigations that utilize an assortment of treatment modalities and contain significant treatment selection bias. In the future, our ability to measure improvements in treatment-related outcomes will depend on the accrual of prospective data so that evidence-based site-, stage-, and tumor-specific therapy can be administered to our patients.

References

1. Lip and oral cavity. In: Greene FL, Page DL, Fleming ID, eds. AJCC Cancer Staging Manual, 6th ed. New York: Springer-Verlag, 2002:23–32

2. Strachan DS. Histology of the oral mucosa and tonsils. In: Avery JK, ed. Oral Development and Histology, 2nd ed. New York: Thieme, 1994: 298–320

3. Werner JA, Dunne AA, Myers JN. Functional anatomy of the lymphatic drainage system of the upper aerodigestive tract and its role in metastasis of squamous cell carcinoma. Head Neck 2003;25:322–332

4. Funk GF, Karnell LH, Robinson RA, Zhen WK, Trask DK, Hoffman HT. Presentation, treatment, and outcome of oral cavity cancer: a National Cancer Data Base report. Head Neck 2002;24:165–180

5. Soo KC, Spiro RH, King W, Harvey W, Strong EW. Squamous carcinoma of the gums. Am J Surg 1988;156:281–285

6. Evans JF, Shah JP. Epidermoid carcinoma of the palate. Am J Surg 1981;142:451–455

7. Campbell BH, Mark DH, Soneson EA, Freije JE, Schultz CJ. The role of dental prostheses in alveolar ridge squamous carcinomas. Arch Otolaryngol Head Neck Surg 1997;123:1112–1115

8. Gupta PC, Mehta FS, Pindborg JJ. Mortality among reverse chutta smokers in south India. Br Med J (Clin Res Ed) 1984;289:865–866

9. Gupta PC, Murti PR, Bhonsle RB. Epidemiology of cancer by tobacco products and the significance of TSNA. Crit Rev Toxicol 1996;26:183–198

10. van der Eb MM, Leyten EM, Gavarasana S, Vandenbroucke JP, Kahn PM, Cleton FJ. Reverse smoking as a risk factor for palatal cancer: a cross-sectional study in rural Andhra Pradesh, India. Int J Cancer 1993;54:754–758

11. Reddy DG, Rao VK. Cancer of the palate in coastal Andhra due to smoking cigars with the burning end inside the mouth. Indian J Med Sci 1957;11:791–798

12. Reddy CR, Ramulu C. Review of carcinoma of hard palate in Visakhapatnam area and its etiopathogenesis. Clinician (Goa) 1972;36:131

13. Chung CK, Rahman SM, Lim ML, Constable WC. Squamous cell carcinoma of the hard palate. Int J Radiat Oncol Biol Phys 1979;5:191–196

14. Barasch A, Gofa A, Krutchkoff DJ, Eisenberg E. Squamous cell carcinoma of the gingiva. A case series analysis. Oral Surg Oral Med Oral Pathol Oral Radiol Endod 1995;80:183–187

15. Mukherji SK, Pillsbury HR, Castillo M. Imaging squamous cell carcinomas of the upper aerodigestive tract: what clinicians need to know. Radiology 1997;205:629–646

16. Lane AP, Buckmire RA, Mukherji SK, Pillsbury HC III, Meredith SD. Use of computed tomography in the assessment of mandibular invasion in carcinoma of the retromolar trigone. Otolaryngol Head Neck Surg 2000;122:673–677

17. Ginsberg LE, DeMonte F. Imaging of perineural tumor spread from palatal carcinoma. AJNR Am J Neuroradiol 1998;19:1417–1422

18. Cady B, Catlin D. Epidermoid carcinoma of the gum. A 20-year survey. Cancer 1969;23:551–569

19. Truitt TO, Gleich LL, Huntress GP, Gluckman JL. Surgical management of hard palate malignancies. Otolaryngol Head Neck Surg 1999;121:548–552

20. Shah JP, Candela FC, Poddar AK. The patterns of cervical lymph node metastases from squamous carcinoma of the oral cavity. Cancer 1990;66:109–113

21. Kimura Y, Hanazawa T, Sano T, Okano T. Lateral retropharyngeal node metastasis from carcinoma of the upper gingiva and maxillary sinus. AJNR Am J Neuroradiol 1998;19:1221–1224

22. Ildstad ST, Bigelow ME, Remensnyder JP. Squamous cell carcinoma of the alveolar ridge and palate. A 15-year survey. Ann Surg 1984;199:445–453

23. Vural E, Hanna E. Extended lateral rhinotomy incision for total maxillectomy. Otolaryngol Head Neck Surg 2000;123:512–513

24. Bell WH. Revascularization and bone healing after anterior maxillary osteotomy: a study using adult rhesus monkeys. J Oral Surg 1969;27:249–255

25. Pepersack WJ. Tooth vitality after alveolar segmental osteotomy. J Maxillofac Surg 1973;1:85–91

26. Stearns JW, Fonseca RJ, Saker M. Revascularization and healing of orthognathic surgical procedures. In: Fonseca RJ, Betts NJ, Turvey TA, eds. Oral and Maxillofacial Surgery: Orthognathic Surgery, vol 2. New York: WB Saunders, 2000:151–168

27. Bell WH, Levy BM. Revascularization and bone healing after posterior maxillary osteotomy. J Oral Surg 1971;29:313–320

28. Bell WH, Fonseca RJ, Kennedy JW, Levy BM. Bone healing and revascularization after total maxillary osteotomy. J Oral Surg 1975;33:253–260

29. Dodson TB, Bays RA, Neuenschwander MC. Maxillary perfusion during Le Fort I osteotomy after ligation of the descending palatine artery. J Oral Maxillofac Surg 1997;55:51–55

30. Apinhasmit W, Methathrathip D, Ploytubtim S, et al. Anatomical study of the maxillary artery at the pterygomaxillary fissure in a Thai population: its relationship to maxillary osteotomy. J Med Assoc Thai 2004;87:1212–1217

31. Turvey TA, Fonseca RJ. The anatomy of the internal maxillary artery in the pterygopalatine fossa: its relationship to maxillary surgery. J Oral Surg 1980;38:92–95

32. Spiro RH, Strong EW, Shah JP. Maxillectomy and its classification. Head Neck 1997;19:309–314

33. Brown JS, Rogers SN, McNally DN, Boyle M. A modified classification for the maxillectomy defect. Head Neck 2000;22:17–26

34. Okay DJ, Genden E, Buchbinder D, Urken M. Prosthodontic guidelines for surgical reconstruction of the maxilla: a classification system of defects. J Prosthet Dent 2001;86:352–363

35. Partially edentulous epidemiology, physiology, and terminology. In: Carr AB, McGivney GP, Brown DT, eds. McCracken's Removable Partial Prosthodontics, 11th ed. St. Louis: Elsevier Mosby, 2005:3–10

36. Denture Base Considerations. In: Carr AB, McGivney GP, Brown DT, eds. McCracken's Removable Partial Prosthodontics, 11th ed. St. Louis: Elsevier Mosby, 2005:127–144

37. Clasp-retained partial denture. In: Carr AB, McGivney GP, Brown DT, eds. McCracken's Removable Partial Prosthodontics, 11th ed. St. Louis: Elsevier Mosby, 2005:11–18

38. Fiebiger GE, Rahn AO, Lundquist DO, Morse PK. Movement of abutments by removable partial denture frameworks with a hemimaxillectomy obturator. J Prosthet Dent 1975;34:555–561

39. Yorozu A, Sykes AJ, Slevin NJ. Carcinoma of the hard palate treated with radiotherapy: a retrospective review of 31 cases. Oral Oncol 2001;37:493–497

40. Chung CK, Johns ME, Cantrell RW, Constable WC. Radiotherapy in the management of primary malignancies of the hard palate. Laryngoscope 1980;90:576–584

41. Koch BB, Trask DK, Hoffman HT, et al. National survey of head and neck verrucous carcinoma: patterns of presentation, care, and outcome. Cancer 2001;92:110–120

42. Clinical and pathologic features. In: Sciubba JJ, Attie JN, eds. Current Problems in Surgery, vol 18. Chicago: Year Book Medical, 1981:66–155

43. Eveson JW, Cawson RA. Tumours of the minor (oropharyngeal) salivary glands: a demographic study of 336 cases. J Oral Pathol 1985;14:500–509

44. Eveson JW, Cawson RA. Salivary gland tumours. A review of 2410 cases with particular reference to histological types, site, age and sex distribution. J Pathol 1985;146:51–58

45. Spiro RH. Salivary neoplasms: overview of a 35-year experience with 2,807 patients. Head Neck Surg 1986;8:177–184

46. Waldron CA, el-Mofty SK, Gnepp DR. Tumors of the intraoral minor salivary glands: a demographic and histologic study of 426 cases. Oral Surg Oral Med Oral Pathol 1988;66:323–333

47. Lopes MA, Santos GC, Kowalski LP. Multivariate survival analysis of 128 cases of oral cavity minor salivary gland carcinomas. Head Neck 1998;20:699–706

48. Spiro RH, Thaler HT, Hicks WF, Kher UA, Huvos AH, Strong EW. The importance of clinical staging of minor salivary gland carcinoma. Am J Surg 1991;162:330–336

49. Spiro RH, Koss LG, Hajdu SI, Strong EW. Tumors of minor salivary origin: a clinicopathologic study of 492 cases. Cancer 1973;31:117–129

50. Jenkins DW, Spaulding CA, Constable WC, Cantrell RW. Minor salivary gland tumors: the role of radiotherapy. Am J Otolaryngol 1989;10:250–256

51. Garden AS, Weber RS, Ang KK, Morrison WH, Matre J, Peters LJ. Postoperative radiation therapy for malignant tumors of minor salivary glands. Outcome and patterns of failure. Cancer 1994;73:2563–2569

52. Tran L, Sadeghi A, Hanson D, Ellerbroek N, Calcaterra TC, Parker RG. Salivary gland tumors of the palate: the UCLA experience. Laryngoscope 1987;97:1343–1345

53. Weisberger E, Luna MA, Guillamondegui OM. Salivary gland cancers of the palate. Am J Surg 1979;138:584–587

54. Mendenhall WM, Morris CG, Amdur RJ, Werning JW, Hinerman RW, Villaret DB. Radiotherapy alone or combined with surgery for adenoid cystic carcinoma of the head and neck. Head Neck 2004;26:154–162

55. Fordice J, Kershaw C, El-Naggar A, Goepfert H. Adenoid cystic carcinoma of the head and neck. Arch Otolaryngol Head Neck Surg 1999;125:149–152

14

Management of the Neck

John W. Werning and
William M. Mendenhall

Since Crile's[1] description of the radical neck dissection (RND) a century ago, the management of regional metastases from head and neck cancer has continued to evolve. Surgery and radiation therapy (RT) continue to be the mainstays of treatment, so clinicians have focused their efforts on refining the application of these modalities to improve control rates and minimize morbidity. Despite these refinements, the indications for and appropriate treatment of the neck remain hotly debated. This chapter examines the quality of the available evidence pertaining to the evaluation and management of regional metastases from the oral cavity.

◆ Cervical Lymph Nodes

Classification

There are approximately 300 lymph nodes in the head and neck region.[2] Historically, the cervical lymph nodes were thought to be organized into "chains" that were named by their proximity to nearby anatomic structures, or by their topographical distribution. For example, the spinal accessory chain was synonymous with the posterior cervical nodes, and the transverse cervical chain was synonymous with the supraclavicular lymph nodes.[2] In 1981, Shah et al[3] suggested that the anatomically based terminology should be replaced by a simpler level-based system that was already being used at Memorial Sloan-Kettering Cancer Center (MSKCC).[3] This system divided the lymph nodes from each side of the neck into seven anatomically defined levels. Since its inception, the classification scheme has been revised so that there are now six recognized lymph node levels, I to VI, and levels I,

II, and V have been subdivided into sublevels A and B (**Tables 14-1** and **14-2**; see **Figs. 14-1** and **14-2** on p. 161).[4] This classification scheme does not include the buccinator and retropharyngeal lymph nodes, which rarely harbor metastases from the oral cavity.[4-6]

The submandibular lymph node group (sublevel IB) includes the *preglandular* and *postglandular* nodes as well as the *prevascular* and *postvascular* nodes. The anatomic relationship of these important lymph nodes to the facial artery and vein and submandibular gland has been clearly described (see **Figs. 14-3** and **14-4** on p. 162).[7] Lymphatic vessels that travel from the floor of the mouth through the mylohyoid muscle and empty into the preglandular submandibular nodes have been histologically documented.[8] It is important to distinguish the prevascular and postvascular nodes from the *facial nodes*, a term that refers to subcutaneous lymph nodes of the face that lie along the course of the facial artery.[7] Two additional groups of submandibular lymph nodes have been described. Although the submandibular gland has no intraparenchymal lymph nodes, *intracapsular submandibular lymph nodes* have occasionally been documented.[7,9] DiNardo[7] has also noted the variable presence of *deep submandibular nodes* along the undersurface of the gland. All six lymph node groups should be removed along with the remainder of the submandibular triangle during neck dissection for cancer of the oral cavity.

Prior classifications have used the boundary of the submandibular triangle to separate sublevel IB from level II, but the posterior belly of the digastric muscle extends across the internal jugular vein into level II. Recent updates of the clinical and radiographic boundaries suggest that the stylohyoid muscle more accurately delineates sublevel IB from level II intraoperatively, and a transverse line drawn

Table 14–1 Lymph Node Groups Found Within the Six Levels and the Six Sublevels (Figs. 14–1 and 14–2)

Lymph Node Group	Description
Submental (sublevel IA)	Lymph nodes within the triangular boundary of the anterior belly of the digastric muscles and the hyoid bone.
Submandibular (sublevel IB)	Lymph nodes within the boundaries of the anterior belly of the digastric muscle, the stylohyoid muscle, and the body of the mandible. It includes the preglandular and the postglandular nodes and the prevascular and the postvascular nodes.
Upper jugular (includes sublevels IA and IB)	Lymph nodes located around the upper third of the internal jugular vein and adjacent spinal accessory nerve extending from the level of the skull base (above) to the level of the inferior border of the hyoid bone (below). The anterior (medial) boundary is the stylohyoid muscle (the radiologic correlate is the vertical plane defined by the posterior surface of the submandibular gland) and stylohyoid muscle (the radiologic correlate is the vertical plane defined by the posterior surface of the submandibular gland) and the posterior (lateral) boundary is the posterior border of the sternocleidomastoid muscle. Sublevel IIA nodes are located anterior (medial) to the vertical plane defined by the spinal accessory nerve. Sublevel IIB nodes are located posterior (lateral) to the vertical plane defined by the spinal accessory nerve.
Middle jugular (level III)	Lymph nodes located around the middle third of the internal jugular vein extending from the inferior border of the hyoid bone (above) to the inferior border of the cricoid cartilage (below). The anterior (medial) boundary is the lateral border of the sternohyoid muscle, and the posterior (lateral) boundary is the posterior border of the sternocleidomastoid muscle.
Lower jugular (level IV)	Lymph nodes located around the lower third of the internal jugular vein extending from the inferior border of the cricoid cartilage (above) to the clavicle below. The anterior (medial) boundary is the lateral border of the sternohyoid muscle and the posterior (lateral) boundary is the posterior border of the sternocleidomastoid muscle.
Posterior triangle group (includes sublevels VA and VB)	This group is composed predominantly of the lymph nodes located along the lower half of the spinal accessory nerve and the transverse cervical artery. The supraclavicular nodes are also included in the posterior triangle group. The superior boundary is the apex formed by convergence of the sternocleidomastoid and trapezius muscles, the inferior boundary is the clavicle, the anterior (medial) boundary is the posterior border of the sternocleidomastoid muscle, and the posterior (lateral) boundary is the anterior border of the trapezius muscle. Sublevel VA is separated from sublevel VB by a horizontal plane marking the inferior border of the anterior cricoid arch. Thus, sublevel VA includes the spinal accessory nodes, whereas sublevel VB includes the nodes following the transverse cervical vessels and the supraclavicular nodes with the exception of the Virchow node, which is located in level IV.
Anterior compartment group (level VI)	Lymph nodes in this compartment include the pretracheal and paratracheal nodes, precricoid (Delphian) node, and the perithyroidal nodes including the lymph nodes along the recurrent laryngeal nerves. The superior boundary is the hyoid bone, the inferior boundary is the suprasternal notch, and the lateral boundaries are the common carotid arteries.

Adapted from Robbins KT, Clayman G, Levine PA, et al. Neck dissection classification update: revisions proposed by the American Head and Neck Society and the American Academy of Otolaryngology–Head and Neck Surgery. Arch Otolaryngol Head Neck Surg 2002;128:751–758, with permission.

on each axial image tangent to the posterior edge of the submandibular gland provides a consistent radiographic boundary between these two levels.[4,10,11]

Radiographically, the inferior bony margin of the jugular fossa defines the location where level II nodes extend to the skull base.[11] A lymph node that lies anterior or lateral to the carotid sheath immediately inferior to the skull base is a high level II node, whereas a node that lies medial to the internal carotid artery is defined as a lateral retropharyngeal node.[11] The junction between level II and III is formed by the bottom of the hyoid body, and the junction between level III and IV is the bottom of the cricoid arch.[11] The lateral border of the sternocleidomastoid muscle defines the posterior or lateral boundary between levels II through IV and the anterior or medial border of level V.[4,10,11] Intraoperatively, the sensory branches of the cervical plexus can also be used to delineate this boundary.[4,11]

The increasing use of highly conformal RT (e.g., intensity-modulated RT, IMRT) has influenced the radiation oncology community to develop consensus guidelines for computed tomography (CT)-based delineation of the lymph node levels that deviate somewhat from the classification scheme sanctioned by the surgical community.[12] For example, radiation oncologists from Brussels contend that lymph node retrieval during neck dissection extends superiorly to the caudal aspect of the transverse process of C1 rather than to the base of the skull. Although the base of the skull is a convenient anatomic and radiographic landmark that has been used to define the superior boundary of level II, the observations of these investigators suggest that RT could also be effectively delivered without including the base of the skull. Consequently, these recently proposed consensus guidelines place the cranial border of level II at the caudal edge of the lateral process of C1. This border, which

Table 14–2 Anatomical Structures Defining the Boundaries of the Neck Levels and Sublevels (Figs. 14–1 and 14–2)

Level	Boundary			
	Superior	**Inferior**	**Anterior (Medial)**	**Posterior (Lateral)**
IA	Symphysis of mandible	Body of hyoid	Anterior belly of contralateral digastric muscle	Anterior belly of ipsilateral digastric muscle
IB	Body of mandible	Posterior belly of muscle	Anterior belly of digastric muscle	Stylohyoid muscle
IIA	Skull base	Horizontal plane defined by the inferior body of the hyoid bone	Stylohyoid muscle	Vertical plane defined by the spinal accessory nerve
IIB	Skull base	Horizontal plane defined by the inferior body of the hyoid bone	Vertical plane defined by the spinal accessory nerve	Lateral border of the sternocleidomastoid muscle
III	Horizontal plane defined by inferior body of hyoid	Horizontal plane defined by the inferior border of the cricoid cartilage	Lateral border of the sternohyoid muscle	Lateral border of the sternocleidomastoid or sensory branches of cervical plexus
IV	Horizontal plane defined by the inferior border of the cricoid cartilage	Clavicle	Lateral border of the sternohyoid muscle	Lateral border of the sternocleidomastoid or sensory branches of cervical plexus
VA	Apex of the convergence of the sternocleidomastoid and trapezius muscles	Horizontal plane defined by the lower border of the cricoid cartilage	Posterior border of the sternocleidomastoid muscle or sensory branches of cervical plexus	Anterior border of the trapezius muscle
VB	Horizontal plane defined by the lower border of the cricoid cartilage	Clavicle	Posterior border of the sternocleidomastoid muscle or sensory branches of cervical plexus	Anterior border of the trapezius muscle
VI	Hyoid bone	Suprasternal	Common carotid artery	Common carotid artery

From Robbins KT, Clayman G, Levine PA, et al. Neck dissection classification update: revisions proposed by the American Head and Neck Society and the American Academy of Otolaryngology–Head and Neck Surgery. Arch Otolaryngol Head Neck Surg 2002;128:751–758, with permission.

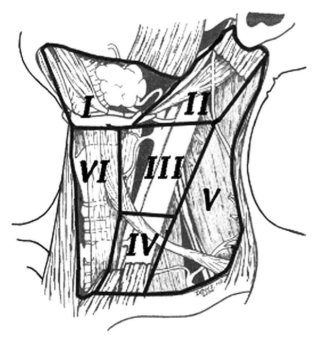

Figure 14–1 The six levels of the neck. (From Robbins KT, ed. Pocket Guide to Neck Dissection Classification and TNM Staging of Head and Neck Cancer, 2nd ed. Alexandria, VA: American Academy of Otolaryngology–Head and Neck Surgery Foundation, 2001, with permission.)

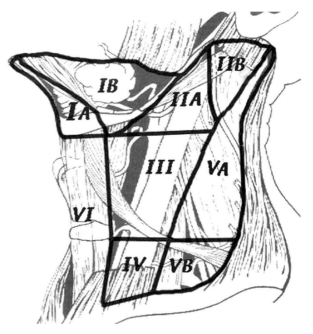

Figure 14–2 The six sublevels of the neck. (From Robbins KT, ed. Pocket Guide to Neck Dissection Classification and TNM Staging of Head and Neck Cancer, 2nd ed. Alexandria, VA: American Academy of Otolaryngology–Head and Neck Surgery Foundation, 2001, with permission.)

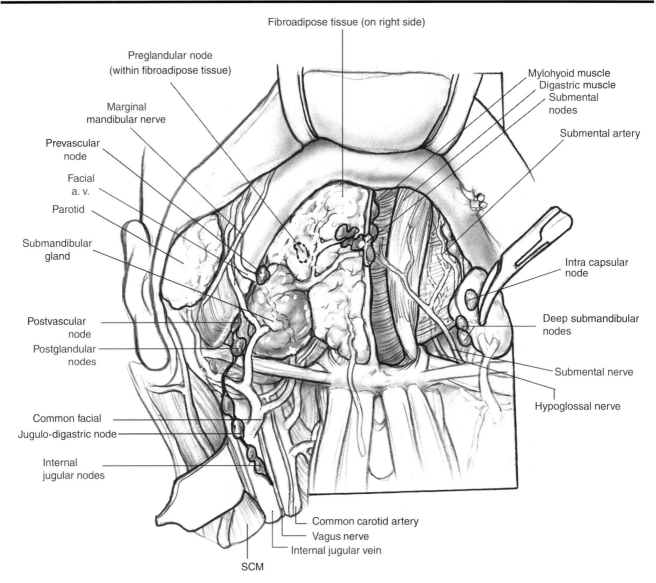

Fibroadipose tissue (on right side)

Preglandular node
(within fibroadipose tissue)

Marginal
mandibular nerve

Prevascular
node

Facial
a. v.

Parotid

Submandibular
gland

Postvascular
node

Postglandular
nodes

Common facial

Jugulo-digastric node

Internal
jugular nodes

SCM

Mylohyoid muscle
Digastric muscle
Submental
nodes

Submental artery

Intra capsular
node

Deep submandibular
nodes

Submental nerve

Hypoglossal nerve

Common carotid artery
Vagus nerve
Internal jugular vein

Figure 14–3 The six groups of submandibular lymph nodes: preglandular, postglandular, prevascular, postvascular, deep, and intracapsular groups. The prevascular node lies anterior to the anterior facial vein on top of the facial artery, whereas the postvascular nodes are located posterior to the anterior facial vein.

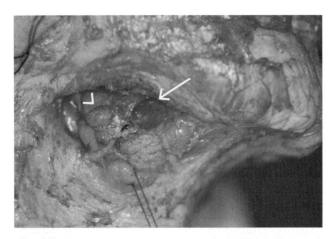

Figure 14–4 Contents of sublevel IB following elevation of the fascia overlying the submandibular gland, illustrating the location of the prevascular node (*arrow*) anterior to the facial vein, and the postvascular nodes (*arrowhead*) posterior to the anterior facial vein.

is lower than the upper limit frequently drawn on conventional portals that extend to the base of the skull, favors maximal conformality in combination with IMRT techniques.[13] For example, if treatment of the contralateral neck with parotid-sparing IMRT is desired, less radiation can be administered to the parotid gland–base of skull region so that salivary function is preserved.

Prognostic Importance of Cervical Lymph Node Metastases

As a group, patients with squamous carcinoma of the upper aerodigestive tract who initially present with regional metastatic disease have a reduction in 5-year survival of approximately 50%.[14] There is a strong association between pathologically proven cervical lymph node metastases and the development of distant metastases that result in poorer survival outcomes.[15–19] Distant metastases occur with greater frequency in patients with multiple lymph node metastases, level IV metastases, and extracapsular spread.[18-20] The development of lung or bone metastases are associated with a median survival of 5 months, and skin metastases are associated with a median survival of only 3 months.[18]

Similarly, regional metastases are associated with worse disease-specific survival (DSS) in patients with cancer of the oral cavity.[21,22] The number of positive lymph nodes also adversely impacts survival.[17,23-26] Patients with oral tongue cancer who have more than one lymph node metastasis demonstrate worse DSS than patients with a single metastatic node.[25] Metastasis to levels III, IV, or V or to the contralateral neck is also an independent predictor of decreased survival.[24,26-28]

Although the presence of occult nodal metastases (ONMs) is associated with worse DSS, the outcome of patients with intranodal micrometastases of 3 mm or less is not as clear.[21,29] Woolgar,[30] for example, was unable to document worse survival in patients with only micrometastases. Additional investigation is necessary to determine the prognostic importance of isolated micrometastatic disease.

Extracapsular spread (ECS) is the most significant predictor of regional recurrence, distant metastases, and survival outcome.[22,25,31] The prognostic importance of ECS is illustrated by two recent retrospective studies from M. D. Anderson Cancer Center (MDACC) that review the treatment outcomes for 266 patients with oral tongue cancer.[22,25] In this series, the 5-year DSS was 88% for pN0 patients and 59% for pN+ patients ($p < .01$).[22] The risk of dying from oral tongue cancer was at least twice as great in patients with pN+ disease with or without ECS than in patients who were pN0 [odds ratio (OR), 3.4; 95% confidence interval (CI, 2.0–5.7). In patients with pathologically node-positive disease, 5-year DSS was 66% in patients without ECS and 48% in patients with ECS ($p = .02$). Although the presence of a single lymph node with ECS was not associated with increased regional failure, involvement of two or more nodes with ECS resulted in a regional recurrence rate of 58.3% and a rate of distant metastases of 33.3%, with a median survival of less than 1 year.[25]

Even though the presence of ECS adversely affects DSS, the impact that the degree of extracapsular spread has on prognosis is less clear.[22,31,32] In one retrospective investigation of patients with oral tongue cancer, there was no significant difference in survival between patients with ECS of ≤2 mm or >2 mm.[25] Similarly, investigators from the Leeds Teaching Hospitals in the United Kingdom were unable to document a difference in DSS or recurrence-free survival between patients with microscopic and those with macroscopic extracapsular spread.[32]

Patterns of Metastasis

Lindberg's[33] classic review of the topographical distribution of clinically palpable lymph node metastases in 1155 patients with head and neck cancer in 1972 provided clinicians with the insight that squamous cell carcinoma of the head and neck metastasizes to the neck in a predictable pattern. Furthermore, he demonstrated that the pattern of lymph node metastases varied in accordance with the location of the primary tumor. Subsequent research by Byers et al[34,35] from MDACC and Shah et al[36,37] from MSKCC that utilized histopathologic assessment to evaluate the lymph nodes that were harvested from neck dissection specimens forms the basis for our present understanding of the patterns of nodal metastastic disease that develop in head and neck cancer. In 1990, Shah[37] published the pathologic findings from 1119 RND specimens, providing us with extensive pathologic data from lymph node levels I through V for different primary tumor sites in the head and neck region.[37] Since then, numerous other investigators have augmented our understanding of metastatic patterns within the neck.[2,7,24,29,31,38-46]

Cancer of the oral cavity most frequently metastasizes to lymph node levels I and II. Shah et al[36] found that ONMs were found in level I and level II in 20% and 17% of 192 elective RND specimens, respectively (**Table 14–3**). In 219 RNDs performed for the cN+ neck, level I and level II were pN+ in 48% and 38% of the specimens, respectively. The prevalence of metastatic disease progressively decreases in levels III, IV, and V in both cN0 and cN+ necks.

The frequency of ONM by neck level for each oral cavity subsite is summarized in **Table 14–4**.[36,47,48] Occult metastases arising from cancers of the floor of mouth, retromolar trigone, buccal mucosa, and the upper and lower alveolar ridges are most commonly located in level I. Level II is the second most frequent location of ONM for each of these sites. Less than 10% of the patients diagnosed with lower lip cancer metastasize to level I or II. Oral tongue cancer, on other hand, metastasizes to levels I, II, or III with similar frequency. The metastatic rate from any oral mucosal region to level V never exceeds 2% in the clinically negative neck.

A prospective investigation of 41 patients with floor of mouth cancer who underwent bilateral submandibular triangle dissection provides insight into the patterns of nodal metastases within sublevel IB.[7] Thirty-nine percent of the patients harbored lymph node metastases in sublevel IB, and 15% of the patients had metastatic disease that was limited solely to sublevel IB. All of the patients with level II metastases had sublevel IB disease. Bilateral metastases were only identified in patients with T4 lesions, and nearly 40% of them had bilateral sublevel IB involvement. The prevascular and retrovascular nodes made up 68% of the nodal metastases detected, and the preglandular and deep submandibular nodes made up 16% of the nodal metastases. No metastases were identified in the postglandular or intracapsular submandibular lymph nodes.[7]

Data pertaining to the pattern of nodal metastasis from cancer of the hard palate is scant. Because most of these malignancies arise from the posterior hard palate and frequently extend onto the maxillary alveolar ridge and soft palate, their metastatic behavior would be expected to be similar. Although soft palate cancers typically metastasize to levels II to IV, metastasis to level I can also occur.[49,50]

During neck dissection, an average of six to nine lymph nodes should be harvested from sublevel IIA, and four or five lymph nodes should be harvested from sublevel IIB, also referred to as the submuscular recess.[39-41] The prevalence of metastases in sublevel IIB is 5% or less in the cN0 neck, approximately 10 to 15% in the cN+ neck, and 5 to

Table 14–3 Prevalence of Nodal Metastasis by Neck Level in Radical Neck Dissection Specimens[36]

Level	cN0 Neck (n = 192)	cN+ Neck (n = 219)
I	20%	48%
II	17%	38%
III	9%	31%
IV	3%	15%
V	0.5%	4%

16% in the pN+ neck.[39–42,51] In neck dissection specimens with level IIA metastases, metastatic disease is also present at level IIB in 8% to 15% of the specimens.[39–41] However, sublevel IIB metastases are typically absent in patients without sublevel IIA involvement.[40,41,51] The authors of these investigations question the necessity to dissect sublevel IIB in the cN0 neck because dissection of this region is associated with spinal accessory neuropraxia from nerve retraction and devascularization. The necessity of dissecting IIB in oral cancer patients that have no clinical nodal disease in sublevel IIA has also been questioned by Robbins et al[4] and others. A recent investigation that evaluated the use of sentinel lymphadenectomy in patients with oral cancer, however, found that 14% of the sentinel nodes were located in sublevel IIB, suggesting that the potential for isolated metastasis to sublevel IIB exists.[52]

Reports on the prevalence of level IV metastasis in patients with oral cancer document significant variability in the cN0 neck, resulting in controversy regarding inclusion of level IV in elective neck dissections.[44,53] Shah et al[36] documented a prevalence of 3% and 15% in the cN0 neck and the cN+ neck, respectively. Crean et al[43] reported a 10% prevalence of level IV metastasis in the cN0 necks of patients with oral cancer from all primary sites, and a 4% frequency of level IV "skip" metastasis. In oral tongue cancer patients with a cN0 neck, Shah et al[36] and Khafif et al[44] documented a frequency of level IV disease in 3% and 4% of dissected necks, respectively. Byers et al,[54] however, documented the presence of isolated skip metastases to levels III and IV in 4% and 7%, respectively, of 270 patients with oral tongue cancer. Woolgar[31] similarly reported the presence of metastases that skipped levels II or

III in 10% of neck dissections. These findings suggest that oral tongue cancer does not consistently metastasize in a predictable manner. It is possible, however, that sampling error during histologic assessment of lymph nodes may have failed to detect micrometastatic disease in the level II or III nodes that were assigned pN0 status.

According to Shah et al's[36] original series, the overall prevalence of level V metastasis in patients with oral cancer is 0.5% in the cN0 neck and 4% in the cN+ neck. However, in a subsequent series from MSKCC, no level V metastases were found in the radical neck dissection specimens of 155 cN0 necks and in only 2.4% of 251 cN+ necks.[45] Furthermore, the prevalence of level V metastases was less than 1% when a metastatic node was present in level I, II, or III. On the other hand, 16% of the neck dissection specimens contained level V disease when an isolated metastatic node was present in level IV. Level V metastasis was found in 40% of the patients with metastases in all of the other four levels. Therefore, level V dissection is not necessary in patients with oral cancer unless lymph node metastases are suspected in multiple levels or in the lower jugular region.

Recently, the need to dissect the apex of level V, which is located above the spinal accessory nerve, has been questioned. In a prospective analysis of 70 consecutive neck dissection specimens, no lymph nodes were found in the apex of level V in 70% of the specimens, and no metastatic nodes were identified in any of the specimens from this region.[55] Avoidance of dissection in this region will minimize shoulder dysfunction when level V dissection is indicated.

Contralateral metastasis are more likely to occur with floor of mouth carcinoma and tumors that extend to within 1 cm of the midline.[46] Oral cancer rarely metastasizes to other nodal groups such as the buccal nodes or the retropharyngeal nodes.[56,57]

In summary, the cN0 neck at risk for ONM should undergo dissection of levels I to III. Dissection of sublevel IIB may not be necessary in the absence of sublevel IIA disease. Dissection of level IV in the cN0 neck remains controversial, particularly for patients with oral tongue cancer. A level V dissection is not indicated in the cN0 neck, but it should be strongly considered in the cN+ neck of patients with multiple levels of nodal involvement or level IV nodal disease. Dissection of level V superior to the spinal accessory nerve

Table 14–4 Frequency of Nodal Metastases by Neck Level in the cN0 Neck for Each Oral Cavity Subsite*

Oral Cavity Site	Neck Level				
	I	II	III	IV	V
Oral tongue[36]	14%	19%	16%	3%	0%
Floor of mouth[36]	16%	12%	7%	2%	0%
Lower lip[†47]	8%	9%	0%	0%	0.1%
Retromolar trigone[36]	19%	12%	6%	6%	0%
Buccal mucosa[36]	44%	11%	0%	0%	0%
Lower alveolar ridge[48]	53%	40%	7%	0%	0%
Upper/lower alveolar ridge[‡36]	27%	21%	6%	4%	2%

*There are insufficient data to detail the pattern of cervical metastasis for the upper lip, hard palate, and upper alveolar ridge.
†No data are available solely for the cN0 neck. These findings summarize the distribution of lymph node metastasis in 968 patients with lower lip cancer.[47] In this series, the rate of occult nodal metastasis (ONM) was 4% and the rate of clinically evident metastases was 5% with an overall rate of cervical nodal metastasis of 9% (85 of 968).
‡Data from both sites were combined in the series published by Shah et al.[36]

should not be performed unless clinical evidence of nodal disease exists. Bilateral neck dissection should be considered whenever the lesion extends to within 1 cm of the midline. Forthcoming prospective research findings from investigations that have used sentinel lymphadenectomy to look for lymph node metastasis in patients with oral cancer should provide additional insight into the patterns of lymph node metastasis.

Determinants of Metastasis

Several characteristics of the primary tumor have been associated with regional metastases and DSS, including T stage, pattern of invasion, angiolymphatic invasion, perineural invasion, and degree of tumor differentiation.[7,21,23,33,47,58–63] Of all the prognostic parameters that have been evaluated, however, tumor thickness and depth of invasion have emerged as the best predictors of ONM in the clinically negative neck (**Table 14–5**).[64–67]

For the purpose of this review, tumor thickness is the measured distance from the surface of the tumor to the base of the tumor, using an optical micrometer.[66,68–73] Depth of invasion is the measured distance from either the surface of the adjacent normal mucosa or the basement membrane to the deepest portion of the tumor, using an optical micrometer (see Fig. 7–1A in Chapter 7).[58,64,65,67,73–76] This distinction is important, because some investigators describe measurements of tumor thickness even though depth of invasion was the end point that was evaluated. We reviewed the

method of histopathologic assessment that was utilized in each of these investigations so that the relationship between tumor thickness or depth of invasion and regional metastatic disease could be accurately portrayed.

O'Brien et al[71] evaluated the relationship among tumor thickness, regional metastasis, and survival in 145 patients with oral cancer. This series did not evaluate any patients with lip cancer. The authors found that a tumor thickness of 4 mm separated tumors into low-risk and high-risk lesions, and that there was a progressive increase in nodal metastasis and death as tumor thickness increased. Lesions <4 mm thick had an 8% prevalence of nodal disease, whereas lesions ≥4 mm in thickness had a prevalence of 48%.

On the other hand, the critical thickness that is associated with an increased risk of metastasis may not be uniform throughout the oral cavity. For example, Woolgar and Scott[73] noted a difference in critical thickness between tongue and floor of mouth cancers. Others have also documented a distinct critical thickness that is associated with higher rates of ONM for cancers of the lip, floor of mouth, and buccal mucosa. De Visscher et al[77] found a metastatic rate of 26% in lower lip lesions of ≥6 mm in thickness and only 5% for lesions <6 mm thick, whereas Onerci et al[68] documented a mean tumor thickness of 3.79 mm in patients without metastasis and 5.6 mm in those with metastasis. Mohit-Tabatabai et al[69] documented a 2% rate of ONM in floor of mouth cancers that were 1.5 mm or less in thickness versus a 33% rate of ONM in patients with lesions greater than 1.5 mm thick. Mishra et al[70] found that buccal carcinoma more than 4 mm in thickness was strongly associated

Table 14–5 Relationship Between Tumor Thickness* (TT) or Depth of Invasion[†] (DI) and Occult Nodal Metastasis (ONM) in Patients with Cancer of the Oral Tongue or Floor of Mouth[‡]

| | Parameter Measured | | Rate of ONM (%) when TT&/DI is: | |
First Author	TT (mm)	DI (mm)	Shallower	Deeper
Lower lip				
de Visscher[77]	5		5	26
Oral tongue				
Spiro[72]	2		2[§]	45[§]
Yuen[66]	3		8	44
Byers[58]		4 (well)[‖]	14	24
		4 (mod)[‖]	29	24
		4 (poor)[‖]	49	64
Kurokawa[75]		4	3	37
Fakih[124]		4	14	73
Fukano[74]		5	6	65
O-charoenrat[76]		5	16	64
Floor of mouth				
Mohit-Tabatabai[69]	1.5		2	33
Spiro[72]	2		2[§]	45[§]

*Tumor thickness is the measured distance from the surface of the tumor to the base of the tumor, using an optical micrometer.
[†]Depth of invasion is the measured distance from either the surface of the normal mucosa or the basement membrane to the deepest portion of the tumor, using an optical micrometer.
[‡]No data are available pertaining to the relationship between tumor thickness or depth of invasion and ONM for the upper lip, buccal mucosa, hard palate, retromolar trigone, and upper and lower alveolar ridges. The presence of masticatory mucosa that overlies bone precludes the development of deep soft tissue invasion at the last four sites.
[§]The results for oral tongue and floor of mouth were not analyzed separately.
[‖]A logistic regression model was utilized to predict the risk of cervical metastases by accounting for clinical N stage, tumor differentiation (well = well differentiated; mod = moderately differentiated; poor = poorly differentiated), and depth of muscle invasion.

with local-regional failure. Urist et al[77a] found that a tumor thickness of greater than 6 mm was associated with the poorest prognosis for buccal carcinoma, whereas depth of invasion was not an independent prognosticator.

Most investigations of tumor thickness or depth of invasion have focused on oral tongue cancer (**Table 14–5**). One study from Hong Kong that measured tumor thickness documented an 8% rate of ONM for oral tongue cancers ≤ 3 mm thick versus a 44% rate of ONM in tumors >3 mm thick.[66] In contrast, Japanese researchers chose to measure depth of invasion, demonstrating a 5.9% rate of ONM in lesions with less than 5 mm of invasion and a 64.7% rate of ONM for lesions with more than 5 mm of invasion.[74] Kurokawa and colleagues[75] found that a depth of invasion of ≥ 4 mm was associated with a higher rate of late cervical metastases and diminished survival. Spanish investigators have found that a depth of invasion of ≤ 3 mm resulted in a 5-year survival rate of 85.7%, whereas invasion of >3 mm was associated with a 5-year survival rate of only 58% ($p < .05$).[65]

Detection of Metastases

The sensitivity and specificity of palpation of cervical lymph node metastases are both in the range of 60 to 70%.[78] Assessment by palpation typically underestimates the size of clinically positive lymph nodes, particularly when the lymph node measures less than 3 cm in diameter.[79] Consequently, radiographic evaluation should be utilized to complement palpation for clinical staging purposes in patients considered at risk for regional metastases.[80,81] In general, 40 to 60% of the "occult" metastases that were not identified via palpation are detected using CT and magnetic resonance imaging (MRI).[78] CT or MRI can provide anatomically precise information that may not be appreciated by palpation, such as size, nodal architecture, focal defects, necrosis, and extracapsular tumor spread.[11]

Although most clinicians and diagnostic radiologists prefer to evaluate the neck by using CT scan, the radiographic modality is typically determined by the imaging method that will optimally evaluate the primary tumor. CT detects nodal necrosis, one of the most reliable criterion for metastatic cervical nodal disease, with greater sensitivity and accuracy than MRI.[82,83] Extracapsular nodal spread is also detected with greater accuracy and sensitivity using CT.[82] Castelijns and Van den Brekel[84] from Amsterdam advocate the application of ultrasonography-guided fine-needle aspiration cytology (FNAC) to exploit the high sensitivity of sonography and the excellent specificity of FNAC. In North America, this diagnostic approach is now the standard of care for the evaluation of thyroid nodules and is gaining impetus as a valuable tool to assess the cervical lymph nodes for metastatic disease.

These advances in diagnostic imaging have markedly improved our ability to identify regional metastatic disease in necks that were previously considered clinically negative, resulting in stage migration that shifts the clinical status of the neck from cN0 to cN+. Although a greater proportion of ONMs is now detectable, some metastatic deposits continue to remain undetected. Twenty-five percent of cN0 necks contain isolated metastatic deposits that are smaller than 3 mm in diameter, and microscopic extracapsular spread is present in nearly 20% of the clinically negative necks.[85–87] Helpful radiographic findings such as necrosis

are infrequently found in smaller lymph nodes. These subclinical metastases may contain up to 10^{11} tumor cells.[88] Our inability to consistently exclude the presence of metastatic disease in the clinically negative neck continues to fuel the controversy that surrounds the management of patients with a cN0 neck.

◆ Rationale for Elective Treatment of the Neck

Elective management of the neck is based on three premises: (1) untreated ONM inevitably progresses to clinically evident regional metastases; (2) persistent ONM is associated with an increased risk of developing additional regional metastases and distant metastases; and (3) regional metastases may be unresectable by the time they are detected.[89] Approximately 10% of otolaryngologists who manage head and neck cancer patients adhere to a policy of watchful waiting, a management philosophy that has been advocated by some authors.[63,90–92] The published experience of several institutions, however, suggests that expectant management of patients at risk for ONM may be imprudent. Yuen et al[93] noted that DSS was significantly worse in patients who were observed than in patients who were treated with elective neck dissection. Furthermore, patients tend to experience regional failure with advanced disease when clinicians observe the neck, and 50% of them are not candidates for salvage treatment.[24,94] The University of Florida experience has similarly shown that, in necks that were initially cN+, salvage treatment after a neck recurrence following RT is approximately 50%.[95] Kowalski[96] documented nearly 90% mortality following salvage therapy for neck recurrences in patients with a cN0 neck that were not initially treated. These findings provide strong indirect evidence for the survival benefit that is derived from elective management of the cN0 neck at risk for occult metastatic disease.

The presence and volume of subclinical metastatic disease in the neck of a patient with oral cancer depends on several factors.[88] The most important factor is the heterogeneity of metastatic potential from tumor to tumor. Metastases can also manifest differential rates of growth that can impact the tumor cell burden. A third factor is the delay that frequently occurs between removal of the primary tumor, the source of metastases, and treatment of metastatic disease. A delay of several weeks can allow for the progression of single-cell metastases to multicellular deposits. This latter issue may also contribute to the increased rate of distant metastases and poor survival in patients with persistent or recurrent disease at the primary site, which is synonymous with subclinical disease that persisted despite treatment. These factors illustrate some of the reasons for heterogeneous tumor behavior that limit our ability to accurately detect or quantify the tumor cell burden in a patient's neck.

Most clinicians who advocate elective management of the cN0 neck believe that treatment is warranted when the probability of ONM exceeds 15 to 20%. This treatment threshold originally evolved from largely empirical recommendations that attempted to achieve a balance between the presumed improvement in survival provided by elective treatment and the calculated risk of morbidity and mortality.[97,98] Decision analysis has been applied to the outcomes of treatment that were published for the cN0 neck between 1971 and 1991, leading to the conclusion that a probability of metastatic disease of more than 20% should be considered the appropriate threshold for elective management of the neck.[99] A recent survey of board-certified otolaryngologists who treat patients with head and neck cancer, however, found that only 50% of the respondents treat patients when the risk of ONM exceeds 15 to 20%.[90] Additional investigation is necessary to evaluate the appropriateness of the treatment thresholds advocated by previous investigators so that guidelines may be provided to further standardize elective management of the cN0 neck.

Elective Treatment of the cN0 neck

Whenever possible, single modality therapy should be used to definitively manage squamous carcinoma of the upper aerodigestive tract. Because surgical resection of the primary tumor is the preferred treatment for oral cancer, the cN0 neck at risk for ONM should be electively dissected (see Chapters 9 to 13). RT remains an option for patients in whom surgery is contraindicated or in those patients who require postoperative RT.

For surgeons who ascribe to the philosophy that a 15 to 20% risk of ONM requires elective management, depth of invasion and other characteristics of the primary tumor should be used to estimate that risk. Intraoperative frozen section analysis following wide resection of superficial malignancies can be used to evaluate depth of tumor invasion with an optical micrometer to determine the need for neck dissection. The measurement of depth of invasion should not be based on the results of an incisional biopsy because the maximal depth of invasion must be ascertained, and sampling error is likely.

Several investigations have indirectly shown that elective irradiation of the cN0 neck provides levels of oncologic control that are comparable to elective neck dissection by documenting marked reductions in the development of delayed nodal metastatic disease. Early studies by Fletcher[100] at MDACC and subsequently by Mendenhall et al[101] and Million[102] at the University of Florida noted a marked decrease in regional failure following elective neck irradiation (ENI), particularly when control was achieved at the primary site. A dose of 50 Gy in 2-Gy fractions achieves a 90% reduction in the incidence of subclinical metastases.[88] In a review of 801 patients with a cN0 neck that were electively irradiated, Bataini and colleagues[103] noted a 3% failure rate in the neck when the primary was controlled, a finding that was reproduced by radiation oncologists at Princess Margaret Hospital in Toronto.[104] A retrospective series of patients with oral cancer treated at Massachusetts General Hospital similarly demonstrated a 3% rate of neck disease following elective neck irradiation versus 31% for those patients who were observed, resulting in a statistically significant difference in 5-year disease-free survival.[105]

Frequently, the decision to electively administer RT to the neck must be made without supporting histopathologic evidence from the primary lesion such as tumor thickness or

Table 14–6 Risk of ONM Based on Clinical Evaluation* (When Histopathologic Assessment of Tumor Thickness or Depth of Invasion Is Not Available or Is Not Applicable)

Group	Estimated Risk of ONM	T Stage	Primary Tumor Site
I: Low risk	<20%	T1	Lower lip, BM, UAR, HP, RMT
		T2	Lower lip
II: Intermediate risk	20–30%	T1	OT, FOM, LAR
		T2	BM, UAR, HP
		T3–T4	Lower lip
III: High risk	>30%	T2–T4	OT, FOM, RMT, LAR
		T3–T4	BM, UAR, HP

*Based on the risk stratification approach proposed by Mendenhall et al.[106] The risk groups have been updated in accordance with findings published in the peer-reviewed literature since 1986.
BM, buccal mucosa; UAR, upper alveolar ridge; HP, hard palate; RMT, retromolar trigone; OT, oral tongue; FOM, floor of mouth; LAR, lower alveolar ridge

depth of invasion that improves our ability to estimate the likelihood of subclinical disease. Mendenhall and Million[106] addressed this dilemma by stratifying patients with a cN0 neck into three categories, thereby estimating the risk of ONM according to primary tumor site and T stage (**Table 14–6**): group I, low risk (<20% chance of ONM); group II, moderate risk (20–30% chance of ONM); and group III, high risk (>30% chance of ONM). There was no difference in regional control rates between low-risk patients who did not receive ENI and those who received ENI, whereas moderate- and high-risk patients who received ENI demonstrated much higher regional control rates than patients who received no treatment, supporting the value of elective irradiation for the cN0 neck in patients at risk for ONM. This risk stratification scheme is useful in situations where RT is being delivered as the sole treatment modality.

◆ The Neck Dissection

Morbidity of the Radical Neck Dissection

Loss of each of the three nonlymphatic structures that are resected during performance of an RND results in some degree of attendant morbidity. Removal of the sternocleidomastoid muscle (SCM) results in cosmetic deformity and loss of coverage of the carotid sheath structures that may become important if flap necrosis or fistula formation occurs. Moreover, preservation of the SCM facilitates dissection in the previously operated or irradiated neck. Preservation of the internal jugular vein (IJV) may facilitate microvascular surgical reconstruction, and indiscriminate sacrifice eliminates its availability if reconstruction is necessary following resection for recurrence. Simultaneous bilateral IJV sacrifice has been associated with serious complications, including increased intracranial pressure, laryngeal edema and airway obstruction, blindness, and death.[107]

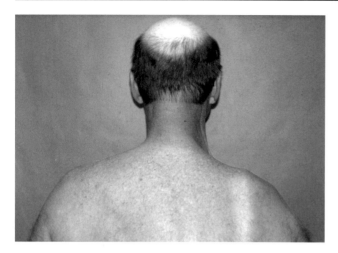

Figure 14–5 Appearance following spinal accessory nerve transection during radical neck dissection. There is prominent atrophy of the trapezius muscle and rotation of the scapula.

Spinal accessory nerve (SAN) sacrifice results in drooping of the shoulder with impairment of lateral shoulder abduction and forward shoulder flexion, abnormal scapular rotation, and pain and stiffness (**Fig. 14–5**). Cervical plexus injury to the cervical motor branches to the trapezius muscle (C2–C4) and the levator scapulae (C3–C5) can exacerbate functional limitations, and damage to the sensitive supraclavicular nerves (C3–C4) can result in neuropathic pain. Neck pain is primarily neuropathic, whereas shoulder pain is predominantly myofascial in origin.[108] These injuries result in biomechanical imbalance between the glenohumeral and scapulothoracic joints, which impairs mobility and increases pain, predisposing the joint to progressive fibrosis and glenohumeral adhesion.[109] Some degree of functional impairment of the SAN inevitably occurs in patients who undergo nerve-sparing neck dissections. Adjuvant RT, however, has no effect on shoulder joint function after surgery.[110]

Classification of the Neck Dissection

Since the original description of the RND in 1906, the neck dissection has undergone several periods of evolution as a consequence of our increased understanding of the patterns of lymph node metastasis and the need to decrease postoperative morbidity.[1] These modifications of the RND were assigned descriptive names that were not widely accepted by the head and neck oncologic community, leading to confusion regarding the difference, for example, between the type III modified RND coined by Medina[111] and the functional neck dissection described by Bocca et al[98] and Suarez.[112] The subsequent introduction of several selective neck dissection (SND) procedures in the literature mandated the need to standardize neck dissection nomenclature. Indeed, the necessity for developing such a widely accepted classification system is illustrated by a publication purporting to evaluate the outcomes of patients treated with bilateral radical neck dissections.[28] In this series, the SAN and IJV were preserved in 40% and 97% of the patients, respectively.

The most recent revision of the neck dissection classification was published in 2002 as a consensus statement proposed by the American Head and Neck Society and the American Academy of Otolaryngology–Head and Neck Surgery, and was primarily driven by the need to refine the SND nomenclature.[4] Research demonstrating the presence of nodal metastatic disease in level IV at a greater frequency than previously documented in patients with oral tongue cancer led many clinicians to extend the supraomohyoid neck dissection (SOHND) into level IV, giving rise to the "extended" SOHND.[54] The realization that additional investigation would likely document the need for further modifications of the selective neck dissection led to the recommendation that selective neck dissections should be designated by the lymph node levels removed. For example, the SOHND should be designated as a SND (I–III) and the "extended" SOHND should be termed a SND (I–IV).[4] This classification system is also intended to facilitate the notation of other regional nodal groups that were removed during neck dissection such as the buccinator or retropharyngeal nodes, that is, SND (I–III, buccinator nodes).

Rationale for the Neck Dissection

Knowledge of the true pathologic stage of the neck can facilitate the management of regional metastatic disease by determining the indications for RT. Elective neck dissection is indisputably effective as a staging procedure for the cN0 neck that provides the clinician with invaluable prognostic information that determines the necessity for postoperative RT. Based on our knowledge of patterns of nodal metastases, a comprehensive neck dissection, which substantially increases the risk of shoulder dysfunction, is not required to pathologically stage the cN0 neck. The selective neck dissection is ideally suited to provide the information necessary to determine the need for RT, and its value as a staging procedure has been widely advocated.[113–119] Recently, the role of sentinel lymph node biopsy as a selective staging procedure to evaluate the need for additional treatment for patients with oral cancer has received a great deal of attention, and a prospective trial sponsored by the American College of Surgeons Oncology Group is underway.[120–123]

Evidence to support the therapeutic value of elective neck dissection has been somewhat more elusive due to the lack of large prospective studies. Two prospective randomized trials from the 1980s that compared elective neck dissection with observation of the cN0 neck in patients with oral cavity cancer were unable to document a difference in disease-free survival, but these findings may have been affected by inadequate sample size.[124,125] A subsequent prospective randomized trial demonstrated improved disease-free survival when elective neck dissection was performed.[126] In addition, several retrospective investigations have documented high rates of regional control and improved survival.[93,127,128]

Therapeutic neck dissection is also preferred over RT to manage the clinically positive neck whenever surgical resection of the primary tumor has been performed. Limited data exist to support the oncologic efficacy of performing a SND without postoperative RT for the clinically negative, pathologically positive neck (cN–, pN+). A single prospective randomized trial demonstrated no difference in recurrence or survival between patients who underwent elective SND (I–III) and those who underwent elective modified RND (MRND) for oral cancer.[129] The patients in this trial were not actually randomized, because patients in the SND arm underwent frozen section analysis of any suspicious lymph node, with conversion to an MRND if frozen section identified nodal metastatic disease. There are several retrospective studies that demonstrate regional control and survival rates that are comparable to elective MRND, but the unmeasured impact of the use of postoperative RT confounds the results of these investigations.[118,130]

The body of literature that addresses the therapeutic efficacy of comprehensive neck dissections and selective neck dissections for the clinically positive, pathologically positive neck (cN+, pN+) largely reports the outcomes of patients with macrometastatic disease. It must be kept in mind that an SND for the cN–, pN+ neck transforms an elective neck dissection into a therapeutic dissection. A therapeutic neck dissection that is performed, for instance, for pN1 disease without ECS or for pN2 disease that contains only micrometastatic deposits likely has a prognosis that differs from the neck that harbors more extensive metastatic disease. Thus, the reported outcomes following neck dissection for macrometastatic disease may not apply to these patients.

A review of the retrospective literature found that MRND was as effective as RND in the management of N1 and N2 disease with less resultant shoulder disability.[131] Despite the lack of prospective evidence supporting the efficacy of MRND for the node-positive neck, there is growing interest in the use of selective neck dissection for node-positive disease.[132] The application of selective neck dissection for node-positive neck disease was first described in 1985 by Byers,[34] who reported a 5% recurrence rate for pN0 disease and a 10% recurrence rate for pN1 disease. Since 2000, numerous investigators have documented their experience with selective neck dissection for the pN+ neck, independently concluding that selective neck dissection with or without postoperative RT provides regional control rates that are comparable to those achieved with MRND or RND with or without postoperative RT.[130,133–136] On the other hand, Byers et al[137] reported that pathologically N1 necks treated with SND (I–III) without postoperative RT at MDACC had a regional failure rate of 35.7%, and that all of the failures occurred in the dissected field. The regional failure rate in this investigation decreased to 5.6% when postoperative radiation was used. These results imply that a comprehensive neck dissection for subclinical disease would be unlikely to improve regional control without the use of adjunctive RT. A large prospective randomized study comparing selective neck dissection with modified radical neck dissection that stratifies subjects by pathologic findings and the use of adjuvant RT would be necessary to definitively answer this contentious issue.

Neck Dissection Technique

Incision Planning for Neck Dissections

An apron incision is performed that extends from the mastoid tip to the submental crease below the mandibular symphysis for unilateral neck dissections and from one

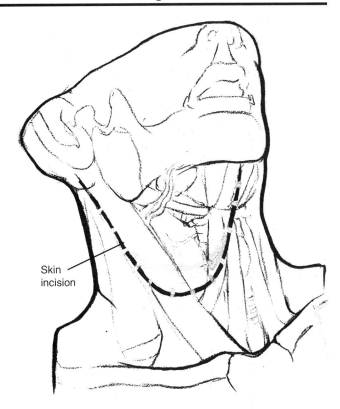

Figure 14–6   Design of unilateral apron incision for neck dissection. Access to sublevel IA is achieved by extension of the incision to the submental crease, and access to levels IV and V can be improved by placing the lower portion of the apron incision more caudally.

mastoid tip to the other for bilateral neck dissections. Extension of the incision to the submental crease facilitates dissection of sublevel IA. The vertical limbs of the incision should gently converge so that the inferior portion of the apron incision runs horizontally to improve vascularization to the distal portion of the flap (**Fig. 14–6**). The apron incision should also extend caudally to the midpoint between the thyroid notch and the cricoid cartilage if dissection of level IV is desired. Application of this incision design optimizes access to the entire neck, obviating the need for a descending limb. A lip-splitting incision can be extended from the submental extent of the unilateral incision and from the midpoint of the apron incision that is performed for a bilateral neck dissection. A tunnel can also be easily developed through the clavipectoral fascia to interpose a pectoralis flap into the neck if necessary. Alternatively, a hockey stick–shaped incision that crosses the midline of the neck can be used. Although this incision may result in improved cosmesis, access to the submental region is compromised.

The Supraomohyoid Neck Dissection (SND I–III) (*Fig. 14–7*)

The technique of supraomohyoid neck dissection described herein is based on the original description provided by Medina and Byers,[138] with some modification. Subplatysmal flap elevation is performed to the inferior border of the mandible immediately superficial to the great auricular nerve and external jugular vein (**Fig. 14–8**). The marginal

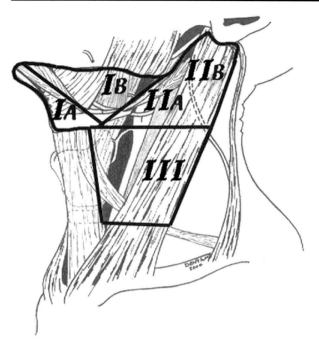

Figure 14–7 The supraomohyoid neck dissection (SND I–III). (From Robbins KT, ed. Pocket Guide to Neck Dissection Classification and TNM Staging of Head and Neck Cancer, 2nd ed. Alexandria, VA: American Academy of Otolaryngology–Head and Neck Surgery Foundation, 2001, with permission.)

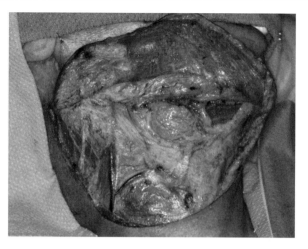

Figure 14–8 Subplatysmal flap elevation to the inferior border of the mandible. The external jugular vein and great auricular nerve have been preserved.

mandibular branch of the facial nerve is preserved. The preglandular/prevascular lymph nodes are reflected inferiorly in concert with division of the facial artery and vein at the inferior border of the mandible as a part of the submandibular triangle dissection.[7] Meticulous dissection of these lymph nodes from the facial artery and vein may be necessary in situations where the facial vessels are preserved for subsequent microvascular reconstruction. The prevascular and postvascular lymph nodes are frequently not addressed when inferior ligation of the facial vein with elevation of the vein and the soft tissues superficial to the vein is employed to preserve the marginal mandibular nerve, so this maneuver should be avoided to improve the nodal harvest from the submandibular region.

Dissection is begun at the anterior belly of the contralateral digastric muscle. The contents of the submental triangle (sublevel IA) are elevated from the surface of the

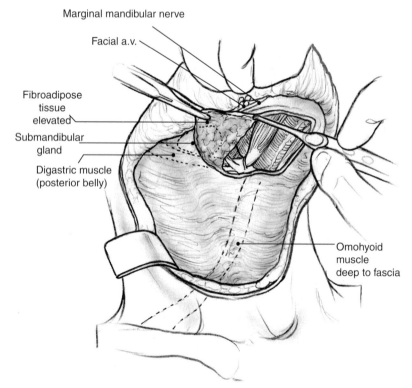

Marginal mandibular nerve

Facial a.v.

Fibroadipose tissue elevated

Submandibular gland

Digastric muscle (posterior belly)

Omohyoid muscle deep to fascia

Figure 14–9 The contents of sublevel IA have been elevated from the surface of the mylohyoid muscle laterally over the anterior belly of the ipsilateral digastric muscle into sublevel IB. The lateral edge of the mylohyoid muscle is visualized immediately above the digastric tendon.

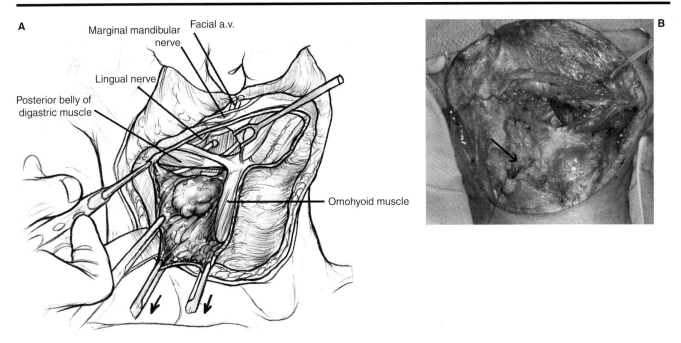

Figure 14–10 The contents of sublevels IA and IB have been reflected inferiorly over the posterior belly of the digastric muscle into level II (denoted by the *arrow* in **B**).

mylohyoid muscle laterally over the anterior belly of the ipsilateral digastric muscle (**Fig. 14–9**). Elevation continues to the lateral aspect of the mylohyoid muscle, which is retracted medially, exposing the lingual nerve and submandibular duct. The contents of the submandibular triangle (sublevel IB) are then elevated inferiorly over the digastric muscle and stylohyoid muscle along with sublevel IA (**Fig. 14–10**).

The fascia overlying the SCM is incised at the anterior border of the muscle and is elevated off the anterior and deep aspects of the muscle. The spinal accessory nerve is identified and preserved. Dissection superficial to the SAN continues anteriorly to the lateral aspect of the IJV. Superior retraction of the stylohyoid muscle and posterior belly of the digastric muscle allows for elevation of the lymph node–bearing tissues of sublevel IIB, the submuscular recess, away from the fascia overlying the splenius capitis and levator scapulae muscles. Sublevel IIB is then rotated underneath the spinal accessory nerve, remaining attached to the contents of sublevel IIA (**Fig. 14–11**). The internal carotid artery is occasionally identified lateral to the deep surface of the internal jugular vein in level IIA caudal to the SAN, and careful dissection is necessary to avoid inadvertent injury (**Fig. 14–12**).

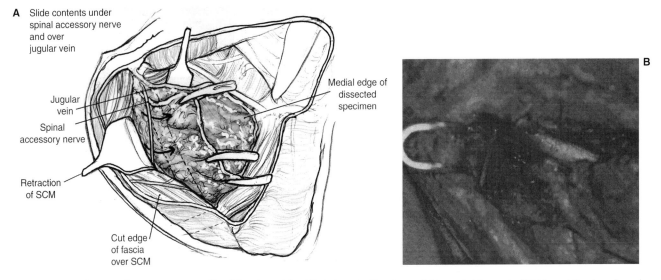

Figure 14–11 The spinal accessory nerve (SAN) has been identified deep to the sternocleidomastoid muscle (SCM), and the lymph node–bearing tissues of sublevel IIB have been rotated underneath the SAN into sublevel IIA.

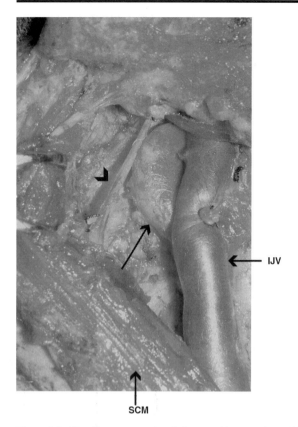

Figure 14–12 Aberrant course of the carotid artery *(arrow)* lateral to the jugular vein. The SCM is retracted laterally, exposing the SAN *(arrowhead)* and the internal jugular vein (IJV). The carotid artery is lateral to the IJV in sublevel IIA.

Dissection is continued along the undersurface of the SCM to the cutaneous branches of the cervical plexus and inferiorly to the omohyoid muscle. The node-bearing fibroadipose tissues of levels II and III are then elevated away from the transverse cervical vessels and the fascia overlying the scalene muscles, phrenic nerve, and brachial plexus. Dissection continues anteriorly to the IJV, where the fascia superficial to the vein is incised, facilitating elevation over the carotid sheath (**Fig. 14–13**). Dissection continues medially to the anterior belly of the omohyoid muscle (**Fig. 14–14**). Inferior to the tendon of the digastric muscle, dissection superficial to the veins overlying the hypoglossal nerve protects the nerve from inadvertent injury. The neck dissection specimen is removed en bloc and divided into levels for histopathologic examination (**Figs. 14–15** and **14–16**).

Extension of the neck dissection to include the contents of level IV does not require transection of the omohyoid muscle, and can be easily performed by retracting the omohyoid muscle inferiorly with a vein retractor (see **Fig. 14–17** on p. 174). Dissection to the level of the subclavian vein can be achieved if the original skin incision was placed low enough and inferior subplatysmal flaps are elevated to the clavicle. Chyle leaks infrequently develop during dissection of this region and are easily controlled with hemostatic clips if they are immediately identified.

Level V can also be completely dissected en bloc with the neck dissection specimen using this incision. The SAN must be identified lateral and medial to the SCM. Although dissection of the apex of level V formed by the SCM and the trapezius is usually not indicated, these tissues can be elevated away from the fascia overlying the deep cervical musculature and rotated underneath the spinal accessory nerve in a fashion similar to mobilization of sublevel IIB. The node-bearing tissues of the posterior triangle are

A

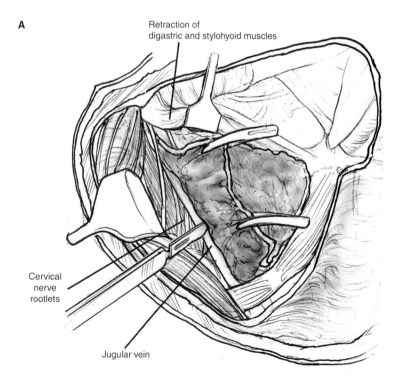

Retraction of
digastric and stylohyoid muscles

Cervical
nerve
rootlets

Jugular vein

B

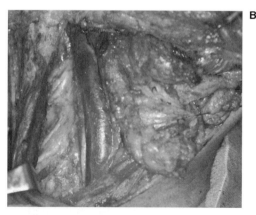

Figure 14–13 The SCM is retracted and the sensory branches of the cervical plexus, which delineate the boundary between level V and levels II through IV, have been identified. The fibroadipose tissues have been elevated medially to the IJV.

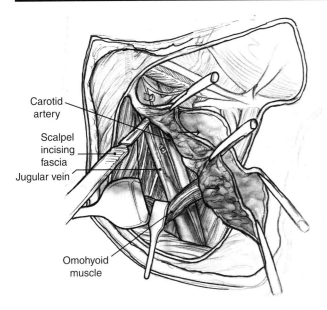

Carotid
artery

Scalpel
incising
fascia

Jugular vein

Omohyoid
muscle

Figure 14–14   Dissection continues medially over the IJV and the carotid sheath to the anterior belly of the omohyoid muscle.

elevated medially from the anterior border of the trapezius underneath the SCM in continuity with levels II, III, and IV. This en bloc dissection is not feasible without the sacrifice of some branches of the cervical plexus.

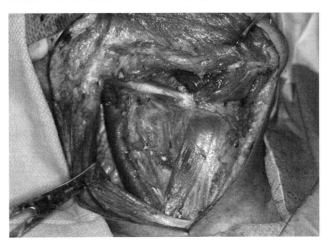

Figure 14–15   Appearance of the neck following completion of the supraomohyoid neck dissection.

Histologic Assessment of Neck Dissection Specimens

The neck dissection specimen provides invaluable information regarding pathologic stage and prognosis that can be utilized to counsel the patient and to determine the potential benefit of administering adjunctive postoperative RT. The specimen should be properly oriented by the surgical oncologist, and the lymph node levels that were removed should be

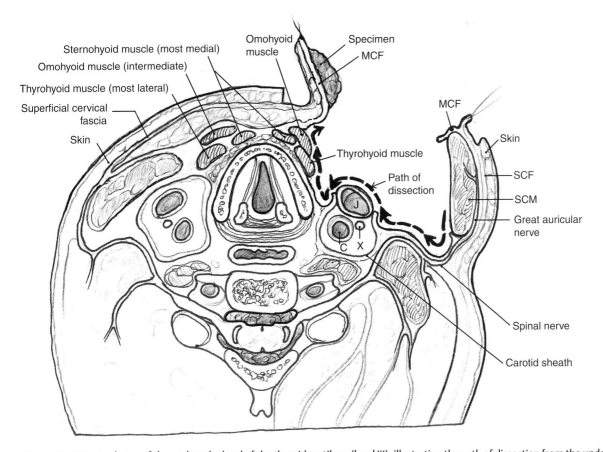

Sternohyoid muscle (most medial)
Omohyoid muscle (intermediate)
Thyrohyoid muscle (most lateral)
Superficial cervical fascia
Skin

Omohyoid muscle

Specimen
MCF

MCF

Skin

SCF

SCM

Great auricular nerve

Thyrohyoid muscle

Path of dissection

Spinal nerve

Carotid sheath

Figure 14–16   Axial view of the neck at the level of the thyroid cartilage (level III), illustrating the path of dissection from the undersurface of the SCM medially over the carotid sheath to the omohyoid muscle. SCF, superficial cervical fascia; MCF, middle cervical fascia.

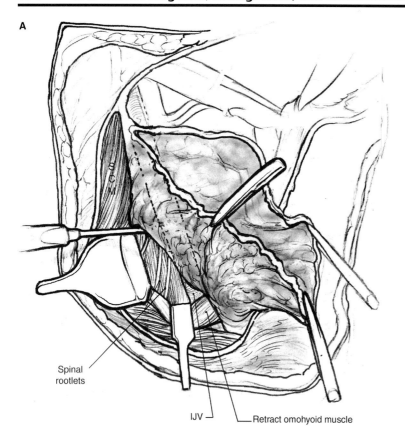

A

Spinal
rootlets

IJV ⎯⎯⎯ Retract omohyoid muscle

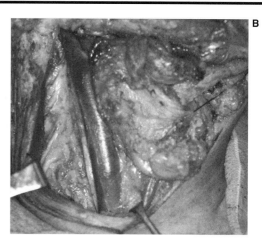

B

Figure 14–17 Inferior retraction of the omohyoid muscle with a vein retractor permits dissection of level IV without difficulty.

communicated to the pathologist. The pathology report should provide detailed information regarding the number of lymph nodes and the number of positive nodes identified in each level, the size of metastases, the presence of extracapsular spread or soft tissue deposits, and the involvement of any nonlymphatic structures (i.e., IJV, SAN) by malignancy.[139] Critical review of the histopathologic findings and a discussion of the findings with the radiation oncologist are an essential step in the decision-making process for every patient.

Several factors can affect nodal yield, including incomplete dissection of the lymph nodes in the specimen by the pathologist, poor surgical technique, and preoperative RT. Meticulous identification of lymph nodes by the surgical pathologist can result in markedly greater lymph node yields.[87] **Table 14–7** summarizes published average lymph node counts for different types of neck dissections.[30,34,37,38,51,115,140,141] The number of lymph nodes harvested during a neck dissection provides important information to the clinician that can influence decision making. For example, an SND (I–IV) specimen that includes 10 uninvolved lymph nodes may not be considered adequate to confidently exclude the presence of ONM, erroneously staging the neck pN0. A review of SND (I–III) performed at MSKCC, however, was unable to document any difference in the pathologic staging value when neck dissections with 15 or fewer nodes were compared with specimens with more than 15 nodes.[115]

The surgical pathologist's approach to the histologic evaluation of cervical lymph nodes varies widely among institutions. Gillies and Luna[139] report that routine processing of each lymph node at the University of Oklahoma and the

MDACC at the University of Texas involves obtaining two hematoxylin and eosin (H&E)-stained slides. Each slide contains four to six ribbons of 3-μm-thick tissue sections, and the tissue sections on the second slide are harvested at a distance of 10 to 20 μm from the tissue on the first slide.[139] Many institutions, however, evaluate a single tissue section from each lymph node. These differences in lymph node processing can affect the histologic findings and the ultimate pathologic stage assigned to the dissected neck. The mathematical probability of identifying a randomly located 2-mm micrometastatic focus with a single tissue section through the center of a 1-cm spherical lymph node is only 37%, whereas the probability increases to 80% when three tissue sections are performed equidistant from each other.[142] Ambrosch et al[64] found that 8% of neck dissections originally designated pN0 based on the evaluation of two to three tissue sections per lymph node were upstaged when serial sectioning was performed at 10-μm intervals, suggesting that performance of more than three tissue sections per node further augments the frequency of micrometastatic detection. Micrometastases 3 mm or less in diameter made up 39% of the "occult" nodal metastases identified in a prospective study by van den Brekel et al.[85] In another prospective analysis of more than 11,000 lymph nodes, one third of the metastatic nodes were 3 mm or less in diameter.[87] Clinicians should understand the approach to the histologic assessment of neck dissection specimens by the surgical pathologists at their institution, because proper interpretation of the pathologic findings and their prognostic significance is otherwise impossible. Because

Table 14–7 Relationship Between Type of Neck Dissection Performed and the Number of Lymph Nodes Harvested from Neck Dissection Specimens

Type of Dissection	Number of Neck Dissections	Mean Number of Lymph Nodes	Institution/Location
Radical neck dissection	1119	39	MSKCC[37]
	384	38	Hong Kong[38]
	58	34	Massachusetts Eye and Ear Infirmary (MEEI)[140]
	25	46	Liverpool[30]
Modified radical neck dissection with preservation of:			
SAN	50	27	MEEI[140]
SAN, IJV	15	31	MEEI[140]
SAN, IJV, SCM	441	31	MDACC[34]
	80	36	Liverpool[30]
	33	22	MEEI[140]
Selective neck dissection			
Levels I–III	302	13*	Brazil[141]
	119	22	Seoul[51]
	75	13	MSKCC[115]
Levels I–IV	129	22	Liverpool[30]

*The median number of lymph nodes was reported.
SAN, spinal accessory nerve; IJV, internal jugular vein; SCM, sternocleidomastoid muscle.

the methodology that is used to evaluate lymph nodes is not uniform, peer-reviewed publications that report the outcomes of therapy for head and neck cancer must be critically reviewed to evaluate the impact that the chosen method of histopathologic assessment had on the findings.

◆ Radiation Therapy

Techniques for irradiation of the neck in conjunction with each primary tumor site were reviewed in Chapters 9 to 13, and the principles of RT are discussed in Chapter 20. The present discussion provides an overview of RT for the management of regional metastatic disease in patients with oral cancer.

Definitive Radiation Therapy

In cases where definitive RT has been chosen to treat the primary tumor and the neck, it is preferable to deliver part of the dose to the primary tumor with interstitial brachytherapy or intraoral cone irradiation to compress the overall treatment time and improve the likelihood of local control. External beam irradiation alone results in suboptimal outcomes and should be avoided if possible. Brachytherapy alone is sufficient for limited superficial tumors of the oral tongue and floor of mouth; external beam irradiation precedes brachytherapy for more advanced tumors. Intraoral cone irradiation should typically precede external beam RT so that the tumor is more easily visualized and intraoral irradiation can be administered before the onset of mucositis.

External beam irradiation is administered with an ipsilateral wedge pair technique for lateralized tumors and with parallel opposed portals for lesions that extend within 1 cm of the midline. The superior border of the fields is 2 cm above the tumor and the inferior border is usually placed at the thyroid notch; the level I and II nodes are included. The low neck (levels III and IV) is treated with an en face portal using a tapered midline laryngeal shield that extends from the top of the field to the bottom of the cricoid cartilage. Care must be taken to ensure that the block does not shield levels III and IV.[143] Similarly, if IMRT is utilized, the IMRT fields should not include the normal larynx when the laryngeal dose would be substantially lower with a technique that shields the larynx in an anterior low-neck field.[144,145] Either 30 Gy in 10 once-daily fractions or 38.4 Gy in 1.6 Gy twice-daily fractions is administered with 6 MV x-rays. Interstitial brachytherapy is performed 1 to 2 weeks following completion of external beam irradiation using iridium 192 (^{192}Ir) via the plastic tube technique to deliver an additional 30 to 40 Gy over 3 to 4 days. If intraoral cone irradiation is selected rather than brachytherapy, the patient is treated with either an orthovoltage or electron beam at 2.5 to 3 Gy/fraction to 20 to 30 Gy depending on the anticipated dose of external beam RT. Patients who are not suitable for brachytherapy or intraoral cone irradiation are treated to 74.4 to 76.8 Gy at 1.2 Gy/fraction using twice-daily fractionation.

Patients who initially present with clinically positive neck nodes must be evaluated for a neck dissection after completing RT; the procedure is mandatory for those who receive lower doses of external beam irradiation (i.e., 30 Gy in 10 fractions), and depends on the response to irradiation for those who receive higher doses (i.e., 74.4 Gy in 62 twice-daily fractions). Regional failure following full-dose irradiation is less likely if clinically positive nodes demonstrate a complete clinical and radiographic response, and neck dissection may be withheld.[146,147] CT that is performed 4 to 6 weeks following completion of RT can be used to predict the likelihood of residual disease and the need for a neck dissection. Independent predictors of residual disease on CT scan include a focal low-attenuation defect and evidence for extracapsular spread.[148] A radiographic complete response, which is defined as the absence of any lymph nodes greater than

1.5 cm or any focally abnormal lymph nodes, results in a negative predictive value of 94%.[149] At the University of Florida, the post-RT CT scan is routinely performed to identify those patients who require neck dissection, thereby avoiding the need to perform planned neck dissections in every patient at risk for persistent nodal disease.

Postoperative Radiation Therapy

Patients are treated with external beam irradiation using the field arrangements previously described. The dose fractionation schedule depends on the surgical margins: negative, 60 Gy in 30 fractions; close (<5 mm), 66 Gy in 33 fractions; and positive, 74.4 Gy in 62 twice-daily fractions. Concomitant cisplatin 30 mg/m^2/wk is administered for high-risk patients with positive margins or ECS.

Preoperative Radiation Therapy

Preoperative irradiation is usually employed for patients with marginally resectable primary tumors or fixed neck nodes. The field arrangements are the same as those previously described. Patients are treated to 50 to 60 Gy at either 2 Gy/fraction once-daily or 1.2 Gy/fraction twice-daily. Fixed nodes may be boosted to higher doses (60 to 70 Gy) using anterior-posterior wedged portals using 6 MV x-rays to avoid additional irradiation to the mucosa and the spinal cord.

Intensity-Modulated Radiation Therapy

Intensity-modulated RT may be used to administer either definitive or adjuvant RT. IMRT results in a more conformal dose distribution, and the dose can be limited to one or both parotid glands to lessen the likelihood of long-term xerostomia. There are several disadvantages associated with IMRT, which include an elevated risk of a marginal miss,

increased labor and expense, and greater total dose due to scatter, which increases the risk of a radiation-induced malignancy in long-term survivors. Thus, IMRT should not be employed unless there is a clear advantage associated with this technique (i.e., salivary sparing where the dose to one or both parotid glands is 26 Gy or less).

◆ Conclusion

A lack of consensus regarding management of the neck for patients with oral cancer persists on many fronts:

1. Is "watchful waiting" an acceptable option for the cN0 neck at risk for metastatic disease?
2. Does a single "critical thickness" exist that can reliably predict the presence of subclinical metastatic disease in patients with cancer of the oral tongue and floor of mouth?
3. Is there a role for sentinel lymph node biopsy in the detection of regional metastatic disease?
4. Is dissection of sublevel IIB or level IV necessary?
5. Does selective neck dissection provide regional control rates that are comparable to comprehensive neck dissections for macrometastatic disease?

These are a few of the many questions that must be addressed through well-designed prospective research. Until these questions are definitively answered, an array of empirical management philosophies will continue to be employed that are based on each clinician's assessment of the best available evidence. It is essential to critically evaluate our approach to the management of oral cancer because local-regional failure continues to be the most frequent location for treatment failure in these patients.

References

1. Crile G. Excision of cancer of the head and neck. JAMA 1906;47:1780–1786
2. Ferlito A, Robbins KT, Medina JE, Shaha AR, Som PM, Rinaldo A. Is it time to eliminate confusion regarding cervical lymph node levels according to the scheme originated at the Memorial Sloan-Kettering Cancer Center? Acta Otolaryngol 2002;122:805–807
3. Shah JP, Strong E, Spiro RH, Vikram B. Surgical grand rounds: neck dissection: current status and future possibilities. Clin Bull 1981;11:25–33
4. Robbins KT, Clayman G, Levine PA, et al. Neck dissection classification update: revisions proposed by the American Head and Neck Society and the American Academy of Otolaryngology–Head and Neck Surgery. Arch Otolaryngol Head Neck Surg 2002;128:751–758
5. Sheahan P, Colreavy M, Toner M, Timon CV. Facial node involvement in head and neck cancer. Head Neck 2004;26:531–536
6. Gross ND, Ellingson TW, Wax MK, Cohen JI, Andersen PE. Impact of retropharyngeal lymph node metastasis in head and neck squamous cell carcinoma. Arch Otolaryngol Head Neck Surg 2004;130:169–173
7. DiNardo LJ. Lymphatics of the submandibular space: an anatomic, clinical, and pathologic study with applications to floor-of-mouth carcinoma. Laryngoscope 1998;108:206–214
8. Abe M, Murakami G, Noguchi M, Yajima T, Kohama GI. Afferent and efferent lymph-collecting vessels of the submandibular nodes with special reference to the lymphatic route passing through the mylohyoid muscle. Head Neck 2003;25:59–66
9. Spiegel JH, Brys AK, Bhakti A, Singer MI. Metastasis to the submandibular gland in head and neck carcinomas. Head Neck 2004;26:1064–1068
10. Robbins KT. Integrating radiological criteria into the classification of cervical lymph node disease. Arch Otolaryngol Head Neck Surg 1999;125:385–387
11. Som PM, Curtin HD, Mancuso AA. An imaging-based classification for the cervical nodes designed as an adjunct to recent clinically based nodal classifications. Arch Otolaryngol Head Neck Surg 1999;125:388–396
12. Gregoire V, Levendag P, Ang KK, et al. CT-based delineation of lymph node levels and related CTVs in the node-negative neck: DAHANCA, EORTC, GORTEC, NCIC, RTOG consensus guidelines. Radiother Oncol 2003;69:227–236
13. Levendag P, Nijdam W, Noever I, et al. Brachytherapy versus surgery in carcinoma of tonsillar fossa and/or soft palate: late adverse sequelae and performance status: can we be more selective and obtain better tissue sparing? Int J Radiat Oncol Biol Phys 2004;59:713–724
14. Hahn SS, Spaulding CA, Kim JA, Constable WC. The prognostic significance of lymph node involvement in pyriform sinus and supraglottic cancers. Int J Radiat Oncol Biol Phys 1987;13:1143–1147
15. Grandi C, Alloisio M, Moglia D, et al. Prognostic significance of lymphatic spread in head and neck carcinomas: therapeutic implications. Head Neck Surg 1985;8:67–73

16. Leemans CR, Tiwari R, Nauta JJ, van der Waal I, Snow GB. Regional lymph node involvement and its significance in the development of distant metastases in head and neck carcinoma. Cancer 1993;71:452–456

17. Pinsolle J, Pinsolle V, Majoufre C, Duroux S, Demeaux H, Siberchicot F. Prognostic value of histologic findings in neck dissections for squamous cell carcinoma. Arch Otolaryngol Head Neck Surg 1997;123:145–148

18. Pitman KT, Johnson JT. Skin metastases from head and neck squamous cell carcinoma: incidence and impact. Head Neck 1999;21:560–565

19. de Bree R, Deurloo EE, Snow GB, Leemans CR. Screening for distant metastases in patients with head and neck cancer. Laryngoscope 2000;110:397–401

20. Vikram B, Strong EW, Shah JP, Spiro R. Failure at distant sites following multimodality treatment for advanced head and neck cancer. Head Neck Surg 1984;6:730–733

21. Hiratsuka H, Miyakawa A, Nakamori K, Kido Y, Sunakawa H, Kohama G. Multivariate analysis of occult lymph node metastasis as a prognostic indicator for patients with squamous cell carcinoma of the oral cavity. Cancer 1997;80:351–356

22. Myers JN, Greenberg JS, Mo V, Roberts D. Extracapsular spread: a significant predictor of treatment failure in patients with squamous cell carcinoma of the tongue. Cancer 2001;92:3030–3036

23. Franceschi D, Gupta R, Spiro RH, Shah JP. Improved survival in the treatment of squamous carcinoma of the oral tongue. Am J Surg 1993;166:360–365

24. Kowalski LP, Bagietto R, Lara JR, Santos RL, Silva JF Jr, Magrin J. Prognostic significance of the distribution of neck node metastasis from oral carcinoma. Head Neck 2000;22:207–214

25. Greenberg JS, Fowler R, Gomez J, et al. Extent of extracapsular spread: a critical prognosticator in oral tongue cancer. Cancer 2003;97:1464–1470

26. Kalnins IK, Leonard AG, Sako K, Razack MS, Shedd DP. Correlation between prognosis and degree of lymph node involvement in carcinoma of the oral cavity. Am J Surg 1977;134:450–454

27. Stell PM, Morton RP, Singh SD. Cervical lymph node metastases: the significance of the level of the lymph node. Clin Oncol 1983;9:101–107

28. Magrin J, Kowalski L. Bilateral radical neck dissection: results in 193 cases. J Surg Oncol 2000;75:232–240

29. Ferlito A, Shaha AR, Rinaldo A. The incidence of lymph node micrometastases in patients pathologically staged N0 in cancer of oral cavity and oropharynx. Oral Oncol 2002;38:3–5

30. Woolgar JA. Micrometastasis in oral/oropharyngeal squamous cell carcinoma: incidence, histopathological features and clinical implications. Br J Oral Maxillofac Surg 1999;37:181–186

31. Woolgar JA. Detailed topography of cervical lymph-note metastases from oral squamous cell carcinoma. Int J Oral Maxillofac Surg 1997;26:3–9

32. Jose J, Coatesworth AP, Johnston C, MacLennan K. Cervical node metastases in squamous cell carcinoma of the upper aerodigestive tract: the significance of extracapsular spread and soft tissue deposits. Head Neck 2003;25:451–456

33. Lindberg R. Distribution of cervical lymph node metastases from squamous cell carcinoma of the upper respiratory and digestive tracts. Cancer 1972;29:1446–1449

34. Byers RM. Modified neck dissection: a study of 967 cases from 1970 to 1980. Am J Surg 1985;150:414–421

35. Byers RM, Wolf PF, Ballantyne AJ. Rationale for elective modified neck dissection. Head Neck Surg 1988;10:160–167

36. Shah JP, Candela FC, Poddar AK. The patterns of cervical lymph node metastases from squamous carcinoma of the oral cavity. Cancer 1990;66:109–113

37. Shah JP. Patterns of cervical lymph node metastasis from squamous carcinomas of the upper aerodigestive tract. Am J Surg 1990;160:405–409

38. Li XM, Wei WI, Guo XF, Yuen PW, Lam LK. Cervical lymph node metastatic patterns of squamous carcinomas in the upper aerodigestive tract. J Laryngol Otol 1996;110:937–941

39. Talmi YP, Hoffman HT, Horowitz Z, et al. Patterns of metastases to the upper jugular lymph nodes (the "submuscular recess"). Head Neck 1998;20:682–686

40. Silverman DA, El-Hajj M, Strome S, Esclamado RM. Prevalence of nodal metastases in the submuscular recess (level IIb) during selective neck dissection. Arch Otolaryngol Head Neck Surg 2003;129:724–728

41. Kraus DH, Rosenberg DB, Davidson BJ, et al. Supraspinal accessory lymph node metastases in supraomohyoid neck dissection. Am J Surg 1996;172:646–649

42. Chone CT, Crespo AN, Rezende AS, Carvalho DS, Altemani A. Neck lymph node metastases to the posterior triangle apex: evaluation of clinical and histopathological risk factors. Head Neck 2000;22:564–571

43. Crean SJ, Hoffman A, Potts J, Fardy MJ. Reduction of occult metastatic disease by extension of the supraomohyoid neck dissection to include level IV. Head Neck 2003;25:758–762

44. Khafif A, Lopez-Garza JR, Medina JE. Is dissection of level IV necessary in patients with T1–T3 N0 tongue cancer? Laryngoscope 2001;111:1088–1090

45. Davidson BJ, Kulkarny V, Delacure MD, Shah JP. Posterior triangle metastases of squamous cell carcinoma of the upper aerodigestive tract. Am J Surg 1993;166:395–398

46. Kowalski LP, Bagietto R, Lara JR, Santos RL, Tagawa EK, Santos IR. Factors influencing contralateral lymph node metastasis from oral carcinoma. Head Neck 1999;21:104–110

47. Zitsch RP III, Lee BW, Smith RB. Cervical lymph node metastases and squamous cell carcinoma of the lip. Head Neck 1999;21:447–453

48. Eicher SA, Overholt SM, el-Naggar AK, Byers RM, Weber RS. Lower gingival carcinoma: clinical and pathologic determinants of regional metastasis. Arch Otolaryngol Head Neck Surg 1996;122:634–638

49. Candela FC, Kothari K, Shah JP. Patterns of cervical node metastases from squamous carcinoma of the oropharynx and hypopharynx. Head Neck 1990;12:197–203

50. Vartanian JG, Pontes E, Agra IM, et al. Distribution of metastatic lymph nodes in oropharyngeal carcinoma and its implications for the elective treatment of the neck. Arch Otolaryngol Head Neck Surg 2003;129:729–732

51. Lim YC, Song MH, Kim SC, Kim KM, Choi EC. Preserving level IIb lymph nodes in elective supraomohyoid neck dissection for oral cavity squamous cell carcinoma. Arch Otolaryngol Head Neck Surg 2004;130:1088–1091

52. Werner JA, Dunne AA, Ramaswamy A, et al. The sentinel node concept in head and neck cancer: solution for the controversies in the N0 neck? Head Neck 2004;26:603–611

53. Ferlito A, Mannara GM, Rinaldo A, Politi M, Robiony M, Costa F. Is extended selective supraomohyoid neck dissection indicated for treatment of oral cancer with clinically negative neck? Acta Otolaryngol 2000;120:792–795

54. Byers RM, Weber RS, Andrews T, McGill D, Kare R, Wolf P. Frequency and therapeutic implications of "skip metastases" in the neck from squamous carcinoma of the oral tongue. Head Neck 1997;19:14–19

55. Hamoir M, Shah JP, Desuter G, et al. Prevalence of lymph nodes in the apex of level V: a plea against the necessity to dissect the apex of level V in mucosal head and neck cancer. Head Neck 2005;27:963–969

56. Tiwari R. Squamous cell carcinoma of the superior gingivolabial sulcus. Oral Oncol 2000;36:461–465

57. Kimura Y, Hanazawa T, Sano T, Okano T. Lateral retropharyngeal node metastasis from carcinoma of the upper gingiva and maxillary sinus. AJNR Am J Neuroradiol 1998;19:1221–1224

58. Byers RM, El-Naggar AK, Lee YY, et al. Can we detect or predict the presence of occult nodal metastases in patients with squamous carcinoma of the oral tongue? Head Neck 1998;20:138–144

59. Lydiatt DD, Robbins KT, Byers RM, Wolf PF. Treatment of stage I and II oral tongue cancer. Head Neck 1993;15:308–312

60. Bradfield JS, Scruggs RP. Carcinoma of the mobile tongue: incidence of cervical metastases in early lesions related to method of primary treatment. Laryngoscope 1983;93:1332–1336

61. Sparano A, Weinstein G, Chalian A, Yodul M, Weber R. Multivariate predictors of occult neck metastasis in early oral tongue cancer. Otolaryngol Head Neck Surg 2004;131:472–476

62. Bundgaard T, Rossen K, Henriksen SD, Charabi S, Sogaard H, Grau C. Histopathologic parameters in the evaluation of T1 squamous cell carcinomas of the oral cavity. Head Neck 2002;24:656–660

63. Umeda M, Yokoo S, Take Y, Omori A, Nakanishi K, Shimada K. Lymph node metastasis in squamous cell carcinoma of the oral cavity: correlation between histologic features and the prevalence of metastasis. Head Neck 1992;14:263–272

64. Ambrosch P, Kron M, Fischer G, Brinck U. Micrometastases in carcinoma of the upper aerodigestive tract: detection, risk of metastasizing, and prognostic value of depth of invasion. Head Neck 1995;17:473–479

65. Gonzalez-Moles MA, Esteban F, Rodriguez-Archilla A, Ruiz-Avila I, Gonzalez-Moles S. Importance of tumour thickness measurement in prognosis of tongue cancer. Oral Oncol 2002;38:394–397

66. Yuen APW, Lam KY, Lam LK, et al. Prognostic factors of clinically stage I and II oral tongue carcinoma—a comparative study of stage, thickness,

shape, growth pattern, invasive front malignancy grading, Martinez-Gimeno score, and pathologic features. Head Neck 2002;24:513–520

67. Asakage T, Yokose T, Mukai K, et al. Tumor thickness predicts cervical metastasis in patients with stage I/II carcinoma of the tongue. Cancer 1998;82:1443–1448

68. Onerci M, Yilmaz T, Gedikoglu G. Tumor thickness as a predictor of cervical lymph node metastasis in squamous cell carcinoma of the lower lip. Otolaryngol Head Neck Surg 2000;122:139–142

69. Mohit-Tabatabai MA, Sobel HJ, Rush BF, Mashberg A. Relation of thickness of floor of mouth stage I and II cancers to regional metastasis. Am J Surg 1986;152:351–353

70. Mishra RC, Parida G, Mishra TK, Mohanty S. Tumour thickness and relationship to locoregional failure in cancer of the buccal mucosa. Eur J Surg Oncol 1999;25:186–189

71. O'Brien CJ, Lauer CS, Fredricks S, et al. Tumor thickness influences prognosis of T1 and T2 oral cavity cancer–but what thickness? Head Neck 2003;25:937–945

72. Spiro RH, Huvos AG, Wong GY, Spiro JD, Gnecco CA, Strong EW. Predictive value of tumor thickness in squamous carcinoma confined to the tongue and floor of the mouth. Am J Surg 1986;152:345–350

73. Woolgar JA, Scott J. Prediction of cervical lymph node metastasis in squamous cell carcinoma of the tongue/floor of mouth. Head Neck 1995;17:463–472

74. Fukano H, Matsuura H, Hasegawa Y, Nakamura S. Depth of invasion as a predictive factor for cervical lymph node metastasis in tongue carcinoma. Head Neck 1997;19:205–210

75. Kurokawa H, Yamashita Y, Takeda S, Zhang M, Fukuyama H, Takahashi T. Risk factors for late cervical lymph node metastases in patients with stage I or II carcinoma of the tongue. Head Neck 2002;24:731–736

76. O-charoenrat P, Pillai G, Patel S, et al. Tumour thickness predicts cervical nodal metastases and survival in early oral tongue cancer. Oral Oncol 2003;39:386–390

77. de Visscher JG, van den Elsaker K, Grond AJ, van der Wal JE, van der Waal I. Surgical treatment of squamous cell carcinoma of the lower lip: evaluation of long-term results and prognostic factors—a retrospective analysis of 184 patients. J Oral Maxillofac Surg 1998; 56:814–820 discussion 820–811

77a. Urist MM, O'Brien CJ, Somg SJ, et al. Squamous cell carcinoma of the buccal mucosa: analysis of prognostic factors. Am J Surg 1987; 154:411–414.

78. van den Brekel MW, Castelijns JA. Imaging of lymph nodes in the neck. Semin Roentgenol 2000;35:42–53

79. Alderson DJ, Jones TM, White SJ, Roland NJ. Observer error in the assessment of nodal disease in head and neck cancer. Head Neck 2001;23:739–743

80. Greene FL, Page DL, Fleming ID. AJCC Cancer Staging Manual, 6th ed. New York: Springer-Verlag, 2002

81. Merritt RM, Williams MF, James TH, Porubsky ES. Detection of cervical metastasis: a meta-analysis comparing computed tomography with physical examination. Arch Otolaryngol Head Neck Surg 1997;123:149–152

82. Yousem DM, Som PM, Hackney DB, Schwaibold F, Hendrix RA. Central nodal necrosis and extracapsular neoplastic spread in cervical lymph nodes: MR imaging versus CT. Radiology 1992;182:753–759

83. Chong VF, Fan YF, Khoo JB. MRI features of cervical nodal necrosis in metastatic disease. Clin Radiol 1996;51:103–109

84. Castelijns JA, Van den Brekel MW. Detection of lymph node metastases in the neck: radiologic criteria [editorial]. AJNR Am J Neuroradiol 2001;22:3–4

85. van den Brekel MW, van der Waal I, Meijer CJ, Freeman JL, Castelijns JA, Snow GB. The incidence of micrometastases in neck dissection specimens obtained from elective neck dissections. Laryngoscope 1996;106:987–991

86. Coatesworth AP, MacLennan K. Squamous cell carcinoma of the upper aerodigestive tract: the prevalence of microscopic extracapsular spread and soft tissue deposits in the clinically N0 neck. Head Neck 2002;24:258–261

87. Jose J, Coatesworth AP, MacLennan K. Cervical metastases in upper aerodigestive tract squamous cell carcinoma: histopathologic analysis and reporting. Head Neck 2003;25:194–197

88. Withers HR, Peters LJ, Taylor JM. Dose-response relationship for radiation therapy of subclinical disease. Int J Radiat Oncol Biol Phys 1995;31:353–359

89. Shasha D, Harrison LB. Elective irradiation of the N0 neck in squamous cell carcinoma of the upper aerodigestive tract. Otolaryngol Clin North Am 1998;31:803–813

90. Werning JW, Heard D, Pagano C, Khuder S. Elective management of the clinically negative neck by otolaryngologists in patients with oral tongue cancer. Arch Otolaryngol Head Neck Surg 2003; 129:83–88

91. Nieuwenhuis EJ, Castelijns JA, Pijpers R, et al. Wait-and-see policy for the N0 neck in early-stage oral and oropharyngeal squamous cell carcinoma using ultrasonography-guided cytology: is there a role for identification of the sentinel node? Head Neck 2002; 24:282–289

92. Khafif RA, Gelbfish GA, Tepper P, Attie JN. Elective radical neck dissection in epidermoid cancer of the head and neck: a retrospective analysis of 853 cases of mouth, pharynx, and larynx cancer. Cancer 1991;67:67–71

93. Yuen AP, Wei WI, Wong YM, Tang KC. Elective neck dissection versus observation in the treatment of early oral tongue carcinoma. Head Neck 1997;19:583–588

94. Andersen PE, Cambronero E, Shaha AR, Shah JP. The extent of neck disease after regional failure during observation of the N0 neck. Am J Surg 1996;172:689–691

95. Mabanta SR, Mendenhall WM, Stringer SP, Cassisi NJ. Salvage treatment for neck recurrence after irradiation alone for head and neck squamous cell carcinoma with clinically positive neck nodes. Head Neck 1999;21:591–594

96. Kowalski LP. Results of salvage treatment of the neck in patients with oral cancer. Arch Otolaryngol Head Neck Surg 2002;128:58–62

97. Lee JG, Krause CJ. Radical neck dissection: elective, therapeutic, and secondary. Arch Otolaryngol 1975;101:656–659

98. Bocca E, Calearo C, de Vincentiis I, Marullo T, Motta G, Ottaviani A. Occult metastases in cancer of the larynx and their relationship to clinical and histological aspects of the primary tumor: a four-year multicentric research. Laryngoscope 1984;94:1086–1090

99. Weiss MH, Harrison LB, Isaacs RS. Use of decision analysis in planning a management strategy for the stage N0 neck. Arch Otolaryngol Head Neck Surg 1994;120:699–702

100. Fletcher GH. Elective irradiation of subclinical disease in cancers of the head and neck. Cancer 1972;29:1450–1454

101. Mendenhall WM, Million RR, Cassisi NJ. Elective neck irradiation in squamous-cell carcinoma of the head and neck. Head Neck Surg 1980;3:15–20

102. Million RR. Elective neck irradiation for TXNO squamous carcinoma of the oral tongue and floor of mouth. Cancer 1974;34:149–155

103. Bataini JP, Bernier J, Jaulerry C, Brunin F, Pontvert D. Impact of cervical disease and its definitive radiotherapeutic management on survival: experience in 2013 patients with squamous cell carcinomas of the oropharynx and pharyngolarynx. Laryngoscope 1990;100:716–723

104. Harwood AR, Beale FA, Cummings BJ, et al. Supraglottic laryngeal carcinoma: an analysis of dose-time-volume factors in 410 patients. Int J Radiat Oncol Biol Phys 1983;9:311–319

105. August M, Gianetti K. Elective neck irradiation versus observation of the clinically negative neck of patients with oral cancer. J Oral Maxillofac Surg 1996;54:1050–1055

106. Mendenhall WM, Million RR. Elective neck irradiation for squamous cell carcinoma of the head and neck: analysis of time-dose factors and causes of failure. Int J Radiat Oncol Biol Phys 1986; 12:741–746

107. Dulguerov P, Soulier C, Maurice J, Faidutti B, Allal AS, Lehmann W. Bilateral radical neck dissection with unilateral internal jugular vein reconstruction. Laryngoscope 1998;108:1692–1696

108. van Wilgen CP, Dijkstra PU, van der Laan BF, Plukker JT, Roodenburg JL. Morbidity of the neck after head and neck cancer therapy. Head Neck 2004;26:785–791

109. Salerno G, Cavaliere M, Foglia A, et al. The 11th nerve syndrome in functional neck dissection. Laryngoscope 2002;112:1299–1307

110. Erisen L, Basel B, Irdesel J, et al. Shoulder function after accessory nerve-sparing neck dissections. Head Neck 2004;26:967–971

111. Medina JE. A rational classification of neck dissections. Otolaryngol Head Neck Surg 1989;100:169–176

112. Suarez O. El problema de las metastasis linfaticas y alejadas del cancer de laringe e hipofaringe. Rev Otorrinolaringol 1963; 23:83–99

113. Spiro JD, Spiro RH, Shah JP, Sessions RB, Strong EW. Critical assessment of supraomohyoid neck dissection. Am J Surg 1988; 156:286–289

114. Kowalski LP, Carvalho AL. Feasibility of supraomohyoid neck dissection in N1 and N2a oral cancer patients. Head Neck 2002; 24:921–924

115. Henick DH, Silver CE, Heller KS, Shaha AR, El GH, Wolk DP. Supraomohyoid neck dissection as a staging procedure for squamous cell

carcinomas of the oral cavity and oropharynx. Head Neck 1995;17:119–123

116. Carvalho AL, Kowalski LP, Borges JA, Aguiar S Jr, Magrin J. Ipsilateral neck cancer recurrences after elective supraomohyoid neck dissection. Arch Otolaryngol Head Neck Surg 2000;126:410–412

117. Kerrebijn JD, Freeman JL, Irish JC, et al. Supraomohyoid neck dissection: is it diagnostic or therapeutic? Head Neck 1999;21:39–42

118. Mira E, Benazzo M, Rossi V, Zanoletti E. Efficacy of selective lymph node dissection in clinically negative neck. Otolaryngol Head Neck Surg 2002;127:279–283

119. Pitman KT, Johnson JT, Myers EN. Effectiveness of selective neck dissection for management of the clinically negative neck. Arch Otolaryngol Head Neck Surg 1997;123:917–922

120. Asthana S, Deo SV, Shukla NK, Jain P, Anand M, Kumar R. Intraoperative neck staging using sentinel node biopsy and imprint cytology in oral cancer. Head Neck 2003;25:368–372

121. Taylor RJ, Wahl RL, Sharma PK, et al. Sentinel node localization in oral cavity and oropharynx squamous cell cancer. Arch Otolaryngol Head Neck Surg 2001;127:970–974

122. Civantos FJ, Gomez C, Duque C, et al. Sentinel node biopsy in oral cavity cancer: correlation with PET scan and immunohistochemistry. Head Neck 2003;25:1–9

123. Civantos FJ. A trial of lymphatic mapping and sentinel node lymphadenectomy for patients with T1 or T2 with clinically N0 oral cavity squamous cell carcinoma. https://www.acosog.org/ studies/ synopses/ Z0360_Synopsis.pdf

124. Fakih AR, Rao RS, Borges AM, Patel AR. Elective versus therapeutic neck dissection in early carcinoma of the oral tongue. Am J Surg 1989;158:309–313

125. Vandenbrouck C, Sancho-Garnier H, Chassagne D, Saravane D, Cachin Y, Micheau C. Elective versus therapeutic radical neck dissection in epidermoid carcinoma of the oral cavity: results of a randomized clinical trial. Cancer 1980;46:386–390

126. Kligerman J, Lima RA, Soares JR, et al. Supraomohyoid neck dissection in the treatment of T1/T2 squamous cell carcinoma of oral cavity. Am J Surg 1994;168:391–394

127. Dias FL, Kligerman J, Matos de Sa G, et al. Elective neck dissection versus observation in stage I squamous cell carcinomas of the tongue and floor of the mouth. Otolaryngol Head Neck Surg 2001;125:23–29

128. O'Brien CJ, Traynor SJ, McNeil E, McMahon JD, Chaplin JM. The use of clinical criteria alone in the management of the clinically negative neck among patients with squamous cell carcinoma of the oral cavity and oropharynx. Arch Otolaryngol Head Neck Surg 2000;126:360–365

129. Brazilian Head and Neck Cancer Study Group. Results of a prospective trial on elective modified radical classical versus supraomohyoid neck dissection in the management of oral squamous carcinoma. Am J Surg 1998;176:422–427

130. Ambrosch P, Kron M, Pradier O, Steiner W. Efficacy of selective neck dissection: a review of 503 cases of elective and therapeutic treatment of the neck in squamous cell carcinoma of the upper aerodigestive tract. Otolaryngol Head Neck Surg 2001;124:180–187

131. Buckley JG, Feber T. Surgical treatment of cervical node metastases from squamous carcinoma of the upper aerodigestive tract: evaluation of the evidence for modifications of neck dissection. Head Neck 2001;23:907–915

132. Gourin CG. Is selective neck dissection adequate treatment for node-positive disease? Arch Otolaryngol Head Neck Surg 2004;130:1431–1434

133. Andersen PE, Warren F, Spiro J, et al. Results of selective neck dissection in management of the node-positive neck. Arch Otolaryngol Head Neck Surg 2002;128:1180–1184

134. Muzaffar K. Therapeutic selective neck dissection: a 25-year review. Laryngoscope 2003;113:1460–1465

135. Kolli VR, Datta RV, Orner JB, Hicks WF, Loree TR. The role of supraomohyoid neck dissection in patients with positive nodes. Arch Otolaryngol Head Neck Surg 2000;126:413–416

136. Chepeha DB, Hoff PT, Taylor RJ, Bradford CR, Teknos TN, Esclamado RM. Selective neck dissection for the treatment of neck metastasis from squamous cell carcinoma of the head and neck. Laryngoscope 2002;112:434–438

137. Byers RM, Clayman GL, McGill D, et al. Selective neck dissections for squamous carcinoma of the upper aerodigestive tract: patterns of regional failure. Head Neck 1999;21:499–505

138. Medina JE, Byers RM. Supraomohyoid neck dissection: rationale, indications, and surgical technique. Head Neck 1989;11:111–122

139. Gillies EM, Luna MA. Histologic evaluation of neck dissection specimens. Otolaryngol Clin North Am 1998;31:759–771

140. Busaba NY, Fabian RL. Extent of lymphadenectomy achieved by various modifications of neck dissection: a pathologic analysis. Laryngoscope 1999;109(2 pt 1):212–215

141. Kowalski LP, Magrin J, Waksman G, et al. Supraomohyoid neck dissection in the treatment of head and neck tumors: survival results in 212 cases. Arch Otolaryngol Head Neck Surg 1993;119:958–963

142. Wilkinson EJ, Hause L. Probability in lymph node sectioning. Cancer 1974;33:1269–1274

143. Mendenhall WM, Parsons JT. Management of the neck and the unknown primary site. In: Gunderson LL, Tepper JE, eds. Clinical Radiation Oncology. New York: Churchill Livingstone, 2000:549–563

144. Mendenhall WM, Parsons JT, Million RR. Unnecessary irradiation of the normal larynx. Int J Radiat Oncol Biol Phys 1990;18:1531–1533

145. Amdur RJ, Li JG, Liu C, Hinerman RW, Mendenhall WM. Unnecessary laryngeal irradiation in the IMRT era. Head Neck 2004;26:257–263

146. Peters LJ, Goepfert H, Ang KK, et al. Evaluation of the dose for postoperative radiation therapy of head and neck cancer: first report of a prospective randomized trial. Int J Radiat Oncol Biol Phys 1993;26:3–11

147. Mendenhall WM, Villaret DB, Amdur RJ, Hinerman RW, Mancuso AA. Planned neck dissection after definitive radiotherapy for squamous cell carcinoma of the head and neck. Head Neck 2002;24:1012–1018

148. Ojiri H, Mendenhall WM, Stringer SP, Johnson PL, Mancuso AA. Post-RT CT results as a predictive model for the necessity of planned post-RT neck dissection in patients with cervical metastatic disease from squamous cell carcinoma. Int J Radiat Oncol Biol Phys 2002;52:420–428

149. Liauw SL, Mancuso AA, Amdur RJ, et al. Postradiotherapy neck dissection for lymph node-positive head and neck cancer: the use of computed tomography to manage the neck. J Clin Oncol 2006;24:1421–1427

15

Reconstruction of the Lips

Peter Neligan,
Patrick J. Gullane, and
John W. Werning

The surgical resection of lip cancer frequently results in alterations of normal lip appearance and function that can profoundly impact the patient's self-image and quality of life. As the principal aesthetic feature of the lower face, subtle changes in the appearance of the vermilion border, labial commissures, or Cupid's bow are easily detected by the casual observer. Neuromuscular injury can lead to asymmetry at rest and during facial expression, and distressing functional disabilities are common. Loss of labial competence may be characterized by impairments in the ability to articulate, whistle, suck, kiss, and control salivary secretions. The significance of the changes that result from surgical resection for cancer of the lip have been appreciated by surgeons for centuries, influencing them to devise creative surgical reconstructive techniques that improve the quality of their patients' lives. These techniques have undergone evolution, and newer procedures have been developed that effectively address small to moderate defects. However, the ultimate reconstructive approach for larger defects of the lip has remained elusive, and presently available methods provide results that are less than optimal. This chapter reviews the reconstructive techniques that are available for various defects of the lips following cancer resection, as well as the limitations that are associated with each of these techniques.

◆ Anatomic and Functional Considerations in Lip Construction

The lip is a trilaminar structure consisting of mucosa, muscle, and skin. Externally, the cutaneous portion of the lip surrounds the mucosal lip. The transition between these two regions is distinguished by the mucocutaneous ridge, or vermilion border. At the midline of the upper lip, there is a V-shaped indentation of the mucocutaneous ridge termed *Cupid's bow*. Above Cupid's bow, the philtrum is a vertical groove-shaped depression that is bordered on either side by elevations known as philtral ridges or columns (**Fig. 15–1**). The vermilion, which is composed of modified mucosa lacking minor salivary glands, forms the major aesthetic feature of the upper and lower lips. The characteristic hue of the vermilion stems from a rich vascular supply that underlies a thin epithelial architecture. Sensation to the upper and lower lips is provided by branches of the maxillary and mandibular divisions of the trigeminal nerve.

The boundaries of the upper lip are defined by the base of the nose centrally and by the melolabial sulcus (nasolabial sulcus) laterally. The inferior margin of the lower lip is defined by the mental crease (labiomental crease).[1] Although the lower lip is composed of only one aesthetic unit, the upper lip is composed of multiple subunits. According to Burget and Menick,[2] each side of the upper lip has two aesthetic subunits: the medial topographic subunit is one-half the philtrum, whereas the lateral subunit is bordered by the philtrum medially, the nostril sill and alar base superiorly, and the melolabial crease laterally. Other authors maintain that the upper lip is composed of three subunits, whereas the entire philtrum constitutes a single subunit (**Fig. 15–1**).[3]

The body of the lip largely results from the underlying orbicularis oris muscle, which forms a functional sphincteric ring. The superficial fibers of the orbicularis oris function to protrude the lips away from the facial plane, whereas the deep and oblique fibers approximate the lips to the alveolar arch.[4] The middle portion of the buccinator muscle travels

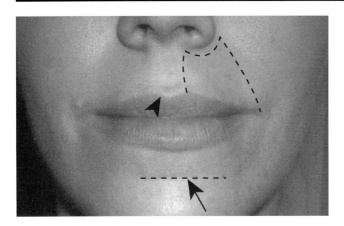

Figure 15–1 Anatomy of the lip and its aesthetic subunits. The upper lip is characterized by the V-shaped Cupid's bow (*arrowhead*) and the philtrum, which is a vertical groove-shaped depression that is bordered on either side by elevations known as philtral ridges. The boundaries of the lateral subunit of the upper lip are defined by the philtral ridge medially, the nostril sill and alar base superiorly, and the melolabial (nasolabial) crease laterally (*dashed line*). The philtrum can be considered as a single medial subunit or can be vertically bisected at the midline into two medial subunits. The lower lip is composed of a single aesthetic subunit, with its inferior boundary located at the mental (mentolabial) crease (*arrow*). (Courtesy of John W. Werning, M.D., D.M.D., University of Florida.)

anteriorly to the angle of the mouth and decussates so that the upper fibers of the mid-buccinator merge with the orbicularis fibers of the lower lip, and the lower fibers merge with the orbicularis fibers of the upper lip.[4] The two most important elevator muscles of the lip include the zygomaticus major and the levator anguli oris; the zygomaticus minor and the levator labii superioris also contribute. The depressor muscles include the depressor anguli oris and the platysma, with minor contributions from the depressor labii inferioris. Variations in the contraction of these muscles result in modification of the shape of the lips associated with facial expression and function. The commissural modiolus is a 1-cm-thick fibrovascular region of muscle fiber intersection of the levator muscles and the depressor muscles that attach firmly to the dermis approximately 1.5 cm lateral to the labial commissure. The modiolus can be located by compressing the skin and mucosa of the commissure using bidigital palpation with the thumb and index finger.[5] The appearance of the labial commissures is significantly impacted by movement of the modiolus on each side, which results from the summation of opposing contractile forces of the levator muscles (zygomaticus major and levator anguli oris) and the depressor muscles (depressor anguli oris and platysma).[6,7] When present, the dimple results from a dermal insertion arising from the inferior muscle bundle of a bifid zygomaticus major muscle.[8,9] The elevators and depressors of the lips are innervated by the buccal and mandibular branches of the lips, respectively. Disruption of the musculature that attaches to the modiolar region (or their neural supply) can alter the appearance of the labial commissure at rest and during function secondary to imbalanced muscular

contraction. Modiolar motion has also been analyzed to measure the success of facial reanimation in patients with facial paralysis.[10]

The arterial supply to the lips is provided by the facial artery, which gives rise to the inferior and superior labial arteries. Anatomic studies have shown, however, that the existence and course of these vessels are variable. The superior labial arteries from each side tend to anastomose in the midportion of the upper lip, coursing between the mucosa and orbicularis muscle in half of the patients and through the muscle in the other half.[11] The inferior labial artery, on the other hand, routinely courses between the mucosa of the inner aspect of the lip and the muscle.[11] Two separate cadaveric studies found that the inferior labial artery was absent on one side in 10% and 64%, respectively, of the cadavers evaluated.[11,12] The bilateral presence of inferior labial arteries was not always predictive of an end-to-end anastomosis between these vessels, and other arterial branches from the facial arteries were frequently identified (e.g., labiomental, sublabial arteries).[11,12] Even though the variable arterial distribution of this region could affect the survival of reconstructive procedures involving the lip, reconstruction with local flaps has been performed for centuries with predictably excellent survival rates.

Although the lips are an important aesthetic feature of the lower face, they also play an important role in facial expression. Oral competence is necessary to effectively consume liquids and foods, and intact neuromuscular function is essential for speech articulation, kissing, and whistling. The lower lip functions as a dynamic "dam" that retains saliva and prevents drooling. The upper lip contributes to oral competence by providing opposition to the lower lip to effect closure.[13] Sensation allows the lips to monitor the texture and temperature of substances prior to oral intake.

◆ Goals of Lip Reconstruction

The goals of lip reconstruction include the following[4,14]:

1. Maintenance of oral competence
2. Maintenance of an adequate oral aperture to accommodate removable dentures
3. Re-creation of the labial vestibule
4. Preservation of labial sensation
5. Maximization of cosmesis

Disruption of the sphincteric function provided by the division of orbicularis oris should be restored. Careful reapproximation of muscle edges with intact motor innervation usually results in complete restoration of dynamic orbicularis function. Although some authors contend that the upper lip functions primarily as a curtain that could be replaced with a static flap reconstruction, we believe that a completely intact sphincter with active function and sensation yields the best functional result.[2,15] In cases where reconstruction of the sphincter is not feasible, an adynamic reconstruction must be pursued that provides some degree of oral competence. Primary closure and local flaps frequently result in microstomia that must be minimized, and patients should be counseled prior to surgery that denture insertion and removal may not be possible. Decreases in the shape or depth of the labial vestibule can exacerbate oral incompetence and drooling, and may preclude patients from wearing a removable prosthesis. Preservation of labial sensation is vitally important to maximize oral competence and to fulfill its other sensory roles.

Reconstruction of the upper lip presents certain aesthetic challenges that are not of concern during lower lip reconstruction. Loss of the philtral ridges and Cupid's bow creates a noticeable cosmetic deformity that presents a significant reconstructive challenge. In profile, the upper lip should protrude anterior to the lower lip, so a reconstruction that results in excisional tightness with reduction or elimination of this relationship is undesirable. In contrast, the lower lip is better able to withstand tissue loss without significant changes in its profile appearance, and can sustain a loss of one third of its breadth before tightness or asymmetry begins to show.

Early lip reconstruction techniques focused primarily on primary closure of the surgical defect, whereas more contemporary techniques attempt to address the importance of an aesthetic, functional result. Reconstruction of the aesthetic subunits as described by Burget and Menick[2] is helpful, and aesthetic features such as Cupid's bow and the philtral columns must be carefully restored. Lack of attention to these principles results in deformity and a patch-like appearance that is immediately recognized by the observer's eye. Surgery that results in asymmetry is typically more noticeable than symmetric alterations; rounding of both commissures is less obvious than rounding of one side. Whenever possible, the height, projection, and relationship between the white and red portions of the lip should also be duplicated. This is most easily achieved by using tissue from the adjacent or opposing lip.[16,17]

◆ Historical Perspective

The first written description of lip reconstruction was provided in 600 B.C. by Sushruta Shamita, an Indian surgeon.[18] Most of the reconstructive techniques in present use are modifications or refinements of techniques that were described in the medical literature over the past two centuries. For instance, Victor von Bruns initially described in 1857 the use of bilateral superiorly based nasolabial flaps for reconstruction of the lower lip.[19] These full-thickness flaps, however, led to denervation of the remaining lower lip as well as the upper lips. Karapandzic[20] refined this technique by eliminating full-thickness extension of the flap through the labial mucosa, emphasizing that "any sensory or motor nerve fibres encountered should be spared." The "fan flap" attributed to Gillies is a refinement of another approach advocated by Von Bruns that employed two quadrilateral, inferiorly based nasolabial flaps.[19,21] It is important for reconstructive surgeons to appreciate the rationale for these technical refinements, because modifications and

variations of these techniques continue to surface in the literature. The historical context of selected reconstructive techniques is highlighted throughout this chapter to illustrate how technical refinements have improved aesthetic and functional outcomes.

◆ Defect-Specific Reconstruction of the Lip

Following surgical resection, the options for reconstruction of the lip are as follows, in order of preference[4,22]:

1. The remaining lip segment
2. The opposite lip
3. The adjacent cheek and nasolabial region
4. The submental and chin region
5. Distant flaps, including free flaps

Defects of the Vermilion

Following vermilionectomy, a labial advancement flap is usually employed to reconstruct the vermilion. The labial mucosa is undermined deep to the minor salivary glands and immediately superficial to the orbicularis oris, preserving the labial artery.[1] The undermined mucosa is advanced forward to reestablish the mucocutaneous junction (see Fig. 9–1 in Chapter 9). Reconstruction of the vermilion may result in excessive thinning of the lip from mucosal retraction or scar contraction, and decreased mucosal sensation.[1,23] Other approaches to reconstruction of the vermilion include the mucosal V-Y advancement flap, the cross-lip mucosal flap, and transposition flaps harvested from the buccal mucosa or the ventral surface of the tongue.[1,24] Buccal mucosal flaps tend to be more erythematous than natural vermilion, resulting in a color mismatch with the remaining vermilion.[23] Mucosal tongue flaps require a second procedure 14 to 21 days later to release and inset the flap. A musculomucosal flap that includes buccal mucosa and buccinator muscle anteriorly pedicled on buccal branches of the facial artery and innervated sensory branches of the infraorbital nerve has been advocated as one option to remedy the loss of sensation in defects that also include loss of orbicularis muscle.[25]

Small Full-Thickness Defects

Primary closure of defects that involve as much as a quarter of the upper lip or one-third of the lower lip can be achieved.[13] Because the upper and lower lips are approximately 7 cm and 8 cm in length, respectively, this approach is limited to T1 lesions.[13] A V-shaped wedge design usually permits closure of smaller defects, whereas an M-plasty placed at the base of the V facilitates the closure of larger defects. An M-plasty incorporated into a lower lip defect results in a W-shaped design (inverse M-plasty). The apex point(s) of the V or the W should be placed in the mental crease for lower lip defects or the melolabial crease

A

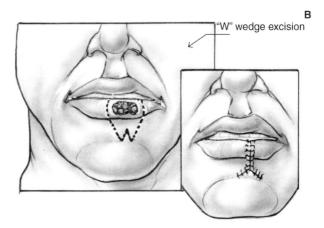

B

Figure 15–2 Wedge-shaped excision followed by primary layered closure. **(A)** V-shaped excision. Whenever possible, the apex of the V should be placed at the level of the mental crease. Extension of the V onto the aesthetic subunit of the chin increases the visibility of the scar. **(B)** An inverse M-plasty, or W, can be incorporated into the V-shaped excision to facilitate closure of larger defects so that the apex of the wedge does not extend onto the chin. The apex points of the W have been placed within the mental crease to disguise the inferior extent of the scar.

for upper lip defects (**Fig. 15–2**). If a larger excision requires extension beyond the mental crease or melolabial crease, the reverse central apex can be placed at the level of the crease. Wedge-shaped defects of the lateral lip should be more obliquely oriented so that the line of closure parallels the relaxed skin tension lines. If an M-plasty is incorporated into a lateral lip defect, the angle formed by the lateral V-shaped subunit of the W should be larger and more obliquely oriented than the medial subunit to properly align the closure (see Fig. 9–2 in Chapter 9).[1,14] Although many authors describe a three-layer closure of the skin, orbicularis oris, and labial mucosa, a four-layer closure that also reapproximates the subcutaneous tissue reduces tension along the closure line. If actinic cheilitis of the adjacent lip is present, vermilionectomy can also be performed in combination with the wedge excision, using a labial mucosal advancement flap to re-create the vermilion border (**Fig. 15–3**). This technique provides an elegant reconstruction of the vermilion, and the cosmetic outcome of this procedure is usually excellent.

The aesthetic result following repair of a V-type excision is often less satisfactory in the upper lip, because the upper lip is able to withstand much less tissue loss before tightness becomes clinically apparent and the normal overhang of upper and lower lip is lost as a consequence of closure-induced tension. In addition, the anchorage of soft tissues around the pyriform aperture to the underlying bony skeleton limits compensatory movement of the remaining lip. This problem can be minimized by using a T excision, which facilitates advancement of the lateral lip elements. The symmetry of Cupid's bow is easily lost with even minor excision in the region of the philtrum. Webster's[26] technique of crescentic perialar cheek excision is an extension of the T-excision technique that increases upper lip movement without disturbing the lateral muscle function (**Fig. 15–4**). If the defect is created lateral to the philtral columns, primary closure may produce deformity and notching. Thus, it is often preferable to use a lip-switch flap from the lower lip, even when the defect makes up less than 30% of the lip's width.

Centrally located upper or lower lip defects constituting less than 40% of the lip that are not amenable to primary closure may be closed by the development of bilateral lip advancement flaps. To improve cosmesis, the horizontal releasing incision can be placed in either the mental crease or along the nasal sill. Removal of a Burow's triangle may be necessary to facilitate flap advancement and to eliminate tissue redundancy that results in a standing cutaneous deformity; this is removed from the chin side of the incision in lower lip reconstructions. In the upper lip, excision of a crescent-shaped piece of skin and subcutaneous tissue lateral to the nasal ala provides the same effect as a Burow's triangle. Closure of the mucosa can usually be

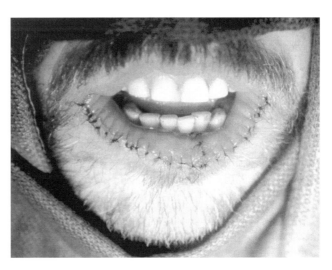

Figure 15–3 Re-creation of the mucocutaneous junction with a labial mucosal advancement flap following vermilionectomy for actinic cheilitis. A superficially invasive carcinoma of the left lower lip was also excised by performing a wedge-shaped excision with primary closure.

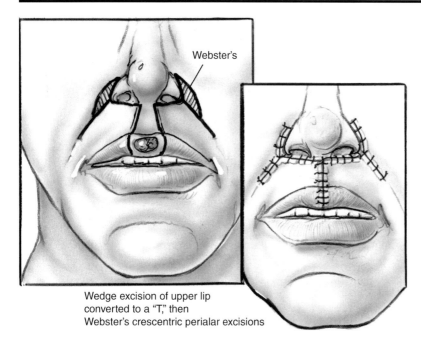

Wedge excision of upper lip
converted to a "T," then
Webster's crescentric perialar excisions

Figure 15–4 Conversion of a wedge excision of the upper lip into a T facilitates medial advancement of the remaining lateral lip and adjacent cheek. Webster's technique of crescentic perialar cheek excision may be used as an extension of the T excision technique to increase the amount of lip advancement so that primary closure can be achieved and the scars can be hidden in the alar creases.

achieved without incising the lateral mucosa. The use of opposing labial advancement flaps preserves sensation and muscular continuity.[1,23]

Intermediate Full-Thickness Defects

For larger defects that involve as much as two thirds of either lip, local flaps are the best reconstructive option. These flaps reconstruct the lip by utilizing three different technical approaches: (1) switching tissue from one lip to the other; (2) rotating tissue from one lip to the other; and (3) advancing cheek tissue into the defect.

The cross-lip (lip-switch) flaps are axial pattern local flaps that transfer labial tissue from the opposing lip based on an arterial pedicle from one of the labial arteries. Cross-lip flaps permit reconstruction with similar tissue from the opposite lip. The *transoral* Abbe flap can be used to reconstruct medial or lateral lip defects with a full-thickness composite flap that reconstructs the mucocutaneous border and the orbicularis oris.[27] Although the Abbe flap is traditionally described as triangular in shape, the flap can also be designed to accommodate wedge- or rectangular-shaped defects. The Abbe flap should measure approximately one-half the width of the defect so that the donor site can be closed primarily, and the flap height should be equal to or slightly greater than the defect to prevent notching (**Fig. 15–5**). Medial lower lip defects should be reconstructed with an Abbe flap that borders the philtrum so that the scar at the donor site is partially camouflaged by the philtral column. Division of the pedicle and revision of the flap is performed 14 to 21 days later. The defect size can occasionally be minimized by Webster's[26] technique of perialar excision that enables significant upper lip advancement, thereby decreasing the size of the lip-switch flap that will be required. This can help to minimize the risk of microstomia.

The *circumoral* Estlander flap is in essence an Abbe flap that is brought *around* the commissure.[28] Once again, the width of the flap is usually one-half the width of the defect and is the same height as the defect (see **Fig. 15–6** on p. 187). Defects that involve the commissure and as much as 50% of the lower or upper lip can be adequately reconstructed with an acceptable functional and cosmetic result. Several modifications of cross-lip flaps have also been described. Burget and Menick,[2] for example, suggested that defects constituting more than half of a topographic subunit of the upper lip necessitate removal of the remaining portions of the subunit so that reconstruction of the entire subunit can be performed by using a foil template of the defect to design the Abbe flap in the lower lip.

There are, however, several limitations to the cross-lip flaps. Blunting of the commissure regularly occurs with the Estlander flap, but this blunting frequently diminishes over time. Thus, commissuroplasty is rarely necessary and should not be considered until at least 6 months following reconstruction. Even though the orbicularis muscle is reconstructed, disruption of the motor supply leads to varying degrees of oral competence. Sensory denervation also occurs that recovers incompletely, and hyperesthesia occasionally develops. "Pin cushioning" frequently develops at the recipient site, and the cross-lip flap tends to appear thicker than the adjacent lip.[1,4,23,27,28]

The *fan flap*, initially described by Gillies and Millard[21] in 1957, is based on a technique described by von Bruns that utilized quadrilateral inferiorly based nasolabial flaps.[19] This flap rotates tissue around the commissure in the same fashion as an Estlander flap, but more tissue from the nasolabial region is included.[4] The flap design was likened to an old-fashioned collapsible hand-held fan, resulting in its name. Unlike a Karapandzic flap, a vertical releasing incision is made in the donor lip.[1] A unilateral flap can be performed to reconstruct a lip defect, but bilateral fan flaps are more frequently employed

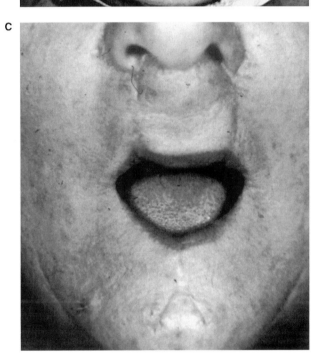

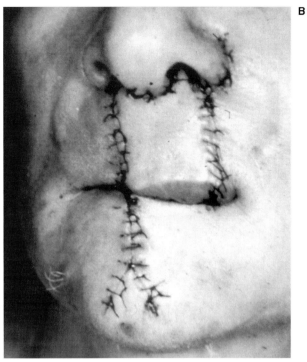

Figure 15–5 The Abbe cross-lip flap. **(A)** The excision involves about 80% of the upper lip. The labial commissures have not been disturbed. The width of the Abbe flap measures approximately one-half the width of the defect so that the donor site can be closed. In contrast, the height of the Abbe flap must equal the height of the defect to prevent notching at the site of closure. To accomplish this, tissue from the chin had to be included in the flap. **(B)** The flap has been inset. The vascular pedicle is still intact. **(C)** Final appearance with the mouth open. Note the lack of microstomia.

to reconstruct total or near-total defects.[4] Although defects involving up to 80% of the lip can be reconstructed with the Gillies fan flap, significant microstomia and vermilion deficiency are frequent sequelae. Denervation can worsen oral incompetence, although partial reinnervation appears to occur within 12 to 18 months.[1,4,29]

The *circumoral advancement-rotation flap* initially described by von Bruns in 1857 utilized full-thickness flaps that resulted in extensive denervation of the orbicularis muscle.[19] Although this ingenious technique effectively closed large composite defects of the lower lip, reconstruction was accomplished at the expense of sensation, motor function, and oral competence. These full-thickness flaps fell into disrepute until 1974, when Miodrag Karapandzic[20] from the University of Belgrade published a modification of von Bruns's technique. The incisional design of the Karapandzic flap, as it is now known, was identical to those advocated by von Bruns, but full-thickness flaps were not created, and the neurovascular

supply to the lip was preserved via meticulous dissection. Although most authors report its use for the closure of lip defects that involve up to two thirds of the lip, others state that the Karapandzic flap can successfully replace 80% of the total lip length.[1,4,17] This flap may be used to reconstruct defects of the upper or lower lip in the following manner (see **Fig. 15–7** on p. 188). Curvilinear circumoral incisions are extended bilaterally from the base of the defect, placing the incisions within the mental crease and the melolabial creases. The incisions are designed to maintain a uniform thickness of the flap bilaterally. Because the melolabial crease closely approximates the commissure, the incision should be placed slightly lateral to the melolabial crease in this region to maintain uniform thickness of the flap. If the defect is eccentrically located, the flap should be designed so that the contralateral lower lip is the longer limb of the flap. Careful dissection of the peripheral muscle fibers and concentric undermining allows advancement without any

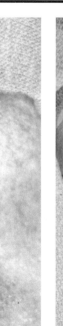

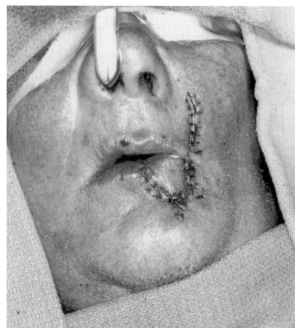

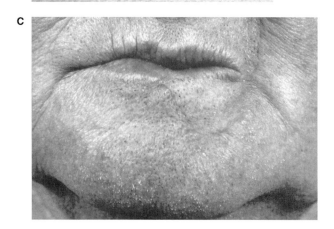

Figure 15–6 The Estlander cross-lip flap. **(A)** V-shaped lower lip defect that extends to the commissure. An Estlander flap has been planned that is the same height and approximately half the width of the defect. **(B)** The flap has been inset and the donor site has been closed. **(C)** Postoperative blunting of the left commissure, which frequently diminishes over time, obviating the need for commissuroplasty.

dissection of the mucosa. Preservation of the neurovascular bundles is imperative. A unilateral flap is adequate for smaller defects, whereas defects that constitute more than 50% of the lip require bilateral flaps. Function is restored because only the peripheral rim of orbicularis oris muscle is incised and the buccinator muscle is preserved. The Karapandzic flap results in blunting or rounding of both commissures, which is usually less noticeable than alteration of only one commissure. Some degree of microstomia is also inevitable, which may preclude the use of dentures. Because the combined width of the upper and lower lips is approximately 15 cm, reconstruction of a 5-cm defect results in a rounded oral aperture with a circumference that is two thirds of the original.[1,4,13,14] Based on the superior functional and cosmetic results that can be achieved, the Karapandzic flap is arguably the flap of choice for most defects.

Frequently, a defect is too wide to close primarily but is not wide enough to require a flap such as the Estlander flap, which interferes with the commissure. The stair-step advancement flap described by Johanson et al,[30] can be used for such defects, and is capable of reconstructing defects that constitute as much as two thirds of the lower lip (see **Fig. 15–8** on p. 189). This technique involves the excision of two to four small rectangles arranged in a stair-step fashion that descends from medial to lateral at a 45-degree angle from either side of the base of the defect. When the defect is located laterally, the step incision is outlined exclusively on the remaining long side of the lip.[31] If the defect is located near the midline or its horizontal length exceeds 20 mm, the staircase pattern is marked on both sides of the lower lip. The first horizontal incision is made parallel to the vermilion border and is approximately half of the width of the resected region. Usually two to four

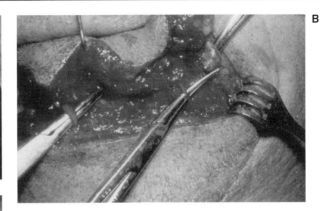

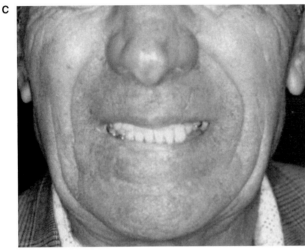

Figure 15–7 The Karapandzic flap. **(A)** Excision defect with the incisional design for the Karapandzic flap. The incisions are placed within the mental crease and the melolabial creases. The incision is placed slightly lateral to the melolabial crease in the region of the commissure to maintain uniform thickness of the flap. **(B)** The neurovascular bundles have been isolated and preserved during dissection of the flap. **(C)** Postoperative appearance.

additional steps are necessary in the vertical direction; the width of each step is approximately one half of its height. Finally, a triangle is excised with its apex located inferiorly. Each of the rectangles and the triangle are excised through the full thickness of the lower lip. This allows advancement of the flap in the direction of the defect with each succeeding higher step in the staircase, and the wound is closed in layers. By placing the step incisions outside of the mental crease, the aesthetic unit of the chin can be preserved. For this reason, the step technique is better than a wedge resection of similar size that would encroach on the chin subunit. The stair-step design allows for closure of the defect and minimizes contracture, but an unnatural-appearing scar usually forms, and loss of sensation occurs.

Ducic and colleagues[4] described the split orbicularis myomucosal flap for the reconstruction of lower lip defects constituting up to 80% of the lower lip. This technique exploits the redundancy of the labial mucosa by performing releasing incisions along the vermilion that split the orbicularis oris at this level. The myomucosal flaps are pulled together to close the superior portion of the defect, and the inferior cutaneous portion of the defect is closed independently. The authors found that separation of the cutaneous from the mucosal portions of the flap reconstruction increased the transverse dimension of the lip.

A variety of other innovative techniques have been developed to reconstruct specific defects of the lower lip. If the vertical component of a full-thickness defect is less than 1.5 cm, V-Y advancement flaps can be used that do not require interruption of the remaining outer ring of orbicularis oris and that minimize microstomia. Bocchi and colleagues[32] from the University of Parma advocate the performance of separate cutaneous and mucosal V-Y advancement flaps that are advanced over the residual orbicularis, preserving its motor innervation. The mucosal V-Y advancement flap can be replaced with a tongue flap to reconstruct the vermilion, but the patient must be maintained in an open-mouthed position with a bite block for 2 weeks, when the pedicle is divided.[33] Defects of the lateral lower lip can be restored with musculocutaneous "depressor flaps" that include the depressor anguli oris and/or platysma muscle. This technique, which has been popularized by Moschella and Cordova[34,35] of the University of Palermo, rotates a triangular piece of cutaneous tissue and underlying muscle that is borrowed from the adjacent cheek into the defect. Reconstruction of the vermilion is achieved by the use of a rotation flap from the buccal mucosa, which should be sutured into position prior to mobilization of the musculocutaneous flap.[35] The underlying marginal mandibular nerve and facial artery are meticulously dissected and preserved, and the vertically oriented depressor muscle fibers are reoriented so that they are parallel to the remaining orbicularis fibers, optimizing labial competence. Microstomia is also minimized by increasing labial tissue volume without modification of the remaining lip. This technique has been used to reconstruct defects that range from 40% of the lower lip to the entire lower lip.

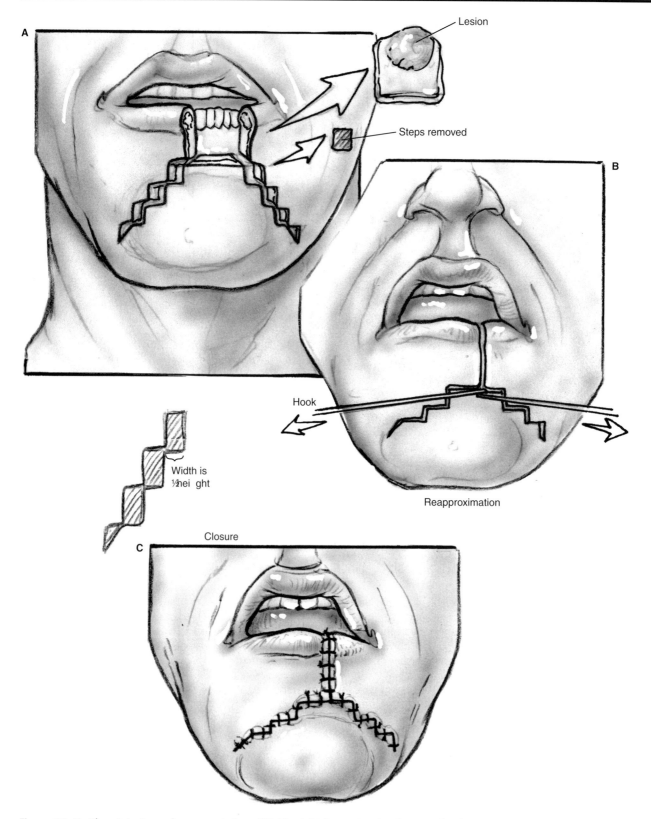

Figure 15–8 The stair-step advancement flap. **(A)** The initial horizontal incision on each side should measure one-half the width of the defect. Three small squares of soft tissue have been excised in a stair-step fashion that descends from medial to lateral at a 45-degree angle from either side of the base of the defect. The width of each step is approximately one half of its height. At the bottom of each stair-step, a triangle is excised with its apex located inferiorly. **(B)** As the flaps are medially advanced, the lateral soft tissue flap "steps" medially onto the stair, filling the corresponding triangular defect in the medial portion of the stair-step defect. **(C)** The defect is primarily closed in multiple layers.

Large Full-Thickness Defects

Defects that involve up to 80% of the total lip length may be reconstructed with bilateral Gillies fan flaps, the Karapandzic flap, or the split orbicularis myomucosal flap.[4] Reconstruction of total or near-total defects constituting more than 80% of the lip typically leads to an inferior aesthetic outcome and compromised labial competence that is largely adynamic.

The current reconstructive methods that employ horizontal cheek advancement flaps have evolved from the techniques described by Dieffenbach (1834), Bernard (1853), von Burow (1855), and von Bruns (1857).[4,19] Bernard and von Burow described the transposition of full-thickness flaps to reconstruct the upper or lower lip, reconstructing the vermilion with a mucosal advancement flap.[4] Transposition of these cutaneous flaps required the excision of four triangular regions of redundant cheek skin to reconstruct the upper lip, and the excision of three cutaneous triangles to reconstruct the lower lip. The reconstructive technique has become known as the "Bernard cheiloplasty" or the Bernard-Burow cheek advancement, and the triangular soft tissue excisions are referred to as Burow's triangles."[1,36] Webster et al,[37] suggested modifications of this technique that align the scars with the relaxed skin tension lines of the face. Although microstomia can be avoided with this approach, there is no functional orbicularis. Consequently, oral competence relies on the development of a tight adynamic lower lip.

Prior to free tissue transfer, nasolabial flaps played a prominent role in total lip reconstruction. Dieffenbach[38] initially described in 1845 the use of nasolabial flaps for upper lip reconstruction. The rectangular-shaped nasolabial flaps that von Bruns described in 1857 for lower lip defects were inferiorly-based.[19] A modification of his technique has also been described by surgeons from Tel Aviv that employs bilateral rectangular superiorly based nasolabial flaps to reconstruct the lower lip.[39] The "gate flap" design, originally published by Fujimori[40] in 1980, rotates two nasolabial island flaps that are based on the angular artery 90 degrees (**Fig. 15–9**). Although Fujimori's technique was fashioned

for the lower lip, modifications of the gate flap have also been proposed for total upper lip reconstruction.[41] Reconstruction with any of these nasolabial flap designs are associated with suboptimal oral competence and aesthetics, and denervation of the flaps routinely occurs.

In an effort to address the limitations of local flaps for large lip defects, some surgeons have employed the use of multiple local flaps. Kroll[42] from M. D. Anderson Cancer Center advocated reconstructing large lower lip defects by reestablishing the oral sphincter with an extended Karapandzic flap, followed by two sequential Abbe flaps 3 weeks apart to augment the central lower lip and a commissureplasty to widen the oral aperture. The Abbe flaps were harvested from a philtral ridge so that the scar was relatively inconspicuous and any notching of the upper vermilion from scar contraction could be disguised as a peak in the Cupid's bow. Using this technique, Kroll noted that the transfer of redundant upper lip tissue improved the appearance and volume of the lower lip, particularly near the midline. In contrast, Williams and colleagues[16,17] reconstruct these defects by simultaneously performing a modified Bernard-Burow cheek advancement flap in combination with a medially based (Abbe) cross-lip flap. In contrast to Kroll's technique, they purport that less microstomia develops, and the orientation of the modiolus is not disturbed. Kroll's technique was described for lower lip defects, whereas Williams et al's approach can be used for upper and lower defects.

The radial forearm flap is the free tissue transfer technique that is most frequently employed for the reconstruction of total lower lip defects. Sakai et al,[43] in 1989 reported the reconstruction of a lower lip defect with a composite radial forearm-palmaris longus tendon free flap. The forearm flap is folded over the tendon sling to resurface the internal and external surfaces of the lip and cheek. A microneural anastomosis between the lateral antebrachial cutaneous nerve and the cut end of the mental nerve can be performed to achieve sensory reinnervation.[44–46] A ventral tongue flap may be used to re-create the vermilion border, although a second procedure is necessary.[44,45] Following flap reconstruction,

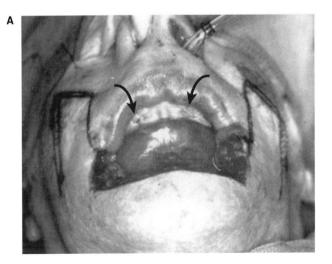

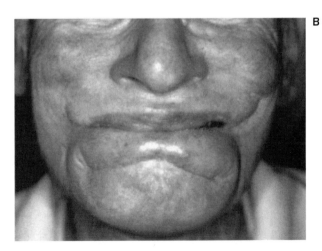

Figure 15–9 The gate flap. **(A)** Total excision of lower lip with gate flaps outlined. Both nasolabial island flaps are rotated inferomedially 90 degrees (*arrows*), so that the superior aspect of each flap restores the medial portion of the defect. **(B)** Postoperative appearance. Although microstomia does not occur, the cosmetic result is frequently suboptimal.

medical tattooing can also be used to create the vermilion with acceptable cosmetic results.[47,48] The radial forearm flap has also been used for total upper lip reconstruction.[48]

Oral competence and aesthetics are optimized by placing the palmaris longus tendon under the appropriate degree of tension. Lip entropion can develop if the palmaris longus tendon is inset too tightly (bow-strung), and ectropion may develop if inadequate tension is placed on the tendon. Sakai et al[43] sutured the palmaris tendon to the orbicularis oris muscle and dermis in the nasolabial region to suspend the reconstruction. Other surgeons have reported good outcomes by suturing the tendon to the periosteum of the malar eminence or to the orbicularis muscle of the upper lip near the philtral columns.[44,49] At the University of Toronto, the palmaris sling is woven through the remaining orbicularis muscle and secured within the muscular tunnel, suturing the tendon to itself (**Fig. 15–10**). We prefer to adjust the tension on the palmaris longus tendon by suturing it to the facial muscles in the region of the modiolus.[46] If adequate tension is placed on the tendon by the facial musculature at the modioli, the muscle action from the remaining facial muscles is transferred to the neolip, resulting in a more dynamic suspension. We believe that suturing the tendon to the malar eminence reduces the amount of adjacent facial muscular activity that can be transferred to the neolip.[46] Other surgeons have similarly chosen the modiolus as the preferred site of anchorage for the tendon.[50]

The design of the radial forearm free flap directly impacts the ultimate functional and aesthetic result. In our experience, optimal suspensory support for the tendon is achieved by slightly overcorrecting the tension. It is important to ensure that the pedicle is not compressed when the flap is folded over the tendon. Adequate suspension of the palmaris tendon will not eliminate lip ptosis and ectropion if the flap is too wide, so the flap should be narrower than the width of the defect (approximately 75%). Because the height of the skin excision and the mucosal resection usually differ, the skin and mucosal elements of the flap must be planned accordingly. Furthermore, fibrosis following surgery and radiation therapy tends to diminish the vertical height of the lip 6 to 12 months after reconstruction, so the vertical height of the reconstruction should be slightly greater than the height of the defect.

The ultimate free flap reconstructive technique of the lip, which would also incorporate muscle between the inner and outer layers and restore the vermilion component, has not been described. Nevertheless, the composite radial forearm-palmaris longus tendon free flap has several advantages over pedicled flaps. This reconstruction allows for a single-stage procedure that results in complete skin coverage and intraoral lining. The large amount of skin that can be used with the radial forearm flap usually results in an adequate stomal size. This technique can also be employed where a segmental mandibulectomy has been performed by incorporating radial bone into the flap, resulting in a very acceptable functional and cosmetic result. Although the color match between the radial forearm flap and surrounding facial tissue is frequently suboptimal, acceptable cosmetic results are attainable by respecting the borders of the aesthetic subunits during surgical resection and reconstructive planning.

In Japan, temporalis, masseter, and depressor anguli oris muscle transfers have been used in place of the palmaris longus tendon to achieve a more dynamic functional result when the lower lip is reconstructed with a radial forearm flap.[51–53] The functional outcomes with these reconstructive approaches have not been rigorously evaluated, and a prospective assessment of oral competence and dynamic function should be conducted to compare the outcomes following the use of palmaris longus tendon and muscle transfer techniques.

Complex Defects that Involve the Lips and Their Adjacent Regions

Locally advanced lip cancer can invade the skin of the chin or the cheek, and may also invade the bone of the mandible or the maxilla. Conversely, cancerous lesions of the buccal mucosa or anterior alveolar ridge are capable of infiltrating the soft tissues of the labial region. Resection of these tumors typically results in an anatomically complex defect that involves the loss of skin, muscle, mucosa, and bone from functionally disparate regions and multiple aesthetic facial subunits. Although reconstruction of a large cheek or intraoral defect can usually be achieved with a single free flap, the restoration of multiple anatomic regions with a single flap frequently results in a poor aesthetic and functional outcome. Because the axes of the cheek and intraoral lining are different, folding a free flap on itself typically leads to an unnatural-appearing, poorly functioning reconstruction. Moreover, a folded flap that does not provide some degree of static suspension will likely result in oral incontinence.[54]

Defects of the lower lip that also involve the chin can frequently be addressed by using a composite radial forearm-palmaris longus tendon free flap, and radial bone can be employed to reconstruct an anterior mandibular defect, as previously discussed.[46] For soft tissue defects of the cheek and the lip that involve the labial commissure, Jeng and colleagues[55] from Taiwan recommend using a circumoral advancement flap in combination with a radial forearm or anterolateral thigh flap. However, if an extensive mandibular defect and a cheek-lip defect coexist, Jeng et al[56] advocate reconstruction with a fibula osteocutaneous flap for the mandibular bone and intraoral lining and an anterolateral thigh flap for the external cheek and lip defects. When more than 60% of the lip has been resected, they utilize a fascia lata graft to reconstruct a complete oral sphincteric ring by weaving it into the remaining orbicularis oris and suturing it into the muscle near the philtral columns. When complex midfacial defects also include the lip, free flap reconstruction should be combined with a lip-switch flap to improve oral competence. For complex midfacial defects of the cheek and maxilla that also involve a substantial portion of the upper lip and labial commissure, Cordeiro and Santamaria[15] restore the oral sphincter with a lip-switch flap from the lower lip and reconstruct the through-and-through cheek defect with a folded rectus abdominis free flap that has a double skin island. The rectus abdominis myocutaneous free flap is the best option for large defects of the midface that require intraoral cheek lining and palatal closure in

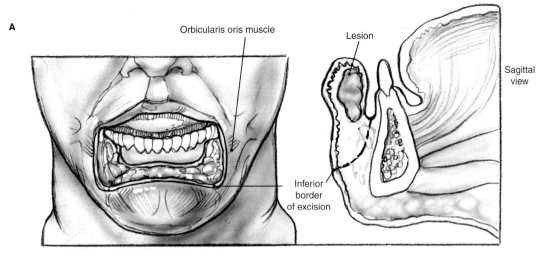

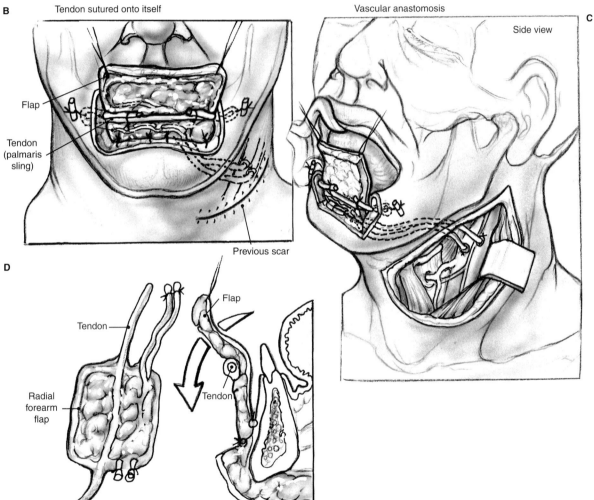

Figure 15–10 The composite radial forearm-palmaris longus tendon free flap. **(A)** (*Left*) Frontal view of a defect encompassing the entire lower lip. (*Right*) Sagittal view, illustrating the disparity between the extent of external skin and internal mucosal resection. **(B)** The palmaris longus tendon is sutured to itself, creating a tendinous sling that is placed under the proper amount of tension to support the radial forearm flap and provide oral competence.

(C) Side view, demonstrating the relationship between the palmaris longus sling and the flap, which is draped over the sling. **(D)** Once the palmaris longus tendon has been placed under the proper amount of tension and the intraoral closure has been completed, the external portion of the flap is draped over the tendon and is sutured to the remaining skin. (*Continued*)

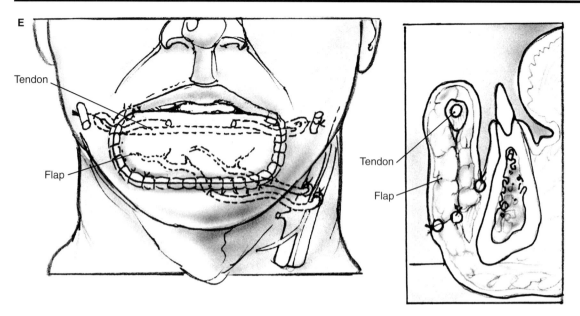

Figure 15–10 (*Continued*) (**E**) Appearance of the completed reconstruction.

combination with the skin and soft tissue of the cheek. Cordeiro and Santamaria emphasize that native labial tissue remains the best option to restore oral competence, and free flap tissue should not be incorporated into the lip reconstruction if another viable option exists.

◆ **Conclusion**

Reconstruction of the lips following surgical resection should be guided by a defect-specific approach that strives to optimize oral competence and re-create natural-appearing lips. A sensate dynamic flap that restores normal lip height, volume, and sphincteric function is preferred, and the

aesthetic subunits of the lip should be respected. Limited defects can be reconstructed by using local flaps from the remaining labial tissue or the adjacent cheek, whereas larger defects may require free tissue transfer or multiple local reconstructive techniques. Because most traditional reconstructive techniques for extensive lip defects have a variety of inherent shortcomings, improved outcomes must be realized by incorporating technical modifications or by employing novel surgical approaches such as the composite radial forearm-palmaris longus tendon free flap. The importance of restoring normal lip appearance and function following cancer resection is undeniable, and surgeons must be able to appreciate the nuances of surgical reconstruction that will make the greatest impact on the ultimate reconstructive outcome.

References

1. Renner GJ. Reconstruction of the lip. In: Baker SR, Swanson NA, eds. Local Flaps in Facial Reconstruction, 1st ed. New York: Mosby, 1995:345–396

2. Burget GC, Menick FJ. Aesthetic restoration of one-half the upper lip. Plast Reconstr Surg 1986;78:583–593

3. Constantinidis J, Federspil P, Iro H. Functional and aesthetic objectives in the reconstruction of lip defects. Facial Plast Surg 1999;15:337–349

4. Ducic Y, Athre R, Cochran CS. The split orbicularis myomucosal flap for lower lip reconstruction. Arch Facial Plast Surg 2005;7:347–352

5. Zufferey J. Anatomic variations of the nasolabial fold. Plast Reconstr Surg 1992;89:225–231

6. Ewart CJ, Jaworski NB, Rekito AJ, Gamboa MG. Levator anguli oris: a cadaver study implicating its role in perioral rejuvenation. Ann Plast Surg 2005;54:260–263

7. Marinetti CJ. The lower muscular balance of the face used to lift labial commissures. Plast Reconstr Surg 1999;104:1153–1162

8. Pessa JE, Zadoo VP, Adrian EK Jr, Yuan CH, Aydelotte J, Garza JR. Variability of the midfacial muscles: analysis of 50 hemifacial cadaver dissections. Plast Reconstr Surg 1998;102:1888–1893

9. Pessa JE, Zadoo VP, Garza PA, Adrian EK Jr, Dewitt AI, Garza JR. Double or bifid zygomaticus major muscle: anatomy, incidence, and clinical correlation. Clin Anat 1998;11:310–313

10. Johnson PJ, Bajaj-Luthra A, Llull R, Johnson PC. Quantitative facial motion analysis after functional free muscle reanimation procedures. Plast Reconstr Surg 1997;100:1710–1719

11. Pinar YA, Bilge O, Govsa F. Anatomic study of the blood supply of the perioral region. Clin Anat 2005;18:330–339

12. Magden O, Edizer M, Atabey A, Tayfur V, Ergur I. Cadaveric study of the arterial anatomy of the upper lip. Plast Reconstr Surg 2004;114:355–359

13. Langstein HN, Robb GL. Lip and perioral reconstruction. Clin Plast Surg 2005;32:431–445

14. Coppit GL, Lin DT, Burkey BB. Current concepts in lip reconstruction. Curr Opin Otolaryngol Head Neck Surg 2004;12:281–287

15. Cordeiro PG, Santamaria E. Primary reconstruction of complex midfacial defects with combined lip-switch procedures and free flaps. Plast Reconstr Surg 1999;103:1850–1856

16. Williams EF, Setzen G, Mulvaney MJ. Modified Bernard-Burow cheek advancement and cross-lip flap for total lip reconstruction. Arch Otolaryngol Head Neck Surg 1996;122:1253–1258

17. Williams EF, Hove C. Lip reconstruction. In: Papel ID, ed. Facial Plastic and Reconstructive Surgery, 2nd ed. New York: Thieme, 2002:634–645

18. Hauben DJ. Sushruta Samhita (Sushruta's collection) (800–600 B.C.?): pioneers of plastic surgery. Acta Chir Plast 1984;26:65–68

19. Hauben DJ. Victor von Bruns (1812–1883) and his contributions to plastic and reconstructive surgery. Plast Reconstr Surg 1985;75:120–127

20. Karapandzic M. Reconstruction of lip defects by local arterial flaps. Br J Plast Surg 1974;27:93–97

21. Gillies HD, Millard DRJ. Principles and Art of Plastic Surgery. Boston: Little, Brown, 1957

22. Wilson JSP, Walker EP. Reconstruction of the lower lip. Head Neck Surg 1981;4:29–44

23. Krunic AL, Weitzul S, Taylor RS. Advanced reconstructive techniques for the lip and perioral area. Dermatol Clin 2005;23:43–53

24. McGregor IA. The tongue flap in lip surgery. Br J Plast Surg 1966;19:253–263

25. Zhao Z, Li Y, Xiao S, et al. Innervated buccal musculomucosal flap for wider vermilion and orbicularis oris muscle reconstruction. Plast Reconstr Surg 2005;116:846–852

26. Webster JP. Crescentic peri-alar cheek excision for upper lip flap advancement with a short history of upper lip repair. Plast Reconstr Surg 1955;16:434–464

27. Abbe RA. A new plastic operation for the relief of deformity due to double harelip. Plast Reconstr Surg 1968;42:481–483

28. Estlander JA. Ene methods aus der einen lippe substanzverluste der Anderen zu ersetzen (English translation of original publication from 1872). Med Rec 1898;53:477

29. Rea JL, Davis WE, Rittenhouse LK. Reinnervation of an Abbe-Estlander and a Gillies fan flap of the lower lip: electromyographic comparison. Arch Otolaryngol 1978;104:294–295

30. Johanson B, Aspelund E, Breine U, Holmstrom H. Surgical treatment of non-traumatic lower lip lesions with special reference to the step technique: a follow-up on 149 patients. Scand J Plast Reconstr Surg 1974;8:232–240

31. Sullivan DE. "Staircase" closure of lower lip defects. Ann Plast Surg 1978;1:392–397

32. Bocchi A, Baccarani A, Bianco G, Castagnetti F, Papadia F. Double V-Y advancement flap in the management of lower lip reconstruction. Ann Plast Surg 2003;51:205–209

33. Yano K, Hosokawa K, Kubo T. Combined tongue flap and V-Y advancement flap for lower lip defects. Br J Plast Surg 2005;58:258–262

34. Moschella F, Cordova A. Platysma muscle cutaneous flap for large defects of the lower lip and mental region. Plast Reconstr Surg 1998;101:1803–1809

35. Moschella F, Cordova A. "Depressor flaps" for large defects of the lower lip and mental region. Plast Reconstr Surg 2005;115:252–256

36. Mazzola RF, Lupo G. Evolving concepts in lip reconstruction. Clin Plast Surg 1984;11:583–617

37. Webster JP, Coffey RJ, Kellcher RE. Total and partial reconstruction of the lower lip with innervated muscle-bearing flaps. Plast Reconstr Surg 1960;25:360–371

38. Dieffenbach JF. Die Operative Chirurgie. Leipzig: F. A. Brockhams, 1845

39. Adler N, Amir A, Hauben D. Modified von Bruns' technique for total lower lip reconstruction. Dermatol Surg 2004;30:433–437

40. Fujimori R. "Gate flap" for the total reconstruction of the lower lip. Br J Plast Surg 1980;33:340–345

41. Aytekin A, Ay A, Aytekin O. Total upper lip reconstruction with bilateral Fujimori gate flaps. Plast Reconstr Surg 2003;111:797–800

42. Kroll SS. Staged sequential flap reconstruction for large lower lip defects. Plast Reconstr Surg 1991;88:620–625

43. Sakai S, Soeda S, Endo T, Ishii M, Uchiumi E. A compound radial artery forearm flap for the reconstruction of lip and chin defect. Br J Plast Surg 1989;42:337–338

44. Serletti JM, Tavin E, Moran SL, Coniglio JU. Total lower lip reconstruction with a sensate composite radial forearm-palmaris longus free flap and a tongue flap. Plast Reconstr Surg 1997;99:559–561

45. Sadove RC, Luce EA, McGrath PC. Reconstruction of the lower lip and chin with the composite radial forearm–palmaris longus free flap. Plast Reconstr Surg 1991;88:209–214

46. Carroll CM, Pathak I, Irish J, Neligan PC, Gullane PJ. Reconstruction of total lower lip and chin defects using the composite radial forearm–palmaris longus tendon free flap. Arch Facial Plast Surg 2000;2:53–56

47. Furuta S, Hataya Y, Watanabe T, Yuzuriha S. Vermilionplasty using medical tattooing after radial forearm flap reconstruction of the lower lip. Br J Plast Surg 1994;47:422–424

48. Eguchi T, Nakatsuka T, Mori Y, Takato T. Total reconstruction of the upper lip after resection of a malignant melanoma. Scand J Plast Reconstr Surg Hand Surg 2005;39:45–47

49. Jeng SF, Kuo YR, Wei FC, Su CY, Chien CY. Total lower lip reconstruction with a composite radial forearm-palmaris longus tendon flap: a clinical series. Plast Reconstr Surg 2004;113:19–23

50. Ozdemir R, Ortak T, Kocer U, Celebioglu S, Sensoz O, Tiftikcioglu YO. Total lower lip reconstruction using sensate composite radial forearm flap. J Craniofac Surg 2003;14:393–405

51. Yamauchi M, Yotsuyanagi T, Yokoi K, Urushidate S, Yamashita K, Higuma Y. One-stage reconstruction of a large defect of the lower lip and oral commissure. Br J Plast Surg 2005;58:614–618

52. Shinohara H, Iwasawa M, Kitazawa T, Kushima H. Functional lip reconstruction with a radial forearm free flap combined with a masseter muscle transfer after wide total excision of the chin. Ann Plast Surg 2000;45:71–73

53. Kushima H, Iwasawa M, Kiyono M, Ohtsuka Y, Hataya Y. Functional reconstruction of total lower lip defects with a radial forearm free flaps combined with a depressor anguli oris muscle transfer. Ann Plast Surg 1997;39:182–185

54. Huang WC, Chen HC, Jain V, et al. Reconstruction of through-and-through cheek defects involving the oral commissure, using chimeric flaps from the thigh lateral femoral circumflex system. Plast Reconstr Surg 2002;109:433–441

55. Jeng SF, Kuo YR, Wei FC, Su CY, Chien CY. Reconstruction of concomitant lip and cheek through-and-through defects with combined free flap and an advancement flap from the remaining lip. Plast Reconstr Surg 2004;113:491–498

56. Jeng SF, Kuo YR, Wei FC, Su CY, Chien CY. Reconstruction of extensive composite mandibular defects with large lip involvement by using double free flaps and fascia lata grafts for oral sphincters. Plast Reconstr Surg 2005;115:1830–1836

16

Reconstruction of the Cheek

Michael E. Budd and
Gregory R. D. Evans

The cheek is a cosmetic and functional vital structure whose loss can affect a multitude of functions essential to a patient's survival and quality of life. It is the primary determinant of emotion and individuality while providing architecture for basic functions such as mastication, deglutition, and communication. Cheek defects result from a multitude of congenital or acquired etiologies, but ablative surgery for oral cancer is by far the most common cause of midfacial deformities. Historically, cancer surgeons were not concerned with the adverse impact that surgical resection might have on postoperative form and function, but such radical surgery has minimally impacted overall survival.[1] Consequently, the surgical focus has shifted to improvements in quality of life by rapidly restoring aesthetics and function. This chapter reviews the reconstruction of defects of the cheek after ablative surgery for oral cancer and the functional outcomes that can be expected following reconstruction.

◆ Goals of Cheek Reconstruction

The boundaries of the buccal mucosa are the inner surface of the lips anteriorly, the pterygomandibular raphe posteriorly, the upper alveolar ridge superiorly, and lower alveolar ridge inferiorly. The tissue layers of the cheek, from medial to lateral, include the buccal mucosa, submucosa, buccinator muscle, buccal space, muscles of facial expression (i.e., risorius, zygomaticus major), facial nerve, parotid duct, and skin (see Fig. 10–1 in Chapter 10).

The primary goal of reconstructive surgery after resection of oral cancer is wound closure with return of form and function by minimizing structural deformity, xerostomia,

anesthesia, and facial paralysis. These deficits may severely affect the patients' quality of life and alter their ability to interact socially, and reconstructive outcomes can profoundly influence patients' ability to cope with their disease.[2] Location of the defect, the extent of tissue loss and of functional loss, and the comorbid medical conditions are the primary determinants for the selection of a reconstruction modality.

There are a variety of techniques and donor materials available to reconstruct the complex three-dimensional defects of the cheek that may involve one or more tissue types, including mucosa, bone, facial mimetic muscles, nerve, and skin. Small mucosal resections not requiring extensive fat or muscle removal should be closed primarily, whereas larger defects need local mucosal flaps or skin grafts for reconstruction.[3] Occasionally, defects involving the entire buccal mucosa, especially after radiation therapy (RT), may necessitate septocutaneous or lubricating free flaps to reduce the incidence of trismus or xerostomia. Full-thickness defects present a significant challenge for the reconstructive surgeon. The creation of a functional oral cavity with internal and external epithelial coverage as well as underlying bone structure must be achieved to reach the primary goal of an aesthetically acceptable closure with resumption of an oral diet and normal verbalization. The conventional reconstruction of cheek defects with pedicle island flaps such as the cervical, upper trapezius, pectoralis major, and latissimus dorsi musculocutaneous flaps accomplishes wound closure with suboptimal aesthetic and functional outcomes relative to modern techniques. Clearly, microvascular free-tissue transfers with radial forearm, scapular-parascapular, anterolateral thigh, rectus abdominis, and latissimus dorsi flaps provide superior

194

aesthetic and functional outcomes. These free flaps provide vastly improved surgical outcomes by reconstructing surgical defects with richly vascularized, nonirradiated, pliable, epithelium-lined soft tissue. Some flaps also have the potential for sensory and motor activity. Large resections sometimes require resection of branches of the facial nerve that necessitate nerve repair with grafting or another reconstructive technique to minimize the morbidity associated with ipsilateral facial paralysis.

◆ Defect-Specific Reconstruction of the Cheek

Defects of the Buccal Mucosa

Primary closure is the preferred method of repair for small, superficial oral cavity wounds. Depending on the extent of the resection, defects larger than 3 cm should be closed with a random local mucosal flap, a skin graft, or a pedicled musculocutaneous flap to minimize the incidence of wound contraction leading to trismus.[3] Defects involving the entire buccal mucosa that are reconstructed with nonlubricating, insensate grafts may develop xerostomia and numbness that impairs food handling, swallowing, and quality of speech.[4,5] These large defects may occasionally require the transfer of sensate or lubricating free grafts to improve function, particularly when significant amounts of underlying soft tissues are resected or metastatic lesions to regional lymph nodes prevent the use of a local flap. In addition, free flaps may be necessary for intraoral contracture release following previous surgery and RT when local tissues are inadequate for reconstruction.

Pedicle Flaps

Even though free flaps clearly have superior aesthetic and functional outcomes, pedicle flaps should be considered in selected patients when comorbid medical conditions preclude the use of free flaps or when surgeons lack the technical skill and equipment to perform free tissue transfers. Cervical pedicle myocutaneous flaps such as the platysma and sternocleidomastoid provide small to medium-sized skin paddles that can cover most buccal defects. These locally obtained flaps readily reach many areas within the oral cavity, and aesthetically acceptable closure of the donor site can usually be achieved. However, these flaps are not acceptable for large tissue defects, or when metastatic tumors, RT, or previous surgery involve the proposed donor sites.[6] Furthermore, the vascular supply to these flaps is often segmental and unreliable. Surgeons should be familiar with reconstruction using platysma and sternocleidomastoid flaps, although other reconstructive options that have fewer limitations are usually available.

The platysma myocutaneous flap has a wide arc of rotation and provides thin, pliable tissue that can replace buccal mucosal defects up to 5 × 7 cm in size.[7] It is simple to harvest, easy to use, and hairless, and its harvest has

minimal aesthetic impact on the neck. However, the dominant vessels are infrequently visualized, and excessive kinking of the pedicle may result after rotating the flap through the 180-degree arc of rotation that is necessary to enter the oral cavity. In addition, the flap must be elevated prior to tumor resection to avoid injury of the facial artery, which is the main blood supply for the upper pedicle. Therefore, the size of the flap may be inadequate if the defect is larger than the preplanned skin paddle.

The sternocleidomastoid myocutaneous flap is also readily available for cheek reconstruction, but it has a variable and tenuous blood supply. This flap derives its blood supply from three sources: the occipital artery, the superior thyroid artery, and a branch of the thyrocervical trunk. The superior-based flap is by far the most commonly employed, because of its more reliable vascular supply from the occipital artery.[8] The sternocleidomastoid flap may be useful in the reconstruction of the mandibular region because of its thicker cylindrical muscle. As a result of its variable blood supply and limited arc of rotation, the sternocleidomastoid flap is considered challenging and tenuous, with a high likelihood of failure.

Free Flaps

Large cheek defects can be reconstructed with free septocutaneous or mucosal flaps that provide epithelium-lined soft tissue with the potential for sensation or lubrication. Unfortunately, no flap currently offers both qualities, and prospective randomized trials have not yet demonstrated improved functional outcomes when sensation is restored earlier with primary neurorrhaphy. As a result, the characteristics of the defect and the desires of the patient are taken into account when determining which flap should be utilized for the reconstruction.

The most reliable septocutaneous free flap for intraoral reconstruction is the radial forearm flap.[9] It is a pliable, thin, and durable flap with a long pedicle and consistent anatomy. The radial forearm tissue may be transferred as a sensate flap by anastomosing the lateral antebrachial cutaneous nerve to the lingual or inferior alveolar nerves.[5,10] Other potential sensate septocutaneous free flaps that can be utilized for intraoral reconstruction include the lateral arm, anterolateral thigh, and dorsal pedis septocutaneous flaps.[11–13] These flaps are associated with several disadvantages such as increased bulk in obese patients with the lateral arm flap, significant donor-site morbidity with the dorsal pedis flap, and high rates of vascular variations with the anterior lateral thigh flap.[12–14] Disadvantages associated with all skin flaps are the lack of mucin-secreting cells and hair follicles.

Mucosal free flaps have been demonstrated to prevent xerostomia in patients with decreased salivary secretion after RT.[9] The preferred mucosal free flap for intraoral reconstruction is the transverse colon because it provides an adequate pedicle and durable, pliable tissue that secretes mucin, even after postoperative RT.[9,15] There are many other mucosal free flaps utilized for intraoral reconstruction, such as the jejunal and gastro-omental flaps.[16,17] However, these two flaps have several disadvantages, including excessive folding, excessive mucous secretion, poor durability, persistent peristalsis, altered gastric motility, and peptic ulceration.[15] The disadvantages of mucosal flaps include numbness, complications associated with intraabdominal procedures, and excessive tissue transplantation that can lead to the formation of redundant pockets, requiring surgical debulking.[9] Excessive mucous secretion can also occur due to the absence of autonomic regulation.

Buccal Fat Pad

The buccal fat pad may be used as a pedicle or free fat graft during the reconstruction of superficial intraoral cheek defects.[18-21] It is located in the pterygomaxillary space and will successfully cover buccal and retromandibular defects up to 7 cm × 5 cm × 2 cm when dissected properly.[22] Frequently, the transferred fat pad will reepithelialize within 12 weeks, minimizing the risk of xerostomia.[23] The disadvantages of using the buccal fat pad include partial flap breakdown, excessive scarring, and infection (16%, 5.4%, and 0.6%, respectively), with the risk of flap breakdown increasing with graft tension.[23] A fully epithelialized buccal fat pad is minimally affected by postoperative RT, although its use as a pedicled flap is not recommended if the donor site was previously irradiated.[23]

Tissue Engineering

Tissue-engineered mucosal grafts may offer another reconstructive option for superficial defects in the future. However, these grafts require a considerable amount of preoperative preparation, and many medical centers do not have facilities that can provide this option. Defects up to 4 × 11 cm have been closed by using engineered cells without long-term complications.[7]

Full-Thickness Defects

Full-thickness cheek defects present unique challenges for the reconstructive surgeon. These defects are frequently associated with loss of oral sensation, lubrication, and facial motor function, and other reconstructive issues such as loss of mandibular continuity must be addressed. Traditional reconstructive techniques using pedicled myocutaneous flaps such as the pectoralis major, trapezius, and latissimus dorsi effectively provide wound coverage, but mandibular defects, facial paralysis, and sensation are not directly addressed with such methods. In comparison, free flaps provide epithelium-lined soft tissue paddles for intraoral reconstruction, bone with sufficient length and strength to restore mandibular continuity, and a skin flap for external coverage. These flaps also regain facial animation and sensation when a neurovascular anastomosis is performed. Despite the variety of available free flaps for reconstruction, the radial forearm, scapular-parascapular, rectus abdominus, latissimus dorsi, and anterolateral thigh flaps are firmly established as reliable options for repairing full-thickness defects of the cheek.

Pedicle Flaps

There is a wide range of pedicled myocutaneous flaps available when tissue bulk is required to reconstruct complex full-thickness cheek defects. The temporalis, upper trapezius, pectoralis major, and latissimus dorsi musculocutaneous flaps may all, with some manipulation, include the cheek and midface within their arc of rotation. However, midface defects are at the limit of their reach, which subjects the distal and most important portions of the flap to relative ischemia, increasing the risk for necrosis and flap loss. Care must be taken with patient selection, because healing deficiencies may cause distal wound breakdown, necrosis, and flap failure. In addition, the pedicle of these flaps must pass through the oral cavity or beneath the cervical and facial skin, creating a significant secondary deformity. This may require multiple operations to debulk these pedicles, lengthening the time required to complete the reconstruction. In the era of free tissue transfer, pedicle flaps should be considered only when free tissue transfer is medically contraindicated, in situations where recipient vessels are not adequate for transfer, or if the surgeon does not have the technical skill or equipment to perform these surgeries.

The temporalis myocutaneous flap may be used to reconstruct moderate-sized defects of the cheek. The primary blood supply is from the internal maxillary artery, which enters the muscle from the deep surface. The arc of rotation may include the contralateral cheek by passing through the ipsilateral buccal soft tissues. In addition, the temporoparietal fascia may be transposed based on the superficial temporal artery with vascularized calvarial bone to reconstruct midface bony defects. A small amount of temporal asymmetry should be anticipated after use of the temporalis flap.

The upper trapezius myocutaneous flap is another option that can be employed for cheek reconstruction because it is thin and pliable. However, limitations in the arc of rotation restrict its use in the anterior head and neck. The upper segments of the trapezius provide uniform thickness and hairless donor tissue, which is excellent for resurfacing the cheek skin or mucosa.[24-26] The flap design allows for primary closure at the donor site with minimal cosmetic impact, and this tissue also falls outside the range of adjuvant RT. The primary blood supply for this partial muscle flap comes from the transverse cervical artery, but the vascular supply is variable. As a consequence, the viability of the skin island is unpredictable, and the use of this flap for intraoral resurfacing may result in fistula formation.[27] The posterior location of the vascular pedicle also predisposes it to compression that could compromise the flap in the postoperative period. Furthermore, the arc of rotation is limited, and the donor site over the acromioclavicular joint is subject to high operative morbidity.

The pectoralis major myocutaneous flap is a simple flap that can be used to cover large defects of the cheek. This flap is easy to dissect and has a reliable vascular supply from the pectoral branch of the thoracoacromial trunk and multiple branches from the lateral thoracic artery. The incidence of total flap necrosis is less then 4% and occurs equally among men and women.[28] On the other hand, partial flap necrosis occurs more frequently in women secondary to the intervening breast tissue.[28] This flap may also be excessively thick with a limited arc of rotation and less reliable viability above the zygomatic arch. There is significant donor-site deformity, especially in women, and variable muscle atrophy with 40 to 50% reduction in bulk.[29] Therefore, its level of coverage within the head and neck and variable bulk severely limits the use of this flap during cheek reconstruction.

The latissimus dorsi is a reliable, flat and broad musculocutaneous flap that provides a large amount of tissue bulk for reconstruction of massive defects. It has a long pedicle and receives its blood supply from the subscapular artery. The thoracodorsal nerve accompanies the vascular pedicle, and its preservation results in preservation of sensory function. Its most common application is the coverage of large orbitomaxillary or lateral skull base defects. The latissimus dorsi flap has limited use in cheek reconstruction secondary to its bulk and may only be used for this purpose in a patient with a lean body habitus. Donor-site morbidity leading to shoulder dysfunction may also occur. Further, the ipsilateral latissimus dorsi flap should be avoided when the spinal accessory nerve has been sacrificed from a radical neck dissection.

Free Flaps

The advent of microvascular free tissue transfer has revolutionized the options for reconstruction of full-thickness cheek defects. Free myocutaneous flaps such as the radial forearm, scapular-parascapular, anterolateral thigh, rectus abdominis, and latissimus dorsi avoid the limitations of pedicle flaps by facilitating a more suitable tissue match, minimal secondary deformities, minimal positional restrictions, and return of neurologic function. The increased vascularity of these flaps enhances wound healing and decreases flap loss. Further, surgeons can more appropriately fit defects due to the unlimited geometric variations by eliminating the fixed pedicle and arc of rotation necessary with local myocutaneous flaps. These grafts can be molded to the defect prior to flap dissection without sacrificing the entire myocutaneous unit. However, some complex defects cannot be reconstructed using a single flap. Therefore, a combination of several flaps and multiple–paddle or folded three-dimensional free flaps can be used for reconstruction.[30–32] Muscle flaps must be adequately suspended or include skin and soft tissues that are not as susceptible to shrinkage. Clearly, a solitary or a combination of free tissue transfers offers superior flexibility, dependability, function, and cosmesis for cheek reconstruction relative to the traditional use of pedicle flaps.

The best choice for reconstruction of a full-thickness cheek defect is probably the radial forearm flap. This flap is easy to harvest and provides thin, pliable tissue with minimal hair and a long vascular pedicle, which is supplied by the radial artery. If bone is required, a portion of the underlying radius may also be harvested, which is dependent on the periosteal blood supply from the radial artery. However, bone stock is limited and the donor site requires long-term casting or prophylactic plating of the radius. Donor-site fractures are not discountable. If the medial and lateral antebrachial cutaneous nerves are harvested, this flap offers the potential for sensation.[33,34] The radial forearm flap also permits creation of two skin "paddles"; the common axis of the flap is de-epithelialized and then folded, creating two epithelial surfaces to reconstruct both the skin and mucosal lining. When facial nerve branches are excised, the palmaris longus tendon may be harvested with the flap and sutured to both the angle of the mouth and zygomatic arch. This technique suspends the facial muscles and prevents droop at the angle of the mouth. Good patient selection is necessary when the radial forearm flap is being considered because it cannot be used in patients with limited ulnar blood flow or if the patency of the palmar arch is in question. The donor site requires meticulous skin grafting to prevent breakdown and exposure of the tendons. In addition, a persistent aesthetic deformity of the donor site routinely occurs.

Like the radial forearm flap, the scapular-parascapular flap may be designed as a bipedicle composite flap of bone and skin, which has two independent arcs of rotation. The transverse and descending branches of the circumflex scapular artery supply two large skin paddles, whereas the thoracodorsal artery supplies branches to the bone. These large skin paddles provide an epithelial layer intraorally and externally, with additional flat cortical bone for maxillary defects. The scapular flap leads to minimal donor-site disfigurement. Flap bulk is usually not limiting and provides good contour for the cheek. Skin color and hair qualities are a closer match than with the radial forearm flap. Difficulties with patient positioning for harvest and ablation, however, limits this flap's desirability.

The lateral thigh septocutaneous flap is ideal for defects that require large amounts of tissue bulk with moderate thickness. It is based on the third perforating branch of the profunda femoris and may regain sensory function by performing a neurorrhaphy with the lateral cutaneous nerve.[35] This flap, usually 2 to 3 cm thick, may be rather bulky in obese patients or contain significant amounts of hair. Good patient selection is required to create a normal cheek contour.

The rectus abdominus flap is perhaps the most versatile and sturdy flap available due to its rich vascularity, but its use is generally limited to the reconstruction of large maxillary defects. The skin and fat may be removed if the myocutaneous flap is too bulky. The fascia can then be used to anchor this flap into the defect while the muscle is subsequently skin grafted. The flap may not fit into a defect in obese individuals, increasing the chance for ischemia and flap failure. This flap is not recommended in patients who have undergone abdominal, intrapelvic, or inguinal hernia surgery, as well as those who have required vascular surgery of the iliac system. Further, the donor site is at risk for ventral hernias or abdominal bulges when not closed properly.

The latissimus dorsi is a thin, flat, broad muscle that will occasionally provide coverage for large cheek defects, but more commonly is used during orbitomaxillary reconstruction for replacement of tissue bulk. The blood supply is provided by the thoracodorsal neurovascular bundle. Donor-site morbidity leading to shoulder dysfunction is the primary disadvantage, but this is usually tolerated fairly well.

Reconstruction of full-thickness cheek defects is not considered completely successful unless oral sphincteric and vermilion sensory functions are reestablished, improving food handling, verbalization, and preventing drooling. It is vital to reestablish orbicularis oris muscle ring continuity to maintain sphincter function by suturing vermilion advancement flaps to the folded aspect of the free flaps, forming a neocommissure.[36] Alternatively, local flaps such as the Estlander flap may be employed to sustain oral muscle competence. This maintains both motor and sensory functions, which are vital for normal oral function. In addition, a split masseter muscle transposition may be performed to reestablish oral sphincter continuity.[37] Caution must be taken when manipulating the masseter muscle because the marginal mandibular branch of the facial nerve lies within close proximity and may be injured.

◆ Facial Nerve Reconstruction

The goal of facial nerve reconstruction is symmetrical, coordinated, and synchronous voluntary and involuntary motion from a normal resting appearance with competent sphincters. However, this goal is not in the realm of our current capabilities. Primary repair or interposition nerve grafts are the best reconstructive options available when ablative surgery interrupts facial nerve continuity.[28] If this is not possible, the best alternative is staged cross-facial nerve reconstruction or hypoglossal-facial nerve transfer.[29] Finally, an innervated and vascularized free-muscle flap can be used to reconstruct facial dynamics if the distal segment of the facial nerve cannot be used.[28]

Direct repair in a clean bed within the first 72 hours after resection offers the best chance for recovery of function.[38] The surgery becomes more challenging with delay, because the distal end of the facial nerve cannot be identified by nerve stimulation after 72 hours.[38] If the patient presents more than 1 year after nerve disruption, the outcome of direct nerve repair is generally poor secondary to severe atrophy of the deinnervated motor muscle end plates.[39]

More proximal resections result in lower numbers of regenerated axons that successfully reach their target receptors, adversely affecting distal motor function.[40] Sade et al observed that regenerating axons tend to deviate from their original spatial orientation when seeking out distal targets.[40] This lessens the possibility for correct localization of the various muscle groups and increases the chances for synkinesis.[41–43]

Interposition nerve grafts are indicated when proximal and distal facial nerve stumps are accessible for dissection and the length of segmental nerve loss precludes a tension-free direct repair. The ideal time of nerve grafting is generally within 30 days of the resection.[39] As with primary repair, patients who present 1 year or longer after nerve disruption generally have poor outcomes secondary to target muscle atrophy.[39]

Minimizing the defect and subsequent nerve graft length while performing a tension-free neurorrhaphy are the most important factors in determining a successful outcome.[40] Overall, 95% of patients should have some return of function; 5% of these patients will have poor function; and 15% will achieve fair results.[44] The remainder usually have good results with resting symmetry, voluntary mouth movement, and complete eyelid closure.[44] Unfortunately, only 15 to 20% of patients regain forehead or lower lip motion.[44] The central face reinnervates first, with increased resting tone usually being the first sign.[44] Return of motion should begin 6 months postoperatively with improvement noted progressively for up to 2 years.[38]

The most common transfer in facial nerve reconstruction is the hypoglossal-facial nerve transfer. The entire hypoglossal nerve distal to the descending branch takeoff and below the digastric muscle is utilized. This nerve may also act as a "baby-sitter" to supply muscle tone and prevent atrophy in paralyzed facial muscles until the regenerating axons in cross-facial nerve grafts reach the motor end plates.[34] This technique takes advantage of reinnervating facial muscles with the same cortical representation. However, the current reported outcomes of cross-facial grafting are poor due to de-innervation atrophy of the target muscles, which is a direct result of the time required for regenerating axons to traverse the lengthy nerve grafts and reach the paralyzed side.[44] The indications for nerve transfers include the absence of a proximal facial nerve stump but an intact distal nerve. Target facial muscles must be functional, and conventional nerve grafting techniques cannot be utilized.

◆ Conclusion

The cheek plays a vital role in oral function and facial appearance that is difficult to reproduce following oral cancer resection. Loss of mucus-secreting buccal mucosa, intact mucosal sensation, buccinator contraction, and normal cheek contours and facial expression cannot be completely restored using the reconstructive options that are currently available. Further advances in free flap technique, tissue engineering, and reinnervation will be needed to achieve reconstructive results that approach the premorbid state. Until then, a defect-specific approach to reconstruction that addresses the most significant functional and cosmetic sequelae of resection should be used to provide patients with aesthetically and functionally acceptable results.

References

1. Schusterman MA, Horndeski G. Analysis of the morbidity associated with immediate microvascular reconstruction in head and neck cancer patients. Head Neck 1991;13:51–55
2. Breitbart W, Holland J. Psychological aspects of head and neck cancer. Semin Oncol 1988;15:61–69
3. Tezel E. Buccal mucosal flaps: a review. Plast Reconstr Surg 2002; 109:735–741
4. Demirkan F, Wei FC, Chen HC, et al. Microsurgical reconstruction in recurrent oral cancer: use of a second free flap in the same patient. Plast Reconstr Surg 1999;103:829–838

5. Santamaria E, Wei FC, Chen CH, et al. Sensation recovery on innervated radial forearm flap for hemiglossectomy reconstruction by using different recipient nerves. Plast Reconstr Surg 1999;103:450–457

6. Zhao Y, Zhang W, Zhao J. Reconstruction of intraoral defects after cancer surgery using cervical pedicle flaps. J Oral Maxillofac Surg 2001;59:1142–1146

7. Lauer G, Schimming R, Frankenschmidt A. Intraoral wound closure with tissue-engineered mucosa: new perspectives for urethra reconstruction with buccal mucosa grafts. Plast Reconstr Surg 2001; 107:25–33

8. Vyas P, Roth D, Perlmutter A. Experience with free grafts in urethral reconstruction. J Urol 1987;137:471–474

9. Lutz B, Wei F. Microsurgical reconstruction of the buccal mucosa. Clin Plast Surg 2001;28:339–347

10. Lutz B, Machens H, Ingianni G. Donor site morbidity after rectus abdominis muscle flaps. Eur J Plast Surg 1997;20:173–180

11. Matloub HS, Larson DL, Kuhn JC, et al. Lateral arm free flap in oral cavity reconstruction: a functional evaluation. Head Neck 1989;11: 205–211

12. Franklin J, Withers E, Madden J, et al. Use of the free dorsalis pedis flap in oral cavity reconstruction: a preliminary report. Plast Reconstr Surg 1979;63:195–204

13. Serafin D. Anterolateral thigh flap. In: Serafin D, ed. Atlas of Microsurgical Composite Tissue Transplantation. Philadelphia: WB Saunders, 1996:421

14. Koshima I, Fukuda H, Utunomiya R, et al. The anterolateral thigh flap; variations in vascular pedicle. Br J Plast Surg 1989;42:260–262

15. Hwang S, Shun Y, Meng C. Primary culture of human gingival tissue cells in vitro. Zhonghua Ya Yi Xue Hui Za Zhi. 1991;10:88–97

16. Panje W, Little A, Moran W, et al. Immediate free gastro-omental flap reconstruction of the mouth and throat. Ann Otol Rhinol Laryngol 1987;96:15–21

17. Sasaki T, Baker H, McConnel D, et al. Free jejunal mucosal patch graft reconstruction of the oropharynx. Arch Surg 1982;117:459–462

18. Tideman H, Bosanquet A, Scott J. Use of the buccal fat pad as a pedicled graft. J Oral Maxillofac Surg 1986;44:435–440

19. Vuillemin T, Raveh J, Ramon Y. Reconstruction of the maxilla with bone grafts supported by the buccal fat pad. J Oral Maxillofac Surg 1988;46:100–106

20. Ho KH. Closure of palatal defects with unlimited buccal fat pad graft. Oral Surg 1988;65:523

21. Ho KH. Excision of cheek leukoplakia and lining the defect with a pedicle buccal fat pad graft. Br Dent J 1989;166:455–456

22. Rapidis A, Alexandridis C, Eleftheriadis E, Angelopoulos A. The use of the buccal pat pad for reconstruction of oral defects: review of the literature and report of 15 cases. J Oral Maxillofac Surg 2000; 58:158–163

23. Close L, Truelson J, Milledge R, Schweitzer C. Sensory recovery in non-innervated flaps used for oral cavity and oropharyngeal reconstruction. Arch Otolaryngol Head Neck Surg 1995;121:967–972

24. McCraw JB, Magee WP, Kalwaic H. Uses of the trapezius and sternocleidomastoid myocutaneous flaps in head and neck reconstruction. Plast Reconstr Surg 1979;63:49–57

25. Papadopoulos O, Tsakoniatis N, Georgiou P, Christopoulos A. Head and neck soft-tissue reconstruction using the vertical trapezius musculocutaneous flap. Ann Plast Surg 1999;42: 457–458

26. Coleman JJ. Midface reconstruction. In: Coleman JJ, ed. Plastic Surgery, vol 3. St. Louis: Mosby, 2000:1409–1424

27. Mathes SJ, Vasconez LO. The cervicohumeral flap. Plast Reconstr Surg 1978;61:7–12

28. Kroll S, Goepfert H, Jones M, et al. Analysis of complications in 168 pectoralis major myocutaneous flaps used for head and neck reconstruction. Ann Plast Surg 1990;25:93–97

29. Shindo M, Sullivan M. Muscular and myocutaneous pedicled flaps. Otolaryngol Clin North Am 1994;27:161–172

30. Rees TD, Liverett DM, Guy CL. The effect of cigarette smoking on skin-flap survival in the face lift patient. Plast Reconstr Surg 1984;73:911–915

31. Webster RC, Dazda G, Hamdan US, Fuleihan NS, Smith RC. Cigarette smoking and face lift: conservative versus wide undermining. Plast Reconstr Surg 1986;77:596–604

32. Goldminz D, Bennett RG. Cigarette smoking and flap and full thickness graft necrosis. Arch Dermatol 1991;127:1012–1015

33. Graham B, Dellon AL. Sensory recovery in innervated free tissue transfers. J Reconstr Microsurg 1995;11:157–166

34. Vriens JP, Acosta R, Soutar DS, Webster MH. Recovery of sensation in the radial forearm free flap in oral reconstruction. Plast Reconstr Surg 1996;98:649–656

35. Yokoo S, Tahara S, Tsuji Y, et al. Functional and aesthetic reconstruction of full-thickness cheek, oral commissure and vermilion. J Craniomaxillofac Surg 2001;29:344–350

36. Demir Y, Latifoglu O, Yavuzer R, Atabay K. Oral commissure reconstruction with split masseter muscle transposition and cheek skin flap. J Craniomaxillofac Surg 2001;29:351–354

37. Aviv J, Urken M. Management of the paralyzed face with microneurovascular free muscle transfer. Arch Otolaryngol Head Neck Surg 1992;118:909–912

38. May M. Facial reanimation and skull base trauma. Am J Otol 1985;suppl:62–67

39. Lee KL, Terzis JK. Management of acute extratemporal facial nerve palsy. In: Terzis JK, ed. Microreconstruction of Nerve Injuries. Philadelphia: WB Saunders, 1987:592

40. Sade J. Facial nerve reconstruction and its prognosis. Ann Otol Rhinol Laryngol 1975;84:695–703

41. Orgel MG, Terzis JK. Epineurial vs. perineurial repair: an ultrastructural and electrophysiological study of nerve regeneration. Plast Reconstr Surg 1977;60:80–91

42. Kline DG, Hudson AR, Bratton BR. Experimental study of fascicular nerve repair with and without epineurial closure. J Neurosurg 1981; 54:513–520

43. Conley J. Perspectives in facial reanimation. In: May M, ed. The Facial Nerve. New York: Thieme, 1986

44. Terzis JK, Schnarrs R. Facial nerve reconstruction in salivary gland pathology: a review. Microsurgery 1993;14:355–367

17

Reconstruction of the Tongue

Jeffrey S. Moyer,
Douglas B. Chepeha, and
Theodoros N. Teknos

Reconstruction of the oral cavity following cancer resection should maximize an individual's ability to chew, swallow, and speak. This reconstruction, however, can be an exceedingly difficult task due to the complexity of the oral cavity, which consists of numerous functional elements that work in concert. Although this chapter focuses on mobile tongue reconstruction, it is critical for reconstructive surgeons to remain cognizant of functional deficits resulting from surgical resection of other contiguous sites within the oral cavity that can adversely impact the functional outcome of their reconstructive efforts.

◆ Anatomic and Functional Considerations in Tongue Reconstruction

The oral and pharyngeal portions of the tongue are dynamic structures whose function is pivotal in achieving optimal deglutition and articulation. The tongue is suspended in the oral cavity by attachments to the hyoid bone, mandible, pharynx, styloid process, and the soft palate. Surgical defects after glossectomy rarely affect one isolated region of the tongue, but frequently involve portions of the floor of mouth, base of tongue, as well as the tonsil and palate. Although the pharyngeal tongue is technically part of the oropharynx, it is difficult to discuss the anatomy and physiology of the oral tongue without addressing the critical role the base of tongue has in the function of this region.

Restoring tongue function after tumor extirpation is a difficult task given the varied functions of individual tongue muscles. The tongue is composed of both extrinsic and intrinsic muscles (**Fig. 17–1**). All are innervated by the hypoglossal nerve, except for the palatoglossus muscle, which is innervated by the vagus nerve. The four paired extrinsic muscles of the tongue each have defined tongue motions. The genioglossus muscle originates from both the genial tubercle and internal mandible. It inserts on the anterior tongue and hyoid bone, thereby allowing tongue protrusion and, when acting together, a side-to-side concavity resulting in cupping of the food bolus. The hyoglossus muscle is a thin, quadrilaterally shaped muscle originating from the upper hyoid. It inserts onto the styloglossus and intrinsic tongue muscles and acts to depress the tongue. Alternatively, the styloglossus muscle extends from the styloid process to intertwine with the hyoglossus muscle. It is responsible for retraction of the tongue upward and backward. The palatoglossus muscle acts to lower the soft palate and elevate the tongue. In contrast to the extrinsic muscles of the tongue, the intrinsic muscles are a complex of indiscrete, interlacing fibers that consist of superior and inferior longitudinal muscles fibers that shorten the tongue during deglutition. The transverse muscle fibers narrow and elongate the tongue, whereas vertical muscle fibers flatten and broaden the tongue.

In addition to the complex interaction of extrinsic and intrinsic tongue musculature, tongue sensation allows for appropriate food bolus positioning within the oral cavity and is necessary for efficient and effective articulation. The sensory supply (touch, pain, and temperature) to the anterior two thirds of the tongue is predominantly from the lingual nerve (trigeminal nerve), and the tactile sensitivity in this region is equivalent to the fingertips. The posterior one third of the tongue is supplied by the glossopharyngeal nerve with small portions of the base of tongue being innervated by the superior laryngeal nerve,

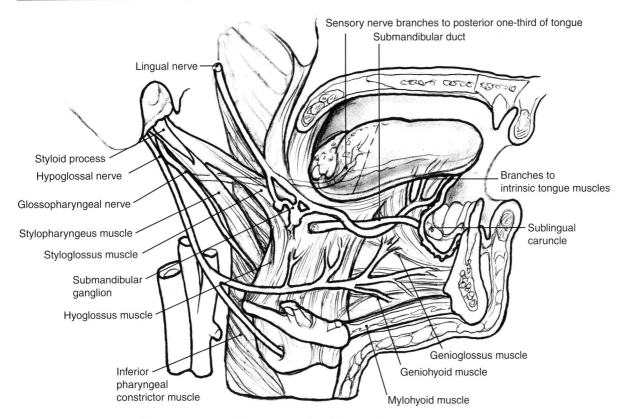

Figure 17–1   Intrinsic and extrinsic muscles of the tongue and their innervation.

a branch of the vagus nerve. The arterial supply to the tongue is from the lingual artery, which is the second branch off the external carotid system and divides into the sublingual and deep lingual arteries at the anterior edge of the hyoglossus muscle (**Fig. 17–2**). Injury to both lingual arteries during tumor extirpation frequently results in necrosis of the remaining tongue and is often an indication for total glossectomy.

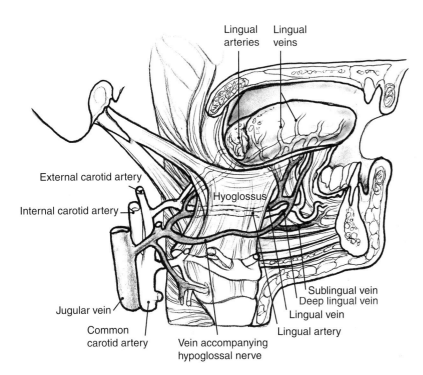

Figure 17–2   Vascular supply of the tongue and floor of mouth.

The extensive interplay between muscle function and sensory input of the oral and pharyngeal tongue makes swallowing an extraordinarily complex event that involves both voluntary and reflex components. The initial act of swallowing is primarily the movement of the tongue against the hard palate with the subsequent movement of the food bolus to the base of tongue. The coordinated function of other oral cavity structures (lips, dentate surfaces, the buccal region) and oropharyngeal structures (soft palate and base of tongue) is also vitally important in this process. When either sensation or muscular motion is absent, localization and manipulation of the food bolus are often inadequate. This can result in significant impairment of the oral preparatory phase as well as the oral phase of swallowing, with increased oral transit times for both solids and liquids. The tongue base is a crucial component of this process, and it is the piston-like motion of the base of tongue that propels food through the oropharynx into the pharyngoesophageal segment. The loss of volume, sensation, and movement in the tongue base not only impairs bolus movement but also contributes to the penetration of material through the laryngeal aditus.

The tongue also plays a central role in articulation by modifying the shape of the oral cavity, causing a change in fundamental resonance characteristics. The complex arrangements of muscles and the high degree of innervation of the tongue facilitate the production of various vowel and consonant sounds that are important for intelligible speech.

◆ Principles and Goals of Tongue Reconstruction

It is a daunting challenge to successfully reconstruct all the functional components of the tongue after partial or total glossectomy. The preservation of functional tongue and adjacent neurovascular structures without compromising oncologic principles is critical to achieving the best reconstructive outcomes. Although any remaining functional tongue can enhance reconstructive results, every effort should be made to preserve the tip of the tongue because of its pivotal role in articulation and swallowing. With this in mind, the primary goal of tongue reconstruction after tumor ablation is to prevent contraction of the remaining tongue and to adequately fill volume deficits created by the excision.

To properly reconstruct the oral tongue, the surgeon must understand how it participates in speech and swallowing. With regard to speech, the tongue is the most important organ of articulation in the oral cavity. Through its appropriate volume and mobility, it allows an individual to form consonants, vowels, and diphthongs, which are the three components of any spoken language. Consonants are produced when the tongue, lip, or palate obstructs to a varying degree the breath stream. On the other hand, vowels are produced by modifying the size and shape of the oral cavity without fully obstructing the breath stream. Finally, diphthongs are made by gliding two vowels together. Therefore, for the purposes of speech production, the tongue should consist of adequate bulk to allow for alteration of the volume of the oral cavity and thus the formation of vowels. In addition, the tongue should be sufficiently

mobile such that the teeth and premaxilla can be reached to adequately obstruct airflow and allow for consonant production. If both of these requirements are met, a patient is able to maintain reasonable articulating ability. This ability may be somewhat improved with a sensate reconstruction as a result of the increased proprioceptive feedback that the tongue provides during speech.

Swallowing, on the other hand, is an equally complex function that is critically dependent on the oral tongue. The oral phase of swallowing consists of oral selection, preparation, control, and delivery to the oropharynx. Based on suitable texture, temperature, and taste (all decided on by a well-innervated tongue), a bolus is allowed to enter the oral cavity to be processed by mastication and lubrication. During this phase, it is imperative that the tongue maintain adequate volume and mobility to completely obliterate the arch under the hard palate and manipulate the bolus for adequate mastication. Subsequently, during the late oral phase of swallowing when the food bolus is delivered to the oropharynx, the dorsal oral tongue protrudes toward the premaxilla, propelling food posteriorly while the base of tongue assumes a vertical position, allowing a passage for food into the oropharynx. If there is inadequate volume in any portion of the tongue, or if the oral tongue is unable to make contact with the hard palate, the bolus may reflux or pool in this dead space. Furthermore, large insensate areas on the tongue may lead to loss of food bolus sensation and the potential for impaired swallowing coordination. Therefore, taken together, the main principles in reconstructing tongue defects of any size are as follows, in order of importance:

1. Maximize function of residual tongue.
2. Maintain adequate volume of the reconstructed oral tongue.
3. Maximize the mobility of the residual tongue.
4. Attempt to retain or restore tactile and motor sensation.

◆ Defect-Specific Reconstruction of the Tongue

One Third or Less Tongue Defect

Defects that consist of less than one third of the tongue (T1 and early T2) can generally be closed primarily. There are a wide variety of anatomic variants of the tongue and surrounding oral cavity structures that facilitate primary closure. However, a particular defect in one patient may be suitable for primary closure, whereas the same-sized defect in another patient with a smaller tongue or limited supporting structures may require free tissue transfer. The surgeon must apply the principles and goals of tongue reconstruction and decide whether these can be met with a simpler reconstruction. Specifically, when deciding which reconstructive modality to utilize, consideration must be given to whether primary closure with recruitment of surrounding normal tongue tissue will affect residual tongue function.

In general, lesions of the lateral tongue should be wedge-excised in a transverse rather than horizontal fashion to improve the ease of primary repair. Defects that cannot be closed in their entirety may be allowed to heal by secondary intention as long as significant contraction will not impact residual function. If the defect extends to the floor of mouth, the use of a split-thickness skin graft or free tissue transfer (radial forearm fasciocutaneous flap) may be necessary to prevent tethering of the tongue to the alveolar sulcus. If a split-thickness skin graft is used instead of free tissue transfer, it is important to use excess skin to compensate for the contraction that will inevitably occur with healing. In addition, the skin graft should have a bolster that is firmly secured with sutures to facilitate healing as well as prevent the aspiration of the bolster. A tracheostomy is frequently recommended in these situations to maintain a secure airway.

Hemiglossectomy Defect

Our general approach for hemiglossectomy reconstruction is to perform an anatomic reconstruction, which re-creates the resected portion of the tongue while maximizing the function of the remaining tongue. To achieve this, we preferentially use free tissue transfer over local or regional tissue mobilization. Our goals for hemiglossectomy reconstruction are as follows:

1. Obliteration of the oral cavity: This is achieved when all oral cavity mucosal surfaces are in contact with one another when the mouth is closed. This goal is important as it should decrease the likelihood of food getting lost in a "dead space" in the oral cavity and improve the handling of secretions by bringing the revascularized free tissue transfer in contact with native mucosa.
2. Maintain premaxillary contact: This is an extension of the goal of obliteration of the oral cavity. Premaxillary contact is particularly important with respect to speech generation of alveolar (n, t, d, ch, j, f, z, 1) sounds. The surgeon needs to ensure that when obliterating the volume of the oral cavity, some of the volume is concentrated anteriorly.
3. Maintain the "finger-like" function of the tongue: Finger-like function is the ability of the tongue to sweep and clear the buccal, labial, and alveolar sulci.
4. Protrusion of the tongue past the plane of the incisors: Protrusion of the tongue is an easier goal to achieve than the maintenance of finger-like function of the tongue in patients with hemiglossectomy defects. Protrusion of the tongue past the plane of the incisors maintains lip contact, which facilitates drinking, handling of secretions, and the production of lingual dental (th) and labial dental (f, v) sounds.
5. Maintain movement of secretions from the anterior to the posterior aspect of the oral cavity.
6. Optimize sensation of the remaining native tissue and the revascularized free tissue transfer.

To achieve these goals in hemiglossectomy reconstruction, we are guided by the following principles:

1. Careful flap selection to restore the volume of the defect. Over-reconstruction of the defect volume is important as

volume is slowly lost over years, particularly in patients who have undergone radiation treatment.
2. Thin tissue should be used to reconstruct thin tissue, and thick tissue should be used to reconstruct thick tissue. Floor-of-mouth tissue should be reconstructed with thin tissue, and tongue tissue should be reconstructed with thicker tissue. This difference of tissue thickness can be achieved by carefully choosing the position of the flap on the donor site or by customizing the flap. The flap can be customized by either thinning the subcutaneous tissue in selected areas or by increasing bulk by folding over de-epithelialized subcutaneous tissue in other selected areas.
3. The volume associated with a mandibular defect or the muscles of the floor of the mouth should be specifically addressed. The volume of these tissues, if resected, must be restored to prevent the tongue reconstruction from contracting inferiorly, which will compromise the goal of obliteration of the oral cavity.
4. The flap design and inset must allow anterior and posterior excursion of the tongue. This facilitates the protrusion of the tongue and its finger-like function.
5. There needs to be a smooth gutter from the anterior floor of mouth to the posterior floor of mouth to facilitate the clearing of secretions. The reconstruction should not block the glossoalveolar, buccal-alveolar, or blunt the labioalveolar sulci.
6. The neural axis of the flap would be oriented in a posterior to anterior axis to facilitate reinnervation of the flap.

Reconstruction is facilitated by performing a safe, 1.5- to 2-cm margin extirpation that runs parallel to the genioglossus, conserves floor-of-mouth mucosa, and respects motor and sensory innervation of the remaining tongue. The volume of the defect is estimated by evaluating three separate areas: the oral tongue defect, the musculature of the tongue deep to the axial plane of the floor of the mouth, and the body of the mandible. Patients differ with respect to tongue size, mandibular height, and dental status, and these varying dimensions all impact the volume required for effective reconstruction.

The *rectangle tongue reconstruction* is our current approach for a hemiglossectomy defect that extends from the tip of the tongue to the glossotonsillar sulcus and includes the oral tongue with or without the base of tongue (BOT). There are, however, other reconstructive approaches for hemiglossectomy defects such as the bilobed-designed flap[1] or the fold and/or roll technique,[2] and the reader should refer to these articles for the specifics of these reconstructive approaches.

In general, three types of vascularized free tissue transfer are used for the reconstruction of hemiglossectomy defects: the radial forearm, which is our flap of choice; the lateral arm, which is the flap of second choice; and the lateral thigh flap. All of these flaps have the advantage of an axial pattern nerve supply to facilitate reinnervation. In a patient with a very low body mass index, a perforator-based rectus flap is a viable option.

Prior to free tissue harvest, the desired flap is sized intraorally by measuring the edges of the defect and a template is generated. The length of the template is determined by

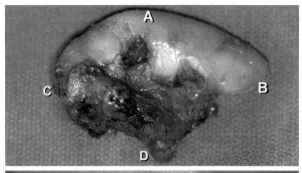

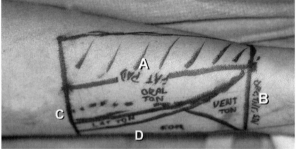

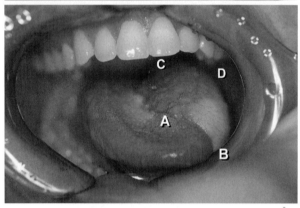

Figure 17–3 Hemiglossectomy defect reconstruction. **(Top)** Representative ex vivo hemiglossectomy specimen. **(Middle)** Rectangle tongue template drawn on the left forearm demonstrating the location of the fad pad (*hashed area*) over the brachioradialis and orientation for a right hemiglossectomy defect. **(Bottom)** One-year result of a left hemiglossectomy defect reconstructed with a radial forearm free tissue transfer using a rectangle tongue template.

measuring from the most dorsal and medial aspect of the defect to the tip of the tongue while the tongue is gently placed on tension in the plane of the midline raphe. This forms the long, medial edge of the rectangle and is usually approximately 8 cm and is side A in **Fig. 17–3**. Next, the width of the rectangle is assessed by measuring from the tongue tip to the most anterior midline portion of the defect when the tongue is gently placed on tension in a superior direction. This forms the shorter, anterior edge of the rectangle (ventral tongue), which is usually approximately 5 cm, and is side B in **Fig. 17–3**. Next, the width is verified on the rectangle by measuring from the most posterior medial aspect of the defect, over the BOT, through the glosso-tonsillar sulcus (GTS) onto the lateral-posterior aspect of the defect. The measurement is side C in **Fig. 17–3** and should be

the same width as side B of the rectangle. Finally, the length of the rectangle is verified by measuring from the most posterior-lateral aspect of the defect, forward along the curvature of the mandible to the anterior midline portion of the defect. This measurement is side D in **Fig. 17–3** and should be the same length as side A of the rectangle.

The template of the rectangle is placed on the donor site and outlined (**Fig. 17–4**). In the forearm donor site, there is a fat pad overlying the brachioradialis with adjacent, thinner skin overlying the flexor carpi radialis and palmaris longus tendons. The line of division between these two different tissue sites can be used as the edge of the lateral tongue reconstruction, with the thinner skin used for floor-of-mouth reconstruction. If more bulk is required for the tongue, additional subcutaneous tissue is harvested adjacent to side A and folded over to bulk up the lateral oral tongue. If additional volume is required for a large volume loss deep to the axial plane of the floor of the mouth or in the area of the body of the mandible, additional subcutaneous tissue can be harvested over the brachioradialis and pedicled off side C. This tissue can be sutured into the defect after microvascular anastomosis to maintain the height of the tongue reconstruction and facilitate oral cavity obliteration.

Depending on the defect created by the resection, there may be two additional subunits that need to be added to the template to achieve an anatomic reconstruction (**Fig. 17–4**). The first is an approximate 2 × 1–cm tab located at the corner between C and D, which is oriented at a 45-degree angle and is used to resurface the retromolar trigone or the anterior tonsillar pillar. The second is an approximate 2 × 1–cm tab that extends parallel to the D side by 2 cm to resurface the anterior floor of mouth.

The inset of the flap is performed in a sequential fashion similar to the method that was used to measure the template. The posterior aspect of the flap is tacked in first. This was on side C at the line of tension to the most inferior portion of the GTS. Next, the corner between side A and side C is tacked to the dorsum of the tongue at the most posterior-superior aspect of the defect. The tongue is kept on gentle tension along the midline raphe. Next, the anterior corner between side A and side B is tacked at the tip. At this point a determination is made as to whether the flap is draping properly into the tongue portion of the defect and adjustments are made. Then, two or three more tacking sutures are placed along the dorsum of the tongue. Next, the line of tension is created from the GTS to the junction between the ventral tongue and anterior floor of mouth along side B. The line of tension is considered appropriate when the tongue portion of the reconstruction is pushed up into the oral cavity and the dorsum of the tongue is aligned in an axial plane. This step should "flip up" the remaining flap tissue that is to be used for reconstruction of the anterior and posterior floor of mouth along side D. This creates a natural-appearing glossomandibular sulcus along the inner table of the mandible. The closure is then completed along side C, side A, side B, and finally side D. Frequently, the anterior and posterior corners along side A need a small amount of trimming to finesse the final result.

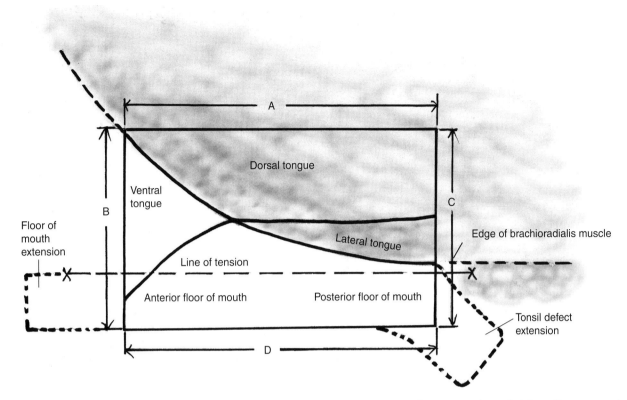

Figure 17–4 Rectangle tongue template placed on the forearm donor site to provide increased bulk to the dorsal and lateral tongue with the inclusion of the forearm fat pad (*shaded area*). The extensions for associated tonsil defects (between angle C and D) and floor of mouth defects (parallel to side D) are also illustrated.

Subtotal or Total Oral Glossectomy Defects

Subtotal or total oral glossectomy defects markedly alter oral function in a variety of ways. First and foremost, resection of the tongue's intrinsic and extrinsic musculature eliminates the "finger-like" mobility of the tongue, altering intraoral food manipulation and severely impairing speech articulation. Furthermore, the inevitable loss of the mylohyoid sling removes the support of the floor of mouth and prevents the elevation of the tongue to the palate.

Although the goals of hemiglossectomy reconstruction focus on the restoration of both the finger-like function and volume of the resected tongue, the primary goal of total glossectomy reconstruction is to restore lost volume. Thus, the reconstruction of subtotal or total oral glossectomy defects must accomplish the following four objectives:

1. Restore the volume of the oral tongue, floor of mouth, and mylohyoid sling.
2. Restore mucosal surfaces of the resected tongue and surrounding structures to preserve the mobility of the residual tongue.
3. Restore and maintain coordinated activity of the tongue to allow tongue elevation to the palate.
4. Restore sensation.

Early attempts at the reconstruction of total glossectomy defects consisted mainly of "plugging-the-hole" approaches that were created by using skin grafts or local flaps. These efforts invariably led to poor functional results due to the lack of volume, increased oral dead space, and pooling of secretions in the oral cavity.

With the advent of pedicled myocutaneous flaps, functional results improved significantly. The bulk provided by myocutaneous flaps allowed surgeons to provide patients with a neo-tongue that had sufficient volume to reach the palate and obliterate dead space, dramatically improving speech and swallowing function. The disadvantages of myocutaneous flaps, however, include the unpredictability of long-term volume restoration as well as the downward-directed scar contracture resulting from muscle atrophy and gravity. Both of these events interfere with the flap-to-palate contact that is necessary for speech and swallowing.

The use of microvascular free tissue transfer ushered in a new era for total glossectomy reconstruction. These versatile flaps provided adequate bulk and the ability to be contoured to complex three-dimensional defects, as well as the potential for sensation. Furthermore, unlike myocutaneous flaps, free flap volume has long-term predictability and is not susceptible to the inferiorly directed contracture seen with the muscle atrophy of pedicled flaps. The exact type of flap used is not nearly as important as choosing a flap that will provide the necessary bulk required for a specific defect. In subtotal or total oral glossectomy defects, we prefer using a rectus abdominus free tissue transfer for reconstruction. The rectus abdominus flap achieves the stated goals of reconstruction, and has the added advantage of providing rectus fascia, which can be transversely fixed to the mandible.

A

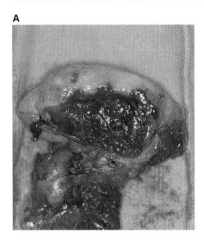

B

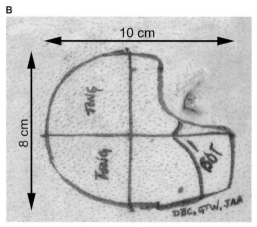

C

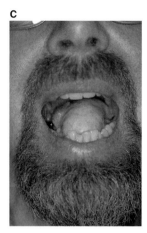

Figure 17–5 Total and subtotal glossectomy reconstruction. **(A)** Representative ex vivo subtotal glossectomy specimen. **(B)** D-shaped template drawn on the abdomen in preparation for a rectus abdominis myocutaneous flap. **(C)** Two-year result of a subtotal glossectomy defect reconstructed with a rectus abdominis myocutaneous flap.

This acts as a neo-mylohyoid sling that supports the reconstruction inferiorly, preventing downward contracture of the reconstruction.

Another important technique to utilize in conjunction with free tissue transfer is a permanent laryngeal suspension suture. The suture not only elevates the larynx under the tongue base but also enlarges the hypopharyngeal inlet. In addition, it also helps support the reconstruction by preventing inferior displacement into the neck, thus complementing the neo-mylohyoid sling of the rectus fascia.

Techniques of Reconstruction for Total Oral Glossectomy Defects

1. The surgeon should adequately assess the volume necessary for restoration and choose the appropriate flap. Most total oral glossectomy patients do well with a rectus abdominus free flap. For subtotal glossectomy patients, the surgeon should also consider the use of an anterolateral thigh or lateral arm free tissue transfer depending on volume requirements.
2. Harvest the flap in a large enough linear dimension to reach from the base of tongue to the anterior velum via a curvilinear path along the soft and hard palate. For total oral glossectomy defects, this is often a D-shaped flap with an 8-cm width and a 10-cm length (**Fig. 17–5**).
3. With methylene blue, tattoo the reference points equidistant along the sides of the flap to allow for symmetric insetting into the oral cavity. This should be performed prior to free flap harvest.
4. Prior to beginning the inset, use a wire passing drill bit to create bilateral symmetric, equally spaced drill holes along the mylohyoid line for flap suspension using the rectus fascia. Typically we drill three holes on each side of the mandible.
5. Inset flap from posteriorly to anteriorly using the appropriate absorbable sutures. During this inset follow the methylene blue tattoo marks to ensure that the flap is being sewn in symmetrically.

6. When the intraoral suturing is complete, suspend the rectus fascia (if available) through the holes previously drilled at the mylohyoid line to prevent flap ptosis with heavy nonabsorbable suture. This step can be performed after the microvascular anastomosis if access to vessels is impaired by the suspension.
7. Suspend the larynx by using a pair of permanent sutures from the paramedian hyoid to holes drilled in the parasymphysis of the mandible. This step can also be performed after the microvascular anastomosis if access to vessels is impaired by the suspension (**Fig. 17–6**).
8. Perform the microvascular anastomosis after the completion of the insetting.

◆ Functional Outcomes

Reconstructive outcome studies are plagued by the lack of a standardized metric for grading resections and reconstructive modalities. No two defects are exactly the same, and reconstructive techniques can rarely be exactly duplicated. There have been very few studies in which solid conclusions can be drawn that definitely prove whether one reconstructive modality is superior to another with respect to functional outcomes. There are, however, some unifying themes that emerge from the literature that suggest which techniques are best suited for particular reconstructive situations.

The single most important factor in functional outcomes after oral tongue reconstruction is the preservation of function of the remaining native tongue as well as the surrounding oral cavity structures. Independent of the technique used for tongue reconstruction, the larger the defect created by tumor extirpation, the worse the swallowing and speech outcomes.[3] The reconstructive modality utilized must prevent tethering of the residual tongue as well as provide sufficient bulk to allow the food bolus to be efficiently propelled into the pharynx.

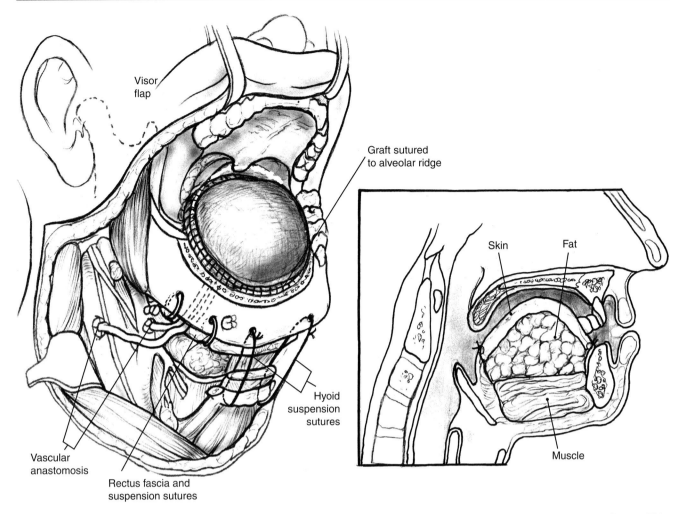

Figure 17–6   Inset of rectus flap with suspension of the rectus fascia to the mandible as well as suspension of the hyoid bone/larynx to the mandible.

Tongue resections that are less than one third the size of the tongue function best when repaired with primary closure. McConnel et al[4] examined patients with small oral tongue defects (<30% of tongue) that were matched for the location of the defect and were reconstructed with primary closure, a pedicled flap, or free tissue transfer. In smaller tongue defects, patients with primary closure had equal to better conversational intelligibility, sentence-articulation, and oropharyngeal swallowing efficiency compared with patients reconstructed with pedicled or free flaps. The adynamic, excess bulk of pedicled or free flaps appeared to adversely impact residual tongue function. A large amount of residual, functioning tongue with normal sensory input that is present in smaller defects may account for the high level of function in this patient population and the lack of significant improvement with more advanced reconstructive modalities.

With larger defects, however, the amount of residual, functioning tongue is much less, and these defects often include surrounding oral cavity and oropharyngeal structures. From a practical point, primary closure is rarely a viable option as there is typically insufficient tissue available to adequately close the larger defects. In addition, the distortion of

surrounding tissue that would be required to close the larger defects would significantly impact what residual tongue function remains.

There is considerable controversy in the literature as to whether free tissue transfer is superior to pedicled flaps for the reconstruction of larger tongue defects when considering speech and swallowing outcomes. Su et al[5] studied the speech and swallowing of 60 patients with carcinoma of the tongue who underwent partial (25%) to total glossectomy with subsequent reconstruction with a radial forearm free tissue transfer or a pectoralis major myocutaneous flap. The authors found higher speech intelligibility scores in patients reconstructed with free flaps when compared with pedicled flaps. Interestingly, the extent of resection was more closely associated with differences in swallowing function than the type of reconstruction (pedicled or free flap).

Haughey et al[2] investigated the use of the radial forearm free tissue transfer for the reconstruction of tongue and floor-of-mouth defects. In this study of 30 oral tongue reconstructions, 86% of patients were able to maintain their nutritional needs by mouth and, on average, 79% of spoken words were understandable to the untrained listener. These results compare favorably to the literature where some studies found oral diet and speech intelligibility rates below 50% for alternative reconstructive techniques.

In a recent study of 12 patients at the University of Michigan with hemiglossectomy defects repaired with a template-based rectangular radial forearm free tissue transfer, all patients taking an oral diet prior to surgery (11/12, 92%) were able to consume a full range of liquids and solids with minimum restrictions after surgery. In addition, most patients (11/12, 92%) had speech that was understandable either most of the time or always.

Supporting the preferential use of free tissue transfer in tongue reconstruction, a large study of patients in which a subset had either a pectoralis major myocutaneous flap ($n = 52$) or free flap ($n = 38$) for oral cavity reconstruction demonstrated that the rates of G-tube dependence and minor complications were greater in the pedicled group compared with the free flap group.[6]

Although some of these differences may be attributable to the inherent differences in healing between free tissue transfer and pedicled flaps (i.e., downward contraction with pedicled flaps), sensation may also play an important role in superior functional outcomes. Recovery of sensation appears to be better in free tissue transfer as compared with pedicled myocutaneous flaps, and this finding correlates with better swallowing and articulation outcomes. Close et al[7] studied 12 patients with either a pedicled flap or free tissue transfer and found only 50% sensory recovery in the pedicled group, whereas 100% of the free tissue transfer group achieved sensory recovery. In addition, some studies of reinnervated free flaps have shown sensation similar to the native tongue.[8]

It is our belief that for hemiglossectomy defects, the more pliable and malleable tissue from free tissue transfer (typically the radial forearm), with its improved sensory capacity (independent of intentional reinnervation), offers a superior result in tongue reconstruction. Similarly for subtotal and total glossectomy defects, the consistent bulk of the rectus free flap offers a greater chance for patients to retain oral function. The reliable bulk, coupled with the ability to support the reconstruction with rectus fascia and a laryngeal suspension, offers a more effective and enduring result.

◆ Conclusion

Even with the significant advances in reconstructive technologies that have been realized over the past 20 years, tongue reconstruction still remains one of the most challenging areas for the reconstructive surgeon. Effective speech and swallowing are highly dependent on the tongue's inherent bulk and "finger-like" function. The goal of all tongue reconstructive approaches should be the repair or replacement of these important functions. The decision of which reconstructive modality to use must be predicated on maximizing tongue function.

Our philosophy has been that smaller defects of the tongue (one third or less) can often be closed primarily, as long as there is not significant distortion of surrounding tissue that affects residual function. For hemiglossectomy defects, we preferentially use the radial forearm free tissue transfer for its ability to replace the bulk after tumor extirpation while preventing tethering, maintaining protrusion, and restoring sensation. For subtotal and total glossectomy defects, we typically use the rectus abdominis free tissue transfer because of its reliable, long-lasting bulk as well as the ability to provide support to the reconstructed tongue.

References

1. Urken ML, Biller HF. A new bilobed design for the sensate radial forearm flap to preserve tongue mobility following significant glossectomy. Arch Otolaryngol Head Neck Surg 1994;120:26–31
2. Haughey BH, Taylor SM, Fuller D. Fasciocutaneous flap reconstruction of the tongue and floor of mouth. Arch Otolaryngol Head Neck Surg 2002;128:1388–1395
3. McConnel FMS, Logemann JA, Rademaker AW, et al. Surgical variables affecting postoperative swallowing efficiency in oral cancer patients: a pilot study. Laryngoscope 1994;104:87–90
4. McConnel FMS, Pauloski BR, Logemann JA, et al. Functional results of primary closure vs flaps in orpharyngeal reconstruction. Arch Otolaryngol Head Neck Surg 1998;124:625–630
5. Su W, Hsia Y, Chang Y, Chen S, Sheng H. Functional comparison after reconstruction with a radial forearm free flap or a pectoralis major flap for cancer of the tongue. Otolaryngol Head Neck Surg 2003;128:412–418
6. Chepeha DB, Annich G, Pynnonen MA, et al. Pectoralis major myocutaneous flap vs revascularized free tissue transfer. Arch Otolaryngol Head Neck Surg 2004;130:181–186
7. Close LG, Truelson JM, Milledge RA, Schweitzer C. Sensory recovery in non-innervated flaps used for oral cavity and oropharyngeal reconstruction. Arch Otolaryngol Head Neck Surg 1995;121:967–972
8. Kuriakose MA, Loree TR, Spies A, Meyers S, Hicks WL. Sensate radial forearm free flaps in tongue reconstruction. Arch Otolaryngol Head Neck Surg 2001;127:1463–1466

18

Reconstruction of the Mandible

Douglas B. Villaret

More than 87% of diagnosed oral cancers arise from mucosal regions that are either in direct contact with, or adjacent to, the mandible.[1,2] As a consequence, the mandible is resected more frequently than any other bone during oral cancer surgery. Defects of the mandible are associated with numerous sequelae, including decreased facial projection, loss of oral competence, and impaired mastication, deglutition, and speech articulation. Fortunately, mandibular reconstruction can reverse the effects of surgical resection by improving facial contours and appearance, masticatory performance, biting force, and tongue and cheek function.[3,4] However, some of the principles that guide the reconstruction of isolated segmental defects resulting from the resection of intramandibular neoplasms such as ameloblastoma or osteosarcoma are not applicable to the reconstruction of more complex "oromandibular" defects created by the resection of malignancies that arise from the oral mucosa and minor salivary glands. Soft tissue losses from the tongue, lips, chin, or cheek that are incurred at the time of surgery may compound or even overshadow the sequelae caused by mandibular resection. This chapter discusses the various options that are available for oromandibular reconstruction by using a defect-based approach, and analyzes the aesthetic and functional outcomes that are achievable with each reconstructive option.

◆ Functional Considerations in Mandible Reconstruction

The contours and projection of the mandible support the soft tissues of the lower face, providing lip support and establishing the facial profile. The mandible also provides support for the tongue and the larynx, and normal mandibular anatomy and function are required for mastication, deglutition, and speech articulation. Thus, mandibular resection can dramatically alter the patient's appearance and functional status, and may have profound consequences for the patient's emotional well-being, health, and quality of life.

Long anterior segmental defects lead to severe retrogenia with lip incompetence and malocclusion, salivary incontinence, speech and swallowing impairment, and possible respiratory compromise from loss of the genial tubercle, which provides a site of anchorage for the musculature of the tongue, floor of mouth, and hyolaryngeal complex.[5] Lateral mandibular defects are associated with less severe deformity and functional morbidity. Because the posterior mandible defines the contour of the posterior lower third of the face, some alteration of appearance is inevitable without reconstruction. Lateral mandibular body defects that spare the symphysis result in a hollowed appearance to the cheek. If the continuity of the mandible is not restored, the mandibular remnants can become displaced by the unopposed contraction of the masticatory muscles that remain attached to the mandible, resulting in mandibular deviation, malocclusion, masticatory dysfunction, and facial asymmetry. Moreover, if a coronoidectomy is not performed at the time of resection, the proximal mandibular segment bearing the condyle will rotate superiorly and medially secondary to unopposed tension of the temporalis muscle.[5] Resection of the condyle results in ipsilateral loss of vertical dimension with a contralateral open bite and gradual mandibular deviation toward the affected side, as well as decrements in bite force and masticatory efficiency.[5] Postsurgical fibrosis can also cause chronic trismus and orofacial pain.

Normal mastication requires manipulation, trituration, and consolidation of the food bolus prior to swallowing. All three components of mastication must be intact for an individual to masticate efficiently. For instance, if the ability to manipulate a food bolus onto the occlusal table is compromised by a loss of tongue volume or sensation, masticatory inefficiency occurs even though the patient can effectively triturate a food bolus.[3] After mandibulectomy, the trituration, or grinding, phase of mastication is frequently affected by the loss of mandibular bone and malocclusion, and biting force is significantly decreased.[3] Sensory and soft tissue deficits may also adversely affect the ability to manipulate a bolus to the occlusal table for trituration and to consolidate the bolus in preparation for deglutition.[3]

◆ Goals of Mandible Reconstruction

The goals of mandibular reconstruction are as follows[5–7]:

1. Restore mandibular continuity.
2. Restore alveolar bone height.
3. Restore osseous bulk.
4. Reconstruct the lower facial contours.
5. Preserve the temporomandibular joint (TMJ) and its relationship within the glenoid fossa.
6. Create a neomandible that is suitable for dental prosthetic rehabilitation.
7. Anatomically and functionally restore adjacent soft tissue defects (i.e., tongue, cheek, lips).

Ultimately, the mandibular reconstruction should be composed of well-vascularized bone of sufficient width that can support a tissue-borne denture or permit the placement of osseointegrated implants.[6] Furthermore, the shape of the re-created mandibular arch should have a natural appearance and provide sufficient lip support and chin projection. Coverage of the newly reconstructed mandible with thin, well-vascularized, moist, sensate, and pliable soft tissue is ideal.[6] Thoughtful reconstruction of defects involving the tongue, lips, and cheek is necessary to reestablish oral competence, and anatomic re-creation of the buccal and lingual sulci improves the stability of dental prostheses and improves manipulation of food material and oral secretions.

◆ Reconstructive Options

Alloplastic Implants

Gap-bridging devices such as mesh cribs may be used to bridge continuity defects of the mandible. This approach employs a fenestrated titanium or polyurethane tray that is contoured to precisely reconstruct the defect and is fixed into position with wires or screws. Particulate bone grafts are then placed into the tray and wrapped in vascularized tissue that allows for revascularization to occur through the fenestrations.[8]

Titanium reconstruction plates are the most frequently used alloplastic material for mandibular reconstruction, and can be employed alone as a gap-bridging device or in combination with a bone graft. The *titanium-coated hollow screw and reconstruction plate* (THORP), introduced in the late 1980s, formed the basis for subsequent innovations in reconstruction plate design.[9] By screwing an expansion bolt into a hollow screw, the screw head becomes rigidly fixed to the THORP plate, avoiding unnecessary pressure on the bone that could cause bone resorption and eventual plate loosening or failure.[9,10] Rigid fixation or locking of the screws to the plate also resulted in higher construct stability and infrequent screw loosening. The locking screw plate systems that are in present use are descendants of the original THORP plate. An additional thread on the head of the screw and in the plate hole allows the screw to be locked into place, obviating the need for an expansion bolt.[10] These locking reconstruction plates (LRPs) are lighter and have a lower profile than the THORP, and an LRP that uses 2-mm screws was recently introduced.[10] Locking reconstruction plates consistently provide excellent stabilization of vascularized bone grafts to the adjacent native mandible.[10,11]

Reconstruction plates have been used to bridge segmental mandibular defects in combination with pedicled musculocutaneous flaps or fasciocutaneous free flaps to reconstruct adjacent soft tissue defects with variable success.[12,13] Most plate failures occur when either anterior or large lateral defects are bridged.[14] Boyd et al[15] from the University of Toronto documented a 21% plate failure rate requiring plate removal following the reconstruction of 40 segmental mandibulectomy defects. Plate failure occurred with only 5% of the lateral defects that were located distal to the canines, whereas 35% of the failures were associated with defects that involved the anterior mandible. Other investigators have reported similarly low rates of plate failure in association with lateral defect reconstruction, whereas failure rates of more than 50% have been documented following anterior reconstruction.[16–18] The likelihood of success also decreases as the length of the defect increases. Arden et al[19] noted a plate complication rate of 81% for segmental defects greater than 5 cm versus only 7% for smaller defects. Thus, the use of an LRP to bridge a mandibulectomy defect should be limited to short lateral defects and patients who have a poor prognosis or cannot tolerate an extended general anesthetic that would allow for osseous mandibular reconstruction.

Most of the failures with bridging reconstruction plates result from soft tissue complications that lead to plate exposure rather than plate loosening or fracture.[13,17] These patients frequently require secondary reconstruction with an osteocutaneous free flap.[13] Boyd et al[15] speculated that failure of anterior alloplastic mandibular reconstructions resulted from (1) progressive ptosis of the lower lip and chin secondary to surgical disruption of the muscles of mastication, scar contracture, and gravity; (2) denervation of the lower lip musculature, increasing the impact of gravity; and (3) superior rotation of the mandibular arch following disruption of the suprahyoid muscular attachments to the anterior mandible, allowing the plate to erode through the soft tissue flap. Blackwell and colleagues[20] suggested that external plate exposure in lateral mandibulectomy defects results from wound contracture with medialization of the overlying cheek skin and eventual pressure necrosis. However, they were able to reduce the incidence of external plate exposure from 30% to only 4% by using a low-profile, rounded-contour LRP.[16,20]

A resected condyle can be replaced with a titanium condylar prosthesis that is stabilized to the distal aspect of the remaining mandible with a reconstruction plate to reestablish the mandibular vertical height and the premorbid occlusion.[21,22] These prostheses, however, have been associated with erosion of the glenoid fossa and migration of the prosthesis into the epitympanum or the middle cranial fossa.[22,23] Alloplastic TMJ prostheses that can be customized and fitted to the patient's unique anatomy are now available (TMJ Concepts, Ventura, CA). These "patient-fitted" condylar prostheses articulate with a polyethylene articular surface that is attached to a glenoid fossa, which is made from titanium mesh and is stabilized to the cranial base with titanium screws. Prosthetic restoration of the glenoid fossa eliminates the risk of condylar migration through the skull base. However, reconstruction with a customized prosthesis at the time of cancer resection is impractical because prosthesis fabrication requires several weeks, and presurgical quantification of the required extent of mandibular resection is usually not possible. This approach, however, could be considered for the definitive reconstruction of a TMJ that was originally reconstructed with a prefabricated titanium condylar prosthesis.

Nonvascularized Bone Grafts

Nonvascularized autogenous bone grafts continue to be a viable option for the reconstruction of nonsegmental defects and some segmental defects of the mandible. A cancellous, cortical, or corticocancellous bone graft may be used, depending on the type and location of the defect. Cancellous bone, which is usually harvested from the posterior ileum, contains marrow and medullary bone matrix, and has the greatest osteoconductive potential. The absence of a cortical component, however, requires the use of a fenestrated tray that provides some structural rigidity. If a resorbable mesh crib was utilized, resorption occurs slowly over the next few years as the cancellous bone consolidates, and a new endosteum and periosteum forms.[24] The cancellous matrix provides a large surface area that allows for rapid revascularization, improving its chances for graft survival.[8] In contrast, osteocyte-containing cortical bone grafts are not as easily revascularized because they are composed of compact lamellar bone and are prone to resorption. Corticocancellous bone grafts, which contain a structurally rigid cortical region and a cancellous region that contains viable osteoblasts, can occasionally be used in lieu of cancellous bone that is supported by a mesh crib.

The success of a nonvascularized bone graft depends on the vascularity of the recipient bed and the quantity of viable osteoblastic cells.[8] Healing occurs through creeping substitution whereby the matrix of the donor graft acts as a framework for new osteoblastic bone deposition. During the first 4 weeks after grafting, osteoblasts form new osteoid, which determines the eventual volume of bone that is formed. Osteogenesis, which involves the transformation of pluripotential stem cells into osteoblastic and osteoclastic cells, occurs for up to 6 months after grafting. This process is mediated by bone morphogenic protein.[8,25]

Nonvascularized bone grafts, however, have several drawbacks that limit their usefulness for mandibular reconstruction following oral cancer resection. Several months are required before these grafts become fully integrated and are able to withstand the forces of mastication. When nonvascularized grafts are used for immediate reconstruction, salivary contamination results in a graft failure rate of at least 50%.[26] The success rate approaches 100% when reconstruction is delayed and an extraoral approach is utilized so that the oral cavity is not entered and salivary contamination does not occur.[27] This approach typically requires a delay of at least 3 months and stabilization with a gap-bridging reconstruction plate during the interim if a continuity defect is present.[28] Such delays may lead to intraoral and extraoral soft tissue contraction, temporarily impair oral function, and exacerbate psychological distress. The success rate of a nonvascularized bone graft is also influenced by the length of the defect that is grafted.[29,30] Investigators from the University of California at San Francisco (UCSF), for example, noted a failure rate of 17% for grafts of 6 cm or less versus 75% for grafts more than 12 cm in length.[29] A pedicled regional flap may also be required to separate the mandibular defect from the oral cavity when a soft tissue deficiency exists. Dental implant placement is not possible at the time of reconstruction, which delays definitive prosthodontic rehabilitation. If a titanium mesh tray has been used for graft stabilization, more than 15% eventually require surgical removal.[31] Finally, placement of the graft into a previously irradiated bed adversely impacts survival, and may require the use of adjunctive hyperbaric oxygen therapy to enhance neovascularization.[32,33]

In the mid-1990s, proponents of cancellous cellular bone grafts were concerned that vascularized bone free flaps such as the fibula would lead to inferior reconstructive outcomes. Carlson and Marx[28] from the University of Miami contended that vascularized bone-containing free flaps are "nonmandibles," which cannot re-create the natural contours of the mandibular arch and lack "the alveolar height and bucco-lingual width critical to denture rehabilitation and normal jaw function." Pogrel and colleagues[29] from UCSF also purported that vascularized bone grafts such as the fibula provide suboptimal mandibular contours and aesthetics, and inadequate bone volume for implant placement. Their skepticism was rationally supported by extensive clinical experience with cancellous bone grafts and limited experience with free tissue transfer. Fortunately, subsequent published research in the otolaryngology and the oral and maxillofacial surgery literature has documented the outcomes with both types of grafts and has clarified their respective niches in mandibular reconstruction. In a subsequent investigation at UCSF that compared vascularized and nonvascularized grafts, for example, successful bony union occurred with 96% and 69% of vascularized and nonvascularized grafts, respectively ($p < .0005$).[34] Furthermore, the mean number of operations that were required to achieve bony union was 1.1 for vascularized grafts versus 2.3 for nonvascularized grafts ($p < .001$). The rate of implant success in this study was 99% in the vascularized group and only 82% in the nonvascularized group ($p < .0001$), with a success rate of 100% in vascularized bone flaps that had previously been irradiated.[34] By the use of serial computed tomography, other investigators have shown that satisfactory mandibular contours can be restored with either type of graft.[35]

In summary, nonvascularized bone can be used to reconstruct mandibular defects that are less than 6 cm in length and have not been irradiated, and in medically compromised patients who cannot tolerate free tissue transfer. Mandibular reconstruction following the resection of benign mandibular pathology may be performed with either vascularized or nonvascularized bone if an extraoral approach is employed and the oral mucosa has not been violated. On the other hand, vascularized bone is usually preferred for immediate reconstruction following resection of malignant disease that results in communication with the oral cavity, in irradiated patients, and in defects greater than 6 cm in length. The success rate and advantages associated with vascularized free tissue transfer have made this surgical modality the treatment of choice for most complex mandibular defects when immediate reconstruction is desired.

Distraction Osteogenesis

Distraction osteogenesis is an established technique that has been used primarily to lengthen long bones and correct certain craniofacial deformities. For instance, a congenitally short tibia may be lengthened by creating an osteotomy through the bone and gradually distracting the bony segments away from each other, resulting in new bone formation. This technique, which results in one focus of bone formation, is known as monofocal distraction osteogenesis. Although monofocal distraction osteogenesis can be used to lengthen a linear bone, this technique is not useful for the correction of segmental skeletal defects. For these circumstances, bifocal or trifocal distraction osteogenesis are more suitable reconstructive options. Bifocal distraction osteogenesis involves the development of a bone transport disk by performing an osteotomy through the bone at one end of a segmental defect. The periosteum and muscular attachments to the bone should be preserved to ensure that the transport disk is richly vascularized. As the bone transport disk is distracted across the segmental defect at a rate of approximately 1 mm/day, a regenerative callus is formed in its wake. Once the bone transport disk "docks" with the native mandible at the other end of the segmental defect, compressive osteosynthesis also occurs. This technique is termed bifocal distraction osteogenesis because there are two sites of bone formation (**Fig. 18–1**).

Trifocal osteogenesis requires the creation of two transport disks from either side of the segmental defect, which are distracted across the defect toward each other. A regenerative callus forms in the wake of each transport disk and a third site of bone formation occurs at the point where the transport disks dock with each other, resulting in compressive osteosynthesis. Once the transport disks have docked, the disks and the adjacent bony segments must be immobilized for consolidation and bony fusion to occur. Trifocal distraction osteogenesis shortens the time required for bone regeneration and also provides a mechanism for curvilinear bone formation.[36,37]

Bifocal and trifocal distraction osteogenesis have been used to reconstruct segmental mandibular defects following tumor resection and traumatic injury. Kuriakose et al[37] reported successful mandibular bone regeneration following bifocal distraction in two segmental mandibular defects, and a 6-cm segmental defect resulting from oral cancer resection has been reconstructed with trifocal distraction in a patient that received preoperative radiation therapy (RT) and chemotherapy.[38] Distraction osteogenesis has also been used to reconstruct curvilinear mandibular regions such as the angle and the symphysis.[39–41] Furthermore, a modified form of monofocal distraction osteogenesis has been employed to increase the vertical height of the partially resected mandible as well as fibular free flap reconstructions so that dental implants can be placed and prosthodontic rehabilitation can be achieved.[42,43]

However, distraction osteogenesis for the reconstruction of segmental mandibular defects will not become widely accepted by the surgical community until several issues are addressed[37]:

1. Curvilinear segments of bone must consistently regenerate.
2. The effect of RT and chemotherapy on distraction osteogenesis and the effect of distraction hardware on RT planning and delivery have to be clarified.
3. The limitations of conventional imaging techniques to monitor bone regeneration must be resolved.
4. The feasibility of distraction under transposed soft tissue flaps must be evaluated.
5. A distraction device that is specifically designed for segmental defects and that addresses the limitations of existing commercial distraction devices should be developed.

Free Tissue Transfer

At most tertiary medical centers, reconstruction with vascularized bone and soft tissue has become the preferred method of restoring segmental mandibular defects. Two large retrospective case series from the Mt. Sinai Medical Center and Memorial Sloan-Kettering Cancer Center, both in New York, NY, report that mandibular continuity with bony union is reestablished in more than 95% of the cases.[7,44] The success rate of dental implant osseointegration with vascularized bone grafts is greater than 90%, and most patients experience a good to excellent aesthetic outcome and are eventually able to consume a soft or regular diet.[7,44,45] In general, the graft survival rate and the aesthetic and functional outcomes that are achieved with vascularized free flap mandibular reconstruction are superior to the results that have been reported for other reconstructive modalities.

The quantity and quality of bone and the amount of skin and soft tissue that must be replaced are the prime considerations that dictate the selection of the donor site (**Table 18–1**).[44] Curvilinear symphyseal defects must be reconstructed with bone that can withstand multiple osteotomies, and the width and height requirements of the bone graft must be anticipated if dental implantation is desired. The unique soft tissue characteristics of each potential donor site must also be considered so that tongue mobility

A

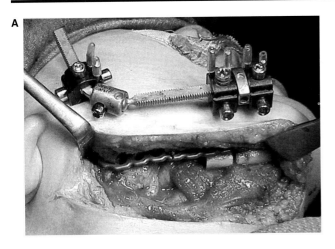

External distraction device

B

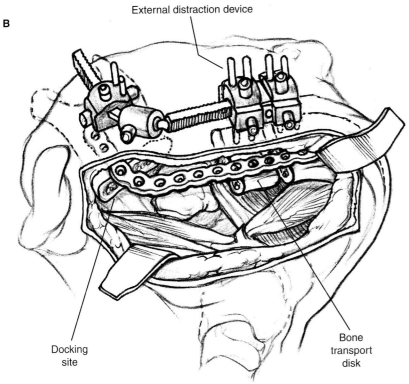

Docking site

Bone transport disk

Figure 18–1 Bifocal distraction osteogenesis. **(A)** There is a segmental defect involving the right mandibular body and angle. An osteotomy has been performed to create a transport disk from the distal end of the defect and an external distraction device has been applied. **(B)** The bone transport disk is distracted away from the osteotomy site toward the docking site at the proximal bone edge. A regenerative callus develops between the transport disk and the distal mandibular segment, and compressive osteosynthesis occurs at the docking site (bifocal osteogenesis).

Table 18–1 Comparison of Various Microvascular Donor Sites with Respect to Quality of Available Bone, Skin, and Vascular Pedicle, and the Ability of the Flap to Accept Osseointegrated Dental Implants

Donor Site	Bone	Skin	Pedicle	Location*	Osseointegration
Fibula	+++	++	++	+++	+++
Iliac crest	+++	+	+	++	+++
Radius	+	+++	+++	++	–
Scapula	++	++	++	–	+

Donor-site characteristics are rated excellent (+++) to poor (+) and negative (–).
*Location refers to donor-site location with respect to a two-team approach for simultaneous tumor ablation and flap harvest.
From Disa JJ, Cordeiro PG. Mandible reconstruction with microvascular surgery. Semin Surg Oncol 2000;19:226–234, copyright © 2000. Reprinted with permission of Wiley-Liss, Inc., a subsidiary of John Wiley & Sons, Inc.

is maintained, the buccal and lingual sulci are reconstructed, and soft tissue losses from the lips, chin, and cheek are optimally replaced.[44] Donor-site selection also depends on the length of the vascular pedicle, the morbidity that occurs with graft harvest, the ease of dissection of the donor site, the ability to reconstruct the defect with a single flap, and the availability and location of the recipient vessels.[44] The vascularized bone-containing free flaps that are most frequently used for mandibular reconstruction include the fibula, radius, scapula, and iliac crest.

Fibula

The fibula free flap, which was originally described as a method of mandibular reconstruction in 1989, has become the free flap of choice for the restoration of most mandibular defects. Indications for the fibular osteocutaneous flap include total or subtotal mandibular defects, bone-only defects, reconstruction of an atrophic mandible, secondary reconstruction of the subcondylar-condylar complex, and pediatric mandibular reconstruction.[7] The technique of flap harvest is relatively straightforward, and the accessibility of the fibular region permits a two-team approach (**Fig. 18–2**).[46] The fibula provides up to 25 cm of bicortical bone that can be osteotomized in multiple locations to create a curvilinear contour in the neomandible without devascularizing individual segments.[44] This graft is considered an excellent recipient site for dental implants even though the average fibular height is only 12 mm.[29,47] This height matches up favorably with an adjacent atrophic edentulous mandible, but the height and volume of bone is markedly less than free iliac crest or native dentate mandibular bone.[7,24] Although a moderate amount of skin and soft tissue can be harvested in the skin paddle with a survival rate of greater than 90%, an extensive soft tissue defect contraindicates the use of this flap.[48] Donor-site morbidity associated with the flap harvest is minimal, and patients are able to continue their daily activities in unhindered fashion. However, isokinetic testing has shown that most individuals have decreased ankle plantar and dorsiflexion and diminution of knee and ankle strength even though patients report that leg strength and overall leg function remain unaffected.[49] The aesthetic result is good to excellent for most patients who undergo fibular reconstruction, and 60 to 70% are able to consume a regular diet.[45,50] Oral continence and intelligible speech are also preserved in the majority of reconstructed patients.[50] Drawbacks of the fibula free flap include its limited pedicle length, the restricted mobility of the skin paddle in relation to the bone, and the risk of distal ischemia of the foot when significant peripheral vascular disease is present.[8] Because of its success and popularity, the fibula free flap has become the standard for comparison when other donor sites are being evaluated for their role in mandibular reconstruction.

Radius

The radial forearm *fasciocutaneous* flap, which is a source of very reliable skin that is thin, pliable, and well vascularized, has evolved into the preferred free flap in most situations where large intraoral soft tissue defects must be restored. In contrast, the poor bone quality provided by the radial forearm *osteocutaneous* flap limits its use for mandibular reconstruction. Unlike the fibula, only 10 to 12 cm of unicortical bone can be harvested, and the bone is easily devascularized when osteotomies are performed. This flap also tends to be a poor recipient for osseointegrated implants. The most significant morbidity results from harvesting the skin paddle, which leads to a cosmetic defect. Although the weakened remaining radius is at risk for pathologic fracture, this concern is essentially eliminated by the prophylactic application of a rigid dynamic compression plate, and arm function appears to remain unaffected.[24,51,52] The indications for the radial osteocutaneous flap are limited to small defects of the mandibular angle, ascending ramus, or the posterior body where a large soft tissue defect of the oropharynx must be restored (see **Fig. 18–3** on p. 218).[24,44,51]

Scapula

The scapula *osteocutaneous* free flap (SOFF), which was originally described for head and neck reconstruction in 1986 by Swartz et al,[53] is a versatile flap that can be used to reconstruct various surgical defects that are missing bone in combination with skin or muscle. Complex three-dimensional defects that require the replacement of bone and soft tissue may be reconstructed with more than one free flap or with a single *multicomponent* free flap. However, the mobility between the individual components of most multicomponent flaps is limited because the tissue components are typically connected by small perforator vessels that limit their arc of rotation.[54] In contrast, the tissue components that are vascularized by the subscapular artery are linked by independent vascular pedicles that permit the harvesting of a multicomponent free flap with highly mobile tissue subunits.[54] The short subscapular artery, which arises from the axillary artery, branches into the circumflex scapular and the thoracodorsal arteries. The circumflex scapular artery supplies three surgically relevant regions via: (1) several periosteal branches that supply the lateral rim of the scapula, (2) a horizontal fasciocutaneous branch to the scapular paddle, and (3) a vertical fasciocutaneous branch to the parascapular paddle.[5,54] The thoracodorsal artery supplies the tip of the scapula via an angular branch and also supplies the serratus anterior and latissimus dorsi muscles. The unique vascular anatomy of this region forms the basis for the *subscapular system* of flaps, which provides the flexibility to independently inset the bony and cutaneous portions of the designed flap, frequently obviating the need to reconstruct with two separate flaps.[8,24] For example, scapular and parascapular skin paddles can be harvested to restore an intraoral soft tissue defect as well as an external cutaneous defect involving the cheek or the chin (see **Fig. 18–4** on p. 219). Likewise, two separate bony defects can be reconstructed by creating a bone flap from the scapular tip, which is supplied by the angular artery, and the lateral scapular border, which is supplied by periosteal branches from the circumflex scapular artery. The tip of the scapula and the latissimus dorsi can also be harvested together, exploiting their common vascular supply from the thoracodorsal artery.

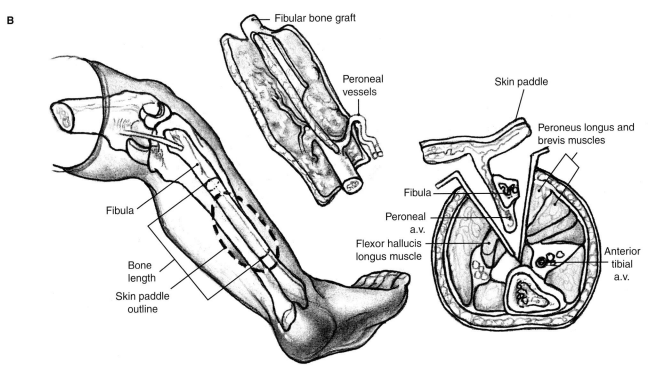

A

Front
of
mouth lesion

1. Inferior alveolar nerve
2. Coronoid process & temporalis m. insertion
3. Masseter m.
4. Ramus of mandible

B

Fibular bone graft

Peroneal
vessels

Skin paddle

Peroneus longus and
brevis muscles

Fibula

Fibula

Peroneal
a.v.

Flexor hallucis
longus muscle

Anterior
tibial
a.v.

Bone
length

Skin paddle
outline

Figure 18–2   Fibula osteocutaneous free flap. **(A)** Anticipated oromandibular defect with loss of the anterior arch, the lateral mandible, and nearby soft tissue (*dashed line*). **(B)** Donor site from the fibula and the harvested flap. Inset: Cross-sectional view. (*Continued*)

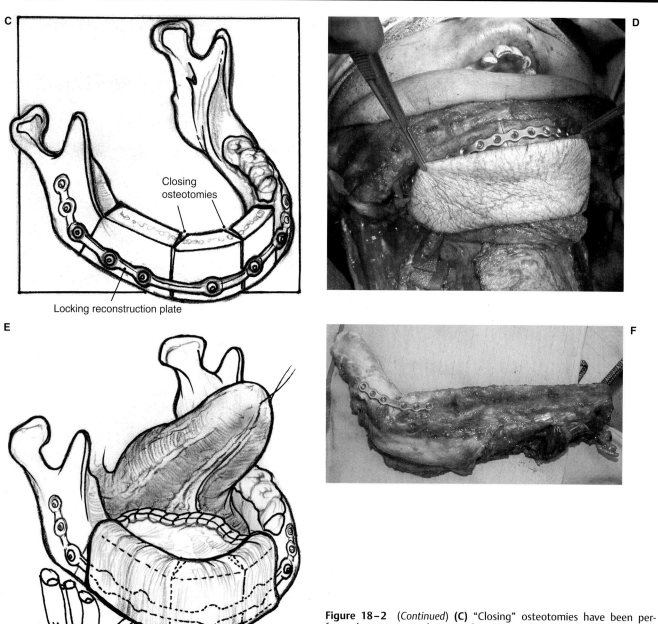

Figure 18–2 (*Continued*) **(C)** "Closing" osteotomies have been performed to re-create the natural contours of the mandibular arch. The fibula has been inset and stabilized to the native mandible with a locking reconstruction plate. **(D)** The inset fibula and its overlying skin paddle. Closing osteotomies have been used to reestablish the mandibular contours. **(E)** Final reconstruction with soft tissue coverage. **(F)** Osteotomies may also be performed to replicate the contour of the mandibular ramus, and the end of the fibula can be rounded to form a condylar head.

The SOFF has a reliable skin flap that provides more soft tissue bulk than the radius and can resurface large intraoral or external cutaneous defects.[44,55] Burkey and Day's group,[55] for example, noted that the mean cutaneous area harvested with the scapula osteocutaneous free flap (110 cm^2) was greater than the mean cutaneous area harvested with either the fibular free flap (55.4 cm^2) or the iliac crest (77.6 cm^2). The lateral scapular border provides 10 to 14 cm of thin bone with a periosteal blood supply that permits osteotomies for bone contouring. Unlike the fibula, however, osteotomies can devascularize the distal segment.[44] The

width of bone that is harvested from the lateral scapula is usually adequate to accommodate the placement of endosteal implants and provides long-term implant stability as evidenced by a rate of peri-implant bone resorption that is similar to the rate observed with implanted native mandibular bone.[56,57] Up to 14 cm of pedicle length is possible when the proximal subscapular vessels are harvested with the flap, whereas the pedicle length ranges from 7 to 10 cm if the circumflex scapular artery is harvested at its takeoff from the subscapular vessels. Donor-site morbidity is subjectively judged by patients as mild in severity, and activities of daily

A

Tonsil

Soft palate

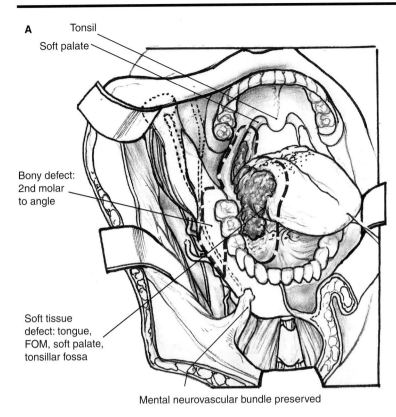

Bony defect:
2nd molar
to angle

Soft tissue
defect: tongue,
FOM, soft palate,
tonsillar fossa

Mental neurovascular bundle preserved

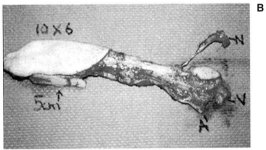

B

C

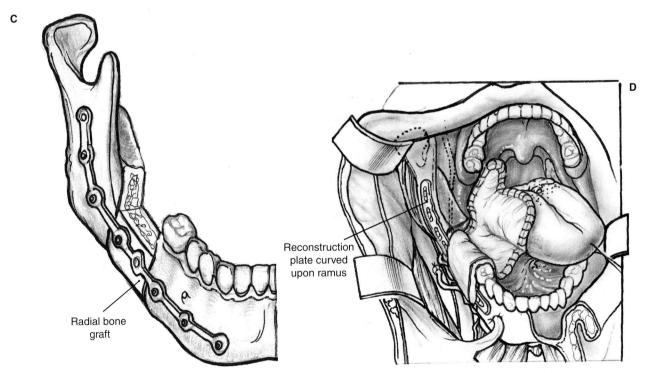

Radial bone
graft

Reconstruction
plate curved
upon ramus

D

Figure 18–3 Radial forearm osteocutaneous free flap. **(A)** Anticipated bony defect of the posterior mandibular body in association with a large soft tissue defect involving the oral cavity and oropharynx. **(B)** Harvested radial forearm osteocutaneous free flap. A smaller skin monitor has been incorporated to assess the viability of the flap because the inset main skin paddle will be inaccessible in the posterior oral cavity and oropharynx. **(C)** Size mismatch between the radial bone and the mandible. **(D)** The bony and soft tissue components have both been inset, completing the reconstruction.

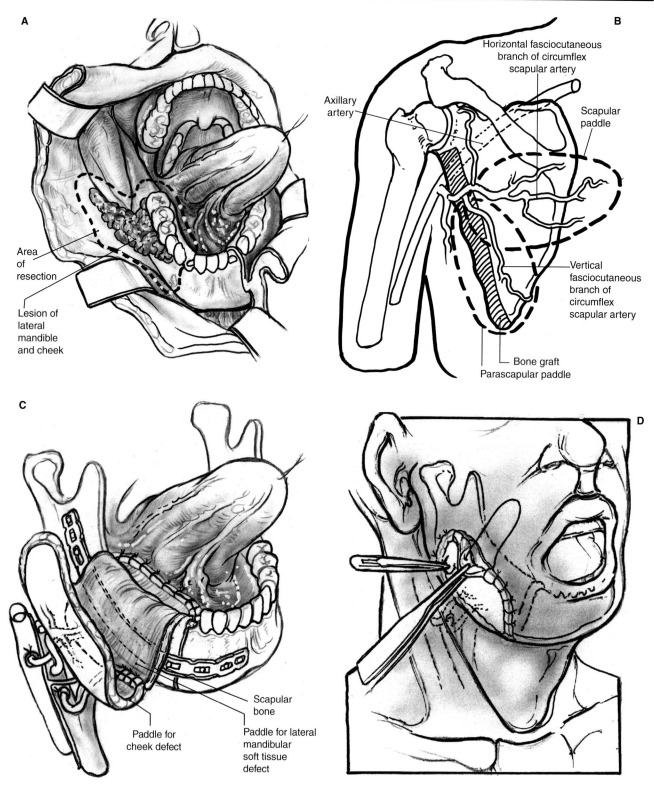

Figure 18–4 Scapula osteocutaneous free flap. **(A)** Planned area of resection will result in a mandibular defect in association with intraoral soft tissue loss as well as a full-thickness defect of the cheek (*dashed line*). **(B)** Illustration of the donor regions supplied by branches of the circumflex scapular artery. **(C)** Insetting the flap, sandwiching the bony component between the internal and external skin paddles. **(D)** Closure of the cutaneous cheek defect.

living and shoulder function are minimally affected.[55] However, the SOFF provides shorter, thinner bone than the fibula or the iliac crest, and the location of the donor site usually precludes a two-team approach, which prolongs the duration of surgery.

The indications for reconstruction of the mandible with a free flap from the subscapular system vary widely at different institutions. At Memorial Sloan-Kettering Cancer Center, mandibular reconstruction with a subscapular flap is generally limited to situations that require a large quantity of skin and soft tissue in combination with a small quantity of bone that does not require osteotomies or endosteal implants.[44] In contrast, surgeons from Vanderbilt University Medical Center have employed scapular osteocutaneous flaps with increasing frequency. In 1998 to 1999, 63.6% of all free flaps performed for head and neck reconstruction at Vanderbilt were scapular flaps, whereas free fibula and iliac crest flaps composed 36.4% and 0% of the total, respectively. Three fourths of these scapular flaps were used to reconstruct the mandible.[55] Urken's group[8] notes that while lateral scapular bone can be used to reconstruct defects of the lateral mandible, the thin bone from the medial scapular tip is more ideally suited for palatal and orbital reconstruction. Combination defects of the palate, retromolar trigone, and mandible may be restored by using the scapular tip to reconstruct the palate and the lateral border to replace the mandible. In this case, scapular and parascapular skin paddles can be designed to reline the palate and gingivobuccal sulcus.[8]

Iliac Crest

The iliac crest *osteomyocutaneous* free flap supplies 14 to 16 cm of corticocancellous bone that is approximately 25 mm in height, which exceeds the average height of fibular grafts by more than a centimeter.[8,24,56] Consequently, mandibular reconstruction with the iliac crest results in a neomandibular height that corresponds more closely with that of adjacent dentate mandibular bone, thereby improving alveolar ridge contours, facilitating dental implant placement and long-term stability, and improving lower lip support and oral competence.[56-58] When the ipsilateral ilium is harvested, the bone flap can be oriented so that the iliac crest reconstructs the lateral inferior mandibular border and the anterior superior iliac spine re-creates the angle.[8] Cordeiro and Hidalgo's group[44] contend that the iliac crest is not suitable for reconstruction of the anterior mandible because contouring osteotomies tend to compromise the bone's blood supply. Urken et al[7] and Genden et al[8] on the other hand, published a series of 137 iliac free tissue transfers that counter their experience, and advocate the use of iliac crest for a variety of oromandibular defects, including the symphyseal region. The experiences of these two surgical groups are also reflected in their divergent recommendations regarding the role that the iliac crest plays in mandibular reconstruction: Urken et al and Genden et al advocate its use in a variety of situations, whereas Cordeiro and Hidalgo's group, who originally described the fibula free flap for mandibular reconstruction, believe that the sole indication for using the iliac crest is when "other free-flap donor sites are unavailable."[44,46]

The iliac crest *osteomyocutaneous* free flap has three tissue components: the iliac crest, the internal oblique muscle, and an overlying skin paddle. Unlike the scapular flap, however, the skin paddle is bulkier and less mobile in relation to the bone. When the bulkiness of the skin paddle precludes its use for intraoral resurfacing, the internal oblique muscle may be used to line the oral cavity, and the skin paddle can be employed to reconstruct an external cutaneous defect, if necessary.[6,59,60] The iliac crest can be used to reconstruct anterior and lateral mandibular defects, and is particularly useful for the complex three-dimensional reconstruction of composite oromandibular defects that result from surgical resection, such as segmental mandibulectomy with subtotal/total glossectomy, oromandibular defects that also include tissue loss from the cheek or chin, or lateral mandibulectomy in combination with infrastructure maxillectomy (**Fig. 18-5**). In the latter case, the internal oblique muscle may be sutured to the edges of the maxillectomy defect to eliminate the need for a palatal obturator.[7,8] Reconstruction of composite defects with the iliac crest flap may obviate the need to reconstruct with multiple free flaps, and a two-team approach is also possible, further shortening the operative time.

There are several limitations associated with the iliac crest free flap, including the short length of the vascular pedicle (approximately 6 cm), and the bulkiness of the skin paddle.[8,24] Donor-site morbidity, however, is its greatest drawback. Patients typically manifest significant gait disturbances for 3 to 4 weeks following surgery, which usually resolve with aggressive physical therapy and mobilization.[24,50] Other complications include persistent hip pain and weakness, femoral nerve injury, and incisional hernias or abdominal wall weakness.[5,50]

◆ Perioperative Considerations

The anticipated cost, complexity, and morbidity of each potential reconstructive option for a particular mandibular defect should be carefully weighed against its potential impact on the patient's quality of life and the patient's prognosis. Patients may be poor candidates for free tissue transfer if they have significant medical comorbidity that contraindicates prolonged general anesthesia or if surgical resection is performed with palliative intent. Risk analysis has shown that patients who have a history of hepatitis or who are preoperatively assigned an American Society of Anesthesiology (ASA) score of either 3 or 4, which are assigned to patients who have severe systemic disease with definite functional limitations (ASA 3) or that is a constant threat to their life (ASA 4), experience more *medical* complications following free tissue transfer.[61,62] On the other hand, an increased rate of *surgical* complications has been linked to greater volumes of intraoperative fluid administration.[62] Furthermore, operative times of greater than 8 to 10 hours have been associated with increased rates of medical and surgical complications.[61,62] Advanced age by itself, however, is not an independent risk factor for postoperative complications and should not be considered a contraindication for free tissue transfer.[61,63]

Immediate reconstruction is usually preferred over delayed reconstruction so that wound contracture is minimized, improvements in quality of life are expedited, and

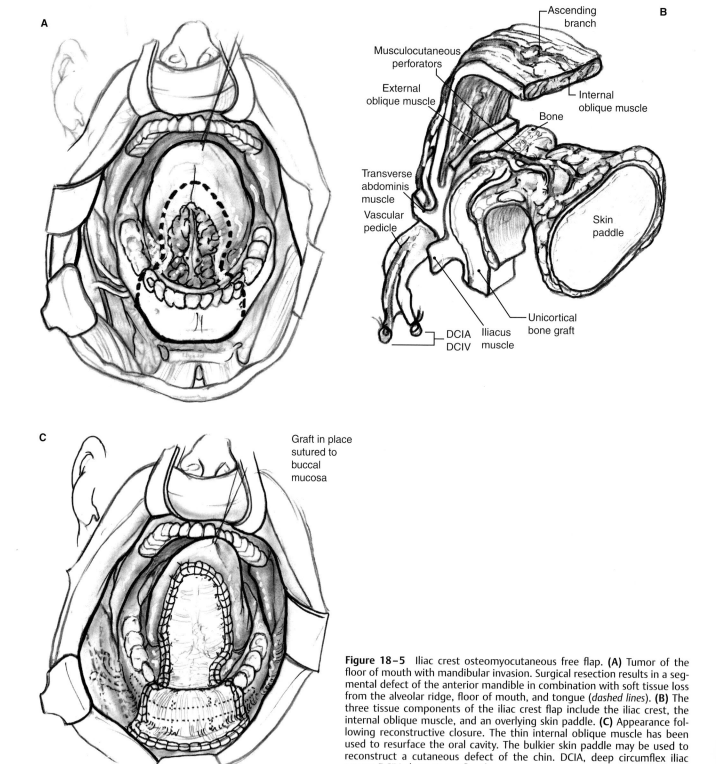

Figure 18–5 Iliac crest osteomyocutaneous free flap. **(A)** Tumor of the floor of mouth with mandibular invasion. Surgical resection results in a segmental defect of the anterior mandible in combination with soft tissue loss from the alveolar ridge, floor of mouth, and tongue (*dashed lines*). **(B)** The three tissue components of the iliac crest flap include the iliac crest, the internal oblique muscle, and an overlying skin paddle. **(C)** Appearance following reconstructive closure. The thin internal oblique muscle has been used to resurface the oral cavity. The bulkier skin paddle may be used to reconstruct a cutaneous defect of the chin. DCIA, deep circumflex iliac artery; DCIV, deep circumflex iliac vein.

the need for additional surgery is avoided. Immediate reconstruction should also be strongly considered if there is an anterior mandibular arch defect or a large adjacent soft tissue defect.[5] Delayed reconstruction may be indicated when a nonvascularized bone graft is preferred, medical comorbidity contraindicates immediate definitive reconstruction, or donor-site morbidity is a concern.

The potential implications of preoperative or postoperative RT on the reconstructive outcome must also be considered. Several investigators have retrospectively evaluated the impact that RT has on the success of mandibular reconstruction plates, with contrasting findings. In one review of 37 patients who underwent mandibular reconstruction with a bridging reconstruction plate at Massachusetts General Hospital, RT was associated with a 33% complication rate requiring revision surgery, whereas revision surgery was required for only 6% of the nonirradiated patients.[18] Furthermore, preoperative as well as postoperative RT have been associated with reduced rates of plate survival.[13,64] Other researchers, however, were unable to demonstrate a link between RT and reconstruction plate failure.[9,17,65] In contrast, there is uniform agreement that RT adversely affects the survival rate of nonvascularized bone grafts.[29,34] Although hyperbaric oxygen therapy or reconstruction of the surrounding soft tissues with a pedicled myocutaneous flap may be used to improve the rate of graft survival, the success of this approach has not been rigorously investigated.[32] The impact of RT on vascularized free tissue remains incompletely characterized. Oral and maxillofacial surgeons from UCSF have documented higher rates of bony union and implant success with vascularized free tissue transfer than with nonvascularized bone grafts when perioperative RT was administered.[34] However, the relationship between perioperative RT and postsurgical complications such as wound breakdown and flap loss has not been defined. In a retrospective review of 100 consecutive patients who underwent mandibular reconstruction with a fibula free flap at the University of Washington, there were no statistical differences in the incidence or severity of complications between patients who received RT and those who did not receive RT.[66] In contrast, a retrospective analysis of 140 fibula free flaps performed at M. D. Anderson Cancer Center found that perioperative RT resulted in a higher complication rate following free tissue transfer.[67]

◆ Classification of the Mandibular Defect

Prior to the era of microvascular reconstruction, surgeons were primarily concerned with achieving closure of large oromandibular defects. The ability to reconstruct sizable complex tissue defects with a single vascularized flap, however, allowed reconstructive surgeons to become more critical of their aesthetic and functional outcomes. Experienced mandibular reconstructive surgeons uniformly agreed that the quality of the soft tissue reconstruction was at least as important as the bony reconstruction, and that functional restoration of the tongue was the most important factor that improved the patient's quality of life.[7,45,59,68] Moreover, descriptions of reconstructive procedures that were solely based on the mandibulectomy defect oversimplified the reconstructive requirements, because identical segmental bone defects could be accompanied by a wide range of soft tissue defects with the loss of mucosa, skin, muscles, and nerves.[59] These insights led to the development of two classification schemes that could be used to standardize descriptive terminology for different oromandibular defects so that defect-specific techniques could be developed and compared among investigators, and the effectiveness of various approaches could be communicated to the surgical community.[59,69]

Urken and colleagues[59] devised a classification scheme that denotes each portion of the segmental mandibular defect by using the following designations: condyle, C; ramus, R; body,

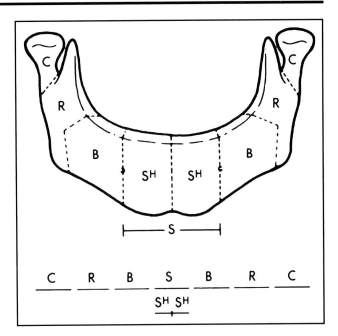

Figure 18–6 Urken's classification of segmental defects. (From Urken ML, Weinberg H, Vickery C, Buchbinder D, Lawson W, Biller HF. Oromandibular reconstruction using microvascular composite free flaps. Arch Otolaryngol Head Neck Surg 1991;117:733–744, copyright © 1991, American Medical Association.)

B; and symphysis, S and S[H] (**Fig. 18–6**).[59] Defects of the symphysis, which describes the region of the mandible between the two canines, are subdivided into full defects (S) and hemisymphyseal defects (S[H]), which stop at the midline. Thus, a hemimandibulectomy defect that includes the condyle, ramus, body, and hemisymphysis is denoted as CRBS[H], and a defect of both mandibular bodies and the symphysis is denoted as BSB. Nomenclature was also proposed to classify various mucosal, cutaneous, and neurologic deficits. In this system, the numbers of possible defect combinations for each tissue type were as follows: bone, 22; soft tissue, 22; and neurologic, at least 8.[68] Consequently, several hundred different oromandibular defects are possible, which makes this classification scheme impractical for its intended use: to improve communication between and among clinicians and investigators.[7,8]

Jewer and Boyd and colleagues[68,69] from Toronto proposed a less complex classification scheme, known as the HCL classification system, which emphasizes the difficulties that are associated with reconstructing a particular oromandibular defect (**Fig. 18–7**). They agreed with Urken et al that defect size was a less critical factor (i.e., small versus large lateral bony defect) than loss of the anterior mandible or the condyle, or the concurrent loss of functionally and aesthetically important soft tissue.[59,68] Central defects of the mandible, containing the canines and the incisors, are designated with a C. The entire segment must be absent to be classified as a C-type defect. Lateral segmental defects of any length that preserved the condyle, including portions of the central segment, are represented by L. Lateral segmental defects that include the condyle are designated by H, for hemimandible, even though such defects are not required to extend to the midline. Subsequent modifications have

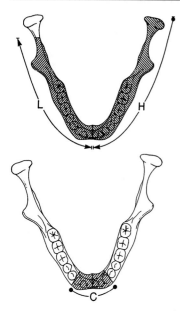

Figure 18–7 HCL classification system. This classification is based on reconstructive difficulty rather than on classic anatomic landmarks. C represents the central segment of the mandible containing the canines and the incisor teeth. For C to be included in the designation, the *whole* segment must be present. L represents a lateral segment of *any length* minus the condyle. It may encroach on the C segment but would only be termed LC if the entire C segment were part of it. H is the same as L except that it includes a condyle. Thus, there are only eight possibilities: C, L, H, CL, CH, LCL, HCL, and HCH. To this bony defect the letters m, s, and ms may be added to signify an additional requirement for mucosa, skin, or both, respectively. (From Boyd JB, Mulholland RS, Davidson J, et al. The free flap and plate in oromandibular reconstruction: long-term review and indications. Plast Reconstr Surg 1995;95:1018–1028, with permission from Lippincott Williams & Wilkins.)

been made that characterize the soft tissue reconstructive needs by adding a lower case m for mucosal defect or an s for external skin defect.[15,68] Hidalgo also suggested that t should be used to indicate the presence of a significant tongue defect. Using this system, a hemimandibulectomy defect that includes the condyle, ramus, body, and hemisymphysis is denoted by an H, whereas a defect of both mandibular bodies and the symphysis is denoted as LCL. The additional loss of oral mucosa and a significant portion of the tongue would be designated by H-mt or LCL-mt, respectively. This classification system offers fewer defect possibilities than Urken et al's classification and has gained wider acceptance by the surgical community.

◆ Defect-Specific Approach to Reconstruction

General Considerations

The countless array of complex oromandibular defects that occur following oral cancer resection prevents an all-inclusive discussion of reconstruction using a defect-based approach. Surgical rehabilitation that is both

defect-specific and patient-specific requires utilization of the entire reconstructive spectrum and close communication between members of the surgical team, the patient, and the maxillofacial prosthodontist. The selection of a particular reconstructive option should be based on the aesthetic and functional losses that result from surgical resection, the ultimate reconstructive goals, and the potential morbidity that may be experienced by the patient. Whenever more than one reconstructive option exists that can provide a comparable rehabilitative outcome, the least morbid surgical approach is preferred. Potential fibular free flap candidates should undergo preoperative assessment of the lower extremity vasculature to evaluate the risk of postoperative lower limb ischemia.[24] Free tissue transfer from the fibula or the iliac crest should not be considered in patients who have an underlying gait disturbance, are extremely athletic, or have significant premorbid weakness and debilitation that may affect ambulation by compounding the functional deficits that result from flap harvest.[7,49] At the same time, the implications of reconstructing with an alloplastic implant, a nonvascularized bone graft, or an alternative source of vascularized tissue that is less suitable for a particular surgical defect must be anticipated.

Lateral Defects with Preservation of the Condyle (L)

Numerous reconstructive options exist for segmental defects of the lateral mandible that preserve the condyle (L). Horizontal sliding osteotomies from the adjacent mandible have been described for segmental defects less than 4 cm in length.[70] Locking reconstruction plates can be used to bridge a segmental defect that involves the body distal to the canine and is less than 5 cm in length if bone grafting is not desired or is contraindicated. Adjacent soft tissue defects should be reconstructed with a pedicled musculocutaneous flap or a fasciocutaneous free flap. Immediate reconstruction with a nonvascularized cancellous bone graft in a resorbable mesh crib can be used for a nonirradiated defect that measures less than 6 cm in length if the mandible has been resected via an extraoral approach and the oral mucosa has not been violated. The fibula is the preferred form of free tissue transfer for most L-type defects when limited soft tissue is needed. Extensive soft tissue defects of the oral cavity or cheek may benefit from reconstruction with a scapular osteocutaneous flap.[55,71] The latissimus dorsi muscle and its neurovascular pedicle have also been harvested with this flap to replace the facial musculature, occasionally achieving dynamic facial reanimation.[7] Complex composite defects may also be replaced with an iliac crest free flap, relining the intraoral surface with the internal oblique muscle and using the bulkier skin paddle to replace extraoral cutaneous tissue loss. Non–tooth-bearing mandibulectomy defects of the posterior body, angle, and ramus can be reconstructed with a radial osteocutaneous free flap when defects of the lateral tongue base or oropharynx are present.[51] When the ramus is resected at the midlevel or higher, precise apposition and stabilization of the bone graft to the condylar remnant is technically challenging. Hidalgo[45,72] uses the condyle as a nonvascularized graft by resecting it from the surgical specimen, fixing the condyle to the distal end of the vascularized bone graft, and repositioning the condyle in the glenoid fossa without repairing the joint capsule. Radiographic evaluation documented the stability of these autotransplanted condylar grafts, and oromandibular function was comparable to patients in whom the joint was not disturbed.[45]

Lateral Defects with Loss of the Condyle (H)

Although lateral mandibular defects that include the condyle may be reconstructed with a pedicled myocutaneous flap or a fasciocutaneous free flap, patients who undergo reconstruction with vascularized bone flaps are more likely to consume a normal diet and dine in public, demonstrate superior speech articulation, and exhibit less deviation of the mandible from the midline.[4] Genden's group[8] designed a new condyle by modifying the proximal end of a fibular graft so that a periosteal cuff is interposed between the fibula and the glenoid fossa, preventing ankylosis and skull base erosion. A temporalis myofascial flap can be used in lieu of the fibular periosteal cuff with the same intent.[73] Prefabricated alloplastic condylar prostheses have been infrequently used in this setting.

Defects of the Central Segment (C)

Central segmental defects should routinely undergo immediate definitive reconstruction. Nonvascularized bone grafts can be used for limited defects of the anterior mandible in accordance with the criteria that were previously discussed. Osteotomized contoured fibular grafts are preferred for most central segment defects that do not require extensive soft tissue replacement. The iliac crest is an excellent choice for full-thickness composite defects that involve the soft tissues of the oral cavity, the central mandibular segment, and the soft tissues of the chin.[7,50,74] Subtotal or total glossectomy in conjunction with central segmental mandibulectomy can also be reconstructed with the iliac osteocutaneous free flap by orienting the bone horizontally and transposing the skin paddle over the bone to reline the oral cavity.[7]

Large Oromandibular Defects

Segmental mandibular defects greater than 16 cm in length, the upper limit of available iliac crest, must be reconstructed with the fibula, which can supply up to 25 cm of bone length. A radial forearm fasciocutaneous flap may also be necessary if an extensive intraoral lining defect coexists.[44] Free tissue from the subscapular system or the iliac crest can be used for composite oromandibular defects as discussed above. Composite oromandibular defects frequently require double free flap reconstruction of massive soft tissue defects with complex three-dimensional requirements, defects of the central segment and the entire lower lip, reconstruction of the mandible and more than half of the tongue, or nonviability of a critical portion of the soft tissue paddle of a composite free flap.[7]

◆ Conclusion

Historically, surgical resection of the oromandibular region often led to defects that had devastating consequences for the patient. The anatomic and functional complexity of the oromandibular region posed innumerable technical challenges for the reconstructive surgeon, and few reconstructive options were available. Fortunately, refinements in alloplastic materials, microvascular surgical technique, and osseointegration have improved the reconstructive outcomes for most of these patients. Superior outcomes have also been realized by defining the role and limitations of nonvascularized bone grafting and free tissue transfer from various donor sites. Despite these innovations, many patients continue to manifest residual sequelae from surgical resection and reconstruction that are constant reminders of their cancer experience. Additional gains in quality of life will require the continued critical assessment of each cancer patient's appearance and function, and a willingness to consider the promise of unproven novel techniques such as distraction osteogenesis.

References

1. Funk GF, Karnell LH, Robinson RA, Zhen WK, Trask DK, Hoffman HT. Presentation, treatment, and outcome of oral cavity cancer: a National Cancer Data Base report. Head Neck 2002;24:165–180
2. Hoffman HT, Karnell LH, Funk GF, Robinson RA, Menck HR. The National Cancer Data Base report on cancer of the head and neck. Arch Otolaryngol Head Neck Surg 1998;124:951–962
3. Curtis DA, Plesh O, Miller AJ, et al. A comparison of masticatory function in patients with or without reconstruction of the mandible. Head Neck 1997;19:287–296
4. King TW, Gallas MT, Robb GL, Lalani Z, Miller MJ. Aesthetic and functional outcomes using osseous or soft-tissue free flaps. J Reconstr Microsurg 2002;18:365–371
5. Colin WB, Haughey B. State of the art techniques for mandibular reconstruction. In: Robbins KT, ed. Advances in Head and Neck Oncology. San Diego: Singular, 1998:133–146
6. Urken ML, Vickery C, Weinberg H, Buchbinder D, Lawson W, Biller HF. The internal oblique-iliac crest osseomyocutaneous free flap in oromandibular reconstruction. Report of 20 cases. Arch Otolaryngol Head Neck Surg 1989;115:339–349
7. Urken ML, Buchbinder D, Costantino PD, et al. Oromandibular reconstruction using microvascular composite flaps: report of 210 cases. Arch Otolaryngol Head Neck Surg 1998;124:46–55
8. Genden EM, Buchbinder D, Urken ML. Mandible reconstruction and osseointegrated implants. In: Papel ID, ed. Facial Plastic and Reconstructive Surgery, 2nd ed. New York: Thieme, 2002:591–600
9. Vuillemin T, Raveh J, Sutter F. Mandibular reconstruction with the titanium hollow screw reconstruction plate (THORP) system: evaluation of 62 cases. Plast Reconstr Surg 1988;82:804–814
10. Militsakh ON, Wallace DI, Kriet JD, Girod DA, Olvera MS, Tsue TT. Use of the 2.0-mm locking reconstruction plate in primary oromandibular reconstruction after composite resection. Otolaryngol Head Neck Surg 2004;131:660–665
11. Kroll S, Reece GP. Aesthetically successful mandibular reconstruction with a single reconstruction plate. Clin Plast Surg 2001;28:273–282
12. Poli T, Ferrari S, Bianchi B, Sesenna E. Primary oromandibular reconstruction using free flaps and THORP plates in cancer patients: a 5-year experience. Head Neck 2003;25:15–23
13. Wei FC, Celik N, Yang WG, Chen IH, Chang YM, Chen HC. Complications after reconstruction by plate and soft-tissue free flap in composite

mandibular defects and secondary salvage reconstruction with osteocutaneous flap. Plast Reconstr Surg 2003;112:37–42

14. Spencer KR, Sizeland A, Taylor GI, Wiesenfeld D. The use of titanium mandibular reconstruction plates in patients with oral cancer. Int J Oral Maxillofac Surg 1999;28:288–290

15. Boyd JB, Mulholland RS, Davidson J, et al. The free flap and plate in oromandibular reconstruction: long-term review and indications. Plast Reconstr Surg 1995;95:1018–1028

16. Blackwell KE, Lacombe V. The bridging lateral mandibular reconstruction plate revisited. Arch Otolaryngol Head Neck Surg 1999;125:988–993

17. Mandpe AH, Singer MI, Kaplan MJ, Greene D. Alloplastic and microvascular restoration of the mandible: a comparison study. Laryngoscope 1998;108:224–227

18. Kim MR, Donoff RB. Critical analysis of mandibular reconstruction using AO reconstruction plates. J Oral Maxillofac Surg 1992;50:1152–1157

19. Arden RL, Rachel JD, Marks SC, Dang K. Volume-length impact of lateral jaw resections on complication rates. Arch Otolaryngol Head Neck Surg 1999;125:68–72

20. Blackwell KE, Buchbinder D, Urken ML. Lateral mandibular reconstruction using soft-tissue free flaps and plates. Arch Otolaryngol Head Neck Surg 1996;122:672–678

21. Daniel E, Browne JD. Minimizing complications in the use of titanium condylar head reconstruction prostheses. Otolaryngol Head Neck Surg 2004;130:344–350

22. Carlson ER. Disarticulation resections of the mandible: a prospective review of 16 cases. J Oral Maxillofac Surg 2002;60:176–181

23. Patel A, Maisel R. Condylar prostheses in head and neck cancer reconstruction. Arch Otolaryngol Head Neck Surg 2001;127:842–846

24. Farwell DG, Futran ND. Oromandibular reconstruction. Facial Plast Surg 2000;16:115–126

25. Axhausen W. The osteogenic phases of regeneration of bone: a historical and experimental study. J Bone Joint Surg. Am 1956;38:593–600

26. Lawson W, Baek S, Loscalzo LJ, Biller HF, Krespi YP. Experience with immediate and delayed mandibular reconstruction. Laryngoscope 1982;92:5–10

27. Tidstrom KD, Keller EE. Reconstruction of mandibular discontinuity with autogenous iliac bone graft: report of 34 consecutive patients. J Oral Maxillofac Surg 1990;48:336–346

28. Carlson E, Marx RE. Mandibular reconstruction using cancellous cellular bone grafts. J Oral Maxillofac Surg 1996;54:889–897

29. Pogrel MA, Podlesh S, Anthony JP, Alexander J. A comparison of vascularized and nonvascularized bone grafts for reconstruction of mandibular continuity defects. J Oral Maxillofac Surg 1997;55:1200–1206

30. Chen YB, Chen HC, Hahn LH. Major mandibular reconstruction with vascularized bone grafts: Indication and selection of donor tissue. Microsurgery 1994;15:227–237

31. Keller EE, Tolman D, Eckert SE. Endosseous implant and autogenous bone graft reconstruction of mandibular discontinuity: a 12-year longitudinal study of 31 patients. Int J Oral Maxillofac Implants 1998;13:767–780

32. Marx RE. Current advances in reconstruction of the mandible in head and neck surgery. Semin Surg Oncol 1991;7:47–57

33. Marx RE, Ames JR. The use of hyperbaric oxygen therapy in bony reconstruction of the irradiated and tissue deficient patient. J Oral Maxillofac Surg 1982;40:412–420

34. Foster RD, Anthony JP, Sharma A, Pogrel MA. Vascularized bone flaps versus nonvascularized bone grafts for mandibular reconstruction: an outcome analysis of primary bony union and endosseous implant success. Head Neck 1999;21:66–71

35. Schliephake H, Schmelzeisen R, Husstedt H, Schmidt-Wondera LU. Comparison of the late results of mandibular reconstruction using nonvascularized or vascularized grafts and dental implants. J Oral Maxillofac Surg 1999;57:944–950

36. Costantino PD, Friedman CD, Shindo M, Houston G, Sisson GA. Experimental mandibular regrowth by distraction osteogenesis. Arch Otolaryngol Head Neck Surg 1993;119:511–516

37. Kuriakose MA, Shnayder Y, DeLacure MD. Reconstruction of segmental mandibular defects by distraction osteogenesis for mandibular reconstruction. Head Neck 2003;25:816–824

38. Sawaki Y, Hagino H, Yamamoto H, Ueda M. Trifocal distraction osteogenesis for segmental mandibular defect: a technical innovation. J Craniomaxillofac Surg 1997;25:310–315

39. Block MS, Otten J, McLaurin D, Zoldos J. Bifocal distraction osteogenesis for mandibular defect healing: case reports. J Oral Maxillofac Surg 1996;54:1365–1370

40. Annino DJ, Goguen LA, Karmody CS. Distraction osteogenesis for reconstruction of mandibular symphyseal defects. Arch Otolaryngol Head Neck Surg 1994;120:911–916

41. Jonsson B, Siemssen SJ. Arced segmental mandibular regeneration by distraction osteogenesis. Plast Reconstr Surg 1998;101:1925–1930

42. Kunkel M, Wahlmann U, Reichert TE, Wegener J, Wagner W. Reconstruction of mandibular defects following tumor ablation by vertical distraction osteogenesis using intraosseous distraction devices. Clin Oral Implants Res. 2005;16:89–97

43. Nocini PF, Wangerin K, Albanese M, Kretschmer W, Cortelazzi R. Vertical distraction of a free vascularized fibula flap in a reconstructed hemimandible: case report. J Craniomaxillofac Surg 2000;28:20–24

44. Cordeiro PG, Disa JJ, Hidalgo DA, Ying Hu Q. Reconstruction of the mandible with osseous free flaps: a 10-year experience with 150 consecutive patients. Plast Reconstr Surg 1999;104:1314–1320

45. Hidalgo DA, Pusic AL. Free-flap mandibular reconstruction: a 10-year follow-up study. Plast Reconstr Surg 2002;110:438–449

46. Hidalgo DA. Fibula free flap: a new method of mandible reconstruction. Plast Reconstr Surg 1989;84:71–79

47. Kildal M, Wei FC, Chang YM, Chen HC, Chang MH. Mandibular reconstruction with fibula osteoseptocutaneous free flap and osseointegrated dental implants. Clin Plast Surg 2001;28:403–410

48. Wei FC, Seah CS, Tsai YC, Liu SJ, Tsai MS. Fibula osteoseptocutaneous flap reconstruction of the composite mandibular defect. Plast Reconstr Surg 1994;93:294–304

49. Anthony JP, Rawnsley JD, Benhaim P, Ritter EF, Sadowsky SH, Singer MI. Donor leg morbidity and function after fibula free flap mandible reconstruction. Plast Reconstr Surg 1995;96:146–152

50. Shpitzer T, Neligan PC, Gullane PJ, et al. The free iliac crest and fibula flaps in vascularized oromandibular reconstruction: comparison and long-term evaluation. Head Neck 1999;21:639–647

51. Villaret DB, Futran NA. The indications and outcomes in the use of osteocutaneous radial forearm free flap. Head Neck 2003;25:475–481

52. Werle AH, Tsue TT, Toby EB, Girod DA. Osteocutaneous radial forearm free flap: its use without significant donor site morbidity. Otolaryngol Head Neck Surg 2000;123:711–717

53. Swartz WM, Banis JC, Newton ED, Ramasastry SS, Jones NF, Acland R. The osteocutaneous scapular flap for mandibular and maxillary reconstruction. Plast Reconstr Surg 1986;77:530–545

54. Germann G, Bickert B, Steinau HU, Wagner H, Sauerbier M. Versatility and reliability of combined flaps of the subscapular system. Plast Reconstr Surg 1999;103:1386–1399

55. Coleman SC, Burkey BB, Day TA, et al. Increasing use of the scapula osteocutaneous free flap. Laryngoscope 2000;110:1419–1424

56. Moscoso JF, Keller J, Genden E, et al. Vascularized bone flaps in oromandibular reconstruction. A comparative anatomic study of bone stock from various donor sites to assess suitability for enosseous dental implants. Arch Otolaryngol Head Neck Surg 1994;120:36–43

57. Schultes G, Gaggl A, Karcher H. Stability of dental implants in microvascular osseous transplants. Plast Reconstr Surg 2002;109:916–921

58. Kovacs AF. Influence of the prosthetic restoration modality on bone loss around dental implants placed in vascularized iliac bone grafts for mandibular reconstruction. Otolaryngol Head Neck Surg 2000;123:598–602

59. Urken ML, Weinberg H, Vickery C, Buchbinder D, Lawson W, Biller HF. Oromandibular reconstruction using microvascular composite free flaps. Report of 71 cases and a new classification scheme for bony, soft-tissue, and neurologic defects. Arch Otolaryngol Head Neck Surg 1991;117:733–744

60. Burkey BB, Coleman JR. Current concepts in oromandibular reconstruction. Otolaryngol Clin North Am 1997;30:607–630

61. Serletti JM, Higgins JP, Moran S, Orlando GS. Factors affecting outcome in free-tissue transfer in the elderly. Plast Reconstr Surg 2000;106:66–70

62. Farwell DG, Reilly DF, Weymuller EA Jr, Greenberg DL, Staiger TO, Futran NA. Predictors of perioperative complications in head and neck patients. Arch Otolaryngol Head Neck Surg 2002;128:505–511

63. Bridger AG, O'Brien CJ, Lee KK. Advanced patient age should not preclude the use of free-flap reconstruction for head and neck cancer. Am J Surg 1994;168:425–428

64. Okura M, Isomura ET, Iida S, Kogo M. Long-term outcome and factors influencing bridging plates for mandibular reconstruction. Oral Oncol 2005;41:791–798

65. Wang ZH, Zhang ZY, Mendenhall W. Postoperative radiotherapy after titanium plate mandibular reconstruction for oral cavity cancer. Am J Clin Oncol 2005;28:460–463

66. Choi S, Schwartz DL, Farwell DG, Austin-Seymour M, Futran ND. Radiation therapy does not impact local complication rates after free flap reconstruction for head and neck cancer. Arch Otolaryngol Head Neck Surg 2004;130:1308–1312

67. Deutsch M, Kroll SS, Ainsle N, Wang B. Influence of radiation on late complications in patients with free fibular flaps for mandibular reconstruction. Ann Plast Surg 1999;42:662–664

68. Boyd JB, Gullane PJ, Rotstein LE, Brown DH, Irish JC. Classification of mandibular defects. Plast Reconstr Surg 1993;92:1266–1275

69. Jewer DD, Boyd JB, Manktelow RT, et al. Orofacial and mandibular reconstruction with the iliac crest free flap: a review of 60 cases and a new method of classification. Plast Reconstr Surg 1989;84:391–403 discussion 404–395

70. Verdaguer J, Soler F, Fernandez-Alba J, Concejo C, Acero J. Sliding osteotomies in mandibular reconstruction. Plast Reconstr Surg 2001;107:1107–1113

71. Deschler DG, Hayden RE. The optimum method for reconstruction of complex lateral oromandibular-cutaneous defects. Head Neck 2000;22:674–679

72. Hidalgo DA. Condyle transplantation in free flap mandible reconstruction. Plast Reconstr Surg 1994;93:770–781 discussion 782–773

73. Pogrel MA, Kaban LB. The role of a temporalis fascia and muscle flap in temporomandibular joint surgery. J Oral Maxillofac Surg 1990;48:14–19

74. Boyd JB, Morris S, Rosen IB, Gullane P, Rotstein L, Freeman JL. The through-and-through oromandibular defect: rationale for aggressive reconstruction. Plast Reconstr Surg 1994;93:44–53

19

Reconstruction of the Maxilla

Christopher D. Lansford,

Neal D. Futran, and

Mark E. Izzard

The structure of the maxilla and the adjacent midface is geometrically and functionally complex, presenting a challenge to those charged with the task of its reconstruction. The maxilla functions as the structural support between the skull base and the occlusal plane, resisting the forces of mastication, anchoring the dentition, separating the oral and nasal cavities, and supporting the globe, face, and its mimetic musculature. As such, the maxilla largely determines the appearance of the face, which serves as an icon for the whole person. The surgical resection of malignancies arising from this region can lead to impairment of mastication, deglutition, and oral hygiene maintenance; alterations in vision, speech, and communication; and adverse effects on self-image, mental health, and social acceptability. Consequently, restoration of the patient's quality of life depends on the degree to which each of these functions is reconstituted through surgical reconstruction and prosthetic rehabilitation. This chapter reviews the reconstruction of the maxilla, applying a defect-specific approach that addresses the unique functional and aesthetic deficits that result from different types of surgical defects.

◆ Anatomic and Functional Considerations in Maxillary Reconstruction

The paired maxillae are the largest and most important bones of the midface, acting as keystones to the facial skeleton. The maxilla consists of a body and its four processes: palatine, alveolar, zygomatic, and frontal. The complex geometric shape of the maxilla may be described as a six-walled structure, or hexahedrium.[1,2] The roof supports the orbital contents, and the floor constitutes most of the hard palate and tooth-bearing upper alveolar ridge. A short segment of the posterior hard palate is also composed of the distinct palatal bone. The medial wall of the maxilla supports the nasolacrimal duct and lateral nasal wall, creating the nasal airway. Part of the lateral wall forms the zygomaticomaxillary complex, which provides facial projection and support of the cheek musculature. The maxillary sinus is housed within the maxilla, and the ethmoid sinuses are located along its superomedial edge.

Masticatory forces are opposed by three vertical buttresses of thickened compact bone that arise from the maxilla. Between these thick buttresses, the maxillary bone becomes quite thin. The zygomaticomaxillary buttress, which lies on the lateral aspect of the anterior face of the hexahedrium and transmits forces to the skull base via the lateral orbital rim, is the strongest vertical buttress. On the anteromedial face of the hexahedrium, the nasomaxillary buttress routes occlusal load to the anterior skull base at the midline. The horizontally oriented inferior orbital rim, which is located between these two vertical buttresses, contributes to orbital support and cheek prominence. The vertical pterygomaxillary buttress is situated along the posterior surface of the maxilla.

The roof of the hexahedrium provides orbital support. Loss of the orbital floor may result in enophthalmos, vertical dystopia, diplopia, and poor eyelid and lacrimal function. Even without bony support, however, the globe's vertical position may be maintained by Lockwood's suspensory ligament as long as its anchoring points, Whitnall's tubercle of the zygoma laterally and the lacrimal crest medially, are preserved.[3] The fascia of the inferior rectus and inferior oblique muscles is included in this suspensory hammock.

The maxilla supports the overlying soft tissues of the midface, including the lower eyelid, cheek, upper lip, and oral commissure, and some of the muscles of facial expression insert directly into the maxilla. Composite resection of the maxilla and facial soft tissues may lead to impairments in facial mimetic function as a direct result of facial nerve or muscle resection, and sensory and autonomic deficits from resection of components of the trigeminal nerve are also frequent sequelae. Loss of eyelid function can result in exposure keratitis, infection, and blindness. Denervation of the orbicularis oris muscle, which normally works in concert with the buccinator muscle to move and hold food between the teeth for chewing, can contribute to oral incompetence.

The hard and soft palate, which separate the oral cavity from the nasal passages, prevent nasal regurgitation of food and regulate nasal air escape during speech. Therefore, palatal disruption can adversely affect speech intelligibility, vocal quality, and normal swallowing function.[4] Preservation of the anterior palate and maxillary incisors is particularly important, because proper consonant production relies on the anatomic integrity of this region.[5]

Loss of the buccal or labial vestibule can restrict lip and cheek movement, which may preclude the use of dentures or prosthetic obturators. Soft tissue reconstruction of the palate and alveolar arch results in blunting of the maxillary arch and the depth of the buccal and lingual sulci, resulting in a "trampoline-like" surface that compromises denture retention. Denture support and retention is most favorable when the soft tissues overlying the load-bearing bone are very thin and immobile, which is typically not achieved using soft tissue reconstruction with a regional or free flap. If soft tissue alone has been used to reconstruct the ipsilateral defect, osseointegrated implants may be placed in the contralateral maxillary arch to support a prosthesis.[6] Alternatively, bony reconstruction partly preserves the three-dimensional ridge and allows the placement of osseointegrated implants when adequate bone stock is replaced.[7–9]

The pliability of the nonkeratinized lining mucosa covering the soft palate, buccal mucosa, and wet vermilion surfaces facilitates speech and swallowing. Reconstruction of the lining mucosa with less pliable tissue that lacks salivary glands such as skin leads to dryness, inspissation, and debris accumulation. Unfortunately, allowing these regions to mucosalize via gradual migration of the native epithelium to the flap periphery is usually impractical, because minimization of postoperative contracture and the expedition of healing take precedence.

Whereas bony defects in the hard palate are well tolerated as long as separation of the oral and nasal cavities is reestablished, the complex functions of the soft palate are usually incompletely restored. In addition to sharing the task of oronasal separation with the hard palate, the soft palate also must occlude the nasopharynx during swallowing and relax to maintain nasopharyngeal airway patency during respiration. The velum and tongue form a proprioceptive unit for speech, chewing, and swallowing. Static and insensate reconstructions abrogate these functions.

◆ Goals of Maxillary and Midface Reconstruction

Prosthetic obturation or surgical reconstruction following maxillectomy should strive to achieve the following goals, in order of importance:

1. Obtain a healed wound.
2. Restore palatal competence and function.
3. Restore normal mastication and deglutition.
4. Support the eye or cosmetically address an exenterated cavity.
5. Maintain a patent nasal airway.
6. Support and suspend adynamic facial soft tissue (e.g., avoidance of ectropion).
7. Restore the midfacial contour.

◆ Classification of the Maxillectomy Defect

Due to the disparate shapes and sizes of tumors affecting the maxilla, and the complex surgical anatomy, the broad category of "maxillectomy" is really a grouping of diverse defects that may range from a small palate oroantral fistula to a large cavity bound by the tongue inferiorly and the anterior skull base superiorly. Tumors requiring maxillectomy are rarely confined by the bony walls of the maxilla itself; thus, resection of adjacent tissues in the velum, palate, midface, and orbits is commonly performed simultaneously. Maxillectomy defects, their reconstructive requirements, and functional and aesthetic outcomes vary greatly.

For this reason, an ideal classification system would succinctly group the wide array of possible tissue losses, help to focus discussion and reconstructive options, and facilitate comparison of results. Attesting to the complexity of these anatomic defects, the medical literature is rife with classification schemes that are neither universally accepted nor comprehensive.[1,10–12] This chapter presents two of these nomenclature systems in detail.

In one classification scheme, Brown and colleagues[10] from Liverpool describe the maxillectomy defect by its vertical and horizontal components. The vertical dimension (classes 1 to 4) designates the extent of unilateral involvement, with emphasis on the orbit. The addition of a letter (a to c) to vertical classes 2 to 4 qualifies the defect in relation to the horizontal aspect of the maxillectomy, accounting for the amount of palate and alveolar ridge that was sacrificed. In general, the vertical component tends to have greater influence on aesthetic results, whereas the horizontal component has much greater functional consequences. This classification system encompasses the deficits resulting from loss of the palate and upper alveolar ridge (dental, masticatory, and articulatory) as well as those resulting from resection of the upper maxilla (aesthetic, sinonasal, and orbital support). The authors have correlated each defect type with the prosthetic and surgical options that most optimally restore the premorbid state (**Fig. 19–1**).

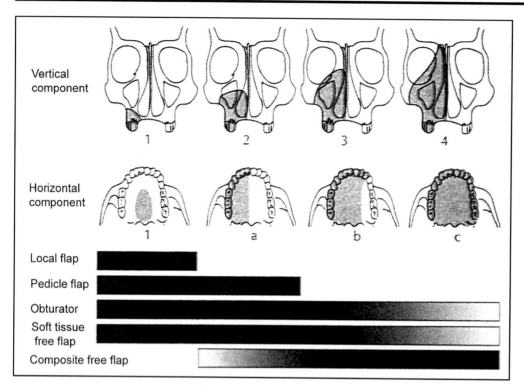

Figure 19–1 Classification scheme for maxillectomy defects proposed by Brown et al. Class 1 through 4 describes the vertical dimension of the maxillectomy. Class 2 to 4 are qualified by the addition of a letter (a to c), which describes the horizontal component. Vertical component class 1: maxillectomy with no oroantral fistula; class 2: low maxillectomy; class 3: high maxillectomy; class 4: radical maxillectomy. Horizontal components: a, unilateral alveolar maxilla and hard palate resected, less than or equal to half the alveolar and hard palate resection not involving the nasal septum or crossing the midline; b, bilateral alveolar maxilla and hard palate resected; includes a smaller resection that crosses the midline of the alveolar bone including the nasal septum; c, the removal of the entire alveolar maxilla and hard palate. Defects of the hard palate that result in an oronasal fistula but preserve the dental-bearing portion of the maxilla are also designated as class 1 defects since the horizontal component has minimal impact on functional and dental outcome (*lower left*). (From Brown JS, Rogers SN, McNally DN, Boyle M. A modified classification for the maxillectomy defect. Head Neck 2000;22:17–26, with permission of John Wiley & Sons, Inc.)

Cordeiro and Santamaria[1] from Memorial Sloan-Kettering Cancer Center (MSKCC) have advocated the use of a maxillectomy defect classification that is a modification of the classification originally proposed by Spiro and colleagues[13] from the same institution (discussed in Chapter 13). In this system, the six-walled geometric structure (hexahedrium) of the intact maxilla has been used to describe four major types of defects. Type I defects include resection of one or two walls of the maxilla, but with preservation of the palate. In this situation, resection of the anterior wall and either the medial wall or orbital floor has usually been performed. Type II defects result from resection of the lower walls of the hexahedrium—the maxillary arch, palate, anterior, and lateral walls, with preservation of the orbital floor. A total maxillectomy is termed a type III defect, in which all six walls of the maxilla are resected, including the orbital floor. Preservation or exenteration of the orbital contents designates a type III defect as either a type IIIa or IIIb defect, respectively. Lastly, type IV defects ("orbitomaxillectomy") involve ablation of the orbital contents and the upper five walls of the maxilla, but with preservation of the palate. The authors used this classification system to estimate the surface area/volume requirement for reconstruction as well as the need for palatal closure and orbital reconstruction, and developed an algorithm to determine the most optimal method of reconstruction for each defect. This scheme, however, does not characterize the quantity of remaining palate and dentition; describing rehabilitation with a dental prosthesis or osseointegrated implant-borne prosthesis would require a more complete depiction of the defect.

◆ Prosthetic Obturation

Predating most surgical reconstructive techniques, restoration of maxillectomy defects has traditionally involved the use of a dental obturative prosthesis.[14] Compared with flap reconstruction, rehabilitation with an obturator shortens the duration and lessens the complexity of the surgical procedure. Dental restoration and effective separation of the sinonasal and oral cavities can be achieved in this manner as long as sufficient maxilla and upper dentition have been preserved. In general, one third of the maxillary alveolar arch is necessary to adequately support and retain a removable prosthesis. The presence of periodontally sound abutment teeth also provides a critical source of additional retention for the prosthesis. Depending on the defect, a prosthesis may be fashioned to restore maxillary as well as nasal, orbital, and ocular defects, and can be used alone or in combination with surgical flaps.[7,15]

Nevertheless, prosthetic rehabilitation has shortcomings that must be considered during the reconstructive decision-making process. Speech and swallowing may be impaired when the prosthesis is not in place, and the prosthesis requires regular removal and cleaning for hygiene, which may be cumbersome and technically difficult, particularly for the elderly, patients with trismus, or those with residual monocular vision.[7,16,17] Failure to obtain a leak-tight seal without irritation frequently accounts for ongoing difficulties with speech and hygiene.[18,19] Larger prostheses must rely on the support and retention provided by the remaining tissues, and a lack of native hard-tissue support limits their utility.

Rehabilitation with a prosthesis does not preclude surgical reconstruction at a later date, but immediate reconstruction simplifies the performance of microvascular dissection and averts the psychologic and emotional impact resulting from disfigurement.[6] Although removable prostheses allow for the direct inspection of surgical defects, the role that direct inspection plays in the early detection of local recurrence has not been proven, and the availability of more sophisticated imaging modalities has diminished the import of clinical examination as the sole means of tumor surveillance. Reconstructive surgeons must carefully compare and contrast the likely outcomes following prosthetic or surgical reconstruction of a particular defect so that the most appropriate rehabilitative option is chosen.

◆ Evolution of Surgical Reconstructive Options

Early techniques of autogenous maxillary reconstruction, described by von Langenbeck[20] in 1862 and further detailed by Gullane and Arena[21] in 1977, began with use of local palatal flaps for small defects. Reconstructive options increased during the mid-twentieth century with the introduction of various local and regional flaps that borrowed tissue from adjacent sites within the oral cavity or areas such as the nose, pharynx, and forehead.[22] In 1948, reconstruction of the maxilla with an iliac bone graft in combination with pedicled soft tissue flaps was successfully used to support a removable denture.[23]

Pedicled myocutaneous flaps that provided larger volumes of well-vascularized soft tissue were developed in the 1960s and 1970s.[24,25] However, these flaps tend to be bulkier than necessary and have limited pliability, often resulting in suboptimal maxillectomy defect reconstruction. The subsequent development of microvascular anastomotic techniques allowed for free tissue transfers, yielding a tremendous breakthrough in the ability to reconstruct defects in a single stage without the limitations of reach and orientation of regional myocutaneous pedicled flaps. This technique allows a wide array of donor tissue types to be used so that the defect can be restored with tissue that matches the original size, shape, and quality of the original soft and hard tissues. A variety of free tissue

transfer donor sites have been described for maxillectomy defects, including radial forearm, rectus abdominis, fibula subscapular system, and iliac crest.[2,6,7,26–38] Flap selection should be determined by a variety of factors. The amount, location, and quality of residual bone of the midface, dentition, and denture bearing alveolar arch largely determine whether a bone-containing flap is necessary. Length of the vascular pedicle; thickness of the skin, muscle, and subcutaneous fat; the volume of the tissue available; the durability and thickness of the bone; and donor-site morbidity are important factors.

Osseointegrated titanium implants, pioneered by Branemark,[39] have extended the reconstructive reach of both prostheses and composite free tissue transfer.[40,41] Free flaps with sufficient bone stock to support osseointegrative implantation include the fibula, iliac crest, and occasionally, the scapula.[8,9] The principles of osseointegration, implantation, and prosthodontic restoration following implantation are discussed in Chapters 22 and 23.

◆ Defect-Specific Reconstruction of the Maxillectomy Defect

Although great technical strides have been made in the field of maxillary and midface reconstruction, the complexity and heterogeneity of the defects that are encountered, in addition to the array of reconstructive methods that are available, have hindered the development of a standardized reconstructive algorithm.[42] Available options for the reconstruction of eight types of maxillectomy defects are reviewed here. Reference to the Brown and MSKCC classification systems is provided when applicable, although some defects are not encompassed by these schemes.

Palate and Alveolar Arch Defects (Brown Class 1)

Small defects involving the alveolar ridge, teeth, and surrounding mucosa with adequate dentition and no oroantral fistula (Brown class 1) have a greater functional than aesthetic consequence, and may be allowed to heal by secondary intention or can be covered with a local flap. Numerous local flap techniques are available, including those from the cleft lip and palate literature.[43–45] Among these, the palatal island flap stands out as a versatile and reliable local flap capable of covering defects up to 15 cm^2. This sensate flap, which is based on the greater palatine vessels, can be elevated away from as much as 90% of the hard palate and rotated up to 180 degrees on its pedicle.[46] Its reach may be extended an additional centimeter by removing the hook of the hamulus, thereby releasing the neurovascular bundle from the greater palatine foramen; this maneuver can lead to eustachian tube dysfunction by disrupting the anterior tendonous insertion of the tensor veli palatini.[46] Irradiated local tissues may limit flap success, and in cases where more conservative therapies fail, use of a thin fasciocutaneous free flap may become necessary.[47] A functional dentition can be restored using a prosthesis supported by retained teeth or osseointegrated implants.

Inferior Maxillectomy (Brown Class 2, MSKCC Type II)

When the defect described above is enlarged to include an oroantral or oronasal fistula, sealing the oral cavity becomes paramount. Restoration of functional dentition and bony support of the anterior arch are also important goals in these defects. If the amount, quality, and location of residual dentition or edentulous alveolar arch are sufficient (i.e., Brown class 2a or 2b), these objectives may be met by using a prosthesis. However, prosthetic replacement of a large anterior arch defect is unlikely to provide adequate support of the upper lip and nasal base.

Even if a prosthesis is used, autogenous soft tissue reconstruction may improve the functional outcome by improving hygiene, increasing tolerance of an imperfectly fitting device, decreasing the size and weight of the obturator, and permanently establishing oronasal separation. Alternatively, autogenous tissue flaps may obviate the need for a prosthesis altogether. A local flap such as the palatal island flap, described above, is often sufficient to seal a palatal fistula.[48] In one published series that reported the use of this flap to reconstruct the palate in 10 patients, eight healed without fistula reformation, and an oral diet was resumed an average of 3.3 days following surgery.[49] A pedicled temporalis flap in combination with skin grafting may provide adequate coverage for a larger defect or in cases where prior irradiation requires the placement of well-vascularized tissue.[50] Choung et al[51] describe the use of ipsilateral or bilateral temporalis muscle with or without a segment of attached calvarial bone. This flap may be passed into the oral cavity by performing anterior and posterior osteotomies of the zygomatic arch and mobilizing the temporalis to its attachments on the coronoid process and deep temporal artery.

Alternatively, Hatoko et al[47] reported success in reconstructing inferior maxillectomies with a fasciocutaneous radial forearm free tissue transfer in three patients who had tolerated obturation poorly. The flap was folded upon itself to provide keratinized epithelium on the oral and nasal surfaces and covered palatal defects up to 20 cm² in size.[47] The patients' articulatory and masticatory function improved, flap drooping was minimal, and two patients were able to wear a denture over the flap.

As the size of the inferior maxilla defect increases and as the quality and quantity of residual alveolar arch and teeth decreases, soft tissue reconstructions may achieve separation of the oral and sinonasal cavities, but they tend to droop into the oral cavity and may provide inadequate support for a denture during functional loading.[7,52] Osseointegrated implants that have been placed into the remaining alveolar arch may partially overcome this problem, but masticatory forces can rotate the attached prosthesis about the stable native maxilla. In contrast, bony reconstruction of the maxillary arch produces a surface that is capable of symmetrically distributing cephalad masticatory forces over a broad, stable surface. However, the alveolar contour, palatal arch, and gingivobuccal sulcus depths are frequently blunted in these reconstructive efforts, so adequate retention for prostheses must by provided by the remaining dentition (**Fig. 19–2**).[7]

Futran and Haller[19] used the radial forearm flap to reconstruct six anterior arch defects requiring thin, pliable tissue with minimal bulk. Improved restoration of the arch contour was achieved in four patients by incorporating vascularized radial bone. Although the partial radius bone stock cannot withstand osseointegrated dental implantation, these patients maintained a regular diet with the use of conventional dentures. In addition, patients had near-normal speech and an acceptable aesthetic result without retraction of the upper lip. Villaret and Futran[53] subsequently expounded on the indications and technical considerations of this osteocutaneous radial forearm flap. The risk of pathologic radial fractures after harvesting this flap may be significantly reduced by rigid titanium fixation of the donor-site radial bone.

Secondary reconstruction of anterior maxillary defects with fibular flaps has been used to provide a stable base for prosthetic rehabilitation.[29] Free osteocutaneous scapula flaps and free tissue transfer using a fasciocutaneous forearm flap followed by secondary iliac crest bone grafting have also been described for patients with defects of the alveolar process, palate, and the anterior or lateral maxillary sinus wall who did not tolerate obturation. Secondary nonvascularized bone grafting appears to confer a greater risk of infection in this setting.[54]

Resections involving the hemipalate and a significant vertical component of the maxilla, not including the orbital floor (Brown class 2a, MSKCC type II), were reconstructed by Futran and Haller[19] with myocutaneous free flaps. Due to the volume of tissue required to refill the midface contour, rectus abdominis and latissimus dorsi flaps were used. The remaining dentition was sufficient to support a conventional prosthesis. The latissimus dorsi free flap is a versatile option for this type of defect that typically provides aesthetic contours to the midface and an effective palatal seal.[55] Cordeiro and Santamaria[1] reconstructed this defect using the abdominis rectus flap in six patients, and the radial forearm osteocutaneous "sandwich" flap in four patients. The latter flap uses the radius to reconstitute the alveolar arch, whereas the large harvested skin surface is folded, covering the bone on the nasal and oral surfaces. All of the patients were able to speak intelligibly, and 46% of the patients had normal speech. Two-thirds of the patients were able to resume a soft diet, and the remaining third were capable of oral intake. Olsen et al[6] successfully used the rectus abdominus flap for these defects, documenting similar postoperative results. These soft tissue reconstructions, however, do not address the defect of the maxillary bony skeleton, particularly the orbit, zygoma, and alveolus. Furthermore, they have the tendency to obliterate the ipsilateral nasal airway when the medial maxillary wall is resected.

Removal of the entire alveolar maxilla and hard palate in combination with a vertical resection that preserves the orbital floor (Brown class 2c), or subtotal resection in patients with minimal or no remaining dentition (Brown class 2b), provides inadequate support and retention for a prosthesis.[10] In a review of 10 patients who underwent osseous free flap reconstructions (nine fibular and one scapular) for reconstruction of the defects described above, Futran and Haller[19] noted that the extensive length of bone used for these larger defects leaves less pedicle length to reach the recipient vessels, and a vein graft was required in eight patients. Six of these patients subsequently underwent full dental restoration using osseointegrated implants.

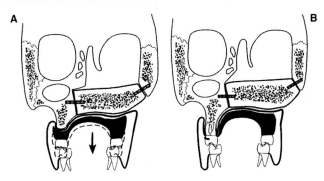

Figure 19–2 (A) Reconstructed maxillary arch with blunted neo-alveolar contour and buccal vestibules provides poor retention of the denture prosthesis in the edentulous patient, and the denture will tend to fall away from the reconstructed roof of the mouth (*arrow*). **(B)** Remaining dental abutments in the residual maxilla serve to retain the denture. The bony reconstruction provides a symmetric, broad distribution of support for the prosthesis during function. (From Funk G, Arcuri MR, Frodel JL. Functional dental rehabilitation of massive palato-maxillary defects: cases requiring free tissue transfer and osseo-integrated implants. Head Neck 1998;20:38–51, with permission of John Wiley & Sons, Inc.)

Osseointegrated implantation should be delayed if the size of the defect and the retention of adequate periodontally healthy teeth provide an environment that is conducive to prosthetic rehabilitation. An interim prosthesis may be used postoperatively to evaluate patient function with a tissue-borne prosthesis. If the patient performs well with the tissue-borne prosthesis, the additional procedure and expense of implantation have been avoided. On the other hand, if the patient exhibits poor masticatory or articulatory function secondary to prosthetic instability, implants can be placed 6 to 8 weeks after flap reconstruction. In situations where a patient is unlikely to function with a tissue-borne prosthesis, immediate implant placement into the bone flap and the adjacent alveolar ridge should be pursued.[7]

Futran et al[32] reported the use of the fibula free flap in 27 patients with defects of the maxilla that were not amenable to the use of a conventional prosthesis. This group consisted of 12 unilateral inferior maxillectomies (Brown class 2b, MSKCC type II), 8 bilateral inferior maxillectomies (Brown class 2c), and 7 total maxillectomies with orbital preservation (Brown class 3b or 3c, MSKCC class IIIa).[1,10] The decision to use a fibula flap was based on the determination by a maxillofacial prosthodontist that insufficient prosthesis-retentive surfaces remained. The fibula was chosen for its ability to support osseointegrative implants, which were placed in 18 patients. All but one flap survived. Wound complications developed in 4 but were successfully managed with local wound care. The cosmetic results achieved following reconstruction of the inferior maxilla were excellent, and the ability to speak intelligibly over the telephone was reported in all of the patients. Fourteen patients enjoyed a regular diet, and the remaining 13 patients used a soft diet. Scapular osteocutaneous free flaps have also been used with some degree of success for a variety of midface defects, including inferior maxillectomies.[56]

Bilateral Inferior Maxillectomy

Complete bilateral inferior maxillectomies—that is, defects in which only the orbital supporting bone and zygomatic arch remain—may be fully reconstructed with a scapular osteocutaneous free flap and osseointegrated implants. Configuring the bony flap so that the biomechanical load of mastication is placed axially on the implants negates the torque on the abutment, thus yielding a durable replacement of the vertical maxillary buttresses (**Fig. 19–3**).[7] The scapula osteocutaneous flap is well-suited to this reconstruction (**Fig. 19–4**). If a prosthesis is used that must bear the entire load of mastication, a minimum of four implants should be placed. In contrast, only two implants are necessary if most of the loading forces are borne by the bony reconstruction; in this case, the implants serve mainly to stabilize the denture prosthesis.[7]

Attaching a prosthesis to osseointegrated implants that have been placed into the remaining superior maxilla in lieu of a load-bearing bony reconstruction of the alveolar arch can be problematic. The unavoidable discrepancy between the axis of the implant and the direction of occlusal forces yields a biomechanically unfavorable support and the potential for fracture. The bone stock of the mid-maxilla is also too thin to accommodate implants, and this area is difficult to reach for routine maintenance of hygiene.[7,57]

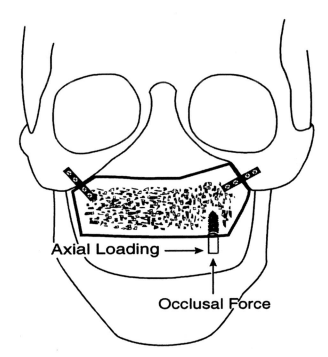

Figure 19–3 Maxilla reconstructed with an implantable bone surface parallel to the occlusal forces. This configuration allows the implants to be placed axial to the loading occlusal forces, which is biomechanically the most favorable orientation for the implants. (From Funk G, Arcuri MR, Frodel JL. Functional dental rehabilitation of massive palatomaxillary defects: cases requiring free tissue transfer and osseointegrated implants. Head Neck 1998;20:38–51, with permission of John Wiley & Sons, Inc.)

Anterior Maxillary Wall with Cutaneous Defect (MSKCC Type I)

Defects limited to the anterior wall of the maxillary sinus with cutaneous loss are usually the result of a skin cancer resection, and are discussed only briefly here. A local skin

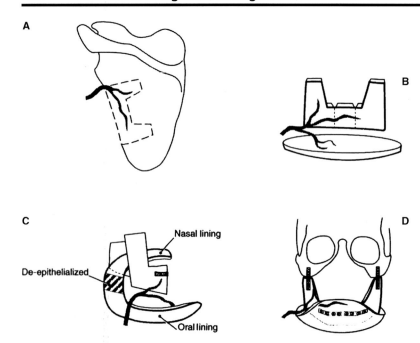

Figure 19–4 Schematic representation of scapular flap contouring and inset for maxillary reconstruction. **(A)** Medial extensions from the lateral border are included to fashion the zygomaticomaxillary buttresses. **(B)** Closing osteotomies to form the maxillary arch. **(C)** Transverse scapula skin paddle covers the lateral border of scapular bone intraorally. **(D)** The skin paddle is used to close the palatal defect posteriorly and reline the nasal floor. The de-epithelialized segment is sutured to the nasal and oral surfaces at the posterior margin of the defect. (From Funk G, Arcuri MR, Frodel JL. Functional dental rehabilitation of massive palatomaxillary defects: cases requiring free tissue transfer and osseointegrated implants. Head Neck 1998;20:38–51, with permission of John Wiley & Sons, Inc.)

flap such as a facial advancement flap with or without skin grafting on the deep surface may suffice for smaller defects not previously irradiated. Tissue from outside an irradiated field, such as the paramedian forehead flap or, for larger defects, the radial forearm or lateral arm free flaps, may become necessary.

Total Maxillectomy with Orbital Preservation (Brown Class 3, MSKCC Type IIIa)

Certain situations involving total maxillectomy in which the orbital structures are preserved may present a technical challenge to the reconstructive surgeon. In addition to the considerable task of restoring oral function and aesthetics, reconstitution of the inferior orbital wall becomes paramount. Without adequate support of the orbit, enophthalmos, vertical dystopia, and diplopia may result.[56] The reconstructive task for this defect is more technically challenging than when the orbital contents are also resected.[1]

Various reconstructive techniques for this defect are available, and rehabilitation with a prosthetic device has been described.[58] Soft tissue pedicled flaps such as the temporalis flap are useful in patients who are not candidates for free tissue transfer.[1,2,55] The addition of vascularized calvarial bone to the temporalis flap can also provide high-quality bone for rigid orbital support[51,59,60] Coleman[2] recommends the use of a vascularized soft tissue flap in combination with primary or secondary nonvascularized bone grafting to re-create the complex three-dimensional structure of regions such as the orbital floor, medial orbital wall, and nasal dorsum. He prefers the free omentum flap for its ability to drape around irregularly shaped bone grafts and the residual skeletal framework. The nasal and external surfaces are easily covered by skin grafting. Latissimus, gracilis, and rectus abdominis muscle flaps also provide an excellent matrix for nonvascularized bone grafts. Cordeiro and Santamaria[1] from MSKCC advocate an approach to reconstruction

following total maxillectomy with orbital preservation that is similar to Coleman's (**Fig. 19–5**). Rigid globe support is maintained by cranial or rib bone graft, whereas the remainder of the defect is filled with fat and muscle supplied by an abdominis rectus free tissue transfer. The skin island is oriented inferiorly to seal the oral cavity. The most notable feature of this reconstructive approach is the use of soft tissue on the inferior surface of the maxilla. This method was also used by Futran and Haller[19] in eight patients who underwent cranial bone grafting to restore the zygomatic bone and orbital floor in addition to the rectus abdominis or latissimus dorsi myocutaneous free flap. Oral function may be restored when adequate support for a tissue-borne prosthesis remains, but bony reconstruction of the alveolar arch offers a superior result in patients who are edentulous or nearly edentulous and in patients who have defects that extend significantly across the midline.

Vascularized osteocutaneous free flaps have the advantage of being more infection resistant than nonvascularized bone-graft reconstructions and are better able to maintain bony volume.[2] For total maxillectomy defects with orbital preservation, the subscapular system of flaps, although technically more complex, offers perhaps the greatest versatility in flap reconstruction.[33,34,37,56] If adequate teeth and retentive surfaces are not available, restoration of mastication requires sufficient vascularized bone to support an implant-borne maxillary prosthesis, which limits flap choices to the subscapular system, fibula, and iliac crest. The iliac crest has a short pedicle and the fibula and iliac crest offer limited soft tissue. Replacement of the alveolar arch inferiorly with the lateral scapula (supplied by the circumflex scapular artery) and the orbital floor and rim with the scapular tip (supplied by the angular branch of the thoracodorsal artery) suits this reconstruction well. The thoracodorsal artery supplies the latissimus dorsi muscle, which may be harvested partially or completely for a wide range of soft tissue reconstructive needs. Furthermore, each of the two components of this flap may be rotated independently of each other.[2,33]

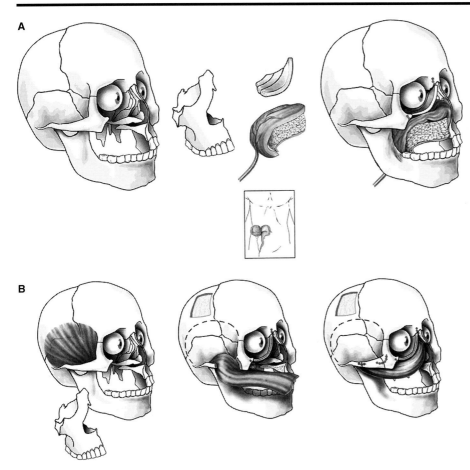

Figure 19–5 **(A)** Memorial Sloan-Kettering Cancer Center (MSKCC) type IIIa defect (Brown class 3 defect). Note resection of all six walls of the maxilla, including the floor of orbit and hard palate. The orbital contents have been preserved (*left*). The resected specimen demonstrates the orbital floor, vertical maxillary buttresses, and palate (*center, left*). This creates a medium surface-area/medium volume defect. Cranial or rib bone graft is used to reconstruct floor of orbit and is covered with single-skin-island rectus abdominis myocutaneous flap (*center, right*). The rectus abdominis myocutaneous flap (donor site depicted in *inset*) provides medium surface area with medium volume. The bone graft is rigidly fixed to reconstruct the floor of orbit. The rectus abdominis myocutaneous flap is inset with the skin island used to close the roof of the palate, soft tissue to fill in the midfacial defect, and muscle to cover the bone graft. Note the extended length of deep inferior epigastric vessels to neck (*right*). **(B)** Patients who are not free-flap candidates may be reconstructed with split calvarial bone grafts, covered with the temporalis muscle, transposed anteriorly. The zygomatic arch should be osteotomized and removed temporarily to increase excursion of the temporalis muscle. (From Cordeiro PG, Santamaria E. A classification system and algorithm for reconstruction of maxillectomy and midfacial defects. Plast Reconstr Surg 2000;105:2331–2346, with permission.)

Schliephake[54] found that although the lateral border of the scapula commonly provides enough bone volume to accommodate dental implants, it is difficult to tailor the bone in a fashion that simultaneously restores the malar prominence, the infraorbital rim, and the maxillary wall, while placing the lateral border of the scapula in an appropriate position for placement of these implants. He concluded that secondary bone grafting for augmentation becomes necessary to provide enough bone stock in the desired location. These techniques have been used with success in the reconstruction of complex midface and skull base defects.[36] The scapular bone, however, may not always be suitable for placement of osseointegrated implants. Further disadvantages in the use of the subscapular system include difficulty in harvesting the flap simultaneously with the extirpative procedure; difficulty in orienting the bone to provide orbit, zygoma, and alveolar reconstruction; and the relatively short pedicle length.

Futran and Haller[19] described the use of a revascularized fibular osteocutaneous free flap in seven patients who had undergone total maxillectomy with orbital preservation. Although superior and inferior bony support was achieved, flattening of the midface occurred. Osseointegrated implants were placed or planned in most of these patients. The bone stock of the fibula is more conducive to implantation than the scapula, whereas the scapula usually yields a superior aesthetic result.

Total Maxillectomy with Orbital Exenteration (Brown Class 4, MSKCC Type IIIb)

When maxillary tumor resection extends to the supraorbital rim, reconstructive options depend on the amount of remaining dentition (**Fig. 19–6A**).[1] When adequate teeth and alveolar arch remain, prosthetic replacement is an option. However, the

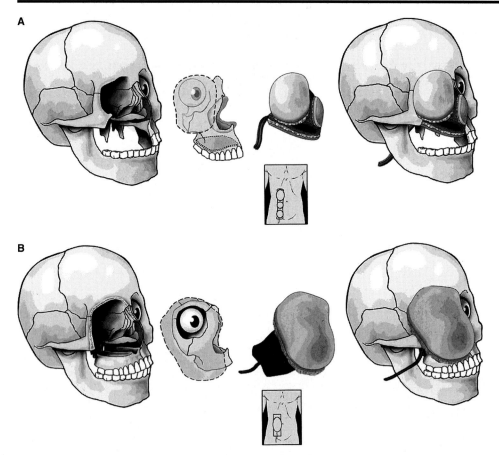

Figure 19-6 **(A)** MSKCC type IIIb defect (Brown class 4 defect). Note resection of all six walls of the maxilla, including the floor of the orbit as well as orbital contents (*left*). Resected specimen demonstrates resection of external eyelid, cheek skin, and orbital contents, in combination with entire maxilla and palate (*center, left*). This creates a large surface area/large volume defect. A three-skin-island rectus abdominis myocutaneous flap design is shown in the *inset*. This flap provides multiple large surface areas with a large volume of soft tissue and muscle to fill in the defect (*center, right*). The rectus abdominis myocutaneous flap (*inset*) demonstrates skin islands to resurface the external skin and palatal defect with muscle and subcutaneous fat used to fill in the soft tissue deficit. If technically feasible, a third skin island can be used to reconstruct the lateral wall of the nose (*right*).

(B) MSKCC type IV (orbitomaxillectomy) defect. Note resection of upper five walls of maxilla, including the orbital contents but sparing the palate (*left*). The resected specimen demonstrates resection of the orbital contents, eyelid, and cheek skin, in continuity with bone (*center, left*). This creates a large surface area/large volume defect. (*Inset*) Design of single-skin-island rectus abdominis myocutaneous flap. This flap provides large surface area with large volume to reconstruct the defect (*center, right*). Rectus abdominis myocutaneous flap in place, demonstrating skin island to resurface the external skin defect with muscle and subcutaneous fat used to fill in the soft tissue deficit (*right*). (From Cordeiro PG, Santamaria E. A classification system and algorithm for reconstruction of maxillectomy and midfacial defects. Plast Reconstr Surg 2000; 105:2331–2346, with permission.)

use of a prosthesis that spans the defect from the oral cavity to the orbit is subject to cheek retraction, poor adaptation of the prosthesis to the contours of the defect, and the distracting appearance of an unblinking, expressionless eye. A superior approach is to replace the palate and alveolar arch with a prosthetic device in conjunction with a bulky myocutaneous flap, such as the abdominis rectus, to fill the midface volume, including the orbit. Cordeiro and Santamaria[1] found that almost half of the patients had an acceptable cosmetic result, 77% regained normal or near-normal speech, and 54% were able to consume a soft diet. To achieve adequate bone volume for both the infraorbital and zygomatic region as well as the alveolar arch, Brown et al[61] advocated the iliac crest myo-osseous flap for midfacial reconstruction. Although they achieved excellent functional and cosmetic results in three patients, others have discouraged the use of this flap in the maxilla because of its excessive bulk, poor skin mobility in

relationship to the bone, and short pedicle length. Use of a scapular free flap to reconstruct the palate and alveolar arch with autogenous vascularized bone may provide an optimal reconstruction by availing ipsilateral osseointegrated implants for prosthesis support and retention as well as adequate bulk for restoration of the cosmetic appearance of the cheek. Of the flaps that have been discussed, the scapula also provides the best skin color match to the midface.

Orbitomaxillectomy (MSKCC Type IV)

Resection of the upper five walls of the maxilla and the orbital contents with preservation of the inferior palatal surface of the maxilla (MSKCC type IV, or orbitomaxillectomy defect) is a somewhat simpler defect to reconstruct than either the total maxillectomy with orbital preservation or the total maxillectomy with orbital exenteration (MSKCC types IIIa and IIIb, respectively) because no horizontal bone must be reconstructed (**Fig. 19–6B**).[1] A single skin-island abdominis rectus flap fills the large volume and large surface area defect appropriately, yielding a fair to good cosmetic result in 75% of the patients.

Infraorbital or Malar Maxillectomy with or Without Exenteration

Supporting an intact globe and functional periocular soft tissue is critical to maintaining functional vision and the normal appearance of this important aesthetic unit. The reconstruction of limited superior maxillectomy defects can be challenging, because the surgeon must locate a source of bone-containing tissue that is small enough to accommodate this type of defect. Prosthetics have no role in this situation, and allografts are prone to extrusion and infection.

The pedicled temporalis and vascularized calvarial bone flap offers appropriately thin and high-quality bone for orbital support.[51,59,60] Access to the orbital floor and infraorbital rim requires resection of at least a part of the lateral maxilla, which may weaken the important zygomaticomaxillary buttress. In addition, this flap places the upper division of the facial nerve at risk, and results in an unnatural appearing temporal depression. Thus, this flap should be reserved for patients who are not candidates for free tissue transfer.

Chepeha et al[62] outlined their approach to orbital restoration in a series of 19 patients with orbital defects. Defects resulting from orbital exenteration with preservation of less than 30% of the bony orbital rim were reconstructed with the osseocutaneous forearm flap. In contrast, orbital exenteration cavities with preservation of the orbital rim were reconstructed with fasciocutaneous forearm flaps. Finally, for defects created by radical orbital exenteration that also included resection of overlying skin and bony malar eminence, osseocutaneous scapula flaps were used. Among 16 patients with greater than 4 months of follow-up, 10 were judged to have minimal or no facial contour deformity, eight frequently engaged in social activities outside the home, and five of nine patients who were employed preoperatively subsequently returned to work. The advantages of autologous tissue reconstruction of the orbit, according to these investigators, include durability, minimization of defect size, avoidance of potential accidental displacement of a patch or prosthesis, and the tendency for attention to be drawn toward the opposite, functional eye instead of a static ocular prosthesis. Additionally, when the eyelids and orbicularis oculi muscles remain unresected, the eyelids may be sewn together, preserving skin color match and facial expression, including the blink reflex. Reconstruction of the infraorbital rim, anterior maxillary wall, and overlying soft tissues has also been successfully performed with the osseocutaneous radial forearm free flap.[27]

◆ Conclusion

Improvements in autogenous tissue reconstruction and prosthetic rehabilitation of the maxilla and midface after cancer resection continue to evolve. The morbidity of maxilla and midface resections remains significant, however, due to the numerous and complex functions of this anatomic region. The current maxillary reconstructive techniques have several limitations, including imperfect restoration of the nasal airway, replacement of mucosa with skin, and the inability to replicate the complex contours of the midfacial bones and their soft tissue coverings. A therapeutic plan should be chosen that addresses the anticipated consequences of a particular surgical defect, optimizes local tissue healing capacity, and takes full advantage of the array of available surgical and prosthetic rehabilitative options. Midface reconstruction demands a thoughtful and multidisciplinary approach by the extirpative surgeon, reconstructive surgeon, prosthodontist, and radiation oncologist to achieve long-term functional and aesthetic success.

References

1. Cordeiro PG, Santamaria E. A classification system and algorithm for reconstruction of maxillectomy and midfacial defects. Plast Reconstr Surg 2000;105:2331–2346

2. Coleman JJ III. Osseous reconstruction of the midface and orbits. Clin Plast Surg 1994;21:113–124

3. Mustarde JC. Repair and Reconstruction in the Orbital Region. New York: Churchill Livingstone, 1991

4. Yoshida H, Michi K, Yamashita Y, Ohno K. A comparison of surgical and prosthetic treatment for speech disorders attributable to surgically acquired soft palate defects. J Oral Maxillofac Surg 1993;51:361–365

5. Mines MA, Hanson BF, Shoup JE. Frequency of occurrence of phonemes in conversational English. Lang Speech 1978;21:221–241

6. Olsen KD, Meland NB, Ebersold MJ, Bartley GB, Garrity JA. Extensive defects of the sino-orbital region. Results with microvascular reconstruction. Arch Otolaryngol Head Neck Surg 1992;118:828–833

7. Funk GF, Arcuri MR, Frodel JL Jr. Functional dental rehabilitation of massive palatomaxillary defects: cases requiring free tissue transfer and osseointegrated implants. Head Neck 1998;20:38–51

8. Moscoso JF, Keller J, Genden E, et al. Vascularized bone flaps in oromandibular reconstruction: a comparative anatomic study of bone stock from various donor sites to assess suitability for enosseous dental implants. Arch Otolaryngol Head Neck Surg 1994;120:36–43

9. Frodel JL Jr, Funk GF, Capper DT, et al. Osseointegrated implants: a comparative study of bone thickness in four vascularized bone flaps. Plast Reconstr Surg 1993;92:449–455

10. Brown JS, Rogers SN, McNally DN, Boyle M. A modified classification for the maxillectomy defect. Head Neck 2000;22:17–26

11. Wells MD, Luce EA. Reconstruction of midfacial defects after surgical resection of malignancies. Clin Plast Surg 1995;22:79–89

12. Triana RJ Jr, Uglesic V, Virag M, et al. Microvascular free flap reconstructive options in patients with partial and total maxillectomy defects. Arch Facial Plast Surg 2000;2:91–101

13. Spiro RH, Strong EW, Shah JP. Maxillectomy and its classification. Head Neck 1997;19:309–314

14. Curtis TA, Beumer J. Restoration of acquired hard palate defects: etiology, disability, and rehabilitation. In: Beumer J, Curtis TA, Marunick MT, eds. Maxillofacial Rehabilitation: Prosthodontic and Surgical Considerations. St. Louis: Ishiyaku EroAmerica, 1996

15. Gliklich RE, Rounds MF, Cheney ML, Varvares MA. Combining free flap reconstruction and craniofacial prosthetic technique for orbit, scalp, and temporal defects. Laryngoscope 1998;108:482–487

16. Brown KE. Peripheral consideration in improving obturator retention. J Prosthet Dent 1968;20:176–181

17. Rahn AO, Boucher U. Maxillofacial Prosthetics: Principles and Concepts. Philadelphia: WB Saunders, 1970

18. Gillespie CA, Kenan PD, Ferguson BJ. Hard palate reconstruction in maxillectomy. Laryngoscope 1986;96:443–444

19. Futran ND, Haller JR. Considerations for free-flap reconstruction of the hard palate. Arch Otolaryngol Head Neck Surg 1999;125:665–669

20. von Langenback B. Die Uranoplastik Mittelst Abosung das Mucosperiostalen Guamenuberzuges. Arch Klin Chir Bd II 1862;Spring:205–287

21. Gullane PJ, Arena S. Palatal island flap for reconstruction of oral defects. Arch Otolaryngol 1977;103:598–599

22. Jackson IT. Local Flaps in Head and Neck Reconstruction. St. Louis: Mosby, 1985

23. Campbell HH. Reconstruction of the left maxilla. Plast Reconstr Surg 1948;3:66

24. Ariyan S. The pectoralis major myocutaneous flap: a versatile flap for reconstruction in the head and neck. Plast Reconstr Surg 1979; 63:73–81

25. Baker SR. Closure of large orbital-maxillary defects with free latissimus dorsi myocutaneous flaps. Head Neck Surg 1984;6:828–835

26. Cordeiro PG, Bacilious N, Schantz S, Spiro R. The radial forearm osteocutaneous "sandwich" free flap for reconstruction of the bilateral subtotal maxillectomy defect. Ann Plast Surg 1998;40:397–402

27. McLoughlin PM, Gilhooly M, Phillips JG. Reconstruction of the infraorbital margin with a composite microvascular free flap. Br J Oral Maxillofac Surg 1993;31:227–229

28. Chepeha DB, Moyer JS, Bradford CR, Prince ME, Marentette L, Teknos TN. Osseocutaneous radial forearm free tissue transfer for repair of complex midfacial defects. Arch Otolaryngol Head Neck Surg 2005;131:513–517

29. Nakayama B, Matsuura H, Ishihara O, Hasegawa H, Mataga I, Torii S. Functional reconstruction of a bilateral maxillectomy defect using a fibula osteocutaneous flap with osseointegrated implants. Plast Reconstr Surg 1995;96:1201–1204

30. Yim KK, Wei FC. Fibula osteoseptocutaneous free flap in maxillary reconstruction. Microsurgery 1994;15:353–357

31. Kazaoka Y, Shinohara A, Yokou K, Hasegawa T. Functional reconstruction after a total maxillectomy using a fibula osteocutaneous flap with osseointegrated implants. Plast Reconstr Surg 1999;103:1244–1246

32. Futran ND, Wadsworth JT, Villaret D, Farwell DG. Midface reconstruction with the fibula free flap. Arch Otolaryngol Head Neck Surg 2002;128:161–166

33. Swartz WM, Banis JC, Newton ED, Ramasastry SS, Jones NF, Acland R. The osteocutaneous scapular flap for mandibular and maxillary reconstruction. Plast Reconstr Surg 1986;77:530–545

34. Schusterman MA, Reece GP, Miller MJ. Osseous free flaps for orbit and midface reconstruction. Am J Surg 1993;166:341–345

35. Shestak KC, Schusterman MA, Jones NF, Johnson JT. Immediate microvascular reconstruction of combined palatal and midfacial defects using soft tissue only. Microsurgery 1988;9:128–131

36. Schmelzeisen R, Schliephake H. Interdisciplinary microvascular reconstruction of maxillary, midfacial and skull base defects. J Craniomaxillofac Surg 1998;26:1–10

37. Uglesic V, Virag M, Varga S, Knezevic P, Milenovic A. Reconstruction following radical maxillectomy with flaps supplied by the subscapular artery. J Craniomaxillofac Surg 2000;28:153–160

38. Brown JS. Deep circumflex iliac artery free flap with internal oblique muscle as a new method of immediate reconstruction of maxillectomy defect. Head Neck 1996;18:412–421

39. Branemark PI. Osseointegration and its experimental background. J Prosthet Dent 1983;50:399–410

40. Jackson IT, Tolman DE, Desjardins RP, Branemark PI. A new method for fixation of external prostheses. Plast Reconstr Surg 1986;77: 668–672

41. Tjellstrom A, Jacobsson M. The bone anchored maxillofacial prosthesis. In: Albrekston T, Zarb G, eds. The Branemark Osseointegrated Implant. Chicago: Quintessence, 1989

42. Ali A, Fardy MJ, Patton DW. Maxillectomy—to reconstruct or obturate? Results of a UK survey of oral and maxillofacial surgeons. Br J Oral Maxillofac Surg 1995;33:207–210

43. Obwegeser HL. Late reconstruction of large maxillary defects after tumor-resection. J Maxillofac Surg 1973;1:19–29

44. Drommer RB, Musgrove B. Skeletal reconstruction in cleft palate patients. Curr Opin Dent 1991;1:282–286

45. Millard DR Jr. Wide and/or short cleft palate. Plast Reconstr Surg 1962;29:40–57

46. Gullane PJ, Arena S. Extended palatal island mucoperiosteal flap. Arch Otolaryngol 1985;111:330–332

47. Hatoko M, Harashina T, Inoue T, Tanaka I, Imai K. Reconstruction of palate with radial forearm flap; a report of 3 cases. Br J Plast Surg 1990;43:350–354

48. Seckel NG. The palatal island flap on retrospection. Plast Reconstr Surg 1995;96:1262–1268

49. Moore BA, Magdy E, Netterville JL, Burkey BB. Palatal reconstruction with the palatal island flap. Laryngoscope 2003;113:946–951

50. Colmenero C, Martorell V, Colmenero B, Sierra I. Temporalis myofascial flap for maxillofacial reconstruction. J Oral Maxillofac Surg 1991;49:1067–1073

51. Choung PH, Nam IW, Kim KS. Vascularized cranial bone grafts for mandibular and maxillary reconstruction. The parietal osteofascial flap. J Craniomaxillofac Surg 1991;19:235–242

52. Beumer J, Nishumura R, Roumanas ED. Maxillary defect: alterations in surgery to enhance the prosthetic prognosis. In: Proceedings of the First International Congress on Maxillofacial Prosthetics. New York: Memorial Sloan-Kettering Cancer Center, 1995:22–26

53. Villaret DB, Futran NA. The indications and outcomes in the use of osteocutaneous radial forearm free flap. Head Neck 2003; 25:475–481

54. Schliephake H. Revascularized tissue transfer for the repair of complex midfacial defects in oncologic patients. J Oral Maxillofac Surg 2000;58:1212–1218

55. Shestak KC. Soft-tissue reconstruction of craniofacial defects. Clin Plast Surg 1994;21:107–111

56. Granick MS, Ramasastry SS, Newton ED, Solomon MP, Hanna DC, Kaltman S. Reconstruction of complex maxillectomy defects with the scapular-free flap. Head Neck 1990;12:377–385

57. Beumer J III, Roumanas E, Nishimura R. Advances in osseointegrated implants for dental and facial rehabilitation following major head and neck surgery. Semin Surg Oncol 1995;11:200–207

58. Wang RR. Sectional prosthesis for total maxillectomy patients: a clinical report. J Prosthet Dent 1997;78:241–244

59. Rose EH, Norris MS. The versatile temporoparietal fascial flap: adaptability to a variety of composite defects. Plast Reconstr Surg 1990;85:224–232

60. McCarthy JG, Zide BM. The spectrum of calvarial bone grafting: introduction of the vascularized calvarial bone flap. Plast Reconstr Surg 1984;74:10–18

61. Brown JS, Jones DC, Summerwill A, et al. Vascularized iliac crest with internal oblique muscle for immediate reconstruction after maxillectomy. Br J Oral Maxillofac Surg 2002;40:183–190

62. Chepeha DB, Wang SJ, Marentette LJ, et al. Restoration of the orbital aesthetic subunit in complex midface defects. Laryngoscope 2004;114:1706–1713

20

Radiation Therapy

Russell W. Hinerman,
Robert Amdur, and
William Mendenhall

◆ General Principles

Treatment Selection

Radiation therapy (RT), much like surgery, is a local-regional treatment modality. RT alone may be used in the management of oral cavity cancer to preserve function and cosmesis and to avoid the morbidity associated with a major operation. In addition, a course of RT is usually less expensive than an operation, although newer radiation techniques such as intensity-modulated RT (IMRT) are generally more costly than older, more conventional treatment regimes. RT may be combined with surgery postoperatively to destroy known or suspected residual cancer. It may also be used pre-operatively to render an advanced, unresectable cancer amenable to complete surgical removal. Finally, a short course of RT may be used to palliate the patient with advanced cancer in whom the possibility of cure is remote.

Radiation Therapy Modalities

Most patients receiving RT for oral cavity cancer are treated with external beam radiation for all or part of their treatment. Megavoltage photon beams are used for management of most cancers arising in the oral cavity; cobalt 60 (^{60}Co) or a 4- to 6-MV linear accelerator is ideal. A megavoltage x-ray beam delivers a relatively low dose to the skin surface and is associated with a high exit dose. As the beam energy increases, the surface dose decreases and the exit dose increases. In contrast, an electron beam delivers a relatively high dose to the skin and subcutaneous tissues; after one to several centimeters, the dose falls off very rapidly, and the exit dose is quite low. As the energy of the electron

beam increases, both the surface dose and the exit dose increase. Orthovoltage x-ray beams, with energies varying from 100 to 250 kV, deliver a maximal dose at the skin surface, and the depth dose falls off less steeply than that of an electron beam. Orthovoltage radiation is used in our department for the treatment of most skin cancers of the head and neck, although an electron beam is preferable for skin cancers on the forehead and the scalp because the dose to the underlying calvarium and the brain may be limited more effectively. The major drawback for using orthovoltage beams is the increased bone absorption compared with megavoltage radiation. Few community-based RT departments still have orthovoltage capabilities, and electrons are used in almost every instance where a megavoltage photon beam is felt to be either too penetrating or lacking sufficient surface dose. Intraoral cone RT is a form of external-beam irradiation given with an orthovoltage or electron beam through a cone placed into the oral cavity to deliver a boost dose to relatively early cancers.

Beams of protons or heavy ions (such as carbon or helium) are produced by a cyclotron and deliver a much more precisely defined high-dose volume with very steep dose falloff in comparison with an x-ray or electron beam. These beams are available for cancer treatment at the Massachusetts General Hospital (Boston, MA) and Loma Linda Medical School (Los Angeles, CA). The University of Florida also recently completed construction on a proton facility in Jacksonville. Neutron beams and pi meson beams have been used experimentally and have no proven advantage over conventional x-ray or electron beams.

Interstitial implants may be used to deliver all or part of the treatment for cancers of the oral cavity. It is necessary to define the tumor precisely and encompass it with the radioactive sources to perform a satisfactory implant. The advantages of interstitial treatment are that the high dose may be limited to a small volume of tissue and the treatment is delivered over a short overall time, producing a high probability of tumor control and a relatively low risk of complications. Cesium needles and iridium seeds or wires are frequently used for implantation in treating oral cavity cancers[1,2] (**Figs. 20–1** to **20–3**). Most oral cavity cancers that are technically suitable for brachytherapy should undergo an interstitial implant for all or part of the treatment because the probability of local control will be improved compared with external beam alone. An alternative to brachytherapy is the intraoral cone.

Radiation Therapy for Oral Tongue Cancer

Early (T1, T2, small T3) oral tongue cancer may be treated with either RT or surgery with an equal likelihood of cure.[3] Although the risk of a significant RT complication is low, surgery is the preferred treatment in the authors' institution because of a smaller risk of bone exposure or soft tissue necrosis that may persist for months or years after RT.[4] Patients are treated primarily with RT if they decline surgery or are at high risk for operative complications. More advanced tumors (large T3, T4) are best treated with a combination of surgery and RT, either pre- or postoperatively.

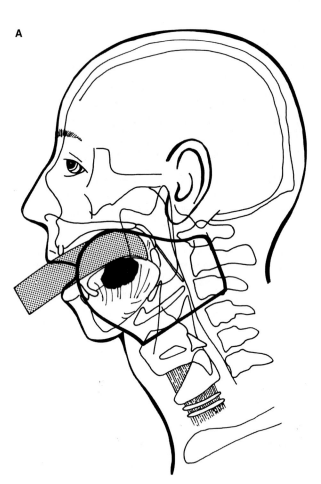

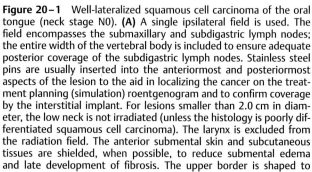

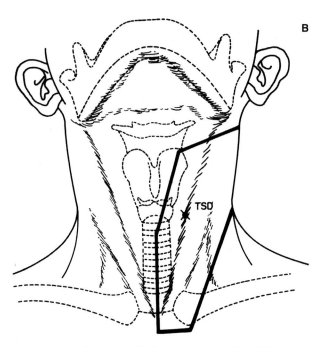

Figure 20–1 Well-lateralized squamous cell carcinoma of the oral tongue (neck stage N0). **(A)** A single ipsilateral field is used. The field encompasses the submaxillary and subdigastric lymph nodes; the entire width of the vertebral body is included to ensure adequate posterior coverage of the subdigastric lymph nodes. Stainless steel pins are usually inserted into the anteriormost and posteriormost aspects of the lesion to the aid in localizing the cancer on the treatment planning (simulation) roentgenogram and to confirm coverage by the interstitial implant. For lesions smaller than 2.0 cm in diameter, the low neck is not irradiated (unless the histology is poorly differentiated squamous cell carcinoma). The larynx is excluded from the radiation field. The anterior submental skin and subcutaneous tissues are shielded, when possible, to reduce submental edema and late development of fibrosis. The upper border is shaped to exclude most of the parotid gland. An intraoral lead block (*stippled area*) shields the contralateral mucosa. The block is coated with beeswax to prevent a high-dose effect on the adjacent mucosa resulting from scattered low-energy electrons from the metal surface. The usual preinterstitial tumor dose is 32 Gy using 1.6 Gy per fraction, twice-a-day fractionation. For larger lesions, which extend near the midline, treatment is applied by means of parallel opposed portals with no intraoral lead block. **(B)** For well-lateralized lesions greater than 2 cm in patients with a stage N0 neck, only the ipsilateral low neck is irradiated. TSD, target-to-skin distance. (From Parsons JT, Mendenhall WM. Million RR, Cassisi NJ. Treatment of tumors of the oropharynx. In: Thawley SE, Panje WR, Batsakis JG, Lindberg RD, eds. Comprehensive Management of Head and Neck Tumors. New York: Elsevier, 1987:692, with permission.)

A

B

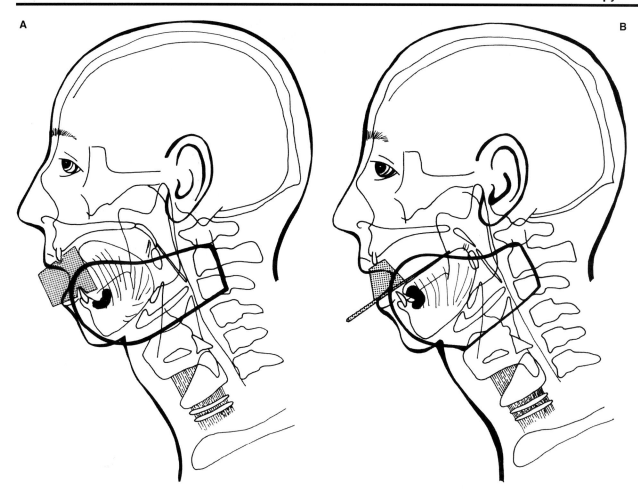

Figure 20–2 Portals for radiation therapy of floor of mouth cancer. **(A)** Limited anterior floor of mouth carcinoma (no tongue invasion and N0 or N1 neck disease). Two notches are cut on a cork so that it can be held in the same position between the patient's upper and lower incisors during every treatment session; the tip of the tongue is displaced from the treatment field. The anterior border of the field covers the full thickness of the mandibular arch. The lower field edge is at the thyroid cartilage, ensuring adequate coverage of the submandibular lymph nodes. The subdigastric lymph nodes will be adequately covered by treating the entire width of the vertebral bodies posteriorly. The superior border is shaped so much of the oral cavity, oropharynx, and parotid glands are out of the portal) with the aid of computer dosimetry. **(B)** Carcinoma of the floor of the mouth with tongue invasion. The tongue is depressed into the floor of the mouth with a tongue blade and cork as shown. (From Parsons JT, Mendenhall WM, Million RR, Cassisi NJ. Radiation therapy of tumors of the oral cavity. In: Thawley SE, Panje WR, Batsakis JG, Lindberg RD, eds. Comprehensive Management of Head and Neck Tumors. New York: Elsevier, 1987:522–523, with permission from Elsevier.)

The actuarial probabilities of local control by T stage at 2 years for patients treated with RT alone at our institution before and after surgical salvage, respectively, are as follows: T1 ($n = 18$), 79% and 93%; T2 ($n = 48$), 72% and 83%; T3 ($n = 29$), 45% and 57%; and T4 ($n = 10$), 0% and 0%. Actuarial cause-specific survival rates for American Joint Committee on Cancer (AJCC) stages I, II, and III at 5 years are 88%, 82%, and 55%, respectively. The risk of severe bone or soft tissue complications necessitating surgical intervention was 6%, 13%, and 3% respectively, for T1, T2, and T3 tumors.[4]

Radiation Therapy for Floor of Mouth Cancer

Until the late 1970s, most early floor of mouth cancers seen at our institution were treated with RT, reserving surgery for radiation failures. With the advent of rim resection, however, it became possible to resect these lesions with relatively little morbidity. Local control and survival rates after rim resection of early-stage cancers are similar to those achieved with RT.[3,5] The late morbidity of RT is greater than that of surgery because mandibular necrosis and soft tissue necrosis, although usually temporary, are not uncommon after treatment with primary radiation. Accordingly, T1 and T2 tumors are now generally treated surgically, particularly if the tumor abuts the gingiva. RT is added only if adverse pathologic factors are present. Patients who decline surgery or are at high risk for operative complications are still treated with primary RT.

The ideal candidate for treatment with radiation alone has a lesion that can be managed by use of an intraoral cone for all or part of the treatment; this produces a low risk of mandibular necrosis. The patient should be edentulous, ideally for several years, resulting in a decreased mandibular height, which facilitates cone placement. Interstitial implantation is essential if intraoral cone therapy is not possible.

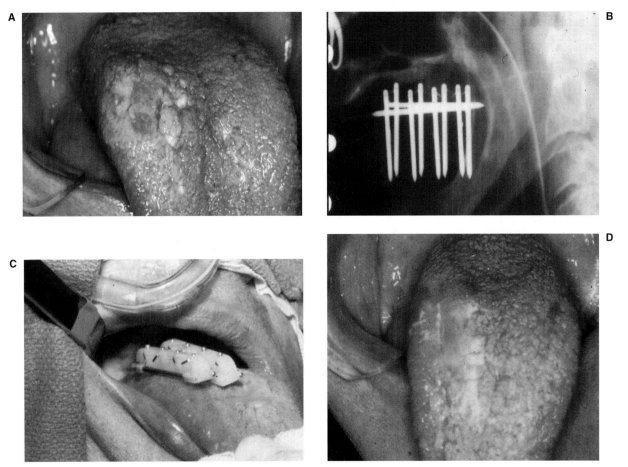

Figure 20–3 A 51-year-old man presented with a 3-month history of a painful sore on the right dorsum of the tongue. The lesion measured 3 × 2 cm and extended near the midline. Biopsy revealed squamous cell carcinoma (T2N0). Treatment plan: (1) opposed lateral portals, 30 Gy over 2 weeks, ^{60}Co; (2) radium needle implant for 45 Gy. **(A)** Squamous cell carcinoma on dorsum of oral tongue. **(B)** Radiograph of radium needles in patient. The needles were mounted in a nylon bar. There were two crossing needles in the lateral bar and one crossing needle in the medial bar. The nylon holder assisted in maintaining the active portion of the needles above the lesion to give an adequate dose to the dorsum of the tongue. **(C)** Radium implant in place. **(D)** Complete healing at 3 months. There was no evidence of disease at 8 years. (*See Color Plate 20–3.*)

The time-dose factors are less critical than with oral tongue lesions, and the required doses are slightly lower. Lesions smaller than 1 cm in diameter and less than 4 mm thick may be treated with intraoral cone or implant alone. Larger tumors have a 20 to 30% risk of subclinical disease in the neck and require external beam irradiation in addition to treatment with oral cone or implantation. The neck and primary site are generally treated to a dose of 45 to 50 Gy, followed by a 25-Gy implant. If an oral cone is used, it should precede the megavoltage portion of treatment to allow for optimal tumor visualization and patient comfort.

The local control rates (direct method) by T stage for patients treated with RT alone at our institution for floor of mouth cancer before and after surgical salvage, respectively, are as follows: T1 ($n = 37$), 86% and 94%; T2 ($n = 36$), 69% and 86%; T3 ($n = 20$), 55% and 65%; and T4 ($n = 5$), 40% and 40%. Actuarial cause-specific survival rates for AJCC stages I, II, III, and IVA at 5 years are 96%, 70%, 67%, and 44%, respectively. The incidence of severe bone or soft tissue complications necessitating surgical intervention was 5% for 117 patients with T1 to T4 primary tumors treated with irradiation alone. Forty-two percent experienced mild to moderate complications.[5]

◆ Conformal Beams/Intensity-Modulated Radiation Therapy

Much information has been published about progressive efforts to achieve increasing dose conformality to tumors and other areas at risk by using computer-generated planning systems.[1,6–15] Such efforts have culminated in increasingly widespread use of new technologies such as three-dimensional (3D) conformal RT (3D-CRT) and IMRT.[16]

Three-dimensional CRT incorporates conventional beams into unconventional, non-coplanar arrangements, with or without standard wedge compensators.[17–20] The result is a highly conformal, isodose pattern around tumor volumes that had not been possible before the computer software innovations of the past decade (**Fig. 20–4**). Though still in

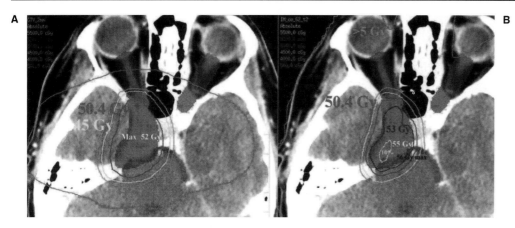

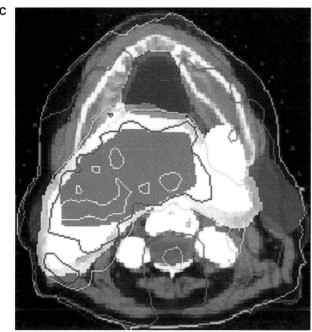

Figure 20–4 (A) Computed tomography from a three-dimensional computer plan for fractionated conformal radiation therapy (3D-CRT) using multiple non-coplanar fields on a cavernous sinus meningioma. Conformality rivals that of intensity-modulated radiation therapy **(B)** in many cases, without the dose inhomogeneities seen with the latter. The absorbed dose to normal structures distant from the target (including total body dose) is also less using 3D-CRT compared with intensity-modulated radiation therapy because of fewer total monitor units needed with 3D-CRT. **(C)** Intensity-modulated radiation therapy is preferable when trying to "wrap around" critical structures, such as the spinal cord. (*See Color Plate 20–4.*)

its relative infancy, IMRT utilizes sophisticated 3D computer-generated planning schemes to optimize dose delivery to specified points, while decreasing the dose to radiosensitive adjacent normal structures such as salivary and neural tissue.[9,16,21–36] Instead of standard wedge compensators, a complex, computer-driven array of lead collimators (multi-leaf collimator) inside the linear accelerator move in and out hundreds of times during a single treatment to achieve this goal.[37] Multiple coplanar or non-coplanar fields are generally used. Although the role of IMRT in head and neck malignancies is primarily to shield parotid and submandibular salivary tissue in an effort to minimize the untoward sequelae of long-term xerostomia, the treatment of various other clinical scenarios in head and neck cancer is aided as well, including tumors adjacent to dose-limiting critical structures (i.e., optic nerves, brain, spinal cord, and orbits). It also holds great promise in re-treating certain patients who have undergone radiation in the past.[38,39]

Ironically, dose inhomogeneity is both a blessing and a curse when using IMRT compared with more conventional techniques. Its advantage has already been stated: the ability to limit dose to normal structures relative to the tumor. Its disadvantage lies in the fact that, to achieve this goal, relative "hot" and "cold" areas must also exist within areas at risk.[40] In practice, this often results in dose inhomogeneities approaching 20% in treated volumes. Although future technologic advances may improve this situation, it is often dealt with in the present by preferentially "aiming" inhomogeneic hot spots to the center of the gross tumor volume (**Figs. 20–5 to 20–8**). An additional disadvantage of IMRT is the risk of a marginal miss if the designated "at-risk" volumes are drawn too tightly.

◆ Dose Fractionation Considerations

Radiation dose is expressed in centigrays (cGy), which are the same as rads (i.e., 5000 cGy = 5000 rad = 50 Gy). The unit of dose specification was changed from "rad" to "Gray" to honor L. H. Gray, a distinguished British physicist. In general, the probability of tumor control and complications increases with increasing dose, dose per fraction,

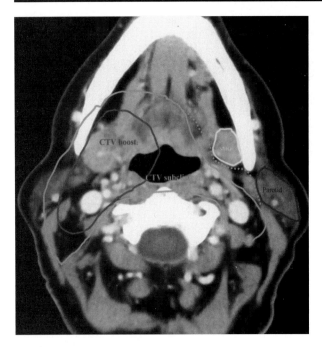

Figure 20–5 Computed tomography from a three-dimensional computer plan for an oropharyngeal cancer. The clinical target volume (CTV) boost includes the primary tumor and involved nodes. The clinical target volume subclinical includes all other areas felt to be potentially at risk for subclinical disease spread. The subclinical disease receives 30 fractions of 1.65 Gy for a total of 49.5 Gy, whereas the gross disease receives 1.8 Gy/fraction for a total of 54 Gy. During the final 12 treatment days, a concomitant boost of 1.5 Gy/fraction is given daily to the gross tumor volume with a minimum 6-hour interval between treatments. The total dose is 72 Gy or more in 30 treatment days. The contralateral submandibular (SMG) and parotid glands are shielded from the high-dose region. (*See Color Plate 20–5.*)

volume irradiated, and decreasing overall treatment time.[7,41] Split-course RT should be avoided because it is associated with a decreased probability of tumor control and does not appreciably lower the risk of late complications.[9,42] Typical conventional fractionation schedules in the United States and France include 75 Gy at 1.8 Gy/fraction over 8 weeks and 70 Gy at 2 Gy/fraction over 7 weeks. Schedules employed in Canada and the United Kingdom tends to be shorter, such as 50 Gy at 2.5 Gy/fraction over 4 weeks. The final dose depends on the volume of tumor irradiated, the radiosensitivity of adjacent normal tissues, and the probability of complications. Acutely responding tissues, such as the normal mucosa and carcinoma, respond similarly to radiation. Therefore, treatment schedules that are associated with a minimum of mucositis and its attendant symptoms have a relatively small chance of eradicating a head and neck cancer.

The probability of late complications is not related to the acute effects of radiation except at the very extremes of acute reactions; it tends to increase with increasing tumor volume because of destruction of normal tissue by the tumor. It is necessary to accept a low risk ($\leq$5%) of severe late complications to have a reasonable probability of disease control with treatment.[43] A very low risk (1%) of severe complications is desirable in the treatment of early cancers for which the chance of cure is high and an acceptable treatment alternative exists (e.g., T1 or T2 vocal cord cancer suitable for a hemilaryngectomy). However, a higher risk of severe complications (5 to 10%) is acceptable for more advanced lesions in which the chance of cure is lower or the surgical alternative is associated with a significant functional or cosmetic deficit.

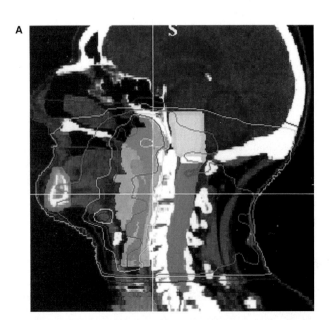
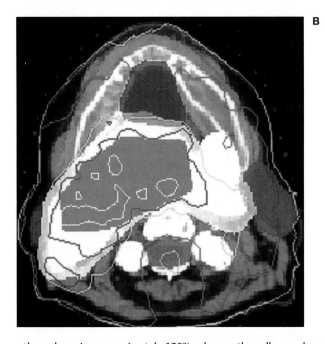

Figure 20–6 Computerized three-dimensional intensity-modulated radiation therapy isodose plan. **(A)** Tissues within the red line receive 100% of the prescribed dose. **(B)** The scattered white lines inside of the red receive approximately 120%, whereas the yellow and green lines receive approximately 90% and 30%, respectively, of the prescribed dose. (*See Color Plate 20–6.*)

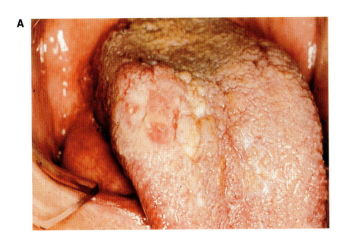

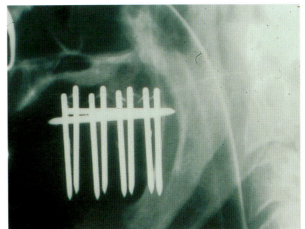

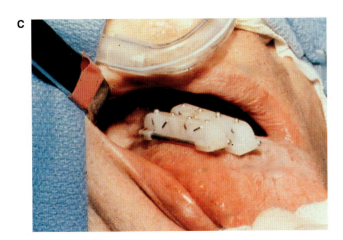

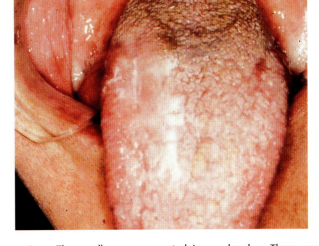

Color Plate 20–3 A 51-year-old man presented with a 3-month history of a painful sore on the right dorsum of the tongue. The lesion measured 3 × 2 cm and extended near the midline. Biopsy revealed squamous cell carcinoma (T2N0). Treatment plan: (1) opposed lateral portals, 30 Gy over 2 weeks, ^{60}Co; (2) radium needle implant for 45 Gy. **(A)** Squamous cell carcinoma on dorsum of oral tongue. **(B)** Radiograph of radium needles in patient. The needles were mounted in a nylon bar. There were two crossing needles in the lateral bar and one crossing needle in the medial bar. The nylon holder assisted in maintaining the active portion of the needles above the lesion to give an adequate dose to the dorsum of the tongue. **(C)** Radium implant in place. **(D)** Complete healing at 3 months. There was no evidence of disease at 8 years. (*See Figure 20–3, p. 240.*)

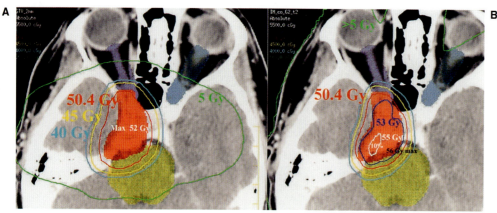

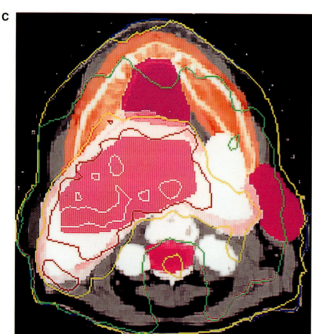

Color Plate 20–4 (A) Computed tomography from a three-dimensional computer plan for fractionated conformal radiation therapy (3D-CRT) using multiple non-coplanar fields on a cavernous sinus meningioma. Conformality rivals that of intensity-modulated radiation therapy **(B)** in many cases, without the dose inhomogeneities seen with the latter. The absorbed dose to normal structures distant from the target (including total body dose) is also less using 3D-CRT compared with intensity-modulated radiation therapy because of fewer total monitor units needed with 3D-CRT. **(C)** Intensity-modulated radiation therapy is preferable when trying to "wrap around" critical structures, such as the spinal cord. (*See Figure 20–4, p. 241.*)

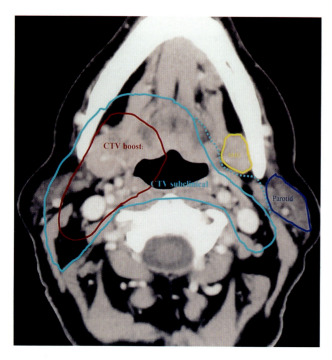

Color Plate 20–5 Computed tomography from a three-dimensional computer plan for an oropharyngeal cancer. The clinical target volume (CTV) boost includes the primary tumor and involved nodes. The clinical target volume subclinical includes all other areas felt to be potentially at risk for subclinical disease spread. The subclinical disease receives 30 fractions of 1.65 Gy for a total of 49.5 Gy, whereas the gross disease receives 1.8 Gy/fraction for a total of 54 Gy. During the final 12 treatment days, a concomitant boost of 1.5 Gy/fraction is given daily to the gross tumor volume with a minimum 6-hour interval between treatments. The total dose is 72 Gy or more in 30 treatment days. The contralateral submandibular (SMG) and parotid glands are shielded from the high-dose region. (*See Figure 20–5, p. 242.*)

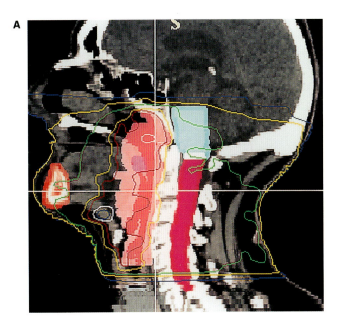

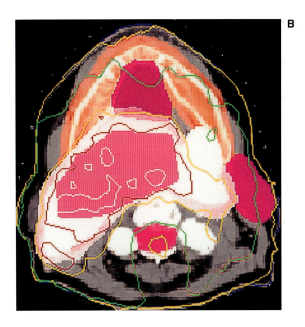

Color Plate 20–6 Computerized three-dimensional intensity-modulated radiation therapy isodose plan. **(A)** Tissues within the red line receive 100% of the prescribed dose. **(B)** The scattered white lines inside of the red receive approximately 120%, whereas the yellow and green lines receive approximately 90% and 30%, respectively, of the prescribed dose. (*See Figure 20–6, p. 242.*)

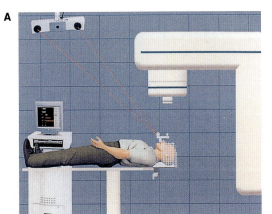

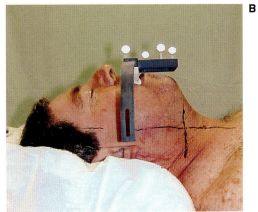

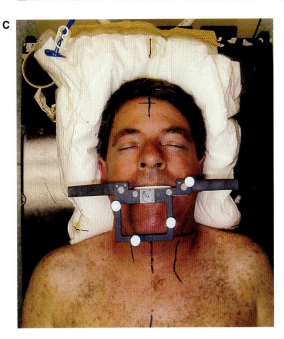

Color Plate 20–7 Immobilization technique for intensity-modulated radiation therapy. **(A)** A custom-made bite block with integrated fiducial markers is localized by ceiling-mounted laser cameras, thereby ensuring reproducibility between daily setups. Treatment is interrupted if excess motion is detected. **(B)** Profile view. **(C)** Frontal view. (*See Figure 20–7, p. 243.*)

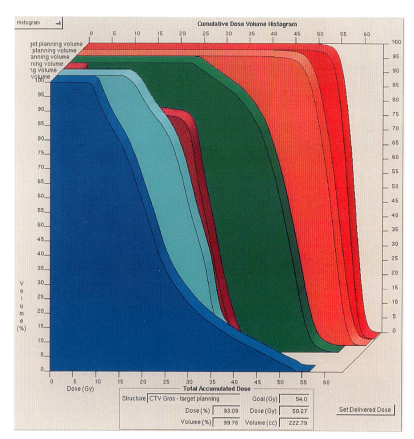

Color Plate 20–8 Dose-volume histogram from an intensity-modulated plan. Percent volume of selected structure is shown on the *y* axis. Dose received is shown on the *x* axis. The dose received by any selected percent volume of a chosen structure can be seen instantly. The dose-volume histogram is used to evaluate normal tissue goals during treatment (e.g., the University of Florida uses a 0.1-cc dose for many structures). (*See Figure 20–8, p. 244.*)

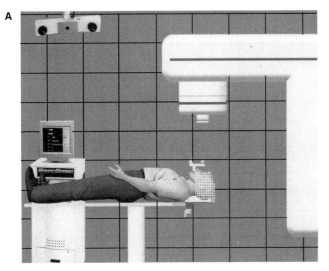

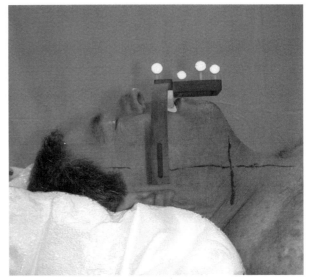

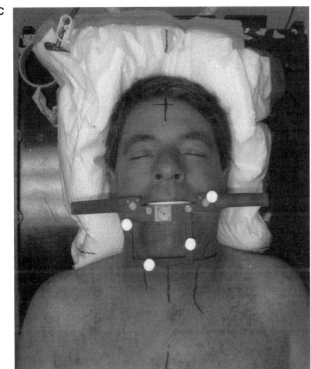

Figure 20–7 Immobilization technique for intensity-modulated radiation therapy. (**A**) A custom-made bite block with integrated fiducial markers is localized by ceiling-mounted laser cameras, thereby ensuring reproducibility between daily setups. Treatment is interrupted if excess motion is detected. (**B**) Profile view. (**C**) Frontal view. (*See Color Plate 20–7.*)

◆ Altered Fractionation

The rationale for altered fractionation is based on the dissociation between acute and late effects. The likelihood of tumor control and acute toxicity increases with increasing total dose and decreasing overall treatment time, and is relatively unrelated to dose per fraction. In contrast, the likelihood of late effects is related to total dose and dose per fraction and is relatively unrelated to overall treatment time. A caveat is that if overall treatment time is shortened to the extent that acute toxicity results in obliteration of an excessive proportion of stem cells, an acute necrosis results, merging into a consequential late complication. In other words, the mucosa or skin becomes so badly denuded that

it never heals. The goals of altered fractionation are to improve the probability of cure or diminish the odds of a late complication.

Common features of altered fractionation schedules include a dose per fraction lower than, or similar to, that used in conventional schedules, two or more fractions administered daily, a higher weekly dose, and a shorter overall treatment time. Altered fractionation schedules may be broadly classified as accelerated or hyperfractionated. *Accelerated fractionation* employs the same total dose, number of fractions, and dose per fraction given over a shorter overall time. An example of a pure accelerated fractionation schedule is 66 Gy in 33 fractions given twice daily over 3 weeks, compared with a conventional course of 66 Gy in

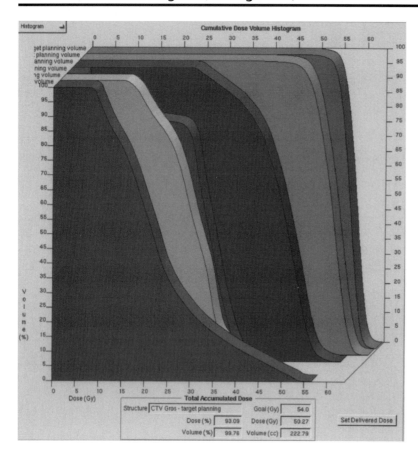

Figure 20–8 Dose-volume histogram from an intensity-modulated plan. Percent volume of selected structure is shown on the *y* axis. Dose received is shown on the *x* axis. The dose received by any selected percent volume of a chosen structure can be seen instantly. The dose-volume histogram is used to evaluate normal tissue goals during treatment (e.g., the University of Florida uses a 0.1-cc dose for many structures). (*See Color Plate 20–8.*)

33 fractions given once daily over 6.5 weeks. *Hyperfractionation* employs an increased total dose and number of fractions, a lower dose per fraction, and the same overall time. An example of a hyperfractionation schedule is 77 Gy in 70 fractions given twice daily over 7 weeks, compared with a conventional course of 70 Gy in 35 fractions given once daily over 7 weeks. In practice, most altered fractionation schedules are a combination of accelerated and hyperfractionated RT. For example, a common "hyperfractionation" schedule employed at our institution (76.8 Gy in 64 fractions twice daily over 6.5 weeks) is actually slightly accelerated because the overall time is reduced by three treatment days. Irradiation is like cooking, and like cooking, altered fractionation schedules may vary, depending on the radiation oncologist. Although mathematical formulae exist that may be used to predict the efficacy of a particular fractionation schedule, it is risky to stray too far from those previously employed lest unanticipated adverse consequences result.

The European Organization for Research and Treatment of Cancer (EORTC) conducted one of the earliest prospective randomized hyperfractionation trials for research and treatment of cancer. A total of 352 patients with T2–T3 N0–N1 squamous cell carcinoma of the oropharynx (excluding base of tongue) received either 70 Gy in 35 fractions once daily or 80.5 Gy at 1.15 Gy per fraction administered twice daily.[44] The overall treatment time was 7 weeks in both arms. Acute effects were increased in those treated with hyperfractionated RT; late effects were equivalent. The 5-year rates of local control (59% vs. 40%, $p = .02$) and survival (40% vs. 30%, $p = .08$) were improved in patients treated with hyperfractionation.

A relatively straightforward method of accelerating RT is to treat once daily more than 5 days a week. Overgaard et al[45] randomized 690 patients to 66 to 68 Gy in 33 to 34 fractions, five fractions per week, over 46 days or the same dose and number of fractions administered six fractions per week over 39 days. All patients received nimorazole, a hypoxic sensitizer. The 3-year results for five fractions per week versus six fractions per week were as follows: local control, 56% vs. 73% ($p = .002$); neck control, 74% vs. 81% ($p > .05$); cause-specific survival, 58% vs. 71% ($p = .08$); and survival, 46% vs. 56% ($p > .05$). In a similar trial recently reported by Skladowski et al,[46] 100 patients with T2-T4 N0-N1 squamous cell carcinoma were randomized to once daily RT administered in either five or seven fractions per week. All patients received 1.8 to 2 Gy per fraction to total doses ranging from 66 to 72 Gy. Patients treated 7 days weekly had improved 3-year rates of local control (87% vs. 37%, $p < .0001$) and survival (78% vs. 32%, $p < .0001$). These differences were larger than many might have predicted. The accelerated RT was also associated with increased EORTC grade 4 mucositis (62% vs. 26%) and grade 3 to 4 late effects (30% vs. 19%). Treatment once daily, six to seven times per week, is an attractive way to accelerate RT in locales where facilities are limited. However, in the United States, where facility availability exceeds that of radiotherapists (technicians trained to run the machines), the likelihood of widespread RT administration over weekends is low. Therefore, to increase the weekly dose while treating 5 days a week without increasing the dose per fraction, it is necessary to treat with two or more fractions per day. The limiting factors influencing the

Table 20–1   Radiation Therapy Alone: Doses and Fractionation Schedules*

| Tumor Stage | Once-a-Day Fractionation | | Twice-a-Day Fractionation |
	1.8 Gy/ Fraction	2 Gy/ Fraction	1.2 Gy/ Fraction
T1	65 Gy	60 Gy	No data
T2	70 Gy	64 Gy	74.4 Gy
T3	70 Gy	70 Gy	76.8 Gy
T4	75 Gy	70 Gy	79.2 Gy

*These are general treatment schedules and will vary with primary site and tumor cell type.
Adapted from Mendenhall WM, Parsons JT, Million RR. Radiation therapy in the management of head and neck cancer. In: Meyerhoff WL, Rice DH, eds. Otolaryngology–Head and Neck Surgery. Philadelphia: WB Saunders, 1992:1011–1025, with permission.

number of fractions that may be administered per day are machine availability and the need to allow enough time between fractions to allow for repair of sublethal damage in normal tissue (6 hours or more).

A landmark study recently conducted by the Radiation Therapy Oncology Group (RTOG) randomized patients to the University of Florida's hyperfractionated schedule (81.6 Gy at 1.2 Gy per fraction twice daily over 7 weeks), the Massachusetts General Hospital's accelerated split-course technique (67.2 Gy at 1.6 Gy per fraction twice daily over 6 weeks), the M. D. Anderson Cancer Center's (MDACC) accelerated concomitant boost (72 Gy at 1.8 to 1.5 Gy per fraction over 6 weeks with twice daily RT given during the last 12 treatment days), and conventional fractionation (70 Gy in 35 fractions over 7 weeks).[47] The 2-year rates of local-regional control were significantly improved for patients treated with either hyperfractionated RT ($p = .045$) or the accelerated concomitant boost technique ($p = .05$) compared with conventional RT. Local-regional control after accelerated split-course RT was similar to that observed after conventional fractionation ($p = .55$). Overall, survival was not significantly improved in any of the experimental arms; it is possible that a modest improvement may be observed with longer follow-up. Acute toxicity was increased in all three altered fractionation schedules; late toxicity at 2 years was not significantly impacted.

Thus, it is apparent that the efficacy of altered fractionation techniques varies with the schedule. Fractionation schedules administering very high weekly doses may necessitate a planned split or lowering the total dose so there is no advantage compared with conventional fractionation. At present, the MDACC's concomitant boost and the hyperfractionated schedules employed by the University of Florida and the EORTC 22791 trial are the most attractive options.[48,49] The advantage of the accelerated concomitant boost technique is that fewer fractions are administered, making it logistically more attractive; the disadvantage is the acute effects take longer to resolve.[47]

Dose-fractionation schedules used at the University of Florida for treatment of various T-stage lesions with external-beam irradiation alone are outlined in **Table 20–1**[50]; these are approximations and vary according to the primary site

and cell type (e.g., lymphoepithelioma may require a lower dose than does squamous cell carcinoma). At our institution, most primary head and neck cancers treated primarily with RT receive hyperfractionated treatment (1.2 Gy twice daily) with a minimum 6-hour interfraction interval. Exceptions to this are low-volume T1 or T2 tumors for which the local control rate is acceptable with once daily fractionation, or in patients for whom two treatments per day is logistically unfeasible. If IMRT is used, a concomitant boost is given during the final 2 weeks of treatment. The subclinical disease receives 30 fractions of 1.65 Gy for a total of 49.50 Gy, whereas the gross disease receives 1.8 Gy per fraction for a total of 54 Gy. During the final 12 treatment days, a concomitant boost of 1.5 Gy per fraction is given daily to the gross tumor volume with a minimum 6-hour interval between treatments. The total dose is 72 Gy or more in 30 treatment days.

◆ Adjuvant Therapy

Chemotherapy

Chemotherapy may be administered in conjunction with RT to improve local-regional control and improve survival. The timing of chemotherapy relative to RT may be categorized as induction (given before RT), concomitant (administered simultaneously with RT), and maintenance (given after RT). In contrast to induction chemotherapy, concomitant chemotherapy appears to result in improved survival. Although most of the data comes from nonoral cavity sites, several important randomized trials pertaining to concomitant chemotherapy and RT for head and neck cancer have been published within the past 8 years.[51–54] However, the optimal combination of chemotherapy and RT is unclear, particularly in light of altered fractionation trials.[47,55]

The question that follows is whether concomitant chemotherapy improves the likelihood of cure for patients treated with altered fractionation. Sanchiz et al[56] reported a prospective randomized trial in which 859 patients with head and neck cancer were randomly assigned to receive 60 Gy in 30 once-daily fractions (group A), 70.4 Gy in 64 twice-daily fractions (group B), or 60 Gy in 30 once-daily fractions with concomitant fluorouracil (FU) (group C). The outcomes for the three treatment groups were as follows: complete response, 68%, 90%, and 96%; average response duration, 25, 51, and 60 months; 10-year disease-free survival, 17%, 37%, and 31%; and 10-year survival, 17%, 40%, and 42%. Thus, both hyperfractionated RT and concomitant FU with once-daily RT resulted in significantly improved progression-free survival ($p < .001$), and overall survival ($p < .001$) compared with conventionally fractionated RT alone. Deficiencies of this early trial are the RT doses were low and the chemotherapy was probably suboptimal.

A single institution study reported by Brizel et al[57] compared a more aggressive RT hyperfractionated schedule with RT and concomitant FU and cisplatin. Patients with locally advanced head and neck cancer who underwent RT alone received 75 Gy in 60 twice-daily fractions; those who underwent concomitant chemotherapy received 70 Gy in 56 twice-daily fractions with a 7-day split. Adjuvant chemotherapy consisted of two cycles of concomitant cisplatin (12 mg/m2) and FU (600 mg/m²) per day for 5 days, followed by two cycles of maintenance chemotherapy. One hundred sixteen patients were included in the study. Patients who received adjuvant chemotherapy had improved 3-year rates of local-regional control (70% vs. 40%, $p = .01$), relapse-free survival (61% vs. 41%, $p = .08$), and overall survival (55% vs. 34%, $p = .07$). Late osteonecrosis or soft tissue necrosis occurred in 20% of those who received hyperfractionated RT and chemotherapy and 15% of those treated with RT alone ($p > .05$).

Jeremic et al[58] reported on 130 patients with advanced cancers of the head and neck who were randomly assigned to receive hyperfractionated RT (77 Gy at 1.1 Gy per fraction, twice daily, in a continuous course) alone or combined with 6 mg/m² concomitant daily cisplatin. Patients who received concomitant chemotherapy had significantly improved 5-year rates of local-regional control (50% vs. 36%, $p = .041$), distant-metastasis-free survival (86% vs. 57%, $p = .001$), and survival (46% vs. 25%, $p = .008$). Treatment splits and hospitalization for acute toxicity occurred in 11% and 9% of patients who received chemotherapy compared with 9% and 6% of those who received RT alone ($p = .99$ and $p = .74$, respectively). The rates of myelotoxicity were significantly higher in those who received concomitant cisplatin: grades 3 to 4 leukopenia (12% vs. 0%, $p = .006$) and grades 3 to 4 thrombocytopenia (8% vs. 0%, $p = .058$).

A multicenter German trial reported by Staar et al[59] randomly assigned 240 patients with stages III and IV squamous cell carcinoma of the oropharynx and hypopharynx to accelerated concomitant boost RT, alone or combined with two cycles of FU and carboplatin. A secondary randomization occurred in both treatment groups to receive or not receive granulocyte colony-stimulating factor (G-CSF) to reduce mucositis. Patients who received concomitant chemotherapy had marginally improved rates of local-regional control ($p = .112$) and survival ($p = .092$); the improvement was observed primarily in patients with oropharyngeal cancers. The administration of G-CSF significantly reduced the probability of local-regional control in both treatment arms. Thus, depending on the altered fractionation schedule that is employed, the addition of concomitant chemotherapy may improve the likelihood of local-regional control and survival for patients with advanced head and neck cancer.

In summary, the optimal combination of RT and concomitant chemotherapy remains unclear and must be defined by future prospective randomized trials. The spectrum of combinations includes protracted split-course RT and very aggressive chemotherapy,[60] conventional continuous-course RT and moderately aggressive chemotherapy,[52] hyperfractionated or accelerated concomitant-boost RT and less aggressive chemotherapy,[58] and RT combined with targeted intraarterial cisplatin.[61] Our current bias is to give the best RT combined with less aggressive chemotherapy consisting of weekly cisplatin or carboplatin and taxol.[62] The disadvantage of the latter chemotherapy regimen is that acute toxicity appears to be more pronounced compared with weekly cisplatin. Patients are usually treated with hyperfractionated or accelerated concomitant-boost RT. The latter is employed if IMRT is used because of logistical considerations. Otherwise, patients are treated with hyperfractionated RT.[48]

Radiation Therapy

Preoperative or postoperative RT is combined with surgery for advanced cancers when the probability for local-regional recurrence is high after surgery or RT alone. Unless a cancer is not completely resectable, postoperative RT is preferred because it is associated with a lower risk of postoperative complications. The rationale for postoperative RT is that it is most likely to be effective against microscopic deposits of cancer cells, which would progress and lead to local-regional recurrence if left unchecked.[63]

The usual indications to give postoperative irradiation at the University of Florida for carcinoma of the oral cavity include one or more of the following pathologic findings related to the primary site: bone invasion or extension of tumor into the soft tissues of the neck (T4 primary); margins that are positive, close (<5 mm), contain carcinoma in situ or dysplasia, or that were initially positive but ultimately negative after re-resection[64–67]; perineural invasion[68–70]; vascular space invasion[71]; or multicentricity (scattered, discontinuous foci or islands of tumor adjacent to the primary site, making margins of resection uncertain).

Factors in the neck specimen for which postoperative irradiation is generally added include multiple positive lymph nodes[72–75] or extracapsular extension (ECE).[71,74,76–79] High risk of occult tumor in an undissected, clinically negative N0 neck is not an adequate reason to add adjuvant RT unless there are additional indications for treatment. The high-risk neck should be electively dissected.

Some of these factors are more ominous than others. For example, early bone erosion of the mandible is not likely to have the same negative prognostic influence as positive margins. Factors thought to be particularly ominous are the presence of positive margins,[65,80,81] multiple indications for administering postoperative irradiation,[80,82,83] and ECE.[75,77–79,81,83–85] Although we have never used poor differentiation as the sole indication for postoperative irradiation, there are data to suggest it may significantly affect local-regional control,[71,75,82] and in otherwise borderline cases, poor differentiation might be a reason to add irradiation postoperatively.

Postoperative radiation doses are generally higher than preoperative doses because residual tumor may be present in a poorly vascularized surgical bed. Hypoxic tumor cells are more resistant to radiation, and a higher dose is required to achieve the same probability of tumor control. The postoperative dose depends on the suspected amount of residual tumor and is selected on the basis of margins of resection and other risk factors. The standard postoperative dose in our department is 60 Gy in 30 fractions. High-risk situations (positive margins, ≥ 3 risk factors present, and so forth) receive a greater dose, often hyperfractionated to 72 to 74.4 Gy in 60 to 62 fractions. Preoperative radiation treatment schedules usually consist of 46 to 50 Gy at 2 Gy per fraction over $4\frac{1}{2}$ to 5 weeks; the dose to fixed nodes is boosted to 60 Gy or more to improve the likelihood of complete resection.

IMRT has been used postoperatively at other institutions.[31,86–89] We currently use IMRT mainly to treat de novo head and neck tumors definitively with irradiation. It is used sparingly in the postoperative setting, mainly because of concerns about the dose distribution to skin and subcutaneous tissues, which may be at more risk after surgery. As the role for IMRT evolves, its use may increase in postoperative situations. We continue to favor more conventional beam arrangements when feasible to optimize dose distributions to the skin and subcutaneous tissues at risk.

In 1989, our results were published on 134 patients who underwent postoperative irradiation for tumors of oral, pharyngeal, or laryngeal sites at the University of Florida.[90] Included were 38 patients with oral cavity cancers. During the time period covered in our initial review, the institutional policy was to use primary irradiation for most oral cavity cancers. In the early 1980s, the approach to oral cavity cancer changed at the University of Florida so that almost all patients were treated initially by operation with postoperative irradiation added as indicated by pathologic findings. The main reason for the change was to avoid the relatively high incidence of bone exposure and soft tissue necrosis observed in patients treated with interstitial implantation for predominantly oral tongue and floor of mouth cancers. The most recent results show statistically significant correlations on univariate analysis between local-regional control and T stage (T1 and T2 versus T3 and T4), pathologic AJCC stage, ECE, perineural invasion, margin status, and the number of indications for postoperative radiation. Multivariate analysis shows T stage, margin status, and the presence of ECE, vascular, or perineural invasion to be independent predictors of local-regional control.[91]

No randomized trials have addressed the efficacy of postoperative adjuvant RT. Some of the best available data are from the Medical College of Virginia, where two groups of surgeons operated on patients with head and neck cancer. The two groups were general surgical oncologists who employed surgery alone and reserved RT for treatment of recurrent disease, and otolaryngologists who routinely sent patients with locally advanced disease for postoperative RT.[81] One hundred twenty-five of 441 patients treated surgically between 1982 and 1988 had ECE or positive margins; 71 were treated with surgery alone, and 54 received postoperative RT. Patients were irradiated at 1.8 to 2.0 Gy per fraction with ^{60}Co or 4-MV x-rays to doses of 50 to 50.99 Gy in 26 patients and to 60 Gy or more in the remainder. Local control rates at 3 years after surgery alone compared with surgery and RT were as follows: ECE, 31% and 66% ($p = .03$); positive margins, 41% and 49% ($p = .04$); and ECE and positive margins, 0% and 68% ($p = .001$). A multivariate analysis of local control was performed evaluating the impact of T stage, N stage, use of postoperative RT, the number of positive nodes, the number of nodes with ECE, primary site, microscopic and macroscopic ECE, and margin status. For the end point of local control, use of postoperative RT ($p = .0001$), macroscopic ECE ($p = .0001$), and margin status ($p = .09$)

were of independent significance. Disease-free survival at 3 years was 25% after surgery alone and 45% after combined modality treatment ($p = .0001$). Cause-specific survival rates at 3 years were 41% for surgery alone and 72% for surgery and postoperative RT ($p = .0003$). Multivariate analysis of cause-specific survival showed that postoperative RT ($p = .0001$) and the number of nodes with ECE ($p = .0001$) significantly influenced this end point. Two irradiated patients experienced mandibular necrosis; one was treated with hyperbaric oxygen treatments and the other with conservative management. Lundahl et al[92] reported a series of 95 patients with node-positive squamous cell carcinoma who were treated with a neck dissection and postoperative RT at the Mayo Clinic. A matched-pair analysis was performed utilizing a series of patients treated with surgery alone; 56 matched pairs of patients were identified. The rates of recurrence in the dissected neck (RR = 5.82; $p = .0002$), recurrence in either side of the neck (RR = 2.21; $p = .0052$), and death from any cause (RR = 1.67; $p = .0182$) were significantly higher for patients treated with neck dissection alone. Thus, it appears that for patients who are at high risk for local-regional failure after surgery, postoperative RT significantly improves disease control above the clavicles as well as survival.

Postoperative irradiation should begin as soon as healing is complete; it can often be started within 3 to 4 weeks of surgery. If irradiation is delayed until gross recurrence has occurred, the chance for successful salvage by irradiation is only 5 to 10%.[65,93,94] If healing is not complete by 6 weeks, data from earlier University of Florida series[95,96] show irradiation can often be safely initiated anyway, and approximately two thirds of patients will heal spontaneously during or after irradiation. Patients at high risk (≥ 3 risk factors) for recurrence and those whose surgery-RT interval has been prolonged (>7 weeks) should be considered for altered dose/fractionation schemes that shorten the length of the RT course, thereby decreasing the overall treatment time.

Chemotherapy and Postoperative Irradiation

The results of two randomized trials (RTOG 9501 and EORTC 22391) were published recently, which showed a statistically significant improvement with concomitant chemotherapy during a course of postoperative radiation in high-risk patients. Both of these trials reported an improvement in local-regional control and disease-free survival with cisplatin (100 mg/m^2) given on days 1, 22, and 43 of the RT regimen. Severe acute effects are seen more frequently with concomitant treatment compared with postoperative radiation alone.[97,98]

References

1. Verhey LJ. Comparison of three-dimensional conformal radiation therapy and intensity-modulated radiation therapy systems. Semin Radiat Oncol 1999;9:78–98
2. Parsons JT, Palta JR, Mendenhall WM, Bova FJ, Million RR. Head and neck cancer. In: Levitt SH, Khan FM, Potish RA, Perez CA, eds. Levitt and Tapley's Technological Basis of Radiation Therapy: Clinical Applications. Baltimore: Lippincott Williams & Wilkins, 1999:269–299
3. Parsons JT, Mendenhall WM, Moore GJ, Million RR. Radiotherapy of tumors of the oral cavity. In: Thawley SE, Panje WR, Batsakis JG, Lindberg RD, eds. Comprehensive Management of Head and Neck Tumors. Philadelphia: WB Saunders, 1999:695–719
4. Fein DA, Mendenhall WM, Parsons JT, et al. Carcinoma of the oral tongue: a comparison of results and complications of treatment with radiotherapy and/or surgery. Head Neck 1994;16:358–365

5. Rodgers LW Jr, Stringer SP, Mendenhall WM, Parsons JT, Cassisi NJ, Million RR. Management of squamous cell carcinoma of the floor of the mouth. Head Neck 1993;15:16–19

6. Grant W III, Woo SY. Clinical and financial issues for intensity-modulated radiation therapy delivery. Semin Radiat Oncol 1999;9:99–107

7. Teh BS, Woo SY. Intensity modulated radiation therapy (IMRT): a new promising technology in radiation oncology. Oncologist 1999;4:433–442

8. Purdy JA. 3D treatment planning and intensity-modulated radiation therapy. Oncology (Williston Park) 1999;13(10, suppl 5):155–168

9. Butler EB, Teh BS, Grant WH III, et al. SMART (simultaneous modulated accelerated radiation therapy) boost: a new accelerated fractionation schedule for the treatment of head and neck cancer with intensity modulated radiotherapy. Int J Radiat Oncol Biol Phys 1999;45:21–32

10. Klein EE, Tepper J, Sontag M, Franklin M, Ling C, Kubo D. Technology assessment of multileaf collimation: a North American users survey. Int J Radiat Oncol Biol Phys 1999;44:705–710

11. Tsien C, Eisbruch A, McShan D, Kessler M, Marsh R, Fraass B. Intensity-modulated radiation therapy (IMRT) for locally advanced paranasal sinus tumors: incorporating clinical decisions in the optimization process. Int J Radiat Oncol Biol Phys 2003;55:776–784

12. Glatstein E. Intensity-modulated radiation therapy: the inverse, the converse, and the perverse. Semin Radiat Oncol 2002;12:272–281

13. Suit H. The Gray Lecture 2001: coming technical advances in radiation oncology. Int J Radiat Oncol Biol Phys 2002;53:798–809

14. Fiveash JB, Murshed H, Duan J, et al. Effect of multileaf collimator leaf width on physical dose distributions in the treatment of CNS and head and neck neoplasms with intensity modulated radiation therapy. Med Phys 2002;29:1116–1119

15. Kuppersmith RB, Greco SC, Teh BS, et al. Intensity-modulated radiotherapy: first results with this new technology on neoplasms of the head and neck. Ear Nose Throat J 1999;78:241–246

16. Cardinale RM, Benedict SH, Wu Q, Zwicker RD, Gaballa HE, Mohan R. A comparison of three stereotactic radiotherapy techniques; ARCS vs. noncoplanar fixed fields vs. intensity modulation. Int J Radiat Oncol Biol Phys 1998;42:431–436

17. Nutting CM, Rowbottom CG, Cosgrove VP, Henk JM. Optimisation of radiotherapy for carcinoma of the parotid gland: a comparison of conventional, three-dimensional conformal, and intensity-modulated techniques. Radiother Oncol 2001;60:163–172

18. Narayan S, Cornblath WT, Sandler HM, Elner V, Hayman JA. Preliminary visual outcomes after three-dimensional conformal radiation therapy for optic nerve sheath meningioma. Int J Radiat Oncol Biol Phys 2003;56:537–543

19. Liu JK, Forman S, Hershewe GL, Moorthy CR, Benzil DL. Optic nerve sheath meningiomas: visual improvement after stereotactic radiotherapy. Neurosurgery 2002;50:950–957

20. Leavitt DD. Beam shaping for SRT/SRS. Med Dosim 1998;23:229–236

21. Wu Q, Manning M, Schmidt-Ullrich R, Mohan R. The potential for sparing of parotids and escalation of biologically effective dose with intensity-modulated radiation treatments of head and neck cancers: a treatment design study. Int J Radiat Oncol Biol Phys 2000;46:195–205

22. Chao KS, Deasy JO, Markman J, et al. A prospective study of salivary function sparing in patients with head-and-neck cancers receiving intensity-modulated or three-dimensional radiation therapy: initial results. Int J Radiat Oncol Biol Phys 2001;49:907–916

23. Kramer BA, Wazer DE, Engler MJ, Tsai JS, Ling MN. Dosimetric comparison of stereotactic radiosurgery to intensity modulated radiotherapy. Radiat Oncol Investig 1998;6:18–25

24. Wu Q, Mohan R, Morris M, Lauve A, Schmidt-Ullrich R. Simultaneous integrated boost intensity-modulated radiotherapy for locally advanced head-and-neck squamous cell carcinomas. I. Dosimetric results. Int J Radiat Oncol Biol Phys 2003;56:573–585

25. Wu Q, Arnfield M, Tong S, Wu Y, Mohan R. Dynamic splitting of large intensity-modulated fields. Phys Med Biol 2000;45:1731–1740

26. Eisbruch A, Ten Haken RK, Kim HM, Marsh LH, Ship JA. Dose, volume, and function relationships in parotid salivary glands following conformal and intensity-modulated irradiation of head and neck cancer. Int J Radiat Oncol Biol Phys 2000;47:1458–1460

27. Mohan R, Wu Q, Manning M, Schmidt-Ullrich R. Radiobiological considerations in the design of fractionation strategies for intensity-modulated radiation therapy of head and neck cancers. Int J Radiat Oncol Biol Phys 2000;46:619–630

28. Chao KS, Low DA, Perez CA, Purdy JA. Intensity-modulated radiation therapy in head and neck cancers: the Mallinckrodt experience. Int J Cancer 2000;90:92–103

29. Hunt MA, Zelefsky MJ, Wolden S, et al. Treatment planning and delivery of intensity-modulated radiation therapy for primary nasopharynx cancer. Int J Radiat Oncol Biol Phys 2001;49:623–632

30. Eisbruch A, Marsh LH, Martel MK, et al. Comprehensive irradiation of head and neck cancer using conformal multisegmental fields: assessment of target coverage and noninvolved tissue sparing. Int J Radiat Oncol Biol Phys 1998;41:559–568

31. Dawson LA, Anzai Y, Marsh L, et al. Patterns of local-regional recurrence following parotid-sparing conformal and segmental intensity-modulated radiotherapy for head and neck cancer. Int J Radiat Oncol Biol Phys 2000;46:1117–1126

32. Eisbruch A, Chao KS, Garden AS. RTOG H-0022: phase I/II study of conformal and intensity-modulated irradiation for oropharyngeal cancer. Radiation Therapy Oncology Group, 2001

33. Nowak PJ, Wijers OB, Lagerwaard FJ, Levendag PC. A three-dimensional CT-based target definition for elective irradiation of the neck. Int J Radiat Oncol Biol Phys 1999;45:33–39

34. Wu Q, Mohan R, Niemierko A, Schmidt-Ullrich R. Optimization of intensity-modulated radiotherapy plans based on the equivalent uniform dose. Int J Radiat Oncol Biol Phys 2002;52:224–235

35. Wang X, Spirou S, LoSasso T, Stein J, Chui CS, Mohan B. Dosimetric verification of intensity-modulated fields. Med Phys 1996;23:317–327

36. Zhou J, Fei D, Wu Q. Potential of intensity-modulated radiotherapy (IMRT) to escalate doses to head and neck cancers: what is the maximum dose? Int J Radiat Oncol Biol Physiol 2003;57:673–682

37. van Dieren EB, Nowak PJ, Wijers OB, et al. Beam intensity modulation using tissue compensators or dynamic multileaf collimation in three-dimensional conformal radiotherapy of primary cancers of the oropharynx and larynx, including the elective neck. Int J Radiat Oncol Biol Phys 2000;47:1299–1309

38. Dawson LA, Myers LL, Bradford CR, et al. Conformal re-irradiation of recurrent and new primary head-and-neck cancer. Int J Radiat Oncol Biol Phys 2001;50:377–385

39. Eisbruch A, Dawson LA. Re-irradiation of head and neck tumors: benefits and toxicities. Hematol Oncol Clin North Am 1999;13:825–836

40. Vineberg KA, Eisbruch A, Coselmon MM, McShan DL, Kessler ML, Fraass BA. Is uniform target dose possible in IMRT plans in the head and neck? Int J Radiat Oncol Biol Phys 2002;52:1159–1172

41. Mendenhall WM, Million RR, Bova FJ. Analysis of time-dose factors in clinically positive neck nodes treated with irradiation alone in squamous cell carcinoma of the head and neck. Int J Radiat Oncol Biol Phys 1984;10:639–643

42. Parsons JT, Bova FJ, Million RR. A re-evaluation of split-course technique for squamous cell carcinoma of the head and neck. Int J Radiat Oncol Biol Phys 1980;6:1645–1652

43. Mendenhall WM, Cassisi NJ, Stringer SP, Tannehill SP. Therapeutic principles in the management of head and neck tumors. In: Souhami RL, Tannock I, Hohenberger P, Horiot J-C, eds. Oxford Textbook of Oncology. Oxford, England: Oxford University Press, 2002:1322–1344

44. Horiot JC, Le Fur R, N'Guyen T, et al. Hyperfractionation versus conventional fractionation in oropharyngeal carcinoma: final analysis of a randomized trial of the EORTC cooperative group of radiotherapy. Radiother Oncol 1992;25:231–241

45. Overgaard J, Hansen HS, Overgaard M, et al. Conventional radiotherapy as primary treatment of squamous cell carcinoma of the head and neck: a randomized multicenter study of 5 versus 6 fractions per week—report from the DAHANCA 7 trial. Int J Radiat Oncol Biol Phys 1997;39(25):88 (abstr)

46. Skladowski K, Maciejewski B, Golen M, Pilecki B, Przeorek W, Tarnawski R. Randomized clinical trial on 7-day-continuous accelerated irradiation (CAIR) of head and neck cancer—report of 3-year tumour control and normal tissue toxicity. Radiother Oncol 2000;55:101–110

47. Fu KK, Pajak TF, Trotti A, et al. A Radiation Therapy Oncology Group (RTOG) phase III randomized study to compare hyperfractionation and two variants of accelerated fractionation to standard fractionation radiotherapy for head and neck squamous cell carcinomas: first report of RTOG 9003. Int J Radiat Oncol Biol Phys 2000;48:7–16

48. Parsons JT, Mendenhall WM, Stringer SP, Cassisi NJ, Million RR. Twice-a-day radiotherapy for squamous cell carcinoma of the head and neck: the University of Florida experience. Head Neck 1993;15:87–96

49. Ang KK, Peters LJ. Concomitant boost radiotherapy in the treatment of head and neck cancers. Semin Radiat Oncol 1992;2:31–33

50. Mendenhall WM, Parsons JT, Million RR. Radiation therapy in the management of head and neck cancer. In: Meyerhoff WL, Rice DH, eds. Otolaryngology–Head and Neck Surgery. Philadelphia: WB Saunders, 1992:1011–1025

51. Adelstein DJ, Lavertu P, Saxton JP, et al. Mature results of a phase III randomized trial comparing concurrent chemoradiotherapy with radiation therapy alone in patients with stage III and IV squamous cell carcinoma of the head and neck. Cancer 2000;88:876–883

52. Calais G, Alfonsi M, Bardet E, et al. Randomized trial of radiation therapy versus concomitant chemotherapy and radiation therapy for advanced-stage oropharynx carcinoma. J Natl Cancer Inst 1999;91:2081–2086

53. Forastiere AA, Berkey B, Maor M, et al. Phase III trial to preserve the larynx: induction chemotherapy and radiotherapy versus concomitant chemoradiotherapy versus radiotherapy alone, Intergroup Trial R91–11. Proc Annu Meet Am Soc Clin Oncol 2001;20:2a(abstr)

54. Pignon JP, Bourhis J, Domenge C, Designé L. MACH-NC (Meta-Analysis of Chemotherapy on Head and Neck Cancer) Collaborative Group. Chemotherapy added to locoregional treatment for head and neck squamous-cell carcinoma: three meta-analyses of updated individual data. Lancet 2000;355:949–955

55. Horiot JC, Bontemps P, van den Bogaert W, et al. Accelerated fractionation (AF) compared to conventional fractionation (CF) improves loco-regional control in the radiotherapy of advanced head and neck cancers: results of the EORTC 22851 randomized trial. Radiother Oncol 1997;44:111–121

56. Sanchiz F, Milla A, Torner J, et al. Single fraction per day versus two fractions per day versus radiochemotherapy in the treatment of head and neck cancer. Int J Radiat Oncol Biol Phys 1990;19:1347–1350

57. Brizel DM, Albers ME, Fisher SR, et al. Hyperfractionated irradiation with or without concurrent chemotherapy for locally advanced head and neck cancer. N Engl J Med 1998;338:1798–1804

58. Jeremic B, Shibamoto Y, Milicic B, et al. Hyperfractionated radiation therapy with or without concurrent low-dose daily cisplatin in locally advanced squamous cell carcinoma of the head and neck: a prospective randomized trial. J Clin Oncol 2000;18:1458–1464

59. Staar S, Rudat V, Stuetzer H, et al. Intensified hyperfractionated accelerated radiotherapy limits the additional benefit of simultaneous chemotherapy: results of a multicentric randomized German trial in advanced head-and-neck cancer. Int J Radiat Oncol Biol Phys 2001;50:1161–1171

60. Kies MS, Haraf DJ, Rosen F, et al. Concomitant infusional paclitaxel and fluorouracil, oral hydroxyurea, and hyperfractionated radiation for locally advanced squamous head and neck cancer. J Clin Oncol 2001;19:1961–1969

61. Robbins KT, Kumar P, Wong FS, et al. Targeted chemoradiation for advanced head and neck cancer: analysis of 213 patients. Head Neck 2000;22:687–693

62. Suntharalingam M, Haas ML, Conley BA, et al. The use of carboplatin and paclitaxel with daily radiotherapy in patients with locally advanced squamous cell carcinoma of the head and neck. Int J Radiat Oncol Biol Phys 2000;47:49–56

63. MacComb WS, Fletcher GH. Planned combination of surgery and radiation in treatment of advanced primary head and neck cancers. Am J Roentgenol Radium Ther Nucl Med 1957;77:397–414

64. Chen TY, Emrich LJ, Driscoll DL. The clinical significance of pathological findings in surgically resected margins of the primary tumor in head and neck carcinoma. Int J Radiat Oncol Biol Phys 1987;13:833–837

65. Huang D, Johnson CR, Schmidt-Ullrich RK, Sismanis A, Neifeld JP, Weber J. Incompletely resected advanced squamous cell carcinoma of the head and neck: The effectiveness of adjuvant vs. salvage radiotherapy. Radiother Oncol 1992;24:87–93

66. Looser KG, Shah JP, Strong EW. The significance of "positive" margins in surgically resected epidermoid carcinomas. Head Neck Surg 1978;1:107–111

67. Scholl P, Byers RM, Batsakis JG, Wolf P, Santini H. Microscopic cut-through of cancer in the surgical treatment of squamous carcinoma of the tongue: prognostic and therapeutic implications. Am J Surg 1986;152:354–360

68. Lydiatt DD, Robbins KT, Byers RM, Wolf PF. Treatment of stage I and II oral tongue cancer. Head Neck 1993;15:308–312

69. O'Brien CJ, Lahr CJ, Soong SJ, et al. Surgical treatment of early-stage carcinoma of the oral tongue: would adjuvant treatment be beneficial? Head Neck Surg 1986;8:401–408

70. Soo KC, Carter RL, O'Brien CJ, Barr L, Bliss JM, Shaw HJ. Prognostic implications of perineural spread in squamous carcinomas of the head and neck. Laryngoscope 1986;96:1145–1148

71. Close LG, Brown PM, Vutich MF, Reisch J, Schaefer SD. Microvascular invasion and survival in cancer of the oral cavity and oropharynx. Arch Otolaryngol Head Neck Surg 1989;115:1304–1309

72. Farr HW, Arthur K. Epidermoid carcinoma of the mouth and pharynx 1960–1964. J Laryngol Otol 1972;86:243–253

73. Franceschi D, Gupta R, Spiro RH, Shah JP. Improved survival in the treatment of squamous carcinoma of the oral tongue. Am J Surg 1993;166:360–365

74. O'Brien CJ, Smith JW, Soong SJ, Urist MM, Maddox WA. Neck dissection with and without radiotherapy: Prognostic factors, patterns of recurrence, and survival. Am J Surg 1986;152:456–463

75. Olsen KD, Caruso M, Foote RL, et al. Primary head and neck cancer. Histopathologic predictors of recurrence after neck dissection in patients with lymph node involvement. Arch Otolaryngol Head Neck Surg 1994;120:1370–1374

76. Cachin Y, Eschwege F. Combination of radiotherapy and surgery in the treatment of head and neck cancers. Cancer Treat Rev 1975;2:177–191

77. Johnson JT, Barnes EL, Myers EN, Schramm VL Jr, Borochovitz D, Sigler BA. The extracapsular spread of tumors in cervical node metastasis. Arch Otolaryngol 1981;107:725–729

78. Johnson JT, Myers EN, Bedetti CD, Barnes EL, Schramm VL, Thearle PB. Cervical lymph node metastases. Incidence and implications of extracapsular carcinoma. Arch Otolaryngol 1985;111:534–537

79. Snyderman NL, Johnson JT, Schramm VL, Myers EN, Bedetti CD, Thearle PB. Extracapsular spread of carcinoma in cervical lymph nodes: impact upon survival in patients with carcinoma of the supraglottic larynx. Cancer 1985;56:1597–1599

80. Amdur RJ, Parsons JT, Mendenhall WM, Million RR, Stringer SP, Cassisi NJ. Postoperative irradiation for squamous cell carcinoma of the head and neck: an analysis of treatment results and complications. Int J Radiat Oncol Biol Phys 1989;16:25–36

81. Huang DT, Johnson CR, Schmidt-Ullrich R, Grimes M. Postoperative radiotherapy in head and neck carcinoma with extracapsular lymph node extension and/or positive resection margins: a comparative study. Int J Radiat Oncol Biol Phys 1992;23:737–742

82. Foote RL, Buskirk SJ, Stanley RJ, et al. Patterns of failure after total laryngectomy for glottic carcinoma. Cancer 1989;64:143–149

83. Peters LJ, Goepfert H, Ang KK, et al. Evaluation of the dose for postoperative radiation therapy of head and neck cancer: first report of a prospective randomized trial. Int J Radiat Oncol Biol Phys 1993;26:3–11

84. Arriagada R, Eschwege F, Cachin Y, Richard JM. The value of combining radiotherapy alone with surgery in the treatment of hypopharyngeal and laryngeal cancers. Cancer 1983;51:1819–1825

85. Bartelink H, Breur K, Hart G, Annyas B, van Slooten E, Snow G. The value of postoperative radiotherapy as an adjuvant to radical neck dissection. Cancer 1983;52:1008–1013

86. Chao KS, Ozyigit G, Tran BN, Cengiz M, Dempsey JF, Low DA. Patterns of failure in patients receiving definitive and postoperative IMRT for head and neck cancer. Int J Radiat Oncol Biol Phys 2003;55:312–321

87. Chao KS, Wippold FJ, Ozyigit G, Tran BN, Dempsey JF. Determination and delineation of nodal target volumes for head and neck cancer based on patterns of failure in patients receiving definitive and postoperative IMRT. Int J Radiat Oncol Biol Phys 2002;53:1174–1184

88. Chao KS, Majhail N, Huang CJ, et al. Intensity-modulated radiation therapy reduces late salivary toxicity without compromising tumor control in patients with oropharyngeal carcinoma: a comparison with conventional techniques. Radiother Oncol 2001;61:275–280

89. Claus F, Vakaet L, De Gersem W, et al. Postoperative radiotherapy of paranasal sinus tumours: a challenge for intensity-modulated radiotherapy. Acta Otorhinolaryngol Belg 1999;53:263–269

90. Mendenhall WM, Parsons JT, Stringer SP, Cassisi NJ, Million RR. Radiotherapy after excisional biopsy of carcinoma of the oral tongue/floor of the mouth. Head Neck 1989;11:129–131

91. Hinerman RW, Mendenhall WM, Morris CG, Amdur RJ, Werning JW, Villaret DB. Postoperative irradiation for squamous cell carcinoma of the oral cavity: 35 year experience. Head Neck 2004;26:984–994

92. Lundahl RE, Foote RL, Bonner JA, et al. Combined neck dissection and postoperative radiation therapy in the management of the high-risk

neck: a matched-pair analysis. Int J Radiat Oncol Biol Phys 1998;40:529–534

93. Ampil RL. Surgery and postoperative external irradiation for head and neck cancer recurrent after surgery alone. Laryngoscope 1988;98:888–890

94. Fletcher GH, Evers WT. Radiotherapeutic management of surgical recurrences and postoperative residuals in tumors of the head and neck. Radiology 1970;95:185–188

95. Isaacs JH Jr, Stiles WA, Cassisi NJ, Million RR, Parsons JT. Postoperative radiation of open head and neck wounds – updated. Head Neck 1997;19:194–199

96. Parsons JT, Mendenhall WM, Stringer SP, Cassisi NJ, Million RR. An analysis of factors influencing the outcome of postoperative irradiation for squamous cell carcinoma of the oral cavity. Int J Radiat Oncol Biol Phys 1997;39:137–148

97. Bernier J, Domenge C, Ozsahin M, et al. Postoperative irradiation with or without concomitant chemotherapy for locally advanced head and neck cancer. N Engl J Med 2004;350:1945–1952

98. Cooper JS, Pajak TF, Forastiere AA, et al. Postoperative concurrent radiotherapy and chemotherapy for high-risk squamous cell carcinoma of the head and neck. N Engl J Med 2004;350:1937–1944

21

Chemotherapy

Maura L. Gillison

Chemotherapy is clinically indicated for patients with newly diagnosed, unresectable, oral cavity carcinoma when administered concurrently with primary radiation therapy (RT) and in the palliation of patients with recurrent, unresectable, or metastatic disease. Apart from these clinical indications, the role of chemotherapy in the management of oral cavity carcinoma is controversial or undefined. The potential for organ preservation therapy in the oral cavity by use of concurrent chemoradiation is largely unexplored, although it is clearly efficacious for laryngeal preservation. A role for chemotherapy in the initial management of early-stage oral cavity carcinoma (T1–T2, N0) is similarly unexplored. A growing body of evidence suggests that there is a role for the administration of concurrent chemoradiation in the adjuvant setting for postoperative patients at high risk for local-regional recurrence.

In a meta-analysis of randomized clinical trials comparing local-regional therapy with and without chemotherapy, chemotherapy significantly improved the survival of patients with previously untreated, nonmetastatic head and neck cancer.[1] This analysis included individual data on over 10,000 patients enrolled in 63 clinical trials. Chemotherapy reduced the risk of death by 10% [hazard ratio (HR), 0.90; 95% confidence interval (CI), 0.85–0.94], which corresponded to an absolute survival benefit of 4% at 5 years. In an analysis of survival by primary site, patients with oral cavity carcinoma derived benefit from chemotherapy (HR, 0.86; 95% CI, 0.79–0.94), but this was not significantly different from patients with primary tumors at other sites. Concomitant chemoradiation therapy (CRT) resulted in a 19% reduction in risk of death (HR, 0.81; 95% CI, 0.76–0.88), which corresponded to an absolute benefit of 8% at 5 years. By contrast, both adjuvant and neoadjuvant chemotherapy

had no effect on overall survival. Chemotherapy regimens that included more than one drug had a greater impact on survival than single-agent chemotherapy, and the benefit to chemotherapy was predominantly in patients under the age of 60 years.[1]

Several additional meta-analyses have reported similar improvements in overall survival in patients receiving concomitantly administered CRT.[2–6] Cisplatin and 5-fluorouracil (5-FU), currently one of the most frequently used and efficacious chemotherapy regimens for head and neck cancer, had the greatest impact on mortality when compared with other regimens.[2] Unfortunately, the administration of chemotherapy is also associated with significant increases in local-regional toxicity that contribute to delays in RT as well as nausea and bone marrow toxicity.[4] This chapter reviews the evidence that is currently available for chemotherapy in the treatment of squamous cell carcinoma of the oral cavity, and provides recommendations for its use that are based on the potential benefit as well as the risk of treatment-associated toxicity.

◆ Established Indications for Chemotherapy

Recurrent or Metastatic Disease

Chemotherapy is indicated for the palliation of symptoms from disease in patients with metastatic oral cavity carcinoma and those with disease that is refractory to local-regional primary therapy. Several single-agent and combination regimens have demonstrated activity in head

251

Table 21–1   Chemotherapeutic Agents with Activity in Metastatic or Recurrent Head and Neck Cancer

Agent	Response Rate	Reference
Cisplatin	28%	11
Carboplatin	22%	11
Paclitaxel	35–36%	54
Docetaxel	Previously treated 17–42%	19–22
	Untreated 57%	
Methotrexate	16–34%	11, 24
Ifosfamide	Previously treated 0–10%	30–34
	Untreated 25–53%	
5-Fluorouracil	15%	25
Irinotecan	21%	37
Gemcitabine	0–13%	20, 36

and neck squamous cell carcinoma (HNSCC). However, few clinical trials of palliative chemotherapy have included quality of life measures. To date, it has largely been assumed, and supported by clinical experience, that clinical response, defined as a greater than or equal to 50% reduction in tumor volume, correlates with palliation of symptoms from disease. Only one randomized clinical trial has demonstrated improved survival following chemotherapy when compared with best supportive care.[7]

When considering the treatment of patients with metastatic or recurrent disease, the performance status of the patient must be considered, and the potential benefit from chemotherapy must be carefully weighed against the possible adverse effects of chemotherapy. In general, response rates to single agent chemotherapy in this setting range from 10 to 25%. Most patients experience disease progression within 2 to 3 months, and median survival is approximately 6 months. The agents with demonstrated activity in head and neck cancers are listed in **Table 21–1**. Most clinical trials have included a heterogeneous group of patients with regard to the primary site. There is no compelling data to suggest that response rates to chemotherapy differ significantly by primary site.

Single-Agent Chemotherapy

The platinum agents cisplatin and carboplatin remain the most commonly used chemotherapeutic agents for head and neck cancer. Cisplatin is a heavy metal that forms interstrand cross-links with DNA and induces arrest in the G2 phase of the cell cycle.[8] Cisplatin is also an effective radiosensitizer that inhibits sublethal damage repair, a hypoxic cell sensitizer, and an inhibitor of tumor neovascularization.[9,10] Cisplatin can be administered on daily, weekly, and every 3-week schedules, and like most chemotherapy agents, is dosed as a function of milligrams per square meter of body surface area (mg/m^2). The response rate to cisplatin is approximately 28% when administered as a single agent in doses of 60 to 120 mg/m^2 every 3 to 4 weeks.[11] In randomized trials, response rates were not significantly improved with higher dose cisplatin, but toxicity was significantly increased.[12,13] Common toxicities from cisplatin include nephrotoxicity, neurotoxicity (peripheral neuropathy), ototoxicity, nausea and vomiting, and cytopenias. Most

patients who receive more than 600 mg/m^2 will experience neurotoxicity, the incidence and severity of which is related to cumulative dose.

Carboplatin is frequently substituted for cisplatin because it is associated with less nephrotoxicity and neurotoxicity. The drug appears to have slightly less activity when compared with cisplatin, with a response rate averaging approximately 22%.[11] Carboplatin is usually dosed as a function of age, gender, and creatinine clearance by use of Calvert's formula, which utilizes a pharmacokinetically targeted end point, the AUC (area under concentration versus time curve, expressed in mg/mL/min), to calculate the dose in milligrams.[14] Common side effects from administration include thrombocytopenia, neutropenia, and anemia.

The microtubule stabilizing agents, docetaxel and paclitaxel, have demonstrated activity in head and neck cancer. By interfering with microtubule assembly, these drugs induce arrest in the G2/M phase of the cell cycle and subsequent cell death by apoptosis.[15,16] In separate phase II studies, the response rate to high-dose continuous infusion paclitaxel (250 mg/m^2 over 24 hours every 3 weeks) appeared higher than when administered as a 3-hour infusion at a lower dose (175 mg/m^2).[17,18] Docetaxel (100 mg/m^2 every 21 days) is also an active agent, with response rates of 17 to 42% in patients with recurrent or metastatic disease and as high as 57% in treatment-naive patients in phase II trials.[19–22] Common toxicities from the taxanes include hypersensitivity reactions, alopecia, neutropenia, arthralgia, peripheral neuropathy, and edema. Initial drug development focused on the maximal tolerated dose of these drugs when administered every 3 weeks. Weekly administration is under active investigation in combination regimens.[23] As taxanes have demonstrated potency as radiation sensitizers, the optimal dose and schedule for concomitant administration with RT are active areas of investigation.

Single-agent methotrexate, a classic antifolate, was the standard of care for metastatic head and neck cancer prior to the development of the platinum agents and taxanes.[11] Weekly administration at 40 to 60 mg/m^2 is well tolerated. Anticipated toxicities at this dose would include mild cytopenias and liver enzyme elevation. Use of the drug is primarily restricted to patients with a poor performance status [Eastern Cooperative Oncology Group (ECOG) 2] and as second- or third-line therapy in patients with taxone- and cisplatin-refractory disease. Response rates of 16 to 31% should be anticipated in patients without prior therapy for metastatic or recurrent disease.[11,24]

5-Fluorouracil (5-FU) is a thymidylate synthetase inhibitor that has demonstrated an approximate 15% response rate in clinical trials when administered as a continuous infusion over 4 to 5 days.[25] The drug has demonstrated synergistic activity with the platinum agents and is rarely used as a single agent. A newer oral prodrug of 5-FU, capecitabine, is preferentially activated in tumor tissue, and sustained drug levels mimic continuous infusion 5-FU.[26] Although response rates to single-agent capecitabine of 24% have been reported in nasopharyngeal cancer, its activity at other head and neck sites appears poor.[27,28] It shows promise, however, in combination with cisplatin as a substitute for 5-FU.[29] Stomatitis, diarrhea, nausea, abdominal pain, and hand-foot syndrome are the principal toxicities of the fluoropyrimidines.

The alkylating agent ifosfamide has demonstrated highly variable response rates in head and neck cancer, from 0 to 10% in patients with prior chemotherapy treatment and 25 to 53% in patients without prior chemotherapy.[30–34] In a randomized phase II trial including 152 patients, response rates to single-agent ifosfamide (1.5 g/m^2 for 5 days together with mesna) and to the combination of ifosfamide and cisplatin (10 mg/m^2 for 5 days) were 53% (31/58) and 66% (50/76), respectively.[35] The principal toxicities of ifosfamide are hematologic, as well as nausea, vomiting, alopecia, and central nervous system toxicity, manifest as confusion and sedation.

Gemcitabine, a deoxycytidine analogue that inhibits DNA synthesis, has yielded a response rate of 13% in 61 patients with metastatic or recurrent head and neck cancer in a single phase II trial, but no activity was observed in a subsequent study.[36,37] The topoisomerase-I inhibitor irinotecan has demonstrated a response rate of 21.2%, but aminocamptothecin (9-AC/DMA) and topotecan have little activity in head and neck cancer.[38–41] Bleomycin, an antitumor antibiotic and intercalating agent, and mitomycin C, an alkylating agent that is an effective hypoxic-cell sensitizer, are older compounds with reported activity in head and neck cancer as single agents and in combination with RT. The cumulative pulmonary toxicity of bleomycin has limited its use, and cisplatin has largely replace mitomycin C as a radiation sensitizer.

Abnormalities of epidermal growth factor receptor (EGFR) signal transduction are common in squamous cell carcinoma of the head and neck. Overexpression of EGFR has been demonstrated in most cancers, and has been associated with poor prognosis.[42] Several inhibitors of EGFR signal transduction have shown promise in preclinical models and modest activity to date in clinical trials.[43] Small molecule inhibitors of EGFR, including OSI-774 and Iressa, have demonstrated 4 to 11% response rates in heavily pretreated patients.[44] A monoclonal antibody to EGFR (C225) has demonstrated 11 to 15% response rates in patients with platinum-refractory disease.[45,46] In a preliminary report of a randomized trial, the addition of C225 to single-agent cisplatin therapy did not significantly affect response rates or survival of patients with recurrent or metastatic disease.[47] The principal toxicities observed to date with EGFR-targeted therapies include rash, diarrhea, and hypersensitivity reactions exclusive to C225.

Multiagent Chemotherapy Regimens

Combination chemotherapy regimens are the standard of care for individuals with recurrent or metastatic head and neck cancer with a good performance status. Combination regimens produce a statistically significant increase in response rates when compared with single-agent chemotherapy. However, improved response rates did not result in improvements in survival in a recent meta-analysis.[48]

A combination regimen of cisplatin and 5-FU has been the standard of care since originally reported by investigators at Wayne State in 1984.[49] This combination has an estimated cumulative response rate of approximately 50% and complete response rate of approximately 5 to 7% in phase II trials.[50] Similar response rates have been reported in a trial exclusive to oral cavity carcinomas.[51] In this regimen,

cisplatin 100 mg/m^2 and continuous infusion 5-FU $1000 \text{ mg/m}^2/\text{d}$ for 4 days are administered intravenously every 21 days. Three large randomized clinical trials have reported improved response rates for this regimen when compared with single-agent therapy, but no improvement in survival.[25,52,53] Response rates in the oral cavity did not significantly differ from tumors at other sites.[25] The substitution of carboplatin for cisplatin reduced response rates.[52]

Both paclitaxel and docetaxel in combination with cisplatin have promising activity in Phase II trials. The docetaxel and cisplatin combination has response rates from 40 to 53%.[22,54,55] In a randomized controlled trial comparing high dose (200 mg/m^2 over 24 hours every 21 days) versus low dose (135 mg/m^2) paclitaxel plus cisplatin (75 mg/m^2 every 21 days), response rates in previously untreated and treated patients were 58% and 32%, respectively.[56] Higher doses did not improve response rates (35% vs. 36%), and no effect of tumor site on response was observed.[56]

Base on these promising results, 194 patients with metastatic or recurrent disease were randomized to receive cisplatin 100 mg/m^2 on day 1 and 5-FU $1000 \text{ mg/m}^2/\text{d}$ on days 1 to 4, or paclitaxel 175 mg/m^2 and cisplatin 75 mg/m^2 on day 1 every 21 days.[57] In preliminary reports, no significant differences in survival (41% vs. 30%, $p = .22$ at 1 year), response (22% vs. 28%, $p = .40$) or quality of life measures between the two regimens were reported. Based on this clinical trial, combined paclitaxel and cisplatin is a reasonable alternative to the cisplatin and 5-FU regimen as first-line therapy for patients with recurrent or metastatic head and neck cancer.[57,58]

Several chemotherapeutic agents have been added to the regimen of cisplatin and 5-FU that have resulted in improved response rates, but improved survival has not been demonstrated. Regimens that include paclitaxel, ifosfamide, and carboplatin (TIC) or cisplatin (TIP) appear promising. Overall response rates of 58% and complete response rates of 17% have been reported in phase II studies in patients with recurrent or metastatic disease. In a separate clinical setting, results for the combination of paclitaxel, 5-FU, and cisplatin appear promising. In a randomized controlled trial including 397 patients, those with untreated disease were randomized to receive cisplatin and 5-FU with or without paclitaxel as induction chemotherapy for locally advanced HNSCC.[59] Patients received three cycles of either cisplatin (100 mg/m^2 on day 1) and 5-FU ($1000 \text{ mg/m}^2/\text{d}$ on days 1 to 5) or the three drug regimen, cisplatin (100 mg/m^2 on day 2), 5-FU ($500 \text{ mg/m}^2/\text{d}$ on days 1 to 5), and paclitaxel (175 mg/m^2 on day 1). Eleven percent of patients had oral cavity carcinoma. The complete response rate was significantly increased with the addition of paclitaxel (33.2% vs. 14.4%, $p < .001$) without increasing toxicity.[59]

Treatment Recommendation for Recurrent or Metastatic Disease

Because none of the currently available chemotherapeutic agents used alone or in combination has been demonstrated to affect patient survival, patients with recurrent or metastatic oral cavity carcinoma and good performance status should be encouraged to participate in clinical trials of new investigational agents. Outside of a clinical trial, the standard of care for patients with a good performance status (ECOG 0 or 1) would include combination chemotherapy with cisplatin (100 mg/m^2 on day 1) and 5-FU (1000 mg/m^2/d as a continuous intravenous infusion on days 1 through 4) every 21 days or cisplatin (75 mg/m^2 on day 1) and paclitaxel (175 mg/m^2 administered intravenously over 3 hours on day 1) every 21 days. Patients with a marginal performance status (ECOG 2) should be treated with single-agent methotrexate (40–60 mg/m^2/week) or with supportive care alone. Patients with an ECOG performance status of 3 should receive supportive care only because they are unlikely to tolerate the side effects of chemotherapy.

Unresectable Disease

Concurrent CRT is the standard of care for patients with unresectable, oral cavity carcinoma and a good performance status. Combined modality regimens have investigated the addition of single or multiagent chemotherapy to standard fractionated, hyperfractionated, accelerated, or split-course RT alternating with chemotherapy. Several studies have demonstrated improvements in survival, disease-free survival, and local control with the addition of chemotherapy.

Single-Agent Chemotherapy

In phase II trials of single-agent cisplatin concurrently administered with external beam RT in patients with advanced stage III and IV HNSCC, a complete response of approximately 70% is achieved, regardless of schedule.[8] The cumulative dose of cisplatin administered, rather than the schedule of administration, appears to be an important factor in randomized trials that have compared RT alone to concurrent cisplatin and radiation (**Table 21–2**). Patients with stage III or IV unresectable disease were randomized to standard fractionation RT (70 Gy total/one fraction per day/2-Gy fractions/35 fractions) with or without weekly cisplatin at 20 mg/m^2 (cumulative dose of 120–140 mg/m^2).[60] Although chemotherapy-treated patients had an improved

complete response rate (73% vs. 59%, $p = .007$), there was no improvement in survival.[60] A subsequent trial clearly demonstrated improved survival when high-dose cisplatin was administered concurrently with RT; 295 patients with unresectable disease were randomized to standard fractionated radiation with or without cisplatin 100 mg/m^2 on days 1, 22, and 43 (cumulative dose 300 mg/m^2) or to a third arm of split-course radiation and three cycles of concurrent combination chemotherapy with cisplatin 75 mg/m^2 and 5-FU 1000 mg/m^2/d on days 1 through 4.[61] With a median follow-up of 41 months, overall survival was significantly improved only in the single-agent cisplatin arm when compared with the radiation-alone arm (37 vs. 23%, $p = .014$).[61] In a third three-arm trial, 159 patients with unresectable stage III or IV disease were randomized to receive standard fractionation radiation alone, or concomitantly with cisplatin 6 mg/m^2/d (cumulative dose 210 mg/m^2) or carboplatin 25 mg/m^2/d.[62] Local-regional control was improved significantly with the addition of either cisplatin or carboplatin (clinical complete response rates of 72% and 68% vs. 38%, $p < .01$). Median survival was significantly longer in both chemotherapy arms of the trial (32 and 30 months vs. 16 months, $p = .02$). Five-year survival was 32% and 29% in the cisplatin and carboplatin arms of the trial, respectively, versus 15% in the radiation alone arm ($p = .02$). Similar favorable outcomes were demonstrated when cisplatin (6 mg/m^2/d) was added to hyperfractionated RT in a trial that included patients with both resectable and unresectable disease.[63]

In a preliminary report of a three-arm trial that included patients with resectable or unresectable disease, 124 patients were randomized to receive either standard fractionation RT alone, concurrently with cisplatin 100 mg/m^2 on days 2, 22, and 42, or concurrently with carboplatin (AUC = 7 mg/mL/min) on days 2, 22, and 42.[64] At 3 years of follow-up, 17.5% of patients were alive in the radiation alone arm versus 52% and 42% in the cisplatin and carboplatin arms, respectively ($p < .001$). Time to progression was also significantly improved in the cisplatin and carboplatin arms when compared with the radiation-alone arm (45.2

Table 21–2 Phase III Trials of Single-Agent Cisplatin Concurrent with Radiation Therapy for Unresectable Head and Neck Cancer

First Author	No. of Patients (% oral cavity)	Chemotherapy	Radiation	Significant Benefit?*			
				CR	LC	PFS DSS	OS
Haselow, 1990[60]	319 (29)	Cisplatin 20 mg/m^2/wk	70 Gy	Yes	NR	NR	No
Adelstein, 2003[61]	295 (13.3)	Cisplatin 100 mg/m^2 on days 1, 22, 43	70 Gy	Yes	NR	Yes	Yes
		or Cisplatin 75 mg/m^2 + 5-FU 1000 mg/m^2/d on weeks 1, 5, 9	60–70 Gy split	No	NR	No	NR
Jeremic, 1997[62]	159 (16.4)	Cisplatin 6 mg/m^2/d	70 Gy	Yes	Yes	No	Yes
		or Carboplatin 25 mg/m^2/d		Yes	Yes	No	Yes
Jeremic, 2000[63]	130 (21)	Cisplatin 6 mg/m^2/d	77 Gy Hfx	Yes	Yes	Yes	Yes
Fountzilas, 2003[64]	124 (NR)	Cisplatin 100 mg/m^2 on days 2, 22, 42	70 Gy	No	NR	Yes	Yes
		or Carboplatin AUC 7 on days 2, 22, 42		No	NR	Yes	Yes

*Compared with radiation alone arm.
NR, not reported; CR, complete response; LC, local-regional confirmed; PFS, progression-free survival; DSS, disease-specific survival; OS, overall survival; Hfx, hyperfractionated radiation therapy.

and 17.7 months vs. 6.3 months, $p = .0002$). Although schedules of cisplatin administration have not been compared in randomized trials in this setting, daily low-dose therapy appears to be associated with decreased toxicity without compromising efficacy. Randomized clinical trials evaluating single-agent mitomycin C have also demonstrated improvements in survival when compared with radiation alone.[65,66]

Multiagent Chemotherapy

Several randomized trials of RT with or without combination chemotherapy and concomitant RT have been completed in patients with unresectable disease. Most of these trials also included patients with resectable disease. The four clinical trials that have included patients with oral cavity carcinoma are displayed in **Table 21–3**. Patients with unresectable head and neck cancer (22% with oral cavity carcinoma) were randomized to hyperfractionated RT administered in three courses of 13 fractions (1.8 Gy twice daily) with or without concomitant cisplatin, 5-FU, and leucovorin.[67] Cisplatin 60 mg/m^2, 5-FU 350 mg/m^2, and leucovorin 50 mg/m^2 were administered on day 2 of each radiation cycle followed by 4 days of continuous infusion 5-FU 350 mg/m^2/d and leucovorin 100 mg/m^2/d. Local-regional control at 3 years (36 vs. 17%, $p < .004$) and overall survival (48 vs. 24%, $p < .0003$) were improved in the chemotherapy arm. Mucositis and radiation dermatitis were made worse by the addition of chemotherapy, but serious late effects of therapy, including xerostomia, fibrosis, and osteoradionecrosis were not different in the two arms. In a smaller trial of 122 patients with resectable and unresectable disease, combination chemotherapy with two cycles of cisplatin (12 mg/m^2/d for 5 days), 5-FU (600 mg/m^2/d as continuous infusion for 5 days), and leucovorin improved local-regional control at 3 years (70 vs. 44%, $p = .01$) when compared with hyperfractionated RT alone, but not overall survival (55 vs. 34%, $p = .07$).[68] Only 5% of patients had oral cavity carcinoma. Disease-free survival and median time to progression were improved in unresectable patients in a small, randomized trial that evaluated the addition of two cycles of cisplatin 100 mg/m^2 on day 1 and 5-FU 1000 mg/m^2/d as continuous infusion on days 1 through 4 to standard fractionation RT.[69] The complete response rate and disease-free survival of unresectable patients was improved with the addition of combination chemotherapy with bleomycin and mitomycin C in a small trial of 49 patients.[70]

Treatment Recommendation for Unresectable Disease

Concurrent CRT is the standard of care for unresectable oral cavity carcinoma. Patients with a good performance status should be encouraged to participate in clinical trials that have been designed to evaluate newer chemotherapeutic agents with potential as radiation sensitizers. Outside of a clinical trial, patients with good performance status (ECOG 0, 1) should receive single-agent cisplatin 100 mg/m^2 administered on days 1, 22, and 42 of standard fractionated RT or administered daily at 6 mg/m^2/d with standard fractionation or hyperfractionated RT. Current data suggest that carboplatin may be less effective than cisplatin, but carboplatin can be substituted for cisplatin in patients with poor renal function. The dose and schedule should be either daily carboplatin at 25 mg/m^2/d of radiation or carboplatin (AUC = 7 mg/mL/min) on days 1, 22, and 42 of standard fractionated RT. Patients with a poor performance status should receive palliative RT alone.

◆ Potential Roles for Chemotherapy that Have Not Been Established

Adjuvant Chemoradiation for Resected High-Risk Disease

Patients with advanced, resectable, stage III or IV oral cavity carcinoma are at high risk for death from local-regional recurrence. Survival at 5 years remains approximately 30 to 35%, and distant metastases develop in approximately 23%.[71] Factors known to increase the risk of local-regional recurrence and distant metastases after surgical resection include positive or close (<5 mm) surgical margins, multiple positive lymph nodes, extracapsular spread of lymph node–positive disease, and perineural, lymphatic, or vascular invasion.[72,73] Extracapsular spread appears to be the single most important factor for local-regional recurrence.[72] The addition of adjuvant chemotherapy, and in particular adjuvant CRT, to the postoperative management of patients with high-risk features on pathologic examination has demonstrated promise in several clinical trials (**Table 21–4**).

In a Head and Neck Intergroup trial, postoperative patients with negative surgical margins were randomized to receive either three cycles of cisplatin and 5-FU prior to postoperative RT or RT alone.[71] Patients with high-risk features, defined as those with extracapsular extension, close margins, or carcinoma in situ at margins, had a trend toward improvement in local control and survival.[71] In a subsequent trial, 88 patients with resected stage III or IV squamous cell carcinoma of the head and neck and pathologically documented extracapsular spread were randomized to receive postoperative RT administered concurrently with or without fixed-dose cisplatin at 50 mg/week.[74] At 5 years, overall survival (36% vs. 13%, $p < .01$), disease-specific survival (45% vs. 23%, $p < .02$), and local-regional disease-free survival (70 vs. 55%, $p = .05$) were improved with the addition of chemotherapy. There was no difference in metastasis-free survival in the two arms [58% vs. 49% at 5 years, $p = NS$ (no significant difference)]. The addition of mitomycin C to postoperative RT has also been shown to improve local control (87% vs. 67%, $p < .015$) and disease-free survival at 5 years (67% vs. 44%, $p < .03$) in postoperative patients with or without positive surgical margins when compared with radiation alone.[75] Overall survival was not improved (48% vs. 42%, $p = NS$).

Based on these promising data, the European Organization for Research and Treatment of Cancer (EORTC) conducted a trial in which 334 postoperative patients were randomized to standard fractionation postoperative RT to a total dose of 66 Gy with or without concurrently administered cisplatin 100 mg/m^2 on days 1, 22, and 43.[76,77] Eligible patients

Table 21–3   Randomized Trials of Multiagent Chemotherapy and Concurrent Radiation Therapy for Unresectable Head and Neck Cancer, Inclusive of Oral Cavity

First Author	No. of Patients (% Oral Cavity)	Tumor Stage	Radiation Therapy	Chemotherapy	CR Rates	Progression-Free Survival	Disease-Specific Survival	Overall Survival	Disease-Free Survival
Smid, 1995[70]	49 (16)	Unresectable	Arms A & B: Standard fractionation 66–70 Gy	Arm B only: Bleomycin 5 U twice a week + Mitomycin C 10–15 mg/m², weeks 1 and 7	Arm A 24% Arm B 63% (p = .005)	Arm A 9% at 18 months Arm B 48% (p = .001)	NR	NR	NR
Weissler, 1992[69]	58 (16)	III or IV Unresectable or high-risk, postoperative patients	Arms A & B: Inoperable patients: Hyperfractionated, split 69 Gy High-risk patients: Positive margins 60 Gy Negative margins 54 Gy	Arm B: Cisplatin 100 mg/m² + 5-FU 1000 mg/m²/d CI×4 days, weeks 1 and 4	NR	NR	NR	NR	Improved in chemotherapy arm
Brizel, 1998[68]	122 (5)	T3, T4, N0–N3, T2N0 BOT Resectable or Unresectable	Arm A: Hyperfractionated 75 Gy Arm B: Hyperfractionated 70 Gy	Arm B only: Cisplatin 12 mg/m²×5 days+5-FU 600 mg/m²/d CI×5 days, weeks 1 and 6+2 cycles adjuvant chemotherapy (cisplatin increased to 16–20 mg/m²)	Arm A 73% Arm B 88% (p = .52)	Arm A 41% at 3 years Arm B 61% (p = .08)	NR	Arm A 34% at 3 years Arm B 55% (p = .07)	NR
Wendt, 1998[67]	270 (22)	Stage III and IV M0 Unresectable	Arms A & B: Hyperfractionated, split 70 Gy	Arm B only: Cisplatin 60 mg/m² on day 1 + 5-FU 350 mg/m² on day 1 + 5-FU 350 mg/m²/d CI on days 2–5 + Leucovorin 50 mg/m² on day 1 + Leucovorin 100 mg/m²/d CI on days 2–5, weeks 1, 3, and 6	NR	Arm A 17% at 3 years Arm B 35% (p < .004) (local-regional)	NR	Arm A 24% at 3 years Arm B 49% (p < .0003)	NR

OC, oral cavity; NR, not reported; CI, continuous infusion; BOT, base of tongue.

Table 21–4 Randomized Trials of Adjuvant Chemoradiation in High-Risk, Postoperative Patients

First Author	High-Risk Features	Radiation	Chemotherapy	Significant Benefit?*		
				LRC	DSS	OS
Bachaud, 1996[74]	Stage III or IV Extracapsular spread	65–74 Gy	Cisplatin 50 mg/week	No	Yes	Yes
Haffty, 1993[75]	Positive margins	60 Gy	Mitomycin C 15–30 mg/m^2	Yes	Yes	No
Bernier, 2004[77]	≥2 involved nodes Extracapsular spread Positive margins Perineural invasion Vascular invasion Positive level IV or V nodes (oral cavity and oropharynx sites)	66 Gy	Cisplatin 100 mg/m^2 on days 1, 22, 43	Yes	Yes	Yes
Cooper, 2004[78]	≥2 involved nodes Extracapsular spread Positive margins	60–66 Gy	Cisplatin 100 mg/m^2 on days 1, 22, 43	Yes	Yes	No

*Compared with radiation-alone arm.
LRC, local-regional control; DSS, disease-specific survival; OS, overall survival.

included those who had two or more positive lymph nodes, extracapsular spread, microscopic positive margins, perineural or vascular invasion, or oral cavity and oropharyngeal tumors with involved nodes in levels IV or V. Twenty-six percent of enrolled patients had oral cavity carcinoma. Patients in the chemotherapy arm of the trial had improvements in 5-year disease-free survival (31% vs. 18%, $p = .07$) and overall survival (53% vs. 40%, $p = .04$) as well as local control (83% vs. 64%, $p = .014$) and progression-free survival (47% vs. 36%, $p = .02$) at a median follow-up of 60 months.[76,77] In a similar Intergroup phase III trial, 459 postoperative patients with high-risk pathologic features (two or more positive nodes, extracapsular spread, or positive margins) were randomized to postoperative radiation with or without cisplatin 100 mg/m^2 on days 1, 21, and 42.[78] The primary outcome for this trial was local-regional control. High-risk features that defined eligibility included N2 or greater nodal involvement, extracapsular extension, and microscopic positive margins of resection. Twenty-seven percent of patients enrolled in this trial had a primary tumor within the oral cavity. Results were reported after a median follow-up of 45.9 months. The rate of local-regional control at 2 years was significantly higher in the combined therapy group than in the group given RT alone (82% vs. 72%, $p = .01$) as was disease-specific survival.[78] There was no difference in overall survival. The results of this trial confirm the outcomes of the EORTC trial, and postoperative CRT with three cycles of high-dose cisplatin is evolving into the standard of care for a selected group of patients at high-risk for recurrence.

Treatment Recommendation for Resected High-Risk Disease

Patients with resected stage III or IV oral cavity carcinoma with pathologic features that place the patient at high risk for local-regional recurrence (positive margins of resection, extracapsular spread, and possibly lymphatic or vascular

invasion) should be referred to a medical oncologist postoperatively to be evaluated for adjuvant concurrent chemoradiation. The current regimen, based on the results of the EORTC and Intergroup trials that were cited earlier, would be for eligible patients to receive three doses of high-dose cisplatin (100 mg/m^2) every 21 days during RT. Participation in clinical trials of alternate regimens should also be encouraged.

Role of Chemotherapy in Resectable Oral Cancer

Induction Chemotherapy Prior to Surgical Resection

No survival advantage has been demonstrated with the addition of "neoadjuvant" or "induction" chemotherapy prior to primary surgical or RT in randomized clinical trials of patients with advanced head and neck cancer.[79] This is despite the fact that these trials have repeatedly demonstrated a reduction in risk of distant metastases as the site of first treatment failure.[80] Based on limited site-specific evidence, neoadjuvant chemotherapy is not indicated for patients with oral cavity carcinoma prior to surgical resection.

A single trial investigating the role of induction chemotherapy prior to surgical resection for oral cavity carcinoma was recently published.[81] In this multicenter, randomized trial, 197 patients with resectable, stage T2–T4, N0–N2, M0 oral cavity squamous cell carcinoma were randomized to three cycles of cisplatin and continuous infusion 5-FU or to immediate surgery. Patients who achieved a partial or greater response to two cycles of chemotherapy received cycle three, whereas those with less than a partial response underwent surgical salvage. All patients received a total of 65 Gy to the tumor bed. Patients with positive margins, invasion of soft tissues, three or more involved nodes, or extracapsular spread received postoperative RT (50 Gy) to the neck and a 15-cGy boost for patients with extracapsular spread. Principal outcomes included disease-free and overall survival. In the chemotherapy arm, 28 (34%) and 34 (41%) of 82 evaluable patients achieved a clinical complete and partial response, respectively. A pathologic complete response was observed in 27%. Individuals in the chemotherapy arm did not have a reduction in risk for local-regional (31% vs. 32%, $p = $ NS) or distant relapse (7% vs. 9%, $p = $ NS). An overall survival of 55% was observed in both arms. Patients in the chemotherapy arm had fewer segmental mandibulectomy procedures (31% vs. 52%, a 21% difference; 95% CI, 7–34%). Fewer individuals in the chemotherapy arm required postoperative RT to the neck (33% vs. 46%, a 13% difference; 95% CI, 0–27%). Individuals who experienced a response to chemotherapy had improved survival, but this is likely a marker for a biologically select group of cancers. Thus, induction chemotherapy has no current defined role in the preoperative setting.

High local control rates have been reported with neoadjuvant chemoradiation prior to surgical resection in oral cavity carcinomas in single-institution phase II studies, but have yet to be evaluated in a randomized trial.[82,83]

Induction Chemotherapy Prior to Primary Radiation Therapy

Results of a large, randomized phase III trial have suggested that four cycles of cisplatin (100 mg/m^2) and 5-FU (1000 mg/m^2/d for 4 days) induction chemotherapy followed by RT may improve disease-free (49% vs. 34%, $p = .04$) and overall survival (30% vs. 24%, $p = .04$) in patients with unresectable head and neck cancer when compared with a control arm of radiation alone.[84] These differences in survival were not confirmed in resectable or unresectable patients by a subsequent randomized trial that evaluated the addition of three, rather than four, cycles of neoadjuvant cisplatin and 5-FU to standard fractionation radiation.[85] It is unclear whether or not this difference is due to chance, or whether the difference can be attributed to the addition of a single cycle of the same chemotherapy regimen, but this is unlikely. At this time, there is no defined role for induction chemotherapy prior to primary radiation-based therapy for patients with oral cavity carcinoma. The potential benefit of the addition of induction chemotherapy to concurrent CRT regimens that are currently the standard of care for patients with unresectable disease is an active area of clinical investigation, but has yet to be addressed in a randomized trial.[86]

Organ Preservation Chemoradiation

The possibility for organ preservation therapy with concurrent chemoradiation for patients with resectable oral cavity carcinoma has not been explored. A single trial has demonstrated that overall survival with primary site preservation can be improved with the addition of two cycles of cisplatin and 5-FU to RT in patients with stage III and IV resectable disease.[87,88] However, only 4% of patients had oral cavity carcinoma, and all were randomized to the chemotherapy arm.

Organ preservation therapy with a combination of concurrent radiation and high-dose cisplatin is currently the standard of care for larynx preservation for patients with T3 N0–N3 disease and low-volume T4 laryngeal carcinomas. Laryngeal preservation is successfully achieved in 88% of surviving patients at 2 years with this approach.[89,90] The trial that defined the new standard of care was Intergroup 91–11, in which 547 laryngeal cancer patients were randomized to receive 70 Gy total of standard fractionation RT alone, standard fractionation RT preceded by three cycles of induction cisplatin and 5-FU, or RT administered concomitantly with three doses of high-dose cisplatin.[89] Although overall survival was not significantly different in the three arms, the concurrent chemoradiation arm was clearly superior with regard to organ preservation when compared with the other two arms of the trial. Induction chemotherapy and concurrent CRT have also shown promise for oropharyngeal and hypopharyngeal preservation.[91,92]

Although advances in reconstructive surgery have improved the quality of life of patients, the morbidity of surgery for advanced oral cavity carcinoma is still considerable. Patients may experience significant alterations in mastication, deglutition, phonation, respiration, and range of motion of the neck and shoulder. Pain, dependency on G-tubes for nutritional supplementation, and alterations in appearance can affect employment and social interaction. Prospective quality of life measures before, during, and after surgery are being applied to oral cancer patients to better understand how surgery affects global measures of quality of life and how these differ by variables such as tumor site and stage.[93–95] The size of the primary tumor, extent of mandibular resection, extent of tongue resection, and percent of soft palate resected are some of the factors associated with functional outcomes and quality of life to date.[95–98] Given these findings, investigators at M. D. Anderson Cancer Center plan to investigate the potential for oral cavity preservation with a combined approach that includes induction followed by concurrent chemoradiation.

Current Treatment Recommendations for Patients with Resectable Oral Cavity Carcinoma

Patients with resectable oral cavity carcinoma with pathologic features indicative of high risk for recurrence (extracapsular spread, microscopic positive margins, two or more involved lymph nodes, level IV or V nodal involvement, or vascular or perineural invasion) and a good performance status (ECOG 0 or 1) should be encouraged to participate in clinical trials evaluating the efficacy of concurrent adjuvant chemoradiation. Outside of a clinical trial, the new standard of care for this patient population includes standard fractionated RT to 66 Gy concurrently administered with three cycles of high-dose cisplatin 100 mg/m^2 on days 1, 12, and 42 of RT. Individuals with a poor performance status should receive radiation alone.

Given the poor 5-year survival of patients with stage III and IV oral cavity carcinoma, patients with resectable disease should be encouraged to participate in clinical trials of novel therapeutic approaches. Promising avenues involving chemotherapy would include neoadjuvant chemoradiation and organ preservation chemoradiation trials. Outside of the context of a clinical trial, there is no role for neoadjuvant chemotherapy or concurrent CRT for organ preservation in the management of resectable oral cavity carcinoma.

◆ Conclusion

The role for chemotherapy in patients with unresectable, recurrent, or metastatic oral cancer is well established. Recent findings suggest that patients with oral cancer who have undergone surgery that manifest high-risk pathologic features should be considered for adjuvant concurrent chemoradiation. There is presently no defined role for induction chemotherapy in the preoperative setting or prior to primary RT for patients with oral cavity carcinoma. The role of chemotherapy in organ preservation therapy for oral cancer remains investigational. Induction chemotherapy or chemotherapy for organ preservation should be administered only within the context of a clinical trial after the patient has been counseled about other available therapeutic options.

References

1. Pignon JP, Bourhis J, Domenge C, Designe L. Chemotherapy added to locoregional treatment for head and neck squamous-cell carcinoma: three meta-analyses of updated individual data. MACH-NC Collaborative Group. Meta-Analysis of Chemotherapy on Head and Neck Cancer. Lancet 2000;355:949–955

2. Browman GP, Hodson DI, Mackenzie RJ, Bestic N, Zuraw L. Choosing a concomitant chemotherapy and radiotherapy regimen for squamous cell head and neck cancer: a systematic review of the published literature with subgroup analysis. Head Neck 2001;23:579–589

3. Bourhis J, Pignon JP. Meta-analyses in head and neck squamous cell carcinoma. What is the role of chemotherapy? Hematol Oncol Clin North Am 1999;13:769–775

4. El-Sayed S, Nelson N. Adjuvant and adjunctive chemotherapy in the management of squamous cell carcinoma of the head and neck region. A meta-analysis of prospective and randomized trials. J Clin Oncol 1996;14:838–847

5. Stell PM. Adjuvant chemotherapy in head and neck cancer. Semin Radiat Oncol 1992;2:195–205

6. Munro AJ. An overview of randomised controlled trials of adjuvant chemotherapy in head and neck cancer. Br J Cancer 1995;71:83–91

7. Morton RP, Rugman F, Dorman EB, et al. Cisplatinum and bleomycin for advanced or recurrent squamous cell carcinoma of the head and neck: a randomised factorial phase III controlled trial. Cancer Chemother Pharmacol 1985;15:283–289

8. Marcu L, van Doorn T, Olver I. Cisplatin and radiotherapy in the treatment of locally advanced head and neck cancer–a review of their cooperation. Acta Oncol 2003;42:315–325

9. Lawrence TS, Blackstock AW, McGinn C. The mechanism of action of radiosensitization of conventional chemotherapeutic agents. Semin Radiat Oncol 2003;13:13–21

10. Yoshikawa A, Saura R, Matsubara T, Mizuno K. A mechanism of cisplatin action: antineoplastic effect through inhibition of neovascularization. Kobe J Med Sci 1997;43:109–120

11. Al-Sarraf M. Head and neck cancer: chemotherapy concepts. Semin Oncol 1988;15:70–85

12. Veronesi A, Zagonel V, Tirelli U, et al. High-dose versus low-dose cisplatin in advanced head and neck squamous carcinoma: a randomized study. J Clin Oncol 1985;3:1105–1108

13. Sako K, Razack MS, Kalnins I. Chemotherapy for advanced and recurrent squamous cell carcinoma of the head and neck with high and low dose cis-diamminedichloroplatinum. Am J Surg 1978;136:529–533

14. Calvert AH, Newell DR, Gumbrell LA, et al. Carboplatin dosage: prospective evaluation of a simple formula based on renal function. J Clin Oncol 1989;7:1748–1756

15. Abal M, Andreu JM, Barasoain I. Taxanes: microtubule and centrosome targets, and cell cycle dependent mechanisms of action. Curr Cancer Drug Targets 2003;3:193–203

16. Blagosklonny MV, Fojo T. Molecular effects of paclitaxel: myths and reality (a critical review). Int J Cancer 1999;83:151–156

17. Forastiere AA, Shank D, Neuberg D, Taylor SGT, DeConti RC, Adams G. Final report of a phase II evaluation of paclitaxel in patients with advanced squamous cell carcinoma of the head and neck: an Eastern Cooperative Oncology Group trial (PA390). Cancer 1998;82:2270–2274

18. Gebbia V, Testa A, Cannata G, Gebbia N. Single agent paclitaxel in advanced squamous cell head and neck carcinoma. Eur J Cancer 1996;32A:901–902

19. Dreyfuss AI, Clark JR, Norris CM, et al. Docetaxel: an active drug for squamous cell carcinoma of the head and neck. J Clin Oncol 1996;14:1672–1678

20. Catimel G, Verweij J, Mattijssen V, et al. Docetaxel (Taxotere): an active drug for the treatment of patients with advanced squamous cell carcinoma of the head and neck. EORTC Early Clinical Trials Group. Ann Oncol 1994;5:533–537

21. Inuyama Y, Kataura A, Togawa K, et al. [Late phase II clinical study of RP56976 (docetaxel) in patients with advanced/recurrent head and neck cancer.] Gan To Kagaku Ryoho 1999;26:107–116

22. Glisson BS. The role of docetaxel in the management of squamous cell cancer of the head and neck. Oncology (Williston Park) 2002; 16(6, suppl 6)83–87

23. Schroeder M, Holzgraefe M. Docetaxel-carboplatin for palliative chemotherapy in recurrent head and neck cancer. Paper presented at the American Society of Clinical Oncology (ASCO), 2003, Chicago

24. Schornagel JH, Verweij J, de Mulder PH, et al. Randomized phase III trial of edatrexate versus methotrexate in patients with metastatic and/or recurrent squamous cell carcinoma of the head and neck: a European Organization for Research and Treatment of Cancer Head and Neck Cancer Cooperative Group study. J Clin Oncol 1995;13: 1649–1655

25. Jacobs C, Lyman G, Velez-Garcia E, et al. A phase III randomized study comparing cisplatin and fluorouracil as single agents and in combination for advanced squamous cell carcinoma of the head and neck. J Clin Oncol 1992;10:257–263

26. Hoff PM. Practical considerations in the use of oral fluoropyrimidines. Semin Oncol 2003;30(3, suppl 6)88–92

27. Chua DT, Sham JS, Au GK. A phase II study of capecitabine in patients with recurrent and metastatic nasopharyngeal carcinoma pretreated with platinum-based chemotherapy. Oral Oncol 2003;39:361–366

28. Wong SJ, Ritch PS, Delzer N, Kidder TM, Campbell BH. Phase II trial of capecitabine in patients with advanced incurable head and neck cancer. Paper presented at the American Society of Clinical Oncology (ASCO), 2003, Chicago

29. Porta R, Carbonell X, del Campo JM, et al. Phase I study of capcitabine in combination with cisplatin in patients with advanced and/or metastatic squamous cell carcinoma of the head and neck. Paper presented at the American Society of Clinical Oncology (ASCO), 2002, Orlando, FL

30. Sandler A, Saxman S, Bandealy M, et al. Ifosfamide in the treatment of advanced or recurrent squamous cell carcinoma of the head and neck: a phase II Hoosier Oncology Group trial. Am J Clin Oncol 1998; 21:195–197

31. Huber MH, Lippman SM, Benner SE, et al. A phase II study of ifosfamide in recurrent squamous cell carcinoma of the head and neck. Am J Clin Oncol 1996;19:379–382

32. Martin M, Diaz-Rubio E, Gonzalez Larriba JL, et al. Ifosfamide in advanced epidermoid head and neck cancer. Cancer Chemother Pharmacol 1993;31:340–342

33. Buesa JM, Fernandez R, Esteban E, et al. Phase II trial of ifosfamide in recurrent and metastatic head and neck cancer. Ann Oncol 1991; 2:151–152

34. Cervellino JC, Araujo CE, Pirisi C, Francia A, Cerruti R. Ifosfamide and mesna for the treatment of advanced squamous cell head and neck cancer. A GETLAC study. Oncology 1991;48:89–92

35. Pai VR, Parikh DM, Mazumdar AT, Rao RS. Phase II study of high-dose ifosfamide as a single agent and in combination with cisplatin in the treatment of advanced and/or recurrent squamous cell carcinoma of head and neck. Oncology 1993;50:86–91

36. Catimel G, Vermorken JB, Clavel M, et al. A phase II study of Gemcitabine (LY 188011) in patients with advanced squamous cell carcinoma of the head and neck. EORTC Early Clinical Trials Group. Ann Oncol 1994;5:543–547

37. Samlowski WE, Gundacker H, Kuebler JP, et al. Evaluation of gemcitabine in patients with recurrent or metastatic squamous cell carcinoma of the head and neck: a Southwest Oncology Group phase II study. Invest New Drugs 2001;19:311–315

38. Murphy BA, Cmelak A, Burkey B, et al. Topoisomerase I inhibitors in the treatment of head and neck cancer. Oncology (Williston Park) 2001;15(7, suppl 8) 47–52

39. Lad T, Rosen F, Sciortino D, et al. Phase II trial of aminocamptothecin (9-AC/DMA) in patients with advanced squamous cell head and neck cancer. Invest New Drugs 2000;18:261–263

40. Murphy BA, Leong T, Burkey B, Langer C, Forastiere A. Lack of efficacy of topotecan in the treatment of metastatic or recurrent squamous carcinoma of the head and neck: an Eastern Cooperative Oncology Group Trial (E3393). Am J Clin Oncol 2001;24:64–66

41. Robert F, Soong SJ, Wheeler RH. A phase II study of topotecan in patients with recurrent head and neck cancer. Identification of an active new agent. Am J Clin Oncol 1997;20:298–302

42. Ford AC, Grandis JR. Targeting epidermal growth factor receptor in head and neck cancer. Head Neck 2003;25:67–73

43. Herbst RS, Langer CJ. Epidermal growth factor receptors as a target for cancer treatment: the emerging role of IMC-C225 in the treatment of lung and head and neck cancers. Semin Oncol 2002;29(1, suppl 4)27–36

44. Cohen EE, Rosen F, Stadler WM, et al. Phase II trial of ZD1839 in recurrent or metastatic squamous cell carcinoma of the head and neck. J Clin Oncol 2003;21:1980–1987

45. Kies MS, Arquetle AM, Nabell L, et al. Final report of the efficacy and safety of the anti-epidermal growth factor antibody Erbitux (IMC-C2245), in combination with cisplatin in patients with recurrent squamous cell carcinoma of the head and neck refractory to cisplatin containing chemotherapy. Paper presented at the American Society of Clinical Oncology (ASCO), 2002, Orlando, FL

46. Baselga J, Triga JM, Bourhis J, et al. Cetuximab (C225) plus cisplatin/carboplatin is active in patients with recurrent/metastatic squamous cell carcinoma of the head and neck progressing on a same dose and schedule platinum-based regimen. Paper presented at the American Society of Clinical Oncology (ASCO), 2002, Orlando, FL

47. Burtness BA, Li Y, Flood W, Mattar BI. Phase III trial comparing cisplatin (C) + anti-epidermal growth factor antibody (EGF-R) C225 in patients with metastatic/recurrent head and neck cancer. Paper presented at the American Society of Clinical Oncology (ASCO), 2002, Orlando, FL

48. Browman GP, Cronin L. Standard chemotherapy in squamous cell head and neck cancer: what we have learned from randomized trials. Semin Oncol 1994;21:311–319

49. Kish JA, Weaver A, Jacobs J, Cummings G, Al-Sarraf M. Cisplatin and 5-fluorouracil infusion in patients with recurrent and disseminated epidermoid cancer of the head and neck. Cancer 1984;53:1819–1824

50. Urba SG, Forastiere AA. Systemic therapy of head and neck cancer: most effective agents, areas of promise. Oncology (Huntingt) 1989;3:79–88

51. Andreadis C, Vahtsevanos K, Sidiras T, Thomaidis I, Antoniadis K, Mouratidou D. 5-Fluorouracil and cisplatin in the treatment of advanced oral cancer. Oral Oncol 2003;39:380–385

52. Forastiere AA, Metch B, Schuller DE, et al. Randomized comparison of cisplatin plus fluorouracil and carboplatin plus fluorouracil versus methotrexate in advanced squamous-cell carcinoma of the head and neck: a Southwest Oncology Group study. J Clin Oncol 1992;10:1245–1251

53. Clavel M, Vermorken JB, Cognetti F, et al. Randomized comparison of cisplatin, methotrexate, bleomycin and vincristine (CABO) versus cisplatin and 5-fluorouracil (CF) versus cisplatin (C) in recurrent or metastatic squamous cell carcinoma of the head and neck. A phase III study of the EORTC Head and Neck Cancer Cooperative Group. Ann Oncol 1994;5:521–526

54. Baur M, Kienzer HR, Schweiger J, et al. Docetaxel/cisplatin as first-line chemotherapy in patients with head and neck carcinoma: a phase II trial. Cancer 2002;94:2953–2958

55. Gedlicka C, Formanek M, Selzer E, et al. Phase II study with docetaxel and cisplatin in the treatment of recurrent and/or metastatic squamous cell carcinoma of the head and neck. Oncology 2002;63:145–150

56. Forastiere AA, Leong T, Rowinsky E, et al. Phase III comparison of high-dose paclitaxel + cisplatin + granulocyte colony-stimulating factor versus low-dose paclitaxel + cisplatin in advanced head and neck cancer: Eastern Cooperative Oncology Group Study E1393. J Clin Oncol 2001;19:1088–1095

57. Murphy BA, Li Y, Cella D, Karnad A, Hussain M, Forastiere A. Phase III study comparing cisplatin (C) and 5-fluorouracil (F) versus cisplatin and paclitaxel (T) in metastatic/recurrent head and neck cancer. Paper presented at the American Society of Clinical Oncology (ASCO), 2001, San Francisco

58. Wells N, Murphy BA, Dietrich M, Forastiere AA, Li Y, Cella D. Quality of life and pain assessment for head and neck cancer patients treated on E1395: a comparison of two different cisplatin-based chemotherapy regimens. Paper presented at the American Society of Clinical Oncology (ASCO), 2002, Orlando, FL

59. Hitt R, Lopez-Pousa A, Rodriguez M, et al. Phase III study comparing cisplatin (P) and 5-fluorouracil (F) versus P, F and paclitaxel (T) as induction therapy in locally advanced head and neck cancer. Paper presented at the American Society of Clinical Oncology (ASCO), 2003, Chicago

60. Haselow RE, Warshaw MG, Oken MM, et al. Radiation alone versus radiation with weekly low dose cis-platinum in unresectable cancer of the head and neck. In: Fee WE, Goepfert H, Johns ME, Strong EW, Ward PH, eds. Head and Neck Cancer, vol 2. Philadelphia: BC Decker, 1990:279–281

61. Adelstein DJ, Li Y, Adams GL, et al. An intergroup phase III comparison of standard radiation therapy and two schedules of concurrent chemoradiotherapy in patients with unresectable squamous cell head and neck cancer. J Clin Oncol 2003;21:92–98

62. Jeremic B, Shibamoto Y, Stanisavljevic B, Milojevic L, Milicic B, Nikolic N. Radiation therapy alone or with concurrent low-dose daily either cisplatin or carboplatin in locally advanced unresectable squamous cell carcinoma of the head and neck: a prospective randomized trial. Radiother Oncol 1997;43:29–37

63. Jeremic B, Shibamoto Y, Milicic B, et al. Hyperfractionated radiation therapy with or without concurrent low-dose daily cisplatin in locally advanced squamous cell carcinoma of the head and neck: a prospective randomized trial. J Clin Oncol 2000;18:1458–1464

64. Fountzilas G, Ciuleanu E, Theophanopoulou M, et al. A randomized study of concomitant radiotherapy with cisplatin or carboplatin versus radiotherapy alone in patients with locally advanced non-nasopharyngeal head and neck cancer. A Hellenic Cooperative Oncology Group (HeCOG) phase III study. Paper presented at the American Society of Clinical Oncology (ASCO), 2003, Chicago

65. Dobrowsky W, Naude J. Continuous hyperfractionated accelerated radiotherapy with/without mitomycin C in head and neck cancers. Radiother Oncol 2000;57:119–124

66. Haffty BG, Son YH, Papac R, et al. Chemotherapy as an adjunct to radiation in the treatment of squamous cell carcinoma of the head and neck: results of the Yale Mitomycin Randomized Trials. J Clin Oncol 1997;15:268–276

67. Wendt TG, Grabenbauer GG, Rodel CM, et al. Simultaneous radiochemotherapy versus radiotherapy alone in advanced head and neck cancer: a randomized multicenter study. J Clin Oncol 1998;16:1318–1324

68. Brizel DM, Albers ME, Fisher SR, et al. Hyperfractionated irradiation with or without concurrent chemotherapy for locally advanced head and neck cancer. N Engl J Med 1998;338:1798–1804

69. Weissler MC, Melin S, Sailer SL, Qaqish BF, Rosenman JG, Pillsbury HC III. Simultaneous chemoradiation in the treatment of advanced head and neck cancer. Arch Otolaryngol Head Neck Surg 1992;118:806–810

70. Smid L, Lesnicar H, Zakotnik B, et al. Radiotherapy, combined with simultaneous chemotherapy with mitomycin C and bleomycin for inoperable head and neck cancer – preliminary report. Int J Radiat Oncol Biol Phys 1995;32:769–775

71. Laramore GE, Scott CB, al-Sarraf M, et al. Adjuvant chemotherapy for resectable squamous cell carcinomas of the head and neck: report on Intergroup Study 0034. Int J Radiat Oncol Biol Phys 1992;23:705–713

72. Peters LJ, Goepfert H, Ang KK, et al. Evaluation of the dose for postoperative radiation therapy of head and neck cancer: first report of a prospective randomized trial. Int J Radiat Oncol Biol Phys 1993;26:3–11

73. Cooper JS, Pajak TF, Forastiere A, et al. Precisely defining high-risk operable head and neck tumors based on RTOG #85–03 and #88–24: targets for postoperative radiochemotherapy? Head Neck 1998;20:588–594

74. Bachaud JM, Cohen-Jonathan E, Alzieu C, David JM, Serrano E, Daly-Schveitzer N. Combined postoperative radiotherapy and weekly cisplatin infusion for locally advanced head and neck carcinoma: final report of a randomized trial. Int J Radiat Oncol Biol Phys 1996;36:999–1004

75. Haffty BG, Son YH, Sasaki CT, et al. Mitomycin C as an adjunct to postoperative radiation therapy in squamous cell carcinoma of the head and neck: results from two randomized clinical trials. Int J Radiat Oncol Biol Phys 1993;27:241–250

76. Bernier J, Domenge C, Eschwege F, et al. Chemo-radiotherapy, as compared to radiotherapy alone, significantly increases disease-free and overall survival in head and neck cancer patients after surgery: results of EORTC Phase III Trial 22931. Paper presented at the American Society for Therapeutic Radiology and Oncology, 2001, San Francisco

77. Bernier J, Domenge C, Ozsahin M, et al. Postoperative irradiation with or without concomitant chemotherapy for locally advanced head and neck cancer. N Engl J Med 2004;350:1945–1952

78. Cooper JS, Pajak TF, Forastiere AA, et al. Postoperative concurrent radiotherapy and chemotherapy for high-risk squamous-cell carcinoma of the head and neck. N Engl J Med 2004;350:1937–1944

79. Adelstein DJ. Induction chemotherapy in head and neck cancer. Hematol Oncol Clin North Am 1999;13:689–698

80. Vokes E. Induction chemotherapy for locoregionally advance head and neck cancer: a concept with continuing promise. In: Perry MC, ed. American Society of Clinical Oncology 2003 Educational Book, vol Spring 2003. Alexandria, VA: American Society of Clinical Oncology, 2003:294–298

81. Licitra L, Grandi C, Guzzo M, et al. Primary chemotherapy in resectable oral cavity squamous cell cancer: a randomized controlled trial. J Clin Oncol 2003;21:327–333

82. Kirita T, Ohgi K, Shimooka H, et al. Preoperative concurrent chemoradiotherapy plus radical surgery for advanced squamous cell carcinoma of the oral cavity: an analysis of long-term results. Oral Oncol 1999;35:597–606

83. Eckardt A, Rades D, Rudat V, et al. [Prospective phase II study of neoadjuvant radiochemotherapy in advanced operable carcinoma of the mouth cavity. 3-year outcome.] Mund Kiefer Gesichtschir 2002;6:117–121

84. Paccagnella A, Orlando A, Marchiori C, et al. Phase III trial of initial chemotherapy in stage III or IV head and neck cancers: a study by the Gruppo di Studio sui Tumori della Testa e del Collo. J Natl Cancer Inst 1994;86:265–272

85. Lewin F, Damber L, Jonsson H, et al. Neoadjuvant chemotherapy with cisplatin and 5-fluorouracil in advanced squamous cell carcinoma of the head and neck: a randomized phase III study. Radiother Oncol 1997;43:23–28

86. Giralt JL, Gonzalez J, del Campo JM, et al. Preoperative induction chemotherapy followed by concurrent chemoradiotherapy in advanced carcinoma of the oral cavity and oropharynx. Cancer 2000;89:939–945

87. Adelstein DJ, Lavertu P, Saxton JP, et al. Mature results of a phase III randomized trial comparing concurrent chemoradiotherapy with radiation therapy alone in patients with stage III and IV squamous cell carcinoma of the head and neck. Cancer 2000;88:876–883

88. Adelstein DJ, Saxton JP, Lavertu P, et al. A phase III randomized trial comparing concurrent chemotherapy and radiotherapy with radiotherapy alone in resectable stage III and IV squamous cell head and neck cancer: preliminary results. Head Neck 1997;19:567–575

89. Forastiere A, Berkey B, Maor MH, et al. Phase III trial to preserve the larynx: induction chemotherapy and radiation therapy versus concomitant chemoradiotherapy versus radiotherapy alone, Intergroup Trial R91–11. Paper presented at the American Society of Clinical Oncology (ASCO), 2001, San Francisco

90. Forastiere A, Gillison ML. Organ preservation in head and neck cancer. In: Ensley JF, Gutkind JS, Jacobs JR, Lippman SM, eds. Head and Neck Cancer: Emerging Perspectives. New York: Academic Press, Elsevier Science, 2003:475–490

91. Lefebvre JL, Chevalier D, Luboinski B, Kirkpatrick A, Collette L, Sahmoud T. Larynx preservation in pyriform sinus cancer: preliminary results of a European Organization for Research and Treatment of Cancer phase III trial. EORTC Head and Neck Cancer Cooperative Group. J Natl Cancer Inst 1996;88:890–899

92. Calais G, Alfonsi M, Bardet E, et al. Randomized trial of radiation therapy versus concomitant chemotherapy and radiation therapy for advanced-stage oropharynx carcinoma. J Natl Cancer Inst 1999;91:2081–2086

93. Rogers SN, Lowe D, Brown JS, Vaughan ED. A comparison between the University of Washington Head and Neck Disease-Specific measure and the Medical Short Form 36, EORTC QOQ-C33 and EORTC Head and Neck 35. Oral Oncol 1998;34:361–372

94. Schliephake H, Jamil MU. Prospective evaluation of quality of life after oncologic surgery for oral cancer. Int J Oral Maxillofac Surg 2002;31:427–433

95. Rogers SN, Lowe D, Patel M, Brown JS, Vaughan ED. Clinical function after primary surgery for oral and oropharyngeal cancer: an 11-item examination. Br J Oral Maxillofac Surg 2002;40:1–10

96. Colangelo LA, Logemann JA, Pauloski BR, Pelzer JR, Rademaker AW. T stage and functional outcome in oral and oropharyngeal cancer patients. Head Neck 1996;18:259–268

97. Pauloski BR, Logemann JA, Colangelo LA, et al. Surgical variables affecting speech in treated patients with oral and oropharyngeal cancer. Laryngoscope 1998;108:908–916

98. Colangelo LA, Logemann JA, Rademaker AW. Tumor size and pretreatment speech and swallowing in patients with resectable tumors. Otolaryngol Head Neck Surg 2000;122:653–661

22

Oral Rehabilitation with Osseointegrated Implants

Daniel Buchbinder and

Hugo St. Hilaire

Osseointegration was first described by Branemark et al,[1] and refers to a direct structural and functional connection between ordered, living bone and the surface of a load-carrying implant. Microscopic examination of a successfully osseointegrated implant shows lamellar bone in direct contact with the fixture. Commercially pure titanium is the most common material used today and allows for osseointegration through its surface oxide layer. Furthermore, it has good mechanical strength and is easily machinable, which makes it an ideal material for dental implantation. Branemark et al successfully applied the principle of osseointegration to the dental restoration of edentulous mandibles more than 30 years ago. The initial success attained in the restoration of edentulous patients led to the use of endosseous osseointegrated implants for single tooth replacement. Dental implants allow for the restoration of a stable, retentive dentition, which is a prerequisite to a successful functional outcome in reconstruction following ablative surgery of the head and neck.

◆ Types of Implants

Transmandibular Implants

Transmandibular implants have been used in the treatment of the severely atrophic edentulous mandible since the mid-1970s.[2] It consists of a baseplate applied to the inferior border of the symphysis through a submental incision, cortical screws, which stabilize the baseplate at the inferior border of the mandible, a transosseous post, and a superstructure. The transosseous post emerges intraorally and supports the superstructure, which retains a removable prosthesis. A period of 12 weeks of osseointegration is required prior to loading. This technology has been applied successfully in patients with oral cancer. August et al[3] reported their retrospective analysis of 18 patients and compared it to a noncancer cohort. Seventeen of the 18 patients underwent radiation therapy (RT) as part of their therapeutic protocol prior to the placement of the transmandibular implant, with two patients undergoing hyperbaric oxygen therapy. There was an increased rate of fistula formation when compared with the noncancer cohort, but no implant needed to be removed. A functional prosthesis was fabricated for each of these patients, resulting in improved aesthetics and comfort.

Subperiosteal Implants

Subperiosteal implants were introduced in the United States in 1949. They are designed to rest directly on the bone in a subperiosteal plane, which avoids injury to important anatomic structures such as the inferior alveolar nerve or the maxillary sinus when significant alveolar resorption is present. They can be used to support a complete or partial maxillary or mandibular prosthesis. Subperiosteal implants are fabricated in two stages. First, the area that will support the implant is exposed and an impression of the bone is taken. The wound is closed and plaster is poured into the impression. The plaster model will be used to fabricate a chrome-cobalt framework that will be inserted at a second surgical procedure. After a healing period of 6 weeks, fabrication of the final prosthesis can be initiated. The use of stereolithography allows for the fabrication of a subperiosteal implant in one surgical step. The success of endosseous dental implants and advances in bone grafting for alveolar augmentation has made the subperiosteal implant mainly of historical interest. Nevertheless, subperiosteal implants have been used in maxillary reconstruction.

Blade Implants

Blade implants have been used since the 1960s. They are endosseous implants that are designed for partially or completely edentulous patients. This design also minimizes the risk of injury to adjacent structures, including the maxillary sinus, nasal cavity, and inferior alveolar nerve, and facilitates placement in thin alveolar bone. They are inserted by exposing the alveolar bone and creating a slot where the implant will seat. A transmucosal connector is present to allow for attachment of a fixed or removable prosthesis. Because the osteotomy is performed at high speed, osseointegration does not occur. Rather, a fibrous tissue interface will be present between the implant and the recipient bone. Similar to the subperiosteal implant, blade implants are mainly of historical interest.

Root Form Implants

Root form dental implants refer to cylindrical fixtures and represent the gold standard in modern oral implantology (**Fig. 22–1**). They are available in a multitude of lengths and diameters. The traditional implant is 3.75 mm in diameter and varies in length from 8 to 18 mm. Fixtures of smaller diameters are available and are used in single-tooth replacement of mandibular or maxillary anterior teeth. Larger diameter implants, also known as wide platform implants, were

initially designed to restore posterior teeth. Fixtures of larger diameter have more surface area that allows for osseointegration and that can withstand greater masticatory loading forces. As a general rule, the longest fixture that will not impinge on important anatomic structures (i.e., maxillary sinus and nasal cavity in the maxilla and the inferior alveolar nerve in the mandible) should be chosen. The dimension of the edentulous area, the availability and quality of the alveolus, and the planned prosthodontic rehabilitation dictates the number of dental implants needed.

Modern dental implants are made of titanium, which have a biocompatible titanium oxide surface layer. Successful osseointegration shows lamellar bone with haversian systems in direct contact with the titanium oxide layer (**Fig. 22–2**). Failed implants show a connective tissue capsule that prevents direct contact and bonding of the implant and bone.[4] Multiple surface modifiers such as etching of the fixture, hydroxyapatite coating, and titanium plasma spray are available. Modification of the implant surface has been performed in an attempt to create an environment more conducive to osseointegration.

◆ Presurgical Planning

A successful dental implant means not only an osseointegrated fixture but also a fixture that can be used for prosthodontic rehabilitation. Fixtures need to be placed in strategic positions that account for the anatomy of the area to be restored. Clinical examination should pay close attention to the condition of the natural dentition and its prognosis. The area to be restored and its opposing dentition are very

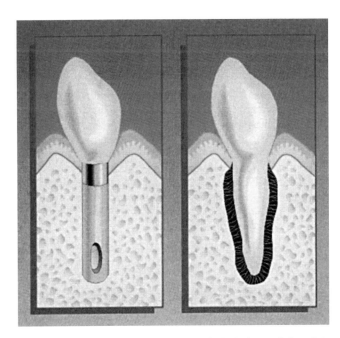

Figure 22–1 Unlike a natural tooth, which (unless ankylosed) is separated from the bone by periodontal ligament space and Sharpey's fibers, the implant surface directly contacts the bone. (From Garg AK, ed. Biology, Harvesting, Grafting for Dental Implants: Rationale and Clinical Applications. Chicago: Quintessence, 2004, with permission.)

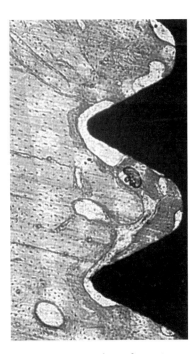

Figure 22–2 Histology of osseointegrated root form implant. Note marrow spaces, some fibrous tissue, and lacunae. (From Weiss CM, Weiss A, eds. Principles and Practice of Implant Dentistry. St. Louis: Mosby. Copyright 2001, with permission from Elsevier.)

important considerations. The degree of mandibular opening, especially in patients who have undergone maxillary or mandibular reconstruction with adjunctive radiotherapy, can become problematic during restoration of posterior edentulous regions. Diagnostic models mounted on an articulator allow the surgeon to evaluate the maxillomandibular relationship. The interarch relationship needs to be evaluated to ensure that adequate space for fabrication of a dental prosthesis exists. Furthermore, if the interarch distance is excessive and the implant to crown ratio is increased, this factor must be considered during the restorative phase. Radiographic examination includes a panoramic radiograph, periapical radiograph, and, when needed, computed tomography (CT). Dental CT reformatting programs such as the DentaScan (GE Medical Systems, Global Center, Milwaukee, WI) allows the clinician to accurately evaluate the amount of bone available for dental implant placement (see Chapter 23). Radiographic examination can be performed with a surgical stent that contains a radiopaque marker at the expected position of the fixture to allow for more precise evaluation of the osseous structures (see Fig. 23–5 in Chapter 23).

◆ Surgical Principles in Dental Implantology

There are three basic surgical principles that should be respected to ensure predictable osseointegration of the fixture:

1. The procedure should be performed in such a way as to minimize contamination of the osteotomy and implant surface. An attempt should be made to avoid saliva at the surgical site and the implant should not be touched in accordance with instructions provided by different implant manufacturers. Topical and systemic antibiotics are recommended in the perioperative period. Chlorhexidine gluconate 0.12% mouth rinse has been shown to decrease the incidence of implant failure and surgical site infection.[5] A course of systemic antibiotic therapy administered in the perioperative period that treats oral flora (i.e., penicillin or clindamycin) has also been associated with higher implant survival.[6]

2. A properly designed full-thickness mucoperiosteal flap must be elevated. Adequate visualization of the surgical site is needed, but periosteal elevation should be kept to a minimum to ensure maintenance of adequate blood supply at the osteotomy site. This will optimize the environment for osseointegration and mucosal coverage of the fixture. With this concept in mind, "flapless" dental implant placement has been developed where the osteotomy is performed by drilling through the gingival tissue. A transmucosal connector is left in place during the osseointegration period. The main drawback of this technique is the absence of visualization of the bony architecture as well as the possible inclusion of epithelial cells at the osteotomy site, which might, in theory, lead to the development of cysts.

3. The generation of heat must be minimized. Eriksson and Adell[7] showed in their study on rabbit bone that a

temperature of 40°C maintained for 7 minutes or 47°C for 1 minute resulted in bone necrosis. The heat that is generated is a function of multiple factors, including bone density, the speed of the drill, and the quality of the burs. Copious sterile cold saline irrigation is used externally (irrigation syringe). Furthermore, most implant systems are designed to allow for internal irrigation of the bur and osteotomy site. The high-speed drill should never exceed 2000 rpm, and the low-speed drill should not exceed 50 rpm.

◆ Surgical Technique for Endosseous Implants

Placement of an endosseous implant is classically performed in two stages: fixture placement (stage I), followed by exposure of the osseointegrated implant and placement of a transmucosal attachment (stage II). Once the surgical site is exposed, the initial osteotomy is created using the pilot drill. The pilot bur is a 2-mm round bur with markings on the shaft that determine the depth of the osteotomy. The osteotomy site is then increased in diameter using a series of guide drills. Up to this point, the hand piece should be set at a speed of 2000 rpm. Depending on the manufacturer and the size of the implants, a different sequence of guide drills will be used. This is usually very well explained by the implant system. When multiple implants are placed, a paralleling post can be inserted in the osteotomy to serve as a guide for implant placement. If a threaded implant is used and the implant is placed in dense bone, the site is tapped at low speed (20–40 rpm). Once osteotomy site preparation is completed, the fixture is mounted on the handpiece and the implant is inserted at low speed or with the use of a ratchet. No threads should be exposed at completion of implant placement, and the fixture should be stable. The cover screw is then applied and the surgical site closed (**Fig. 22–3**).

An osseointegration period of 4 months in the mandible and 6 months in the maxilla is classically allowed. The site is then reentered, the cover screw is removed, and a transmucosal attachment (healing abutment) is screwed to the fixture platform. Allowing 2 weeks to ensure adequate healing of the periimplant soft tissue, the prosthodontist then can change the healing abutment to a final abutment, which will serve to support a dental restoration (**Fig. 22–4**). A sequential photographic depiction of surgical implantation in conjunction with the use of DentaScan imaging software is provided in Fig. 23–5 in Chapter 23.

◆ Timing of Implant Placement in Maxillary and Mandibular Reconstruction

The use of vascularized bone-containing free flaps has facilitated the placement of dental implants at the time of osseous reconstruction. This is based on the premise that bone-containing flaps retain viable osteoprogenitor cells

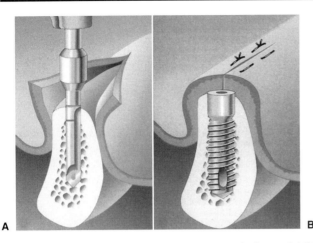

Figure 22–3 **(A)** Creation of the osteotomy using a high-speed drill. Sharp burs and copious cold saline irrigation are necessary to minimize heat generation. **(B)** The implant fixture is inserted at low speed (≤50 rpm), and a cover screw is placed in the top of the fixture (not shown) prior to mucoperiosteal flap closure. The cover screw will be removed so that the transmucosal attachment can be screwed into the fixture platform in Stage II. (From Garg AK, ed. Biology, Harvesting, Grafting for Dental Implants: Rationale and Clinical Applications. Chicago: Quintessence, 2004, with permission.)

that enable osseointegration.[4] Primary placement of dental implants reduces the time for completion of the final dental prosthesis and also eliminates a surgical procedure.[8] It also facilitates surgical access to the bone[9] and enables the coordination of plate and screw fixation with implant placement so that the hardware does not need to be removed for implant placement.[10] Furthermore, the primary placement of dental implants avoids the need for hyperbaric oxygen in patients who will undergo RT postoperatively.[11] A major drawback of primary dental implant placement is the unavailability of a surgical stent as a guide for fixture placement. This might result in unfavorable positioning of dental implants by an inexperienced surgeon. Some may argue that primary implant placement increases

surgical time, but four fixtures can be easily inserted in less than 1 hour. In complex reconstructions where multiple osteotomies are to be performed and several dental implants are to be placed, secondary implantation may be advisable.[9]

Primary implant placement can be performed in situations where postoperative RT will be administered, but stage II surgery should be performed 6 months following implantation to ensure that osseointegration has been achieved. If this is necessary, the duration of time from stage I surgery to placement of the final prosthesis will be approximately 8 months (**Fig. 22–5**).

Urken et al[12] reported on a series of 360 fixtures primarily placed in 81 patients. They found an overall success rate of 92%, with success being defined as a clinically stable fixture without evidence of periimplant infection and radiographic pathology. Eighty-one fixtures were subjected to RT, with an 86% success rate. Updates of this series from the Mt. Sinai Medical Center (New York, NY) group were published in 2000.[13] They reported data on 728 fixtures that were placed primarily in 183 patients. The overall success rate was 95%, with a success of 88% in subsequently irradiated implants. Sclaroff et al[14] reported similar results but with a much smaller cohort.

A modification of the concept of primary dental implant placement is seen in prefabricated flaps. Rohner et al[15] reported their experience with the use of prefabricated flaps in maxillofacial reconstruction. They use dental models for fabrication of a template that is used to implant the fibula 4 to 6 weeks prior to the free fibula transfer for maxillofacial reconstruction. The final dental prosthesis is fabricated prior to the free tissue transfer and can be used as a guide for fixation of the fibula. Furthermore, the prosthesis is left in place to allow for immediate function. Flap survival was 92% and implant survival in successful flap was 95%.

Delayed implant placement has the main advantage of allowing for the use of a precise surgical stent to guide the placement of the implant fixture in a more favorable location for prosthodontic rehabilitation.[11] On the other hand, delaying the insertion of fixtures increases the time period before reconstruction. Furthermore, in cases where the patient is

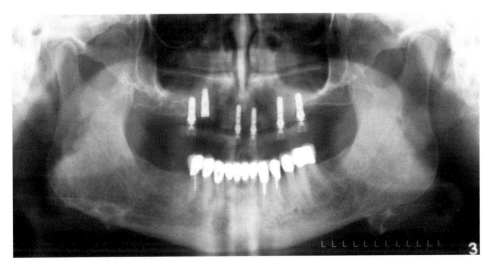

Figure 22–4 Panoramic radiograph demonstrating multiple osseointegrated root form implants in the upper alveolar ridge. Transmucosal attachments (abutments) have been inserted into five of the six implant fixtures. The cover screw remains in the second implant fixture from the patient's right. (Courtesy of James C. Pettigrew, Jr., D.M.D., Department of Oral and Maxillofacial Radiology, University of Florida.)

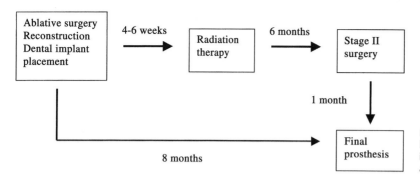

Figure 22–5 Schematic representation of the time line used for reconstruction of patients when dental implants are placed primarily and postoperative radiation therapy is delivered.

found to need adjunctive RT, the implants must be placed into irradiated bone. This means that hyperbaric oxygen therapy may be required, significantly increasing the time period required for final dental rehabilitation.

◆ Dental implantation in Different Bone-Containing Free Flaps

Iliac Crest

The iliac crest is the most uniformly implantable donor site,[4] with the area nearest to the anterior superior iliac spine being less implantable. Kovacs[16] reported on the stability of the bone stock in patients who had undergone mandibular reconstruction using a vascularized iliac crest bone graft with delayed placement of dental implants. No patient underwent RT. He found a horizontal bone loss that stabilized at 2 mm after 2 years in function. There was no significant difference between implant retained and implanted supported prosthesis. The overall implant success was 97.6%.

Scapula

The scapula has the second best bone stock for the placement of dental implants. The distal scapula (nearest the inferior angle) offers the greatest quantity of bone. Disa et al[17] indirectly followed changes in the bone mass of osseous free flaps used in mandibular reconstruction with radiologic evaluation, and found that there was less than 10% loss of bone over a period of 24 to 76 months. Furthermore, no significant difference was found in implanted or nonimplanted free flaps.

Fibula

The fibula has been found to provide less implantable bone than the iliac crest or the scapula,[4] particularly in females. The fibula, however, offers thick cortical shelves, which ensure better primary stability of the implants. Retrieval studies by Sumi et al[18] led them to conclude not only that the fixture should engage the superior and inferior cortices, but also that an effort should be made to engage the lateral cortical bone by using fixtures of large diameter. To increase the amount of bone available when a reconstruction is performed with a fibular free flap, "double barrel" or distraction osteogenesis can be performed.

Radius

The radius is the least implantable donor site. The cavaderic study by Moscoso et al,[18a] showed that none of the female specimens and only half of the male specimens met the criteria for placement of dental implants (minimum of 10 mm in height and 5 mm in width). This makes the radius inadequate when considering a reconstruction with dental implant placement.

◆ Preprosthetic Procedures

Soft Tissue Management

After an adequate period of time is allowed for osseointegration, adjunctive soft tissue procedures may be required to enhance the prosthetic rehabilitation. The soft tissue coverage of the fixture should be kept to a minimal thickness, which will allow for a shorter transmucosal connector, easier maintenance of oral hygiene, and more favorable interarch space. This can be achieved by a "debulking" procedure at the time of stage II surgery. Great care should be taken to avoid injury to the vascular pedicle. A split-thickness skin graft or acellular dermis might be used to reline the neoalveolus. Fabrication of an acrylic stent will permit easy stabilization of the graft and prevent development of a hematoma. The stent may be fixated using the titanium fixtures or transalveolar screws. The oral cavity should also be evaluated for any lip or buccal mucosal adhesion to the alveolus, which can be addressed by performing a vestibuloplasty at the time of stage II surgery.

Free Bone Grafting

Augmentation of the osseous structure of the maxilla and mandible can be performed when inadequate bone is present for placement of dental implants. Because the success of a free bone graft relies solely on the recipient site, augmentation is contraindicated in irradiated fields unless hyperbaric oxygen therapy has been used. Augmentation in width is much more predictable than in height. It is performed using an onlay graft that should be cortical in nature to allow for rigid fixation. Following a healing period of 4 to 6 months, the site is reentered and dental implants are placed. Multiple donor sites have been used, including the mandibular symphysis and ramus, the calvarium, ribs, the tibia, and the anterior and posterior iliac crest.

Special attention to the maxillary sinus must be made when considering dental implant placement in the posterior maxilla. A combination of alveolar atrophy and pneumatization of the maxillary sinus often lead to a situation where inadequate bone is present for predictable dental implant placement. A maxillary sinus lift can be performed to address this problem. Osteotomies are performed along the lateral antral wall that is in-fractured. The schneiderian membrane is elevated from the sinus wall and floor. Bone graft material is then packed on the floor of the maxillary sinus, effectively increasing the amount of bone available to place a dental implant. If enough bone is present to provide primary stability (5 mm), the implant can be placed simultaneously.

Distraction Osteogenesis

In situations where bone height is found to be inadequate, distraction osteogenesis has been used to enhance the reconstruction. It allows for an increase in the available bone stock for the eventual placement of longer endosseous fixtures with a more favorable implant-to-restoration ratio. Furthermore, distraction osteogenesis allows for expansion of the soft tissue. Its use has been reported for mandibular fibular reconstruction.[19–21] The surgical procedure is straightforward. The neomandible is exposed through an intraoral vestibular incision. The plates and screws used to fixate the transplant are removed. Great care is taken to leave the lingual tissue undisrupted. The alveolar distractor device is adapted in position and the screw hole drilled. The distractor is removed, and a horizontal osteotomy is made using a sagittal saw, a fissure bur, or an osteotome. The horizontal osteotomy is made in such a way as to ensure a minimum of 6 mm of bone on the cephalic segment.[22] Vertical osteotomies are also performed at the lateral extent of the segment to be distracted, parallel to or slightly divergent from each other. The appliance is then repositioned and activated to ensure completion of the osteotomy. The appliance is then deactivated and the wound is closed. The activation arms are exposed intraorally. The surgical procedure is followed by a latency period of 5 days, which allows for the formation of a bony callus. The activation phase follows whereby the appliance is activated by increments of 0.5 mm twice a day, until the desired alveolar height is obtained. This is followed by a consolidation phase of 3 to 4 months, after which the alveolar distractor can be removed and dental implants placed. Simultaneously, a vestibuloplasty can be performed if deemed necessary. Finally, new appliances have been developed that include the dental implants as part of the distractor devices. This decreases the number of surgical procedures needed for reconstruction, but limited experience with this new device is available.[23]

◆ Dental Implant Placement Following Radiation Therapy

Radiation therapy is frequently used as an adjunct in the treatment of oral cancer. The effect of radiation on the tissues of the head and neck is well documented. The hypocellular, hypovascular, and hypoxic environment created by RT appear, at first glance, to be a hostile environment for dental implants. Significant controversy is found in the literature with respect to this subject. When evaluating the literature, careful attention must be paid to the amount of radiation used, the use of hyperbaric oxygen therapy, the length of follow-up, as well as the timing of implant placement with respect to RT.

Goto et al[24] reviewed their experience in the placement of dental implants following ablative surgery of the maxilla and mandible. They reported a success rate of 79.7% when fixtures were placed in irradiated native or neoalveolus, with most of the failures associated with short (10 mm and less) fixtures. The latter was confirmed by Niimi et al,[25] but the radiation dose delivered was only 30 Gy. These results cannot be extrapolated to patients undergoing higher dose RT of 50 to 60 Gy.

Visch et al[26] evaluated the survival rate of dental implants placed following RT. They found a 10-year survival rate of 84% in patients who had received less that 50 Gy and of 71% in patients treated with 50 Gy or more. Of interest is the poor performance of dental implants in the irradiated maxilla (55% anterior and 62% posterior), which makes implant location the most dominant variable influencing implant survival.

Barber et al[27] reported on their experience in placement of dental implants in mandibular reconstruction using vascularized fibular transfer. All 20 patients underwent adjunctive RT (more than 50 Gy) and hyperbaric oxygen therapy, as described by Marx and Ames,[28] prior to dental implant placement. They found that all fixtures were osseointegrated at 6 months.

The type of osseous reconstruction should also be considered when evaluating the effect of radiation on dental implants. This is well exemplified by the work of Werkmeister et al,[29] who prospectively followed implants secondarily placed in delayed mandibular reconstruction using nonvascularized bone graft without adjunctive hyperbaric oxygen therapy for a period of 3 years. The cohort that underwent RT showed a statistically significant increase in soft tissue complication (infection and dehiscence) and implant failure. The latter group had a success rate of 74.3%, whereas the nonirradiated group had a success rate of 85.3%.

It is clear that if dental implant placement is to be performed after RT, hyperbaric oxygen therapy should be strongly considered. The recommended protocol includes 20 dives of 100% oxygen at 2.4 atm for 90 minutes presurgically followed by 10 dives postoperatively. Furthermore, Larsen[30] suggests delaying implantation until 6 months after completion of RT and increasing the integration period by 3 months.

◆ Effects of Chemotherapy on Dental Implants

Antineoplastic drugs cause severe acute side effects in multiple organ systems, including hematopoietic tissue, the kidney, and the digestive system (i.e., mucositis of the oral cavity). Late side effects of chemotherapy include vasculitis, which can lead to altered blood supply to the skeleton of the maxillofacial region and affect bone metabolism. With this premise in mind, Kovacs[31] studied dental implants placed in native bone of patients previously treated with cis- or carboplatin and 5-fluorouracil. He followed 106 fixtures, placed following resolution of the acute side effects of chemotherapy, in 30 patients. The survival of these implants was compared with 54 fixtures placed in 17 patients. No patient in either of these cohorts was treated with adjunctive radiotherapy. No significant difference was noted in survival of the dental implant placed in either group of patients. This is consistent with the limited literature on this topic, which consists mainly of case reports.[32,33]

Karr et al[34] reported their experience with complications of dental implants subjected to chemotherapy. Most complications that were encountered occurred with subperiosteal and blade implants ($n = 4$). These were mainly infectious in nature, and required the removal of the fixture with delays in administration of chemotherapy. They also reported painful mucositis associated with an endosseous and a staple implant, which required interruption of the chemotherapy. None of these patients had undergone a dental evaluation prior to the initiation of chemotherapy. This emphasizes the importance of a thorough dental examination prior to chemotherapy. Professional dental prophylaxis to remove plaque, calculus, and debris around the fixture should be performed. This will reduce periimplant gingival inflammation as well as the level of mucositis during chemotherapy. Furthermore, when the fixture supports a removable prosthesis, it should be relined with a tissue conditioner, which will be gentler to the tissue on which it rests. When subperiosteal or blade implants are present and are potential sources of infection, they should be removed prior to chemotherapy.

◆ Maintenance of Dental Implants

Similar to any type of prosthodontic rehabilitation, the success of an implant-retained or supported prosthesis depends greatly on the patient's compliance with oral hygiene and routine dental hygiene visits. Patients suffering from oral cancer have been shown to have poorer oral hygiene than the general population. This is attributed not only to a lack of willingness but also to the presence of more complex intraoral anatomy following reconstruction.[35] The patient should be instructed at the time of placement of the transmucosal attachment to initiate gentle brushing of the area to avoid accumulation of dental plaque and debris. An appropriate recall interval should be determined according to the patient's needs. A dental hygienist or a dentist must use specially designed instruments that will not affect the titanium fixture. Plastic, gold plated, or graphite instruments are used to remove the calculus that might form at the abutment. At home, the patient should perform conventional tooth brushing and flossing four times a day to clean the implant site as well as the native dentition. This can be supplemented with an end-tufted brush or heavier flosses to access difficult to reach areas. Removable

prostheses should be removed every night and cleaned thoroughly. The dentist should remove fixed prostheses at appropriate intervals where oral hygiene measures are more complex.

◆ Craniofacial Implants

The experience in oral implantology has been applied to the craniofacial skeleton since the late 1970s for the bone-anchored hearing aid (BAHA) and for the retention of maxillofacial prostheses. The fixtures used for this purpose are endosseous threaded implants, similar to the ones used in oral implantology, but of shorter length. Tjellstrom and Granstrom[36] reported on their first 100 craniofacial implants placed to support the BAHA. They found a success rate of 90% with a follow-up of 8 to 16 years. Despite the initial belief that the skin/implant interface would be problematic, adverse skin reactions were not found to be a problem, with minimal erythema being the most common observation.

Craniofacial implants can be used to retain auricular, nasal, orbital, and facial prostheses. Following placement of the fixtures in strategic position and after an osseointegration period of 6 months, the surgical site is reentered and a transepithelial attachment is placed. This abutment will support a framework that will retain the prosthesis. The success of these implants is very predictable, with reported success rates of up to 95% in nonirradiated sites.[37] When implantation in a previously irradiated site is being considered, hyperbaric oxygen therapy is recommended.

◆ Implant Failure

Criteria for successful osseointegration of a dental fixture have been established, and multiple clinical tests can be used to evaluate dental implants. The recommended minimum criteria for dental implant success are as follows: (1) an individual, unattached implant is immobile when tested clinically; (2) radiographic examination does not reveal any periimplant radiolucency; (3) radiographic vertical bone loss is less than 0.2 mm/yr after the first year of functioning; (4) the individual implant performance is characterized by an absence of signs and symptoms such as pain, infections, neuropathies, paresthesia, or violation of the dental canal; and (5) at a minimum, the implant should fulfill the above criteria with a success rate of 85% at the end of a 5-year observation period, and a success rate of 80% after 10 years.[38]

Clinical periodontal probing is performed to evaluate the epithelial-connective attachment and marginal bone level. A periodontal probe is inserted into the gingival sulcus, and the distance from the depth of the sulcus to the free gingival margin is measured and recorded. An increase in sulcular depth is indicative of marginal bone loss and should be less than 0.2 mm/yr after the first year after implantation. Furthermore, bleeding on probing (indicative of inflammation, or periimplantitis) and the presence of suppuration should be noted.

Periapical radiographs of good quality are also used to follow marginal bone height. No periimplant radiolucency should be present. When bone loss is present, mobility of the fixture should be evaluated. Mobility of a fixture is an indication of disintegration or fibrous encapsulation of the implant and represents implant failure. Because manual testing is subjective, a Periotest device, which measures the dampening characteristics of the tissues, should be used. Finally, the neutral proteolytic enzyme activity test is characterized by a high negative predictive value, which can serve as an indicator of stable periimplant conditions.[39]

◆ Conclusion

Osseointegrated implants have dramatically improved the functional stability and cosmetic result of prosthetic therapy following treatment for oral cancer. Careful preoperative planning, meticulous intraoperative technique, and fastidious postoperative hygiene are critical to successful osseointegration. Implantation into previously irradiated bone and osseous free flaps are viable options in many patients, but the narrower margin for technical error reemphasizes the importance of adhering closely to the principles that enable osseointegration to occur.

References

1. Branemark PI, Hansson BO, Adell R, et al. Osseointegrated implants in the treatment of the edentulous jaw: experience from a 10-year period. Scand J Plast Reconstr Surg Suppl 1977;16:1–132

2. Bosker H, Jordan RD, Sindet-Pedersen S, Koole R. The transmandibular implant: a 13-year survey of its use. J Oral Maxillofac Surg 1991; 49:482–492

3. August M, Bast B, Jackson M, Perrott D. Use of the fixed mandibular implant in oral cancer patients: a retrospective study. J Oral Maxillofac Surg 1998;56:297–301

4. Urken ML, Buchbinder D, Weinberg H, Vickery C, Sheiner A, Biller HF. Primary placement of osseointegrated implants in microvascular mandibular reconstruction. Otolaryngol Head Neck Surg 1989; 101:56–73

5. Lambert PM, Morris HF, Ochi S. The influence of 0.12% chlorhexidine digluconate rinses on the incidence of infectious complications and implant success. J Oral Maxillofac Surg 1997;55:25–30

6. Laskin DM, Dent CD, Morris HF, Ochi S, Olson JW. The influence of preoperative antibiotics on success of endosseous implants at 36 months. Ann Periodontol 2000;5:166–174

7. Eriksson RA, Adell R. Temperatures during drilling for the placement of implants using the osseointegration technique. J Oral Maxillofac Surg 1986;44:4–7

8. Chang YM, Santamaria E, Wei F-C, et al. Primary insertion of osseointegrated dental implants into fibula osteoseptocutaneous free flap for mandible reconstruction. Plast Reconstr Surg 1998; 102:680–688

9. Kildal M, Wei FC, Chang YM, Chen HC, Chang MH. Mandibular reconstruction with a fibula osteoseptocutaneous free flap and osseointegrated dental implant. Clin Plast Surg 2001;28:403–410

10. Foster RD, Anthony JP, Sharma A, Pogrel MA. Vascularised bone flaps versus nonvascularized bone grafts for mandibular reconstruction: an outcome analysis of primary bony union and endosseous implant success. Head Neck 1999;21:66–71

11. Marunick MT, Roumanas ED. Functional criteria for mandibular implant placement post resection and reconstruction for cancer. J Prosthet Dent 1999;82:107–113

12. Urken ML, Buchbinder D, Costantino PD, et al. Oromandibular reconstruction using microvascular composite flaps: report of 210 cases. Arch Otolaryngol Head Neck Surg 1998;124:46–55

13. Samouhi P, Buchbinder D. Rehabilitation of oral cancer patients with dental implants. Curr Opin Otolaryngol Head Neck Surg 2000; 8:305–313

14. Sclaroff A, Haughey B, Gay WD, Paniello R. Immediate mandibular reconstruction and placement of dental implants at the time of ablative surgery. Oral Surg Oral Med Oral Pathol 1994;78:711–717

15. Rohner D, Jaquiery C, Kunz C, Bucher P, Maas H, Hammer B. Maxillofacial reconstruction with prefabricated osseous free flaps: a 3-year experience with 24 patients. Plast Reconstr Surg 2003; 112:748–757

16. Kovacs AF. Influence of the prosthetic restoration modality on bone loss around implants placed in vascularized iliac bone grafts for mandibular reconstruction. Otolaryngol Head Neck Surg 2000; 123:598–602

17. Disa JJ, Hidalgo DA, Cordeiro PG, Winters RM, Thaler H. Evaluation of bone heights in osseous free flap mandible reconstruction: an indirect measure of bone mass. Plast Reconstr Surg 1999; 103:1371–1377

18. Sumi Y, Hasegawa T, Miyaishi O, Ueda M. Interface analysis of titanium implants in a human vascularized fibula bone graft. J Oral Maxillofac Surg 2001;59:213–216

18a. Moscoso JF, Keller J, Genden E, Weinberg H, Biller HF, Buchbinder D, Urken ML. Vascularized bone flaps in oromandibular reconstruction: a comparative anatomic study of bone stock from various donor sites to assess suitability for endosseous dental implants. Arch Otolaryngol Head Neck Surg 1994;120:36–43

19. Levin L, Carrasco L, Kazemi A, Chalian A. Enhancement of the fibula free flap by alveolar distraction for dental implant restoration: report of a case. Facial Plast Surg 2003;19:87–93

20. Marchetti C, Degidi M, Scarano A, Piattelli A. Vertical distraction osteogenesis of fibular free flap in mandibular prosthetic rehabilitation: a case report. Int J Periodontics Restorative Dent 2002;22:251–257

21. Chiapasco M, Brusati R, Galioto S. Distraction osteogenesis of a fibular revascularized flap for improvement of oral implant positioning in a tumor patient: a case report. J Oral Maxillofac Surg 2000; 58:1434–1440

22. Klesper B, Lazar F, Siebegger M, Hidding J, Zoller JE. Vertical distraction osteogenesis of fibula transplants for mandibular reconstruction: a preliminary study. J Craniomaxillofac Surg 2002;30:280–285

23. Zhang C, Zhang Z. Reconstruction of mandible with fibular flap and dental implant distractor: a new approach. Chin Med J (Engl) 2002; 115:1877–1880

24. Goto M, Jin-Nouchi S, Ihara K, Katsuki T. Longitudinal follow-up of osseointegrated implants in patients with resected jaws. Int J Oral Maxillofac Implants 2002;17:225–230

25. Niimi A, Fujimoto T, Nosaka Y, Ueda M. A Japanese multicenter study of osseointegrated implants placed in irradiated tissues: a preliminary report. Int J Oral Maxillofac Implants 1997;12:259–264

26. Visch LL, Van Waas MAJ, Schmitz PIM, Levendag PC. A clinical evaluation of implants in irradiated oral cancer patients. J Dent Res 2002;81:856–859

27. Barber HD, Seckinger RJ, Hayden RE, Weinstein GS. Evaluation of osseointegration of endosseous implants in radiated, vascularized fibula flaps to the mandible: a pilot study. J Oral Maxillofac Surg 1995;53:640–644

28. Marx RE, Ames JR. The use of hyperbaric oxygen therapy in bony reconstruction of the irradiated and tissue-deficient patient. J Oral Maxillofac Surg 1982;40:412–420

29. Werkmeister R, Szulczewski D, Walteros-Benz P, Joos U. Rehabilitation with dental implants of oral cancer patients. J Craniomaxillofac Surg 1999;27:38–41

30. Larsen PE. Placement of dental implants in the irradiated mandible: a protocol involving adjunctive hyperbaric oxygen. J Oral Maxillofac Surg 1997;55:967–971

31. Kovacs AF. Influence of chemotherapy on endosteal implant survival and success in oral cancer patients. Int J Oral Maxillofac Surg 2001;30:144–147

32. McDonald AR, Pogrel MA, Sharma A. Effects of chemotherapy on osseointegration of implants: a case report. J Oral Implantol 1998; 24:11–13

33. Steiner M, Windchy A, Gould AR, Kushner GM, Weber R. Effects of chemotherapy in patients with dental implants. J Oral Implantol 1995;21:142–147

34. Karr RA, Kramer DC, Toth BB. Dental implants and chemotherapy complications. J Prosthet Dent 1992;67:683–687

35. Kovacs AF. The fate of osseointegrated implants in patients following oral cancer surgery and mandibular reconstruction. Head Neck 2000;22:111–119

36. Tjellstrom A, Granstrom G. Long term follow-up with bone-anchored hearing aid: a review of the 100 patients between 1977 and 1985. Ear Nose Throat J 1994;73:112–114

37. Jacobsson M, Tjellstrom A, Fine L, Andersson H. A retrospective study of osseointegrated skin-penetrating titanium fixtures used for retaining facial prostheses. Int J Oral Maxillofac Implants 1992;7:523–528

38. Albrektsson T, Zarb G, Worthington P, Eriksson AR. The long-term efficacy of currently used dental implants: a review and proposed criteria of success. Int J Oral Maxillofac Implants 1986;1:11–25

39. Duyck J, Naert I. Failure of oral implants:aetiology, symptoms and influencing factors. Clin Oral Investig 1998;2:102–114

23

Dental Implant Imaging

James J. Abrahams and
Parminder Deol

Before the development of dental computed tomography (CT) reformatting software, preoperative radiographic assessment of the mandible and maxilla prior to dental implant placement was performed by evaluating plain radiographs. Panoramic radiographs are not optimal for this type of evaluation because the width of the mandible cannot be accurately assessed, and image distortion can be as high as 25%.[1] Axial CT provides limited information because much of the bony anatomy runs parallel to the plane of the scan. Furthermore, direct coronal CT imaging is often not useful because of streak artifact created from dental restorations and because the degree of hyperextension required of the patient cannot always be achieved. The development of CT image reformatting software has overcome the limitations of conventional CT, markedly improving the sophistication of presurgical planning for dental implant placement. This chapter reviews the applications of CT image reformatting software for dental implantation, using DentaScan to illustrate the power of this imaging tool.

◆ DentaScan

The use of CT in implant dentistry and oral and maxillofacial surgery grew significantly with the introduction of DentaScan (GE Medical Systems, Global Center, Milwaukee, WI) in the 1980s.[2,3] DentaScan, a CT software program, is an extension of CT technology that assists oral-maxillofacial surgeons with pretreatment planning for endosseous implantation. DentaScan uses thin axial scans parallel to the mandibular occlusal plane to produce new reformatted images in two unique views: panelliptical and parasagittal.

Reformatting images allows for close inspection of the buccal and lingual cortices. An updated version, DentaScan Plus, has recently become available.

Technical Considerations

Axial images are obtained with 1×1–mm slice thickness and table increment, with the exception of images obtained on the multislice scanner, where thickness and table increment can be 1.25 mm. Images are acquired using a bone algorithm without intravenous contrast (**Figs. 23–1** and **23–2**).[4] Because the scan angle of the maxilla and mandible is slightly different, separate scans must be performed.

The acquired axial images are then processed with the dental CT reformatting program. A curved line is superimposed on an axial image that shows the curve of the mandible or maxilla at the level of the roots of the teeth by positioning the cursor on approximately six different points along the curve of the jaw (**Figs. 23–1A** and **23–2A**). The DentaScan program then automatically connects these points, resulting in a smooth curve that is superimposed on the jaw. The curved line defines the location and plane of the reformatted panoramic images (**Figs. 23–1B** and **23–2B**). The distance between reformatted cross-sectional images can be varied, but they are usually 1 to 2 mm apart.

At completion, there are approximately 30 to 50 axial images, 40 to 100 cross-sectional images, and five panoramic images. Life-size (one to one magnification) cross-sectional and panoramic images are preferred, and a millimeter scale displayed on the films can be used to verify the degree of magnification. Streak artifact that degrades visualization of bone

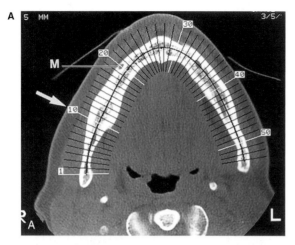

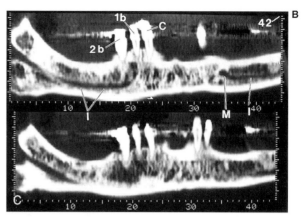

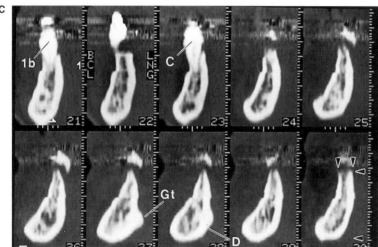

Figure 23–1 Computed tomography (CT) scan (DentaScan) of the mandible. The anatomy identified on the mandibular anatomic specimen is represented on these CT images. **(A)** Axial image of mandible with a superimposed curve. The curve defines the plane and location in which the panoramic images in **B** are reformatted. Numbered lines drawn perpendicular to this curve (*arrow*) define the plane and location in which the cross-sectional images viewed in **C** are reformatted. **(B)** Panoramic views. The numbered tick marks along the bottom of the images correspond to the numbered perpendicular lines displayed on the axial image in **A**. The tick marks along the side of the image correspond to the axial images that were used to reformat these images. Note that there were 42 axial images acquired and thus 42 tick marks along the side of this image. **(C)** Cross-sectional views of the right side of the mandible mesial to the mental foramen (see perpendicular lines 21 through 30 in **A**). Image 21 shows the first bicuspid (premolar) just mesial to the mental foramen, which is located at tick mark 20 on the axial and panoramic views. Image 27 corresponds with the midline, where the genial tubercle is located. The height of the mandible distal to the mental foramen is measured from the top of the alveolar process to the top of the mandibular canal (not shown), whereas mesial to the foramen it is measured from the top of the alveolar process to the bottom of the mandible (arrowheads in image 30). Measurement of the width is also demonstrated in image 30. C, canine; D, digastric fossa; Gt, genial tubercle; I, inferior alveolar canal; M, mental foramen; 1b, first bicuspid (premolar); 2b, second bicuspid (premolar). (From Abrahams JJ. Anatomy of the jaw revisited with a dental CT software program: pictorial essay. AJNR 1993;14:979–990, with permission. Copyright by American Society of Neuroradiology.)

on direct coronal images does not degrade the reformatted cross-sectional images because the artifact is projected at the level of the crowns of the teeth rather than the bony alveolus.

Interpretation of Dental Computed Tomography Program Images and Measurements

Each CT view can be related to the others by a series of scale marks that appear on the films. The marks that run along the side of the panoramic and cross-sectional images (**Fig. 23–1B,C**) correspond to the axial slices that were used to reformat the images.

The mandibular height distal to the mental foramen is measured from the top of the alveolar process to the top of the inferior alveolar canal, whereas the mandibular height mesial to the mental foramen is measured from the top of the alveolar process to the bottom of the mandible (**Fig. 23–1C**, arrowheads in image 30). In the distal maxilla, height is measured from the top (inferior surface) of the alveolar ridge to the floor of the maxillary sinus (**Fig. 23–2C**, arrows in image 7), whereas height in the mesial maxilla is measured from the top of the alveolar process to the nasal floor.

The inferior alveolar canal is usually readily identified on cross-sectional images. In situations where the canal cannot be seen, several methods can be used to identify the location of the canal: (1) the cortical niche sign, which is an indentation of the inner or medullary aspect of the lingual cortex of the mandible; (2) triangulation, using the scale marks on the panoramic and axial films to identify the canal on cross-sectional views; and (3) extrapolation of the location of the canal from the images in which it is visualized or from its location on the opposite side of the mandible.[5,6]

The DentaScan program enables the surgeon to visualize the bony structures preoperatively, eliminating the need to make strategic decisions at the time of surgery. DentaScan also provides surgeons with information about the internal structure of the jaw that cannot be gained by direct intraoperative inspection. The CT scans are photographed in true life-size format with a vertical scale in millimeters that runs along the side of the images.

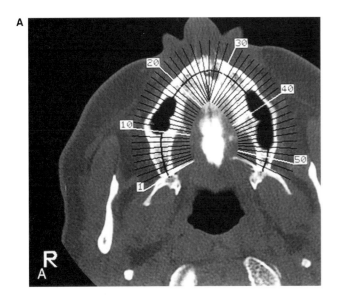

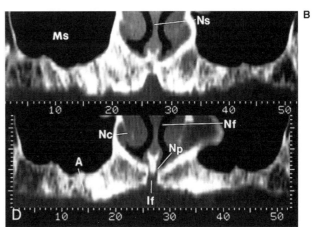

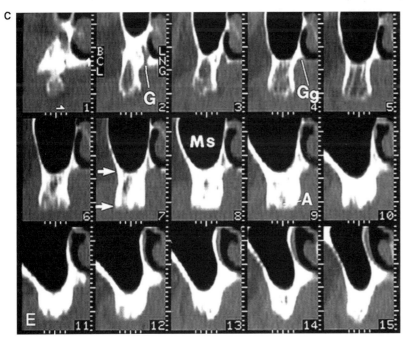

Figure 23–2   CT (DentaScan) scan of maxilla. **(A)** Axial image with superimposed curve. The curve defines the plane and location in which the panoramic images seen in **B** are reformatted. Numbered lines drawn perpendicular to this curve define the plane and location in which the cross-sectional images viewed in **C** are reformatted. **(B)** Panoramic view. **(C)** Cross-sectional views. Images 1 to 15 are through the posterior right maxilla (see perpendicular lines 1 through 15 in **A**). The arrows in image 7 indicate how the height of the distal alveolar process is measured from the floor of the maxillary sinus to the top of the alveolar process. A, alveolar process; G, greater palatine foramen; Gg, groove for greater palatine nerve; If, incisive foramen; Ms, maxillary sinus; Nc, nasal concha; Nf, nasal fossa; Np, nasopalatine canal; Ns, nasal septum. (From Abrahams JJ. Anatomy of the jaw revisited with a dental CT software program: pictorial essay. AJNR 1993;14:979–990, with permission. Copyright by American Society of Neuroradiology.)

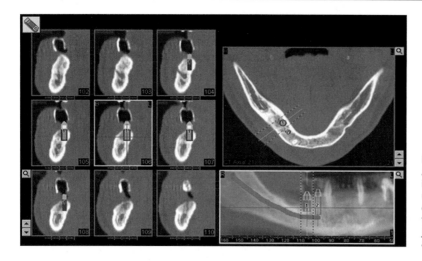

Figure 23–3 Presurgical planning using SimPlant. Axial, panoramic, and reformatted cross-sectional images are displayed. The images have been enhanced using the interactive tools supplied by SimPlant to outline the planned placement of the implants and the location of the inferior alveolar canal. (Courtesy of James C. Pettigrew, Jr., D.M.D., Department of Oral and Maxillofacial Radiology, University of Florida.)

It is preferable to have 1 to 1.5 mm of bone on either side of the implant and 1 to 2 mm of bone between the bottom of the implant and adjacent vital structures such as the maxillary sinus, nasal floor, and the inferior alveolar canal.[1] The anatomic features of the mandible that are most important to the implant surgeon include (1) the location of the inferior alveolar nerve canal (**Fig. 23–1B**), (2) the contour of the alveolar ridge (**Fig. 23–1C**), and (3) the height of the alveolar ridge (**Fig. 23–2C**).

Early long-term studies with osseointegrated (root-form) implants reported a success rate of 91% in the mandible and 81% in the maxilla.[7] Later, with the advent of DentaScan, a success rate for osseointegrated implants approaching 100% has been reported.[8] This rate of success has been made possible in part by a comprehensive appraisal of the morphologic features of the proposed implantation site: the quality and quantity of available bone, the presence of intrabony pathology, the inclination of the alveolar process, and the location of important anatomic structures in relation to the site of planned implantation.

The potential applications of DentaScan have evolved from its original use for dental implantation to the evaluation and localization of intrabony pathology of the maxilla or mandible.[9–12] DentaScan has also been investigated as a diagnostic modality for the detection of mandibular invasion (see Chapter 12).

◆ Interactive Dental Computed Tomography Reformatting Programs

SimPlant (Columbia Scientific Inc., Glen Burnie, MD) is another CT reformatting program that permits implant surgeons to create a virtual treatment plan for implantation using interactive software. SimPlant utilizes raw data from the CT scan in concert with computer graphics to perform presurgical planning for dental implant placement.[13] The program allows the surgeon to vary the display of the reformatted CT images so that bony anatomy can be assessed, and bone dimensions can be measured from one point to another. There is also a feature that facilitates visualization of the inferior alveolar canal, and the angulation and position of the planned implant can be modified on the screen to simulate its position at the time of surgical placement. The surgeon can use these tools to determine the proper diameter and length of the implant, and to insert the implant at the proper location and angulation (**Fig. 23–3**).

Other innovations that employ reformatted CT images to improve the accuracy of dental implantation have recently been introduced. High-quality three-dimensional imaging of the maxilla or mandible can be achieved with cone-beam CT. Cone-beam CT systems such as the NewTom 9000 (NewTom AG, Marburg, Germany) provide images of high contrast structures such as bone that are comparable to conventional CT with reduced radiation exposure.[14] Surgical navigation systems such as IGI (DenX America, Boynton Beach, FL) are also available that facilitate image-guided implantation. The IGI system, for example, utilizes an infrared tracking system that provides the real-time position of the dental handpiece as well as the patient to optimize the location and orientation of implant placement. Critical structures such as the inferior alveolar canal can be marked preoperatively so that precise intraoperative localization is possible. The system also provides an implant menu, which enables the surgeon to choose specific implants and sizes from several commercially available vendors so that accurate preoperative planning and intraoperative placement can be performed. Conventional image-guidance systems that are used for surgical procedures in otolaryngology or neurosurgery employ an instrument tracking device, whereas the IGI system utilizes separate tracking devices for the dental handpiece and the patient. This avoids imprecise placement of an implant resulting from patient repositioning that can occur as a result of head movement or mandibular opening (**Fig. 23–4**).[15]

◆ Dental Implants

A variety of implants can be used for prosthodontic rehabilitation, including transmandibular, subperiosteal, and blade implants. Cylindrical titanium root form implants that are capable of osseointegration are now considered the gold

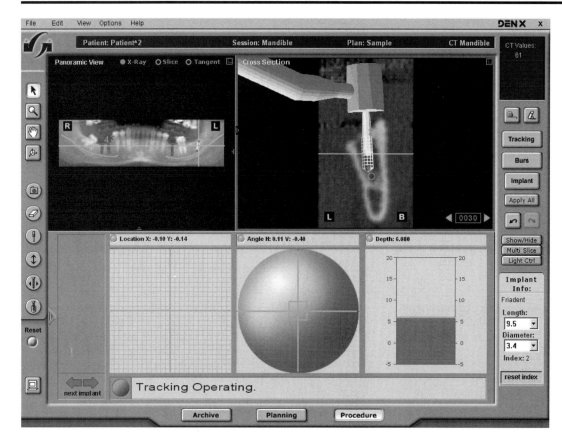

Figure 23–4 Image-guided implantation using the IGI system. A panoramic image demonstrates the planned location for the implants and the marked inferior alveolar canal (*upper left*). A reformatted cross-sectional image simulates the handpiece position (*upper right*). The location of the inferior alveolar canal is highlighted in red. At the bottom of the computer image, three indicators (from left to right) illustrate the position, angle, and depth of drilling in real time. (From DenX America, Boynton Beach, FL, with permission.)

standard in oral implantology. Numerous implant systems are commercially available, and prosthodontic techniques have been refined to provide durable, biologically sound, cosmetic results. The use of CT image reformatting software adds another level of sophistication to the implantation process that directly impacts the long-term functional and cosmetic outcome.

Endosseous implantation is performed in two stages: fixture placement (stage I), followed by exposure of the osseointegrated implant and placement of a transmucosal attachment (stage II). The implant site can be predetermined radiographically by (1) measuring the desired location of implantation from an existing tooth; (2) measuring from a stable anatomic landmark that can be identified radiographically and intraorally at the time of surgery; (3) using an acrylic stent with markers that establish radiographic and intraoral points of reference; or (4) using a computerized virtual stent that is created preoperatively with an image guidance system. The use of an acrylic stent in combination with DentaScan will be discussed to illustrate how dental implantation is performed.

Intraoral placement of an acrylic stent with radiopaque markers at the time of image acquisition allows the surgeon to verify the desired location for implantation intraoperatively by reinserting the stent and correlating the intraoral location of the markers with the cross-sectional DentaScan images (**Fig. 23–5B–D**). These radiographic templates can also be used to ensure the proper angle of insertion of the implant. The location and vertical angulation of the implant are critical considerations that not only optimize eventual prosthodontic restoration, but also avoid cortical perforations when implant sites are thin buccolingually.[13,16] The process of anatomic localization using a surgical stent and DentaScan followed by the surgical stages of implant placement are described in **Fig. 23–5**.

◆ Conclusion

Osseointegrated dental implants have enabled clinicians to improve the masticatory function, speech articulation, and cosmetic appearance of patients who have been treated for oral cancer. Dental CT reformatting programs have provided surgeons with sophisticated imaging tools that improve the accuracy of implant placement, ensure implant longevity, and minimize the surgical morbidity associated with implantation. The introduction of other refinements such as cone-beam CT and surgical navigation are likely to provide even greater rates of surgically precise implantation and lower rates of iatrogenic injury.

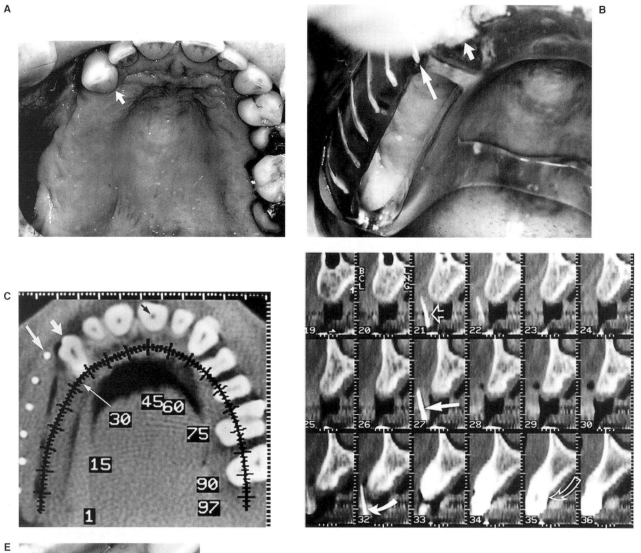

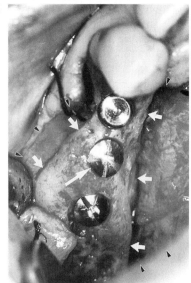

Figure 23–5 Surgical implant procedure. **(A)** This patient, being evaluated for dental implants, is edentulous distal to the right maxillary canine (*arrow*). **(B)** A stent with six vertical markers has been placed over the alveolar ridge and residual teeth. The sixth marker (*long arrow*) is adjacent to the right canine (*short arrow*) and will be demonstrated on the CT images. This marker appears as a dot on the axial image next to perpendicular line 32 **(C)** and as a line on cross-sectional image number 32 **(D)**. **(C)** Axial view demonstrating the sixth marker (*long thick arrow*) at perpendicular line 32 (*thin arrow*) and adjacent to the right canine (*short white arrow*). Note the radiolucent pulp in the center of the teeth (*black arrow*). **(D)** Cross-sectional views demonstrating markers 4 (*open arrow*), 5 (*straight arrow*), and 6 (*curved arrow*) of the stent. Note that marker 6 is adjacent to the right canine (*open curved arrow*). By placing the stent on the patient during surgery, the surgeon knows that the bone under marker 6 is as depicted by cross-sectional image 32. **(E)** An incision is made, and the gingival and periosteal flap (*arrowheads*) is held back with sutures. This exposes the bone of the alveolar process (*short arrows*). Holes are drilled, and three titanium implants are inserted into the bone. Note that the implants are flush with the bone, and their openings are covered with healing screw caps (*long arrow*). The incision is sutured closed and permitted to heal for 4 months in the mandible and 6 months in the maxilla. (*Continued*)

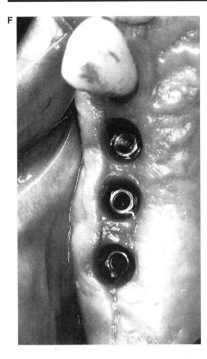
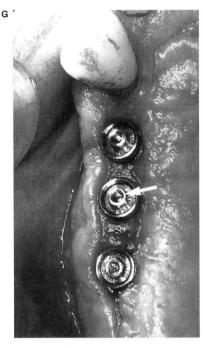
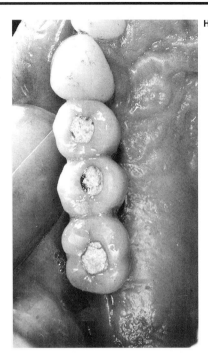

Figure 23–5 (*Continued*) **(F)** Before this photograph was taken, a small incision was made to remove the healing caps. Healing abutments, which were attached to the implants, have been removed. The threaded opening of the implant is visualized. **(G)** The permanent abutments, which raise the fixture above the gingival surface, have now been attached. The screw hole (*arrow*) in the center of the abutment will accommodate the screw that fixes the prosthesis. **(H)** The prosthesis is now attached to the three implants. (From Abrahams JJ. The role of diagnostic imaging in dental implantology. Radiol Clin North Am 1993;31:163–180, with permission from Elsevier.)

References

1. Reddy MS, Mayfield-Donahoo T, Vanderven FJ, Jeffcoat MK. A comparison of the diagnostic advantages of panoramic radiography and computed tomography scanning for placement of root form dental implants. Clin Oral Implants Res 1994;5:229–238

2. McGivney GP, Haughton V, Strandt JA, Eichholz JE, Lubar DM. A comparison of computer-assisted tomography and data-gathering modalities in prosthodontics. Int J Oral Maxillofac Implants 1986;1:55–68

3. Wishan MS, Bahat O, Krane M. Computed tomography as an adjunct in dental implant surgery. Int J Periodontics Restorative Dent 1988; 8:30–47

4. Brockenbrough JM, Petruzzelli GJ, Lomasney L. DentaScan as an accurate method of predicting mandibular invasion in patients with squamous cell carcinoma of the oral cavity. Arch Otolaryngol Head Neck Surg 2003;129:113–117

5. Abrahams JJ, Hayt MW, Rock R. Dental CT reformatting programs and dental imaging. In: Som PM, Curtin HD, eds. Head and Neck Imaging. St. Louis: Mosby, 2003:907–918

6. Abrahams JJ. CT assessment of dental implant planning. Oral Maxillofac Surg Clin North Am 1992;4:1–18

7. Adell R, Lekholm U, Rockler B, Branemark PI. A 15-year study of osseointegrated implants in the treatment of the edentulous jaw. Int J Oral Surg 1981;10:387–416

8. Frederiksen NL. Diagnostic imaging in dental implantology. Oral Surg Oral Med Oral Pathol Oral Radiol Endod 1995;80:540–554

9. Abrahams JJ. The role of diagnostic imaging in dental implantology. Radiol Clin North Am 1993;31:163–180

10. Abrahams JJ, Oliverio PJ. Odontogenic cysts: improved imaging with a dental CT software program. AJNR Am J Neuroradiol 1993;14:367–374

11. Fagelman D, Huang AB. Prospective evaluation of lesions of the mandible and maxilla: findings on multiplanar and three-dimensional CT. AJR Am J Roentgenol 1994;163:693–698

12. Yanagisawa K, Friedman CD, Vining EM, Abrahams JJ. DentaScan imaging of the mandible and maxilla. Head Neck 1993;15:1–7

13. Mupparapu M, Singer SR. Implant imaging for the dentist. J Can Dent Assoc 2004;70:32

14. Schulze D, Heiland M, Blake F, Rother U, Schmelzle R. Evaluation of quality of reformatted images from two cone-beam computed tomographic systems. J Craniomaxillofac Surg 2005;33:19–23

15. User Manual IGI. Jerusalem: DenX Advanced Dental Systems, 2004

16. Rosenfeld AL, Mecall RA. The use of interactive computed tomography to predict the esthetic and functional demands of implant-supported prostheses. Compend Contin Educ Dent 1996;17: 1125–1132

24

Oral Prosthetic Rehabilitation

Jack W. Martin,

James C. Lemon, and

Mark S. Chambers

Following oral cancer resection, reconstruction and rehabilitation are of a paramount importance to the patient's ultimate aesthetic and functional outcome. Mastication, swallowing, vocal quality and speech articulation, freedom from pain and deformity, and self-esteem are all reliant on the perioperative and postoperative treatment decisions that are made. Innovations such as microvascular surgery and osseointegration have dramatically improved the reconstructive and rehabilitative options for many patients who were previously subjected to permanent disability and deformity. Prosthetic rehabilitation has evolved along with these developments, providing oral cancer patients with unprecedented levels of cosmesis and function that translate into an improved quality of life and reintegration into society. This chapter reviews the techniques of prosthetic rehabilitation for patients with oral cancer, and offers several suggestions to the surgeon that enable the maxillofacial prosthodontist to fabricate a removable fixed dental prosthesis that is functionally and aesthetically superior.

◆ Pretreatment Dental Evaluation and Management

Dental problems in head and neck cancer patients typically mirror those seen in the general population: moderate to advanced periodontal disease, dental caries, and poor dental hygiene.[1-3] Prior to cancer treatment, every patient should undergo a comprehensive radiographic and clinical examination by a dentist who is familiar with the impact of treatments such as radiation therapy and surgery on the dentition. The individual prognosis of each tooth is evaluated, and the patient's history of and motivation to comply with recommended dental hygiene measures and follow-up dental visits are factors that determine the fate of their dentition. It is frequently prudent to extract teeth whenever patients demonstrate a lack of compliance with prior dental care, because periodontal inflammation or unaddressed dental caries can lead to disastrous consequences following radiotherapy, such as osteoradionecrosis or extensive recurrent caries and endodontic complications. On the other hand, careful consideration must be given to preserving periodontally sound teeth that could improve posttreatment function and that may serve as important abutment teeth for fixed or removable prostheses. Teeth that are deemed worthy of salvage should undergo disease removal prior to initiation of cancer treatment. Plaque and calculus removal is performed, carious lesions are removed and restored, and endodontic therapy is completed. Patients are also thoroughly educated regarding the need to meticulously follow recommended plaque control and fluoride regimens, and should be reevaluated following completion of cancer treatment on a regular basis (see Chapter 8).

Maxillofacial prosthodontics is the specialty of dentistry concerned with the prosthetic rehabilitation of intraoral and extraoral structures that have been affected by disease, injury, surgery, or congenital malformation. Patients should be referred to the maxillofacial prosthodontist early in their treatment workup to evaluate the oral/dental status and to discuss the options of prosthetic rehabilitation. Stone casts obtained from impressions of the maxillae and mandible during the initial dental visit may be useful if intraoral or extraoral surgical prostheses are planned.[4-7] During the treatment planning phase, the maxillofacial prosthodontist must also consider the cost, longevity, and ability of the patient to tolerate treatment. Patient care and outcomes are improved by using a team approach to the management of patients with head and neck cancer. This team includes the head and neck surgeon, radiation oncologist, medical oncologist, prosthodontist, speech pathologist, nutritionist, reconstructive surgeon, and nursing staff. Careful planning among the maxillofacial prosthodontist, radiation oncologist, and surgeon facilitates proper patient education and pretreatment planning, which improves the coordination and delivery of care. The results of this evaluation can then be integrated into the overall treatment plan by the primary surgeon. Miscommunication or lack of communication between the surgeon and the maxillofacial prosthodontist is responsible for most avoidable posttreatment complications associated with prosthetic rehabilitation of the head and neck patient.[1,4,5,8]

Head and neck cancer surgeons should have thorough knowledge of dental anatomy to facilitate accurate communication with the prosthodontist who is responsible for the patient's rehabilitation.[5] For example, it is important for the prosthodontist to know which teeth will be removed during surgical resection so that an immediate or postoperative prosthesis can be appropriately planned and fabricated. Teeth should be identified by using the universal dental numbering system, where the maxillary right third molar is tooth 1, the maxillary left third molar is tooth 16, the mandibular left third molar is tooth 17, and the mandibular right third molar is tooth 32. The use of descriptive terms such as "mandibular left second molar" for tooth 18 provides additional clarification in cases where erroneous extraction of a critical abutment tooth would significantly impact the prosthetic result.

Surgeons must also appreciate how surgical resection of certain anatomic structures can profoundly impact prosthesis function, or may prevent rehabilitation with a prosthesis altogether. For example, the upper alveolar ridge, maxillary tuberosity, and hard palate are major supporting tissues for maxillary prostheses, whereas the lower alveolar ridge, retromolar pad, and buccal shelf provide support for mandibular prostheses.[4,5,9,10]

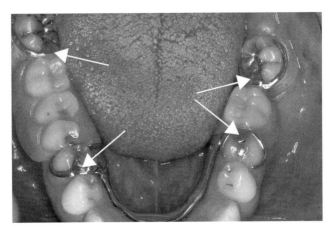

Figure 24–1 Tooth-supported mandibular removable partial denture (RPD) with bilateral mesial and distal abutment teeth. Clasp arms engage undercuts of the abutment teeth to provide retention. Vertical support is provided by occlusal rests (arrows), which "rest" on the occlusal surface of abutment teeth. (Courtesy of John W. Werning, M.D., D.M.D., University of Florida.)

extends distally to replace missing posterior teeth, which is referred to as a *distal extension partial denture*. The *distal extension RPD* lacks the support and retention that is achieved with a *tooth-supported* RPD, so a distal abutment tooth should be preserved whenever possible.[11] Maxillary obturators can be completely tissue-supported or tooth-tissue supported. Osseointegrated implants also allow for the use of implant-supported prostheses (**Fig. 24–2**).

Several factors determine the functionality of a maxillary or mandibular denture or obturator. The degree to which each of these factors can be addressed during resection, reconstruction, and prosthesis fabrication will directly impact the final result. Prosthetic rehabilitation with a maxillary obturator will be used as an example to characterize the interrelationship between surgical tissue loss, prosthesis design, and patient function.

Support is the resistance to movement of a prosthesis toward the tissue. The primary areas available for support in the residual maxilla include the residual teeth, upper alveolar ridge, and hard palate. When teeth are present, occlusal rests that contact the occlusal surface of an

◆ Principles of Prosthetic Rehabilitation

Prosthodontic rehabilitation can be achieved by using fixed dental prostheses that can be cemented to abutment teeth, or fixed to implant abutments using either adhesive cement or screws. There are two types of removable prostheses: (1) *complete dentures*, which are completely tissue-supported prostheses that rehabilitate an edentulous dental arch; and (2) *removable partial dentures* (RPDs), which are used to restore the partially edentulous dental arch. A *tooth-supported* RPD is supported by teeth both mesially and distally, and is not reliant on support from the tissues overlying the alveolar ridge (**Fig. 24–1**). *Tooth-tissue supported* prostheses, however, derive their support from the teeth as well the tissues of the alveolar ridge. In some cases, the denture base of a tooth-tissue supported prosthesis

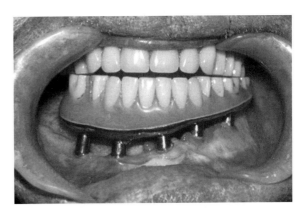

Figure 24–2 Implant-supported complete denture used to rehabilitate a reconstructed edentulous mandible.

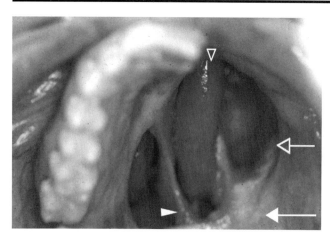

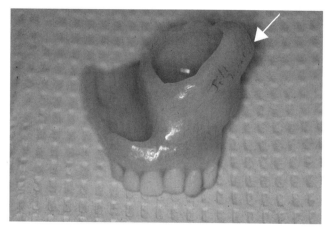

Figure 24–3 Maxillectomy defect involving the left hemimaxilla and most of the contralateral hard palate. The soft palate and some of the premaxilla have been preserved. Support for the obturator is provided by the remaining teeth and alveolar ridge, as well as the pterygoid plates *(arrow)* and nasal septum *(arrowhead)*. Retention of the obturator is provided by engaging the nasopharyngeal surface of the soft and the superior surface of the hard palate as well as the lateral scar band *(open arrow)*. Retention will also be achieved through surface adhesion, surface tension, and the incorporation of metal clasps or bars into the metal framework that engage undercuts of tooth surfaces. Removal of the inferior turbinate *(open arrowhead)* will eliminate contact between the turbinate and the prosthesis that can lead to mucosal irritation and patient discomfort. (Courtesy of John W. Werning, M.D., D.M.D., University of Florida.)

Figure 24–4 Maxillary obturator for a large defect in an edentulous patient. The absence of teeth mandate the need to gain enough support and retention from the remaining alveolar ridge, hard palate, and the residual defect. The obturator bulb *(arrow)* is hollow, which reduces the weight of the prosthesis, minimizing the impact of gravity on vertical displacement. (Courtesy of John W. Werning, M.D., D.M.D., University of Florida.)

abutment tooth can be integrated into the metal framework of the prosthesis, minimizing movement toward the underlying alveolar mucosa. As the number of remaining teeth decreases, the importance of the amount and form of residual alveolar ridge increases. Preservation of the anterior alveolar ridge and maxillary tuberosity are particularly useful anatomic regions that provide support. Within the defect, the bony orbital floor, pterygoid plates, and nasal septum can also be used to support the obturator. The pterygoid plates are a useful location for posterior support that is frequently exploited, whereas the orbital floor and nasal septum are used less commonly (**Fig. 24–3**).[11–13]

Retention is the resistance to vertical displacement of the prosthesis. In addition to the usual forces that cause vertical displacement, the force of gravity can vertically displace the maxillary obturator. Periodontally sound teeth are an excellent source for prosthesis retention. Direct retention can be achieved by employing metal clasps or bars that engage undercuts of tooth surfaces.[14–17] Retention of the obturator, however, is more challenging when the residual maxilla is edentulous. When a large defect is obturated, the obturator bulb should be hollow to reduce its weight, minimizing the effect of gravity on retention (**Fig. 24–4**).[18] Indirect retention is also possible by making design modifications that prevent rotational displacement of the prosthesis around its *fulcrum line*, which is the axis about which the denture rotates when subjected to various forces (**Fig. 24–5**).[11] Resistance to vertical displacement can also be provided by the defect itself through the exploitation of adhesion, interfacial surface tension, and tissue undercuts. The prosthesis can engage the nasopharyngeal surface of the soft palate or an undercut along the line of hard palate resection (**Fig. 24–3**). The lateral

scar band that develops where the skin graft joins with the residual buccal mucosa can also be utilized so that the prosthesis is retained by the tautness of the scar band (**Fig. 24–6**). The height of the lateral wall of the defect is another source of indirect retention; extending the height of the lateral wall of the obturator minimizes rotation of the prosthesis around the fulcrum line into the defect.[12,19] *Stability* is the resistance to prosthesis displacement by functional, horizontal, or rotational forces. Stability is provided by some of the structures and prosthetic design principles that

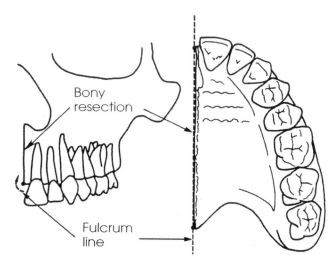

Figure 24–5 Standard midline resection creates a defect unfavorable for obturation because of potential prosthesis movement around a fulcrum line located at the defect margin. (From Taylor TD, LaVelle WE, Arcuri MR. Dental management and rehabilitation of tumors of the oral cavity. In: Thawley SE, Panje WR, Batsakis JG, Lindberg RD, eds. Comprehensive Management of Head and Neck Tumors, vol 1, 2nd ed. Philadelphia: WB Saunders, 1999:720–721, with permission.)

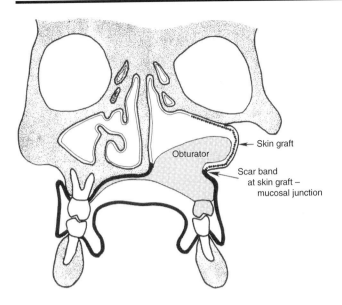

Figure 24–6 The contour of the lateral defect wall at the skin graft–mucosal junction can be engaged successfully by an obturator prosthesis. The palatal mucosa has been reflected over the midline palatal bone cut to facilitate mucosal healing. (From Taylor TD, LaVelle WE, Arcuri MR. Dental management and rehabilitation of tumors of the oral cavity. In: Thawley SE, Panje WR, Batsakis JG, Lindberg RD, eds. Comprehensive Management of Head and Neck Tumors, vol 1, 2nd ed. Philadelphia: WB Saunders, 1999:720–721, with permission.)

have already been discussed. Teeth can provide resistance to movement in all directions, and maximal extension of the borders of the prosthesis into the buccal vestibule improves horizontal stability.[12,20] Equal distribution of occlusal forces along the maxilla from the opposing mandibular teeth can also enhance stability.[12]

These principles also pertain to prosthetic rehabilitation of the mandible, including the support, retention, and stability provided by the teeth, and maximal extension of the denture borders into the buccal and lingual vestibules and onto the retromolar pad. Osseointegrated implants have provided us with another method by which improved support, retention, and stability can be achieved.

◆ Timing of Definitive Removable Prosthesis Fabrication

When dental extractions, tumor resection, or other preprosthetic surgical procedures have been performed, definitive tissue-supported removable partial or complete dentures should not be fabricated until the denture-bearing surfaces are completely mucosalized and bony remodeling is complete, which usually occurs within 3 months. Premature insertion can lead to wound complications and an unstable, nonretentive denture if subsequent bony remodeling occurs, because the alveolar ridge contours and vestibular borders no longer correspond to those of the denture. Temporary interim prostheses that are placed after surgery frequently require modification to provide the patient with a comfortable, functional prosthesis until the definitive prosthesis can be made.

Following radiotherapy to the oral cavity region, the most appropriate time for removable prosthesis insertion has not been established. In a recent retrospective review of 190 patients, Gerngross et al[21] noted that patients who were treated with greater than 50 Gy were more likely to experience complications before and after denture insertion; 92% of these patients underwent prosthesis insertion more than 90 days after radiotherapy. Irradiated patients were 1.7 times more likely to have a postprosthesis insertion complication than a preprosthesis insertion complication [odds ration (OR), 1.71; 95% confidence interval (CI), 1.03–2.80]. However, there was no difference in the complication rate between the group of patients who received their dentures within 180 days of radiotherapy and those who underwent denture insertion more than 180 days after treatment. Therefore, it appears that patients who require irradiation can be managed in a similar fashion to nonirradiated individuals.

◆ Maxillectomy Defects

Classification

As discussed above, the support, stability, and retention of an obturator are determined by the size and location of the surgical defect, status of the dentition, and the supporting surface area of the remaining palate and within the defect.[3–6,8,10] Maxillectomy defect classification systems have been developed that can be used to ascertain the most effective means of prosthetic rehabilitation for a particular type of maxillectomy defect. The classification by Aramany[22] from 1978 focused on obturator design alone, whereas a later classification system proposed by Okay and colleagues[10] from Mt. Sinai Medical Center (New York, NY) provides rehabilitative options for defects that also account for the increasing role of local flaps and free tissue transfer. Based on a retrospective review of 47 consecutive palatomaxillary restorations, they devised a classification scheme that incorporated design considerations for surgical reconstruction and prosthodontic rehabilitation that focused on four objectives: (1) closure of the oral cavity, (2) provision of a stable base for the restoration of function, (3) restoration of midface symmetry, and (4) support of orbital structures. The size and location of the defect, remaining dentition, and palate were found to influence the choice and design of the free tissue transfer or prosthodontic rehabilitation. These findings were used to describe four major classes of maxillary defects[10]:

Class Ia defects involve any portion of the hard palate, but not tooth-bearing maxillary alveolus (**Fig. 24–7**). Such defects could be rehabilitated with an obturator, a local advancement flap, or a fasciocutaneous free flap. Prosthetic obturation was generally stable and well tolerated.

Class Ib defects involve the premaxilla or any portion of maxillary alveolus and dentition posterior to the canines (**Fig. 24–8**). Because these defects involved a limited portion of the dental arch, movement of an obturator

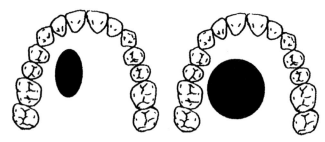

Figure 24–7 Class Ia defects involve any portion of hard palate but not tooth-bearing maxillary alveolus. (From Okay DJ, Genden E, Buchbinder D, Urken M. Prosthodontic guidelines for surgical reconstruction of the maxilla: a classification system of defects. J Prosth Dent 2001;86:352–363, with permission from the editorial council of the *Journal of Prosthetic Dentistry*. Copyright 2001.)

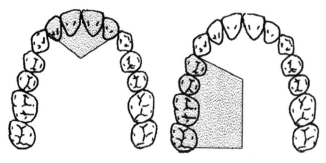

Figure 24–8 Class Ib defects involve premaxilla or any portion of maxillary alveolus and dentition posterior to canines. (From Okay DJ, Genden E, Buchbinder D, Urken M. Prosthodontic guidelines for surgical reconstruction of the maxilla: a classification system of defects. J Prosth Dent 2001;86:352–363, with permission from the editorial council of the *Journal of Prosthetic Dentistry*. Copyright 2001.)

around the fulcrum line could be stabilized by the remaining palate and dentition. A fasciocutaneous free flap (e.g., radial forearm) could be used to separate the oral cavity from the nose and/or maxillary sinus, but such a reconstruction prevented extension of the obturator bulb into the defect to engage retentive anatomic undercuts.

Class II defects include (1) any portion of the hard palate and tooth bearing maxillary alveolus and only one canine, where the anterior margin of the defect was located within the premaxilla; or (2) anterior transverse palatectomy defects that involved less than one half of the palatal surface (**Fig. 24–9**). Prosthetic rehabilitation of these defects is less stable because the dental arch size and form is reduced, palatal support is diminished, and there are fewer teeth for clasping. Some of these defects can be successfully reconstructed with vascularized bone-containing free flaps (VBCFFs) that reestablish the bony dental arch and allow placement of osseointegrated implants.

Class III defects include (1) any portion of the hard palate and tooth-bearing maxillary alveolus that includes both canines,

or (2) total and transverse palatectomy defects that involve more than 50% of the hard palate (**Fig. 24–10**). These defects are characterized by minimal remaining palate or dentition, making obturation a poor choice. Vascularized bone-containing free flaps provide better restoration of these defects than soft tissue free flaps, because they provide bone that can support implantation as well as a stable base that can oppose the mandible during function.[10]

The authors also subclassified defects based on loss of the orbital floor or zygomatic arch. Although microvascular reconstruction of the maxilla can provide excellent functional and cosmetic results, imprecise reconstruction may lead to worse outcomes than obturation. Thus, the decision to perform free flap transfer depends in large part on the clinical scenario as well as the expertise of the reconstructive surgeon.

Technical Considerations

Resection of the maxillary sinus, hard palate, and upper alveolar ridge may leave the patient with significant postoperative speech and swallowing problems.[4–6] These problems can be reduced or eliminated by careful planning between surgeon and dentist. The dental stone casts obtained at the initial dental visit can be used to review the expected horizontal component of the defect with the surgeon and to fabricate the prosthesis.[4–6] The vertical component of the maxillary defect, which can range from a limited resection with no oroantral/oronasal communication to extensive defects of the maxilla and orbit that may require a combination prosthesis (intraoral prosthesis and facial prosthesis), should also be discussed.

There are several surgical techniques that can be incorporated into a maxillectomy procedure to improve prosthetic rehabilitation[4–6]:

1. Make the alveolar cuts through the socket of an extracted tooth (or an edentulous space) in a dentate patient. This prevents iatrogenic bone loss and ensures the longevity of the tooth next to this cut (**Fig. 24–11**).[6]

2. When making the palatal cut, as much of the premaxilla as possible should be spared. The premaxilla is very important for the support and retention of a prosthesis

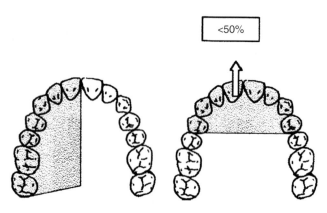

Figure 24–9 Class II defects involve any portion of hard palate and tooth-bearing maxillary alveolus and only one canine. Anterior margin of defect lies within premaxilla. This class includes transverse palatectomy defects that involve less than 50% of hard palate. (From Okay DJ, Genden E, Buchbinder D, Urken M. Prosthodontic guidelines for surgical reconstruction of the maxilla: a classification system of defects. J Prosth Dent 2001;86:352–363, with permission from the editorial council of the *Journal of Prosthetic Dentistry*. Copyright 2001.)

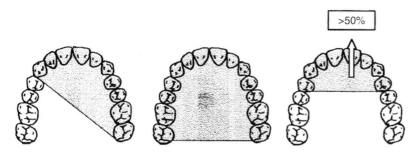

Figure 24–10 Class III defects involve any portion of hard palate and tooth-bearing maxillary alveolus, including both canines. This class includes total and transverse palatectomy defects that involve over 50% of hard palate. (From Okay DJ, Genden E, Buchbinder D, Urken M. Prosthodontic guidelines for surgical reconstruction of the maxilla: a classification system of defects. J Prosth Dent 2001;86:352–363, with permission from the editorial council of the *Journal of Prosthetic Dentistry*. Copyright 2001.)

(**Fig. 24–11**). If the cancer is located in the anterior region of the maxilla, it may be possible to spare the maxillary tuberosity on the defect side, which would also increase prosthetic support (**Fig. 24–12**).

3. As a general rule, a split-thickness skin graft (STSG) should be placed in the maxillary defect.[23] The skin graft provides an excellent scar band for retention of the prosthesis and decreases mucus secretion and crust formation in the ablated sinus, making hygiene of this area easier for the patient (**Figs. 24–3** and **24–6**).

4. If the palatal mucosa is not affected by disease, it can be retained and wrapped around the midline portion of the palatal cut (**Fig. 24–6**).[4–6]

5. Removal of the inferior and middle turbinates allows extension of the prosthesis into the defect area. If the turbinates are not removed, they often become irritated by the prosthesis (**Fig. 24–3**).[6]

6. Consideration should be given to removing the mandibular molar teeth on the side of the maxillectomy as they can become a hygiene problem and are essentially nonfunctional after a maxillectomy.[4–6]

7. The modified Weber-Ferguson incision is generally used to gain access for the maxillectomy. It is preferable for

a cosmetic and functional outcome to perform the maxillectomy intraorally, if possible, eliminating the facial incision. This makes manipulation of the lip and cheek less painful for the patient during postoperative prosthetic procedures.[3–7,23,24]

8. A surgical obturator prosthesis should be placed to restore the oral contour for immediate function and aesthetics postoperatively.[4–6] This prosthesis will support the surgical packing and can be fixated to the remaining teeth with surgical wire or retained with a bone screw in the edentulous patient. The obturator may negate the use of a nasogastric tube and decrease the time of rehabilitation postoperatively. It will maintain proper lip and cheek support during healing, helping to reduce the contracture of scar tissue. When the surgical packing is removed (usually within 3 to 5 days of the procedure), the surgical obturator can be converted into an interim prosthesis. Use of a surgical prosthesis can also improve the patient's mental outlook.[4–7,23,24]

Some clinicians suggest that maxillary defects should be closed completely using free-tissue grafts.[4–6,25,26] Function and cosmesis can be effectively restored with surgical

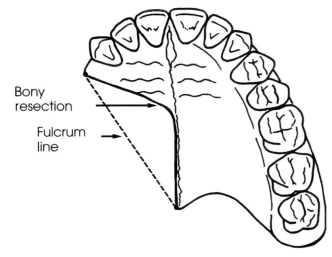

Figure 24–11 Preservation of the premaxillary segment shifts the fulcrum line favorably for prosthesis retention, stability, and support. The line of resection through the alveolar ridge should preserve adequate alveolar bone around the adjacent retained tooth. (From Taylor TD, LaVelle WE, Arcuri MR. Dental management and rehabilitation of tumors of the oral cavity. In: Thawley SE, Panje WR, Batsakis JG, Lindberg RD, eds. Comprehensive Management of Head and Neck Tumors, vol 1, 2nd ed. Philadelphia: WB Saunders, 1999:720–721, with permission.)

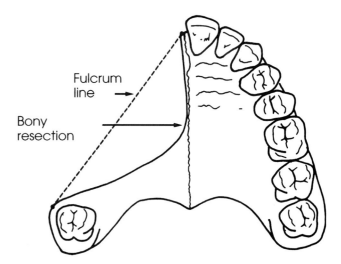

Figure 24–12 Preservation of a portion of the posterior maxilla also improves prosthesis retention, stability, and support. (From Taylor TD, LaVelle WE, Arcuri MR. Dental management and rehabilitation of tumors of the oral cavity. In: Thawley SE, Panje WR, Batsakis JG, Lindberg RD, eds. Comprehensive Management of Head and Neck Tumors, vol 1, 2nd ed. Philadelphia: WB Saunders, 1999:720–721, with permission.)

reconstruction. This method can occlude the surgical defect but may preclude prosthetic rehabilitation and complicate oral rehabilitation if fistulation develops or flap bulkiness is present. Free tissue transfer, however, is an excellent reconstructive option for carefully selected defects and may be an alternative for patients who do not desire a prosthesis (see Chapter 19).[4–6,10]

There are three distinct phases of maxillary obturator rehabilitation: surgical, interim, and definitive. The surgical obturator prosthesis is placed at the time of surgery, and is used to establish oronasal separation and lip and cheek support so that the patient can effectively speak and swallow during the postoperative period. This prosthesis also minimizes postoperative deformity and allows the defect to be packed, providing a pressure dressing for the skin graft. Three to five days after surgery, the surgical obturator is relined and modified to optimize extension of the borders in the buccal vestibule and along the residual palate to improve the seal between the prosthesis and the adjacent tissues, and the obturator can also be modified to adapt to the surgical defect. The definitive obturator prosthesis is fabricated several months after radiation therapy has been completed to allow for stabilization of the defect, which progressively heals and remodels over time.[4,6,18,27] The definitive prosthesis can usually be safely inserted 3 to 6 months after completion of radiotherapy.[21]

Assessment of Obturator Function

A properly functioning obturator can markedly improve quality of life after maxillectomy. According to Kornblith and colleagues[28] from Memorial Sloan-Kettering Cancer Center, the most significant predictors of superior obturator function include resection of one third or less of the soft palate and one fourth or less of the hard palate. Improved psychosocial adaptation following obturation is associated with the ability to pronounce words, mastication, deglutition, and minimal changes in vocal quality.[28] Continued fibrosis of the tissues bordering the prosthesis may lead to nasal reflux and hypernasal speech, which occurs due to leakage of air from the oral cavity into the nasal cavity. To evaluate for the presence of hypernasal speech, the patient is asked to say several words beginning with the *b* sound. If the *b* sound is not distinguishable from the *m* sound, then air escape is occurring. The patient should also say the word *beat* with and without occlusion of the nares. If the sound quality changes, hypernasality is present. Functional modification of the borders of the prosthesis using an autopolymerizing acrylic resin typically corrects the problem. Hypernasal speech may also result from inadequate elevation or shortening of the soft palate secondary to fibrosis following resection of the anterior soft palate. In this case, a pharyngeal obturator extension may be required.[18]

◆ Soft Palate Defects

When the soft palate is resected, the surgeon must consider whether the remaining soft palate will be functional. It is frequently easier to rehabilitate a patient's speech and swallowing if the soft palate is completely removed, particularly when one third or less of the posterior soft palate remains following tumor resection.[4–6,29] If the remaining soft palate is nonfunctional, rehabilitation can be difficult or even impossible. However, a thin strip of soft palate may be useful for prosthesis retention in a patient with limited supporting tissue.[4,5,8,23] Intraoperative consultation with the maxillofacial prosthodontist at the time of surgical resection is often helpful to decide whether retention of the residual soft palate will be helpful or detrimental.

Immediate surgical obturation is most beneficial in dentate and edentulous patients where the entire soft palate is to be resected, although some edentulous patients may require delayed obturation.[29] Speech evaluation following obturator placement is extremely important in optimizing prosthetic rehabilitation of soft palatal defects.[3–6,8,23] Surgical and prosthetic treatment may provide the patient with the capability of controlling nasal air emission and resonance, but articulatory disorders can persist. Evaluation of articulation errors and inappropriate nasal resonance by a speech pathologist can guide optimal modification of the obturator to address these deficits.[3–6,8,23]

Palatopharyngeal (or velopharyngeal) incompetence is defined as normal anatomy with ineffective or absent motor function, whereas palatopharyngeal insufficiency is caused by abnormal anatomy such as cleft palate or resection of the soft palate or lateral pharyngeal wall. In general, palatopharyngeal insufficiency is treated with a pharyngeal prosthesis, whereas palatopharyngeal incompetence is treated with a palatal lift.[18] Primary radiation treatment of the soft palate may cause palatopharyngeal insufficiency due to fibrosis and tumor necrosis that can lead to nasal regurgitation and hypernasal speech (**Fig. 24–13**).[6] Effective prosthetic rehabilitation of this deficiency is frequently challenging and of limited benefit.

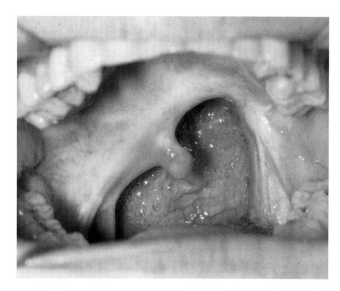

Figure 24–13 Palatopharyngeal insufficiency secondary to soft palate fibrosis from surgical resection and postoperative radiotherapy.

◆ Mandibulectomy Defects

Marginal mandibulectomies can be reconstructed primarily with an STSG (**Fig. 24–14**).[5,24] If the tongue or floor of mouth is sutured to the buccal or labial mucosa for mandibular coverage, prosthetic rehabilitation is difficult, if not impossible.[5,8] Skin grafts provide a sound tissue base for a prosthesis and separate the tongue and floor of the mouth from the buccal mucosa. Often, revascularization of the skin graft by the underlying mandibular bone is achieved by suturing a bolster dressing over the graft. This technique, however, does not reestablish the original depth of the buccal and lingual vestibules, which decreases the retention and stability of a removable prosthesis. This dilemma can be addressed by fabricating an immediate surgical stent from a stock plastic impression tray lined with tissue-conditioning material that uniformly contours the skin graft over the residual alveolar ridge and extends the borders into the depth of the buccal and lingual vestibules.[30] The stent can be stabilized to adjacent tissues and teeth using silk sutures and steel ligature wire, or by the placement of circummandibular wires. A form-fitting customized stent can also be fabricated with self-curing acrylic resin lined with tissue-conditioning material. Use of such a stent allows the maxillofacial prosthodontist to take advantage of the residual alveolar ridge and caudally positioned vestibules during fabrication of the prosthesis. Mandibular reconstruction that has resulted in a deficient vestibular depth and excessive soft tissue covering the reconstructed neoalveolar ridge frequently prevents fabrication of a retentive, stable prosthesis.[4–6] Vestibuloplasty with placement of an STSG or placement of dental implants is an effective way to address this problem.[4–6,8]

Following mandibulectomy, surgical stents or arch bars may be necessary to reposition the mandibular segments in their proper position before surgical reconstruction.[4–6] The maxillary teeth opposing the mandibular reconstruction require removal to minimize trauma to bone and soft tissue flaps. If

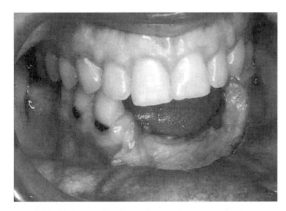

Figure 24–14 Healed split-thickness skin graft covering residual mandible following marginal mandibulectomy. Because there are no abutment teeth in the left posterior mandibular region, prosthetic restoration requires fabrication of a tooth-tissue supported distal extension RPD with less retention, support and stability. Placement of a surgical stent at the time of skin grafting increases the surface area of the residual alveolar ridge and reestablishes the buccal and lingual vestibule so that the borders of the denture base can be extended, thereby augmenting support.

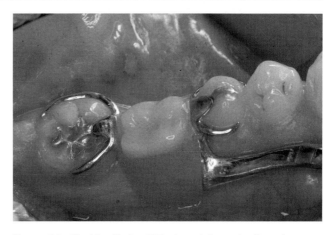

Figure 24–15 Mandibular RPD viewed from the lingual aspect, replacing tooth 19. Occlusal rests support the RPD on the mesio-occlusal surface of tooth 18 distally and the disto-occlusal surface of tooth 20 mesially. Retentive clasp arms engage tooth surface undercuts on these teeth. The metal framework is composed of a chromium-cobalt alloy and the tissue-colored denture base is made of acrylic resin. (Courtesy of John W. Werning, M.D., D.M.D., University of Florida.)

reconstruction is not contemplated in a mandibulectomy patient, removal of the condyle and ramus on the affected side will prevent migration of these structures toward the maxilla, simplifying prosthetic rehabilitation.[5]

Free-tissue transfer has revolutionized mandibular reconstruction, providing predictable results, even in irradiated patients.[4–6,31–35] The three most common types of osseous free-tissue transfer into mandibulectomy defects include the scapula, iliac crest, and fibula.[31] From the perspective of rehabilitation potential, the fibula appears to be the most adaptable graft, supplying bone of adequate length and quality to reconstruct most mandibular defects.[31–35] The fibula is also an excellent recipient for dental implants and prosthesis support.[4–6,36–40]

Prosthesis fabrication following marginal mandibulectomy in dentulous patients is based on the principles of framework design used for RPDs. Support can be provided by the incorporation of occlusal rest seats, and retention can be gained through the employment of clasps or bars that engage tooth undercuts (**Fig. 24–15**). Retention and stability of tissue-supported prostheses are also provided by the contour of the remaining alveolar ridge and its mucosal extensions distally in the retromolar pad region and the buccal and lingual vestibules. More extensive mandibular reconstructions frequently rely on osseointegrated implants that compensate for the loss of native tissue.

◆ Tongue Defects

Tumors involving the oral tongue often require extensive resection of bone and soft tissue resulting in functional and cosmetic morbidity.[3–6,8,23] The degree of speech impediment depends on the extent to which the tongue function is compromised. The resection of large portions of the tongue impairs its mobility and prevents its apposition with other oral structures, compromising articulation and deglutition.[23]

Palatal augmentation prostheses that are approximated to the maxilla conform to postoperative tongue movements and help normalize speech (improving specific sounds) and swallowing.[4–6] Tongue prostheses can be fabricated, but in general have poor function and patient acceptance. Several types of flaps can be used to restore the tongue; although nonfunctional, they reduce space in the oral cavity and make prosthetic fabrication easier and more effective.[5,23,41,42]

◆ Osseointegrated Implants

Dental implants are often used to provide improved support, retention, and stability to fixed and removable prostheses.[4,5,43–45] Osseointegration is a direct structural and functional connection between ordered, living bone and the surface of an implant that results in a stable implant that can bear the load resulting from mastication and parafunction.[43,44] The root form implant is the most commonly used endosseous implant. Once osseointegration of an endosteal dental implant occurs, abutments can be connected to the implant that allow for the attachment of a superstructure and, eventually, a dental prosthesis.[44–47] Principles of osseointegration and techniques of implantation were reviewed in Chapters 22 and 23.

The fibula free flap, which may be harvested as an osteomyocutaneous flap or a purely osseous flap, is an excellent recipient site for implants.[36–40] As much as 26 cm of the fibula can be harvested without affecting leg function. Patients who have osseointegrated implants placed in a fibula graft can reestablish near-normal mastication and speech.[36] However, stable implants that support fixed prostheses or removable overdentures can also be placed into iliac crest and scapula free flaps.[48–50] Implants placed into the native mandible have a documented lower failure rate than implantation into the maxilla or vascularized bone grafts.[51] Implant *survival*, however, does not translate into implant *success*, which is realized after successful prosthetic rehabilitation has been achieved.[52] Approximately three quarters of the implants that are placed in head and neck cancer patients can eventually be used as abutments for functional dental prostheses.[51]

Implants may be placed during or after the primary reconstructive procedure, but implantation must be delayed if a surgical stent will be required to optimize implant positioning and alignment.[5] Desirable prosthetic results require careful presurgical planning among the cancer surgeon, the implant surgeon, and the maxillofacial prosthodontist to ensure that the timing, location, and number of implants are optimized. In general, the prosthesis is fabricated so that it can be easily removed by the patient and allow for the maintenance of good oral hygiene. Most irradiated head and neck cancer patients are restored using removable prostheses. Implants can be restored with an overlying removable prosthesis using ball abutments and O-ring

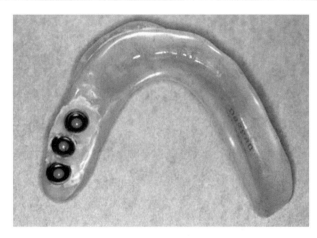

Figure 24–16 Tissue surface of mandibular implant-retained removable overdenture revealing O-ring attachments that snap on to ball-shaped implant abutments.

attachments that are embedded in the prosthesis (**Fig. 24–16**). Extracoronal resilient attachment (ERA) implant abutments have also been successfully used in fabricating implant-supported overdentures. This system employs short, vertically resilient abutments that may be used for patients who have trismus. Crowns and bridges can be retained on implant abutments through the use of a screw or by cementation to the abutments.

◆ Conclusion

Dental status has a persistent impact on quality of life in patients who have been successfully treated for head and neck cancer. Patients who become edentulous as a consequence of cancer treatment report more severe pain and score worse on validated measures that assess chewing, swallowing, speech, eating in public, and physical well-being.[53] Thus, rehabilitation with functional, aesthetic dental prostheses after cancer treatment is a critical component of patient management that focuses on improving their quality of life. Thoughtful collaboration among the maxillofacial prosthodontist, radiation oncologist, surgical oncologist, and implant surgeon optimizes the delivery and timing of dental care, ensures that critical abutment teeth are preserved and dental implants are strategically placed, and provides an opportunity to review intraoperative measures that will improve the quality of the ultimate prosthetic result. To achieve these goals, each member of the multidisciplinary team must have working knowledge of the principles of prosthetic rehabilitation and appreciate the potential adverse impact that a suboptimal prosthesis could have on the patient's functional, aesthetic, and emotional outcome.

References

1. King GE, Jacob RF, Martin JW. Oral and dental rehabilitation. In: Johns ME, ed. Complications in Otolaryngology–Head and Neck Surgery. Philadelphia: BC Decker, 1986:131

2. Blashchbe DP, Osborn AG. The mandible and teeth. In: Bergeron RT, Osborn AG, San PM, eds. Head and Neck Imaging. St. Louis: CV Mosby, 1984:279

3. Chambers MS, Toth BB, Martin JW, Fleming TJ, Lemon JC. Oral and dental management of the cancer patient: prevention and treatment of complications. Support Care Cancer 1995;3:168–175

4. Chambers MS, Lemon JC, Martin JW, Garden AS, Toth BB. Oral rehabilitation of patients with head and neck cancer. In: Myers EN, Suen JY, Myers JN, Hanna E, eds. Cancer of the Head and Neck. Philadelphia: WB Saunders, 2003

5. Martin JW, Lemon JC, Chambers MS. Surgical techniques to enhance prosthetic rehabilitation: oral and dental oncologic principles. In: Bailey BJ, ed. Head and Neck Surgery–Otolaryngology, 3rd ed. Philadelphia: Lippincott-Raven, 2001:1597–1606

6. Martin JW, Lemon JC, King GE. Maxillofacial restoration after tumor ablation. Clin Plast Surg 1994;21:87–95

7. Martin JW, Jacob RF, Larson DL, King GE. Surgical stents for the head and neck cancer patient. Head Neck Surg 1984;7:44–46

8. Lemon JC, Martin JW, Jacob RF. Prosthetic rehabilitation. In: Weber RS, Miller MJ, Goepfert H, eds. Basal and Squamous Cell Skin Cancers of the Head and Neck. Philadelphia: Williams & Wilkins, 1996:305–312

9. Martin JW, Lemon JC, King GE. Oral and facial restoration after reconstruction. In: Kroll S, ed. Reconstructive Plastic Surgery for Cancer. St. Louis: Mosby, 1996:130–138

10. Okay DJ, Genden E, Buchbinder D, Urken M. Prosthodontic guidelines for surgical reconstruction of the maxilla: a classification system of defects. J Prosthet Dent 2001;86:352–363

11. Carr AB, McGivney GP, Brown DT, eds. McCracken's Removable Partial Prosthodontics, 11th ed. St. Louis: Elsevier Mosby, 2005

12. Desjardins RP. Obturator prosthesis design for acquired maxillary defects. J Prosthet Dent 1978;39:424–435

13. Parr GR, Tharp GE, Rahn AO. Prosthodontic principles in the framework design of maxillary obturator prostheses. J Prosthet Dent 1989;62:205–212

14. Firtell DN, Grisius RJ. Retention of obturator-removable partial dentures: a comparison of buccal and lingual retention. J Prosthet Dent 1980;43:212–217

15. Martin JW, King GE. Framework retention for maxillary obturator prostheses. J Prosthet Dent 1984;51:669–672

16. King GE, Gay WD. Application of various removable partial denture design concepts to a maxillary obturator prosthesis. J Prosthet Dent 1979;41:316–318

17. Schwartzman B, Caputo A, Beumer J. Occlusal force transfer by removable partial denture designs for a radical maxillectomy. J Prosthet Dent 1985;54:397–403

18. Taylor TD, ed. Clinical Maxillofacial Prosthetics. Chicago: Quintessence, 2000

19. Brown KE. Peripheral consideration in improving obturator retention. J Prosthet Dent 1968;20:176–181

20. Carr AB, McGivney GP, Brown DT. Partially edentulous epidemiology, physiology, and terminology. In: McCracken's Removable Partial Prosthodontics, 11th ed. St. Louis: Elsevier Mosby, 2005:3–10

21. Gerngross PJ, Martin CD, Ball JD, et al. Period between completion of radiation therapy and prosthetic rehabilitation in edentulous patients: a retrospective study. J Prosthodont 2005;14:110–121

22. Aramany MA. Basic principles of obturator design for partially edentulous patients. Part I: classification. J Prosthet Dent 1978;40:554–557

23. Curtis TA, Beumer J. Restoration of acquired hard palate defects: etiology, disability, and rehabilitation. In: Beumer J, Curtis TA, Firtell DN, eds. Maxillofacial Rehabilitation: Prosthodontic and Surgical Considerations. St. Louis: CV Mosby Co,1979:188–243

24. Teichgraeber J, Larson DL, Castaneda O, Martin JW. Skin grafts in intraoral reconstruction. A new stenting method. Arch Otolaryngol 1984;110:463–467

25. Olsen KD, Meland NB, Ebersold MJ, Bartley GB, Garrity JA. Extensive defects of the sino-orbital region. Results with microvascular reconstruction. Arch Otolaryngol Head Neck Surg 1992;118:828–833

26. Kuriloff DB, Sullivan MJ. Revascularized tissue transfers in head and neck surgery. In: Bailey BJ, ed. Head and Neck Surgery Otolaryngology. Philadelphia: Lippincott-Raven, 1998:2345–2387

27. Martin JW, Austin JR, Chambers MS, Lemon JC, Toth BB. Postoperative care of the maxillectomy patient. ORL Head Neck Nurs 1994;12:15–20

28. Kornblith AB, Zlotolow IM, Gooen J, et al. Quality of life of maxillectomy patients using an obturator prosthesis. Head Neck 1996;18:323–334

29. Curtis TA, Beumer J. Restoration of acquired hard palate defects: etiology, disability, and rehabilitation. In: Beumer J, Curtis TA, Marunick MT, eds. Maxillofacial Rehabilitation: Prosthodontic and Surgical Considerations. St. Louis: Ishiyaku EroAmerica, 1996

30. Tomsett KL, Chambers MS, Martin JW, Gillenwater A, Lemon JC. A technique for the fabrication of an intermediate mandibular surgical stent securing a skin graft. J Prosthet Dent 2005;93:395–397

31. Schusterman MA, Reece GP, Miller MJ, Harris S. The osteocutaneous free fibula flap: is the skin paddle reliable? Plast Reconstr Surg 1992;90:787–793 discussion 794–788

32. Ioannides C, Fossion E, Boeckx W, Hermans B, Jacobs D. Surgical management of the osteoradionecrotic mandible with free vascularised composite flaps. J Craniomaxillofac Surg 1994;22:330–334

33. Lydiatt DD, Lydiatt WM, Hollins RR, Friedman A. Use of free fibula flap in patients with prior failed mandibular reconstruction. J Oral Maxillofac Surg 1998;56:444–446

34. Shaha AR, Cordeiro PG, Hidalgo DA, et al. Resection and immediate microvascular reconstruction in the management of osteoradionecrosis of the mandible. Head Neck 1997;19:406–411

35. Ang E, Black C, Irish J, et al. Reconstructive options in the treatment of osteoradionecrosis of the craniomaxillofacial skeleton. Br J Plast Surg 2003;56:92–99

36. Winslow CD, Wax MK. Tissue transfer: Fibula. Emedicine.com. August 28, 2003

37. Anthony JP, Rawnsley JD, Benhaim P, Ritter EF, Sadowsky SH, Singer MI. Donor leg morbidity and function after fibula free flap mandible reconstruction. Plast Reconstr Surg 1995;96:146–152

38. Disa JJ, Cordeiro PG. The current role of preoperative arteriography in free fibula flaps. Plast Reconstr Surg 1998;102:1083–1088

39. Hidalgo DA. Fibula free flap mandibular reconstruction. Clin Plast Surg 1994;21:25–35

40. Urken M, Cheney ML, Sullivan MJ. Fibula free flaps. In: Urken ML, ed. Atlas of Regional and Free Flaps for Head and Neck Reconstruction. New York: Raven Press, 1995

41. Godoy AJ, Perez DG, Lemon JC, Martin JW. Rehabilitation of a patient with limited oral opening following glossectomy. Int J Prosthodont 1991;4:70–74

42. Cantor R, Curtis TA. Prosthetic management of edentulous mandibulectomy patients. II. Clinical procedures. J Prosthet Dent 1971;25:546–555

43. Branemark PI, Zarb G, Albrektsson T. Tissue-integrated prostheses. In: Branemark PI, ed. Osseointegration in Clinical Dentistry. Chicago: Quintessence, 1985:1–50

44. Scortecci GM. Introduction to oral implantology in restorative dentistry. In: Scortecci GM, Misch CE, Benner KU, eds. Implants and Restorative Dentistry. New York: Martin Dunitz, 2001:1–25

45. Eckert SE, Desjardins RP. The impact of endosseous implants on maxillofacial prosthetics. In: Taylor TD, ed. Clinical Maxillofacial Prosthetics. Chicago: Quintessence, 2000:145–153

46. Lee MB. Implants. Webmaster@cincinnati-oralsurgery.com. April 2003

47. Astrand P, Engquist B, Dahlgren S, Engquist E, Feldmann H, Grondahl K. Astra Tech and Branemark System implants: a prospective 5-year comparative study: results after one year. Clin Implant Dent Relat Res 1999;1:17–26

48. Kovacs AF. Influence of the prosthetic restoration modality on bone loss around dental implants placed in vascularized iliac bone grafts for mandibular reconstruction. Otolaryngol Head Neck Surg 2000;123:598–602

49. Schultes G, Gaggl A, Karcher H. Stability of dental implants in microvascular osseous transplants. Plast Reconstr Surg 2002;109:916–921

50. Gurlek A, Miller MJ, Jacob RF, Lively JA, Schusterman MA. Functional results of dental restoration with osseointegrated implants after mandible reconstruction. Plast Reconstr Surg 1998;101:650–655

51. Shaw RJ, Sutton AF, Cawood JI, et al. Oral rehabilitation after treatment for head and neck malignancy. Head Neck 2005;27:459–470

52. Kovacs AF. The fate of osseointegrated implants in patients following oral cancer surgery and mandibular reconstruction. Head Neck 2000;22:111–119

53. Duke RL, Campbell BH, Indresano AT, et al. Dental status and quality of life in long-term head and neck cancer survivors. Laryngoscope 2005;115:678–683

25

Xerostomia and Mucositis

Mark S. Chambers,
Adam S. Garden,
Ellen F. Manzullo, and
Jack W. Martin

Oral complications following radiation therapy (RT) or chemotherapy can profoundly impact the head and neck cancer patient's quality of life (QOL). These complications arise directly from treatment-induced tissue injury, which results in acute and chronic sequelae. Xerostomia and mucositis are the most common clinical manifestations of tissue injury caused by nonsurgical therapy for oral cancer. An appreciation for the mechanism and type of injuries that cause these complications is critical so that appropriate preventive measures are implemented and cause-specific therapy can be administered. This chapter reviews the pathophysiologic and histopathologic alterations that are associated with treatment-induced xerostomia and mucositis, and discusses the prevention and management of these debilitating complications using the best available evidence from the peer-reviewed literature.

◆ Xerostomia

The paired major salivary glands (parotid, submandibular, and sublingual) have a basic anatomic structure composed of acini with a specialized row of myoepithelial cells and a ductal system. The acinar cells are the secretory end piece and are responsible for the initial transport of fluid into the glandular ductal system. The parotid gland consists of mainly serous acinar cells (highly radiosensitive), whereas the submandibular gland has both mixed mucous and serous cells. The sublingual gland has mainly mucinous cells (highly radioresistant). The ductal cells of each gland form a branching system that moves saliva into the

respective glandular duct within the oral cavity. Saliva is a complex bodily fluid composed of 94% water and an array of immunoglobulins, proteins, enzymes, and small organic molecules that help to protect, repair, and moisturize the oral cavity. The major salivary glands produce up to 90% of salivary secretions, with the average daily output of saliva in healthy humans being 1000 to 1500 mL.[1] The paired parotid glands produce the majority of stimulated saliva, whereas the submandibular glands contribute mainly to resting salivary flow. Salivary secretion may be decreased by several disease processes and other factors. Xerostomia has been estimated to affect 22 to 26% of the general population, but occurs more commonly in the elderly and patients with advanced cancer (29 to 77%).[2,3] Xerostomia has also been reported in association with some immunotherapies, chemotherapy, and RT involving the major salivary glands.[4–7]

In therapy for head and neck cancer, the appropriate daily and total radiation doses are based on tumor size and individual clinical situations. Typically, daily radiation doses are 1.8 to 2 Gy, with subclinical microscopic cancer requiring at least 50 Gy over a 5-week period: smaller lesions (T1), 60 to 66 Gy; intermediate lesions (T2), 66 to 70 Gy; and large tumors (T3–T4), more than 70 Gy.[8] RT frequently involves delivery of high doses to the salivary glands bilaterally, with radiation portals often including the parotid and submandibular glands, and, in some cases, a large proportion of minor salivary glands.[9,10] Clinically, xerostomia has been reported with as little as two or three doses of 2 Gy, although many changes occurring with less than 60 Gy are reversible.[11] However, doses greater than 30 Gy can cause permanent xerostomia.[9] The mean radiation doses that have been associated with permanent impairment of parotid gland saliva secretion are approximately 24 Gy for unstimulated and 26 Gy for stimulated saliva.[12]

The extent of glandular change is generally directly related to the dose of radiation to the salivary glands, with the most severe and irreversible forms of salivary dysfunction resulting from damage to or loss of salivary acinar cells.[11] However, the pathogenesis of radiation-induced xerostomia involves more than damage to the salivary glands. A lack of wetting medium reduces the ability of chemoreceptors on the tongue and palate to accept stimuli presented with foods or liquids, resulting in failure of the salivary response. The minimal and thickened mucinous saliva that is produced may form a barrier to dietary, thermal, and mechanical stimulation of the taste buds.

Methods for assessing radiation-induced xerostomia include clinical examination; subjective measures, such as patient self-report instruments and visual analogue scales; and objective measures, such as assessment of stimulated and unstimulated salivary flow rates.[13] The correlation between objective salivary flow measurements and subjective measurements, however, is somewhat weak.[14] Scoring systems that grade the severity of acute and late radiation-induced salivary hypofunction have been published by several organizations, including the Radiation Therapy Oncology Group (RTOG), the European Organization for Research and Treatment of Cancer (EORTC), and the National Cancer Institute (NCI) (**Tables 25–1 to 25–3**).[15,16]

Xerostomia is associated with an increased risk of "radiation caries," which results from an increased number of caries-forming bacteria in the oral cavity, low salivary pH with loss of buffering capacity, decreased mechanical flushing, and decreased production of salivary proteins, immunoglobulins (i.e., IgA, IgG), lysozymes, and peroxidases.[11] Xerostomia may result in mucositis; oral pain or discomfort; and difficulty with mastication, deglutition, and articulation. It is also associated with the development of dysgeusia, ageusia, soft tissue breakdown, bone loss, and chronic infection.[7,17] When not monitored and controlled, xerostomia may lead to accumulation of plaque and other debris on teeth and periodontal tissues.[13] Cariogenic plaque buildup on teeth may lead to tooth decay, gingivitis, and periodontitis (see Figs. 8–1 and 8–2 in Chapter 8). According to Berger and Kilroy,[18] elevated plaque matrix resulting from xerostomia may pose the greatest risk of osteoradionecrosis. Ill-fitting removable prostheses in patients with xerostomia that cause tissue irritation can compound mucositis and result in fenestration of supporting mucosa and posttreatment

osteoradionecrosis. In addition, recent evidence suggests a potential link between oral and dental disease and systemic illnesses, such as atherosclerosis, coronary heart disease, and cerebrovascular ischemia.[19]

Minimizing Xerostomia: Preemptive Interventions

Oral and Dental Care

To minimize the severity of xerostomia and oral complications, it is important to begin aggressive oral care before RT.[13] Appropriate nutritional intake, effective oral hygiene, and early detection of oral lesions are important pretreatment practices. Evaluation by a dental team experienced in oral oncology, ideally weeks in advance of therapy, is essential to determine oral health status, perform necessary dental and oral interventions, and to allow time for healing from any invasive procedures that are required. In particular, attention should be given to mucosal lesions, dental caries and endodontic disease, periodontal disease, ill-fitting dentures, orthodontic appliances, temporomandibular dysfunction, and salivary abnormalities. A stringent oral hygiene program is critical and should be continued before, during, and after therapy.

Radiation Therapy Protectants

Agents have been developed to ameliorate or eliminate toxicities associated with chemotherapy and RT.[20] Amifostine, an

Table 25–1 Radiation Therapy Oncology Group (RTOG) Scoring Criteria for Acute Radiation-Induced Salivary Gland Morbidity[15]

Grade	Criteria
0	No change over baseline
1	Mild dryness, slightly thickened saliva, and slightly altered or metallic taste
2	Moderate to complete dryness, thick sticky saliva, and markedly altered taste
3	Not defined for acute xerostomia
4	Acute salivary gland necrosis

Table 25–2 Radiation Therapy Oncology Group (RTOG)–European Organization for Research and Treatment of Cancer (EORTC) Scoring Criteria for Late Radiation-Induced Salivary Gland Morbidity[15]

Grade	Criteria
0	None
1	Slight dryness of mouth with good response to stimulation
2	Moderate dryness of mouth with poor response to stimulation
3	Complete dryness of mouth with no response to stimulation
4	Fibrosis

Table 25–3 National Cancer Institute Scoring Criteria for Xerostomia[16]

Grade	Criteria
0	None
1	Symptomatic (dry or thick saliva) without significant dietary alteration; unstimulated saliva flow >0.2 mL/min
2	Symptomatic and significant oral intake alteration (e.g., copious water, other lubricants, diet limited to purees and/or soft, moist foods); unstimulated saliva 0.1 to 0.2 mL/min
3	Symptoms leading to inability to adequately aliment orally; IV fluids, tube feedings, or total parenteral nutrition (TPN) indicated; unstimulated saliva <0.1 mL/min

agent studied for its selective protection of normal tissue from damage induced by radiation and chemotherapy, was approved by the U.S. Food and Drug Administration (FDA) as a cytoprotective agent with cisplatin-based chemotherapy for ovarian cancer and later for prevention of xerostomia in patients treated with RT for head and neck cancer.[21] This recommendation was based on the results of a phase III multi-institutional study reported by Brizel and colleagues.[22] Some concern has been expressed regarding the possibility that this agent could also protect tumor tissue from the effects of radiation, thereby reducing the biologically effective radiation dose to the tumor.[21] In an attempt to address this concern, a 2-year follow-up of the above-mentioned phase III trial was recently published, which documented no difference in local-regional control or survival between the amifostine group and the control group.[23]

Clinical practice guidelines of the American Society of Clinical Oncology, published in 1999, indicate that amifostine may be considered for use in patients who undergo fractionated RT in the head and neck region to decrease the incidence of acute and late xerostomia. The recommended dose of amifostine is 200 mg/m^2/d given as a slow intravenous infusion over 3 minutes, 15 to 30 minutes before each fraction of RT. Patients require close monitoring for side effects, including hypotension and nausea, and some patients may require antiemetics.[20] Investigations using a subcutaneous administration of amifostine are ongoing, as this form of administration may be more practical and may lower the toxicity of the drug.

Parotid Gland–Sparing Techniques

Recent efforts have focused on the use of conformal or other newer RT techniques to spare a portion of the major salivary glands.[9,24,25] Reddy and colleagues[26] investigated the use of parotid-sparing irradiation techniques in patients with cancer of the oral cavity, specifically a two-dimensional (2D) technique sparing at least one parotid gland versus bilateral opposed photon beams including both parotid glands.[26] Patients treated with the parotid-sparing technique were able to maintain nutritional intake and baseline body weight during and after irradiation. In contrast, those treated with a bilateral technique had poor nutritional intake and lost more than 10% of their body weight, which was not regained during the 2 years after treatment.

An emerging parotid-sparing technique, three-dimensional (3D) intensity-modulated radiation therapy (IMRT), involves the manipulation of beam intensity across each treatment field, providing a dose distribution that conforms more accurately to the 3D configuration of the target volume than conventional 3D conformal RT. This technique delivers a higher dose to the tumor target without increasing the dose to normal tissues, delivers a higher dose per fraction, and offers an improved physical and biologic therapeutic ratio.[27] Intensity-modulated radiation therapy can potentially deliver a lower dose of radiation to the parotid glands compared with conventional beam arrangements, and thus offers the greatest potential for patients with mucosal primary tumors that require bilateral neck irradiation.

A phase II study that evaluates the use of IMRT in combination with amifostine to augment salivary gland sparing has also been initiated.[28]

Other possible techniques in salvaging salivary tissue during RT include salivary gland transfer techniques and gene therapy.[29–35] Research is currently revealing promising results for both of these therapies.

Treating Xerostomia: Pharmacologic Options

Current therapies for the pharmacologic management of radiation-induced xerostomia include the use of prescription fluoride agents to maintain optimal oral hygiene, antimicrobials to prevent dental caries and oral infection, saliva substitutes to relieve dryness, and sialogogic agents to stimulate saliva production from remaining intact salivary gland tissues.[13,17,36] Proper oral care before, during, and after RT is essential, with use of topical 0.4% stannous fluoride gel once daily to minimize dental caries.[13] Oral antimicrobial agents may also be beneficial to prevent oral infection. Chlorhexidine gluconate, for example, provides broad-spectrum activity in vitro against gram-positive, gram-negative, and fungal pathogens, and binds well to oral surfaces (minimizing gastrointestinal absorption).[13] Saliva substitutes containing hydroxyethyl-, hydroxypropyl-, or carboxymethylcellulose may be beneficial as palliative agents to relieve the discomfort of xerostomia by temporarily wetting the oral mucosa.[37] Other new saliva substitutes (moisturizing gels) with enzymatic and protein components (i.e., glucose oxidase and lactoperoxidase), which present prospective antibacterial effectiveness and increased oral moisture, are under study.[13] The use of chewing gums made with noncariogenic sweeteners may help to stimulate saliva secretion and reduce oral mucosal friction.[38]

For patients with residual salivary gland function, cholinergic agonists may produce symptomatic improvement.[10] Pilocarpine is currently the only sialogogic agent approved by the FDA for radiation-induced xerostomia. Pilocarpine functions primarily as a muscarinic-cholinergic agonist with mild β-adrenergic activity. Muscarinic agonists in sufficient dosage can increase secretion of exocrine glands, such as salivary and sweat glands, and the tone of smooth muscle in the gastrointestinal and urinary tracts. Studies have shown oral pilocarpine to have efficacy in patients with Sjögren's syndrome, radiation-induced xerostomia, and opioid-induced xerostomia, as well as increasing salivary flow and restoring salivary composition in those with graft-versus-host disease due to allogeneic bone marrow transplantation.[4,11,37,39–43] Pilocarpine therapy has been shown to reduce the counts of the cariogenic bacterium *Streptococcus mutans* in xerostomic cancer patients.[44] Pilocarpine is contraindicated in patients with uncontrolled asthma, acute iritis, or narrow-angle glaucoma. It should be used with caution in patients with controlled asthma, chronic bronchitis, chronic obstructive pulmonary disease, or cardiovascular disease.[45]

Other cholinergic agents with sialogogic properties, such as cevimeline hydrochloride, may prove beneficial for cancer patients with xerostomia. Cevimeline is a newer and more selective muscarinic agonist with documented safety and efficacy in the treatment of xerostomia associated with Sjögren's syndrome, and has received FDA approval for that use.[46,47] Most recently, two multicenter double-blind trials demonstrated that cevimeline 30 to 45 mg administered three times per day increased mean unstimulated salivary flow in patients with xerostomia following RT for head and neck cancer.[48]

◆ Mucositis

The oral cavity, as the first part of the digestive tract, is the portal of entry and the site for mastication of food and contains the taste organs. The oral cavity is lined throughout by its mucous membrane, which is composed of two layers: the surface epithelium and the lamina propria.[49] The epithelium consists of several layers of cells that flatten as they approach the surface. Regeneration of epithelial cells, lost at the surface, occurs by mitotic division of cells in the deeper layers.[13,49] A basement membrane separates the lamina propria from the stratified squamous epithelium. The mucous membrane is attached to the underlying structures by a layer of connective tissue, the submucosa, which varies in thickness and density. The morphologic structure of the mucous membrane varies in different areas of the oral cavity in accordance with the functions of specific zones and the mechanical influences that bear on them, and these morphologic differences impact the sequelae that develop following treatment with chemotherapy or RT.[13,49]

Oral mucositis, the most common acute complication of RT and chemotherapy, affects the quality of life of cancer patients by causing pain and impaired mastication, deglutition, and speech. The symptomatology associated with mucositis can also lead to disruptions in treatment, which may affect ultimate disease outcomes.[50]

Effects of Radiation Therapy on Oral Mucosa

Therapeutic administration of ionizing radiation to the head and neck produces several oral changes, including mucosal thinning, salivary gland atrophy and vascular fibrosis, and damage to the taste buds. These complications are generally of one of two types: acute (e.g., treatment-related mucositis or infectious stomatitis) or long-term (e.g., xerostomia, dental decay, trismus, hypovascularity, and osteoradionecrosis). Clinically, the severity of the morbidity is related to radiation dose, fractionation regimen and length of therapy, volume of tissue treated, and age of the patient when treated.[51]

Mucositis is the acute clinical manifestation of radiation toxicity to the rapidly proliferating cells in the basal regions of the epithelium.[52] Decreased cell regeneration leads to epithelial atrophy and mucosal thinning. All intraoral sites may be affected, although nonkeratinized surfaces are most severely affected. Erythema is the initial manifestation, followed by the development of white desquamative patches that are painful on contact. Epithelial sloughing and fibrinous exudate lead to the formation of a pseudomembrane and ulceration. Epithelial cell loss results

in the exposure of the richly innervated underlying connective tissue stroma, which contributes to the pain associated with severe mucositis.[52] The severity of mucositis induced by RT depends on several factors, including the administered dose, the dose fraction, the volume of tissue radiated, type of radiation given, and administration of a concomitant boost.[52] Other factors such as smoking, over-the-counter mouthwashes, collagen vascular disease, and HIV infection may contribute to the severity of mucositis.[52,53] Mucosal healing occurs, on average, 3 to 4 weeks after completion of conventionally fractionated RT.

In contrast, cancer chemotherapeutic drugs are cytotoxic, and their use often directly and adversely affects the rapidly replicating oral mucosa. This direct effect results in thinning, denudation, and ulceration of the buccal mucosa, tongue, gingivae, and pharynx. The severity of the mucositis varies with the type and dose of chemotherapeutic agents administered, the patient's ability to tolerate the drug, and the status of the oral environment (i.e., salivary function, oral hygiene, presence of caries).[54] Many drugs, including analgesics, antidepressants, antihypertensives, and antihistamines, that cause dry mouth can intensify the degree of mucositis through their anticholinergic or antiadrenergic properties.

Effects of Chemotherapy on Oral Mucosa

Mucositis denotes the cytotoxic reaction of the oral mucosal tissues to chemotherapy. The contribution of other factors such as infection, trauma, and factitious injury, must be considered before grading such a mucosal effect. Mucosal reactions that are mistakenly attributed to chemotherapy can cause effective therapy to be delayed, chemotherapy dosage to be reduced, or chemotherapy/RT to be completely discontinued. Thus, oral care must include microorganism assays by culture to evaluate the incidence of mucositis versus infection.[51,55] The patient must report any mucosal changes or increased sensitivity. Mucosal toxicity depends on the cytotoxic agent, therapeutic regimen, duration of treatment and dose intensity, intercurrent illnesses, concomitant medications, and previous treatment.[56] The risk of developing mucositis increases with the number of chemotherapeutic cycles. The most pronounced mucosal effects are exhibited by drugs affecting DNA synthesis (e.g., 5-fluorouracil, methotrexate, cytarabine).[13,56]

In general, mucositis begins as erythema of the nonkeratinized mucosa accompanied by increased sensitivity, which is a result of the thinning of the protective lining that follows decreased replication of the oral epithelium.[13,55] The mucositis can become local, as in the case of irradiated oral tissues, or diffuse, as in the case of mucosal denudation following chemotherapy, especially in areas where mucosal surfaces continually rub against another surface. In chemotherapy, direct stomatotoxicity is caused by the treatment-induced reduction in basal cell renewal resulting in mucosal atrophy, similar to that induced by RT.[52] The mucosal atrophy is noted within 5 to 7 days following administration of a cytotoxic drug.[53] The most consistent symptom of mucositis is extreme pain. Examination usually demonstrates erythema and ulceration of some or all mucosal surfaces.

Ulcerative areas may appear grayish white with central areas of necrosis. If the patient's bone marrow is relatively unaffected by the chemotherapy, the mucositis is self-limiting and tends to heal spontaneously in approximately 14 days or longer, according to the chemotherapy cycle.[53]

Considerable interpatient variability exists in the tolerance to chemotherapy regimens and the development of mucositis. Some chemotherapy agents, including antimetabolites, antibiotics, and, to a lesser degree, alkylating agents and vinca alkaloids, will produce mucositis in a dose- and duration-dependent manner. However, any agent that is given at an intensified dose or of sufficient duration will produce direct or secondary mucosal toxicities that will be dose-limiting.[56,57] Treatment factors that influence the frequency and severity of oral mucositis induced by chemotherapy include the chemotherapeutic agent used, dosage, delivery schedule, and combination with RT.[52] Thus, it is exceedingly important to be cognizant of the relationship between the time of chemotherapy administration and the development of any mucosal reactions. One would expect mucosal toxicity (i.e., mucositis) to occur soon after the initiation of chemotherapy. An exception to this is the development of mucosal herpes simplex virus infection that can be seen early in the chemotherapy cycle as confirmed by microbiologic assessment. Such an occurrence may be misdiagnosed as mucositis and may result in failure to treat the underlying infectious process. Furthermore, mucosal reactions that occur in association with a hematology nadir could be related to infectious stomatitis. Culturing is critical at this point to differentiate chemotherapy-induced mucosal toxicity from mucosal neutropenic infectious complications caused by bacterial, fungal, or viral micro-organisms.

Oral complications in cancer patients receiving chemotherapy can potentially lead to systemic involvement, so infections must be recognized, properly diagnosed, and treated quickly and aggressively.[53] In fact, the mouth is the most frequently documented source of sepsis in the granulocytopenic cancer patient.[53,58,59] The role that routine pretreatment oral examination and dental treatment play in minimizing the development of chemotherapy-associated mucositis cannot be overemphasized.[51,55,57]

Pathophysiology and Grading

Analyses of mucositis have been largely based on observational data. Although there have been suggestions as to how mucositis develops, the pathophysiology of this condition is, for the most part, undefined.[60] Although different potential therapeutic agents sometimes modify outcome, they do so in a way that is not always reproducible or consistent.[56,60] Sonis et al[60] described a logical hypothesis as to the mechanisms by which drug-induced mucositis develops and heals, based on animal and clinical data. They reported that mucositis is a complex biologic process that occurs in four successive phases: (1) inflammatory/vascular, (2) epithelial, (3) ulcerative/infective, and (4) healing. Each phase is interdependent and is the consequence of a series of actions mediated by cytokines, the direct effect of the chemotherapeutic drug on the epithelium, the oral bacterial flora, and the status of the patient's bone marrow.[60] As demonstrated

by observations in models of graft-versus-host disease, injury to host tissues elicited by RT or chemotherapy is capable of causing the release of cytokines from the epithelium and connective tissues. The final phase of mucositis is related to healing and consists of a renewal of epithelial proliferation and differentiation, normalization of the peripheral white blood cell count, and reestablishment of the local microbial flora.[60]

An important effect of treatment-related toxicity is the loss of rapidly proliferating epithelial cells in the oral cavity, gut, and the bone marrow. Within the oral cavity, the loss of these cells leads to mucosal atrophy, necrosis, and ulceration. Accurate and reproducible evaluation of this mucosal toxicity is important to monitor patient toxicity during therapy, to document the toxicity of conventional therapy, and to critically assess the effects of alternative therapies.[52] Several oral toxicity scoring systems have been described, although scant data exist regarding their inter- and intra-user reliability [e.g., World Health Organization (**Table 25–4**), NCI common toxicity criteria (CTC) (**Table 25–5**), RTOG].[13,16,52,54,61,62] Despite the desire for a universally accepted, validated, and reliable scoring scheme to assess oral mucositis and critically appraise the effects of new cancer treatment modalities, diverse treatments and differing assessment end points make the formulation of such a scale difficult.[52] A sensitive, objective, and reproducible scoring system that can be widely applied is greatly needed. One system, the Oral Mucositis Assessment Scale (OMAS), has been evaluated in a multicenter trial for validation purposes. It grades the ulceration and pseudomembranous reaction as well as erythema.[63]

Treatment

There is no universally accepted standard therapy for the prophylaxis or treatment of cancer therapy-induced oral mucositis. Numerous local and systemic approaches to the treatment of mucositis are available.[56] The range of treatments that have been recommended for mucositis includes topical antimicrobials, marrow-stimulating cytokines, vitamins, inflammatory modifiers, palliative rinses, amino acid supplements, cryotherapy, and laser treatment.[52,60] In addition, hygiene rinses, containing antidotal concoctions of antibiotics, antifungals, and narcotic analgesics in a coating suspension, are administered for treatment palliation.[63–66] Other agents such as leucovorin, vitamins, cryotherapy, and growth factors have been tried for the prevention of chemotherapy-induced mucositis.[67–71] To date, none of the aforementioned items have shown a significant impact. A recent phase III trial that evaluated iseganan

Table 25–4   World Health Organization (WHO) Mucositis Scale[61]

Grade	Clinical Features
0	—
1	Soreness/erythema
2	Erythema, ulcers but able to eat solids
3	Ulcers but requires liquid diet
4	Oral alimentation not possible

Table 25–5 National Cancer Institute Scoring Criteria for Mucositis[16]

Grade	Clinical Examination	Functional/Symptomatic
1	Erythema of the mucosa	Minimal symptoms, normal diet; minimal symptoms but not interfering with function
2	Patchy ulcerations or pseudomembranes	Symptomatic but can eat and swallow modified diet; respiratory symptoms interfering with function but not interfering with activities of daily living (ADL)
3	Confluent ulcerations or pseudomembranes; bleeding with minor trauma	Symptomatic and unable to adequately aliment or hydrate orally; respiratory symptoms interfering with ADL
4	Tissue necrosis; significant spontaneous bleeding, life-threatening consequences	Symptoms associated with life-threatening consequences
5	Death	Death

hydrochloride (HCl), a synthetic peptide with broad-spectrum antimicrobial activity, failed to document a reduced risk of developing RT-induced ulcerative oral mucositis.[72] Some evidence suggests that locally applied cytoprotectants (e.g., allopurinol, glutamine, prostaglandin E_2, and vitamin E) and hematopoietic growth factors [e.g., granulocyte-macrophage colony-stimulating factor (GM-CSF), granulocyte colony-stimulating factor (G-CSF)] can reduce the severity and incidence of mucositis.[56] Other promising approaches include systemically administered cytoprotectants (e.g., amifostine, glutamine, azelastine, uridine) that have demonstrated a marked reduction of mucositis as compared with controls in randomized, controlled trials.[56]

Comprehensive care should be focused on the prevention of complications by eliminating known and predictable factors that initiate pathology and by promoting good hygiene and nutrition, thereby minimizing the risks of infection, bleeding, and pain. Prophylaxis of mucositis is essential to alleviate symptoms and avoid secondary complications.[13,55] To avoid such sequelae, the patient should be advised of the importance of brushing with a soft toothbrush and a mild dentifrice, keeping the oral mucosa moist and clean, and selecting and maintaining an appropriate diet during the period following chemotherapy. The fear that brushing will increase the chances of oral complications has always been a concern for practitioners. Yet the benefits of brushing outweigh the drawbacks. Even in healthy mouths, a certain degree of bacteremia can be associated with normal function (e.g., eating).[73] However, any threat of persistent bacteremia in a compromised host is cause for concern.[74–76] Thus, the benefits of controlling bacteremia-promoting plaque through appropriate hygiene—swishing fluids is a poor substitute for thorough oral care by brushing—far exceeds the drawback of a potential increase in oral complications. Indeed, with careful oral care that includes brushing, chemotherapy-induced sequelae can be kept to a minimum or even eradicated.

Compliance with oral care procedures is the key to maintaining the relative health of the mucosal tissues and the effectiveness of locally applied topical oral agents. Such topical medications should be nonirritating and nondehydrating.

Mouth rinses are frequently recommended as therapy for mucositis in both dentate and edentulous patients. These rinses cleanse the mouth, hydrate the mucosa, and treat the mucositis. Any oral medications that contain alcohol, thymol, eugenol, or phenol, which are part of most commercial mouthwashes, should be avoided because they can irritate and desiccate inflamed, compromised xerostomic tissues.[77] Such rinses can lead to further compromise of the mucosa, prolonging the healing of the oral wounds. Rinsing with bland preparations such as sodium bicarbonate solution (1 tsp of sodium bicarbonate in 10 oz of water) alkalinizes the oral cavity environment and adequately cleanses the tissues of debris, bacteria, and mucus.[13,57]

Topical coating agents can be most effective in promoting mucosal wound healing, yet the sequence of delivery to the compromised oral soft tissues is important.[13,55] Initially, the tissue must be cleansed of mucoid debris before the application of the agents. If decontamination is necessary, a troche or lozenge form of the agent should be taken, as it provides a longer and more constant application of the medicine to the tissue.[51,56] An oral liquid suspension can be used if the mouth is dry, even though the liquid will be in contact with the tissue and any organisms for only a limited time. All prostheses are to be removed during the oral-mucosal treatment.[13] If a mucosal coating agent is to be used, it must be used last so as not to neutralize the effects of the topical antimicrobial agents. Thirty minutes should elapse between the applications of the agents. In providing the treatment described above, an oral-care schedule for patients receiving chemotherapy can be very useful to the practitioner. Again, it must be emphasized that appropriate assessment and therapy depends on constant vigilance of oral mucosal wounds with appropriate cultures.

Finally, topical anesthetics in addition to systemic analgesia therapy may be necessary for reduction of upper aerodigestive tract pain related to dysphagia and odynophagia.[13,56] Compounding a solution with a mucoprotectant, diphenhydramine, and lidocaine can be most beneficial when all other topical medications have had no benefit. The suppressive effect on the gag-cough reflex leading to possible aspiration must be explained to the patient before using such topical anesthetic solutions.

◆ Conclusion

Xerostomia and mucositis are common, potentially serious, complications of treatment for oral cancer that mandate the need to minimize their incidence and reduce their severity. Consequently, careful evaluation of the oral cavity should be routinely performed prior to treatment for oral cancer, and meticulous oral hygiene must be emphasized after completion of treatment. Preventing and treating the oral complications of cancer are important responsibilities of the practitioner, and anticipating primary and secondary mucosal insults and promptly recognizing oral complications can decrease the incidence of complications or ameliorate their morbid side effects. Rigorous evaluation of potential therapeutic modalities through clinical trials is essential to establish evidence-based therapeutic approaches for the management of these morbid complications.

References

1. Seikaly H, Jha N, McGaw T, Coulter L, Liu R, Oldring D. Submandibular gland transfer: a new method of preventing radiation-induced xerostomia. Laryngoscope 2001;111:347–352

2. Davies AN, Broadley K, Beighton D. Xerostomia in patients with advanced cancer. J Pain Symptom Manage 2001;22:820–825

3. Narhi TO. Prevalence of subjective feelings of dry mouth in the elderly. J Dent Res 1994;73:20–25

4. Nagler RM, Gez E, Rubinov R, et al. The effect of low-dose interleukin-2-based immunotherapy on salivary function and composition in patients with metastatic renal cell carcinoma. Arch Oral Biol 2001;46:487–493

5. Sreebny LM, Valdini A, Yu A. Xerostomia. Part II: relationship to nonoral symptoms, drugs, and diseases. Oral Surg Oral Med Oral Pathol 1989;68:419–427

6. Kies MS, Haraf DJ, Rosen F, et al. Concomitant infusional paclitaxel and fluorouracil, oral hydroxyurea, and hyperfractionated radiation for locally advanced squamous head and neck cancer. J Clin Oncol 2001;19:1961–1969

7. Logemann JA, Smith CH, Pauloski BR, et al. Effects of xerostomia on perception and performance of swallow function. Head Neck 2001;23:317–321

8. Shaha AR, Patel S, Shasha D, Harrison LB. Head and neck cancer. In: Lenhard REJ, Osteen RT, Gansler T, eds. Clinical Oncology. Atlanta, GA: American Cancer Society, 2001:297–330

9. Eisbruch A, Kim HM, Terrell JE, Marsh LH, Dawson LA, Ship JA. Xerostomia and its predictors following parotid-sparing irradiation of head-and-neck cancer. Int J Radiat Oncol Biol Phys 2001;50:695–704

10. Jellema AP, Langendijk H, Bergenhenegouwen L, et al. The efficacy of Xialine in patients with xerostomia resulting from radiotherapy for head and neck cancer: a pilot-study. Radiother Oncol 2001; 59:157–160

11. Leek H, Albertsson M. Pilocarpine treatment of xerostomia in head and neck patients. Micron 2002;33:153–155

12. Eisbruch A, Ten Haken RK, Kim HM. Dose, volume, and function relationships in parotid salivary glands following conformal and intensity-modulated irradiation of head and neck cancer. Int J Radiat Oncol Biol Phys 1999;45:577–587

13. Chambers MS, Toth BB, Martin JW, Fleming TJ, Lemon JC. Oral and dental management of the cancer patient: prevention and treatment of complications. Support Care Cancer 1995;3:168–175

14. Fox PC, Busch KA, Baum BJ. Subjective reports of xerostomia and objective measures of salivary gland performance. J Am Dent Assoc 1987;115:581–584

15. Cox JD, Stetz J, Pajak TF. Toxicity criteria of the Radiation Therapy Oncology Group (RTOG) and the European Organization for Research and Treatment of Cancer (EORTC). Int J Radiat Oncol Biol Phys 1995;31:1341–1346

16. National Cancer Institute. Common Terminology Criteria for Adverse Events (CTCAE) v3.0. http://www.fda.gov/cder/cancer/toxicity frame.htm. Accessed February 14, 2006.

17. Criswell MA, Sinha CK. Hyperthermic, supersaturated humidification in the treatment of xerostomia. Laryngoscope 2001;111:992–996

18. Berger AM, Kilroy TJ. Oral complications of cancer therapy. In: Berger AM, Portenoy RK, Weissman DE, eds. Principles and Practice of Supportive Oncology. Philadelphia: Lippincott-Raven, 1998:223–236

19. Slavkin HC, Baum BJ. Relationship of dental and oral pathology to systemic illness. JAMA 2000;284:1215–1217

20. Hensley ML, Schuchter LM, Lindley C, et al. American Society of Clinical Oncology clinical practice guidelines for the use of chemotherapy and radiotherapy protectants. J Clin Oncol 1999;17:3333–3355

21. Lindegaard JC, Grau C. Has the outlook improved for amifostine as a clinical radioprotector? Radiother Oncol 2000;57:113–118

22. Brizel DM, Wasserman TH, Henke M, et al. Phase III randomized trial of amifostine as a radioprotector in head and neck cancer. J Clin Oncol 2000;18:3339–3345

23. Wasserman TH, Brizel D, Henke M, et al. Influence of intravenous amifostine on xerostomia, tumor control, and survival after radiotherapy for head-and-neck cancer: 2-year follow-up of a prospective, randomized, phase III trial. Int J Radiat Oncol Biol Phys 2005;63:985–990

24. Chao KS, Deasy JO, Markman J, et al. A prospective study of salivary function sparing in patients with head-and-neck cancers receiving intensity-modulated or three-dimensional radiation therapy: initial results. Int J Radiat Oncol Biol Phys 2001;49:907–916

25. Chao KS, Majhail N, Huang CJ, et al. Intensity-modulated radiation therapy reduces late salivary toxicity without compromising tumor control in patients with oropharyngeal carcinoma: a comparison with conventional techniques. Radiother Oncol 2001;61:275–280

26. Reddy SP, Leman CR, Marks JE, Emami B. Parotid-sparing irradiation for cancer of the oral cavity: maintenance of oral nutrition and body weight by preserving parotid function. Am J Clin Oncol 2001; 24:341–346

27. Webb S. IMRT: general considerations. In: Webb S, ed. Intensity-Modulated Radiation Therapy. Philadelphia: Institute of Physics Publishing, 2001:1–34

28. Rosenthal DI, Chambers MS, Weber RS, Eisbruch A. A phase II study to assess the efficacy of amifostine for submandibular/sublingual salivary sparing during the treatment of head and neck cancer with intensity modulated radiation therapy for parotid salivary sparing. Semin Oncol 2004;31:25–28

29. Spiegel JH, Deschler DG, Cheney ML. Microvascular transplantation and replantation of the rabbit submandibular gland. Arch Otolaryngol Head Neck Surg 2001;127:991–996

30. Spiegel JH, Zhang F, Levin DE, Singer MI, Buncke HJ. Microvascular transplantation of the rat submandibular gland. Plast Reconstr Surg 2000;106:1326–1335

31. Greer JE, Eltorky M, Robbins KT. A feasibility study of salivary gland autograft transplantation for xerostomia. Head Neck 2000;22:241–246

32. Nagler RM, Baum BJ. Prophylactic treatment reduces the severity of xerostomia following radiation therapy for oral cavity cancer. Arch Otolaryngol Head Neck Surg 2003;129:247–250

33. Delporte C, O'Connell BC, He X, et al. Increased fluid secretion after adenoviral-mediated transfer of the aquaporin-1 cDNA to irradiated rat salivary glands. Proc Natl Acad Sci U S A 1997;94:3268–3273

34. Epperly MW, Gretton JA, DeFilippi SJ, et al. Modulation of radiation-induced cytokine elevation associated with esophagitis and esophageal stricture by manganese superoxide dismutase-plasmid/liposome (SOD2-PL) gene therapy. Radiat Res 2001;155 (1 pt 1):2–14

35. Chambers MS. Clinical commentary on prophylactic treatment of radiation-induced xerostomia. Arch Otolaryngol Head Neck Surg 2003;129:251–252

36. Epstein JB, Robertson M, Emerton S, Phillips N, Stevenson-Moore P. Quality of life and oral function in patients treated with radiation therapy for head and neck cancer. Head Neck 2001;23:389–398

37. LeVeque FG, Montgomery M, Potter D, et al. A multicenter, randomized, double-blind, placebo-controlled, dose-titration study of oral pilocarpine for treatment of radiation-induced xerostomia in head and neck cancer patients. J Clin Oncol 1993;11:1124–1131

38. Olsson H, Spak CJ, Axell T. The effect of a chewing gum on salivary secretion, oral mucosal friction, and the feeling of dry mouth in xerostomic patients. Acta Odontol Scand 1991;49:273–279

39. Mercadante S, Calderone L, Villari P, et al. The use of pilocarpine in opioid-induced xerostomia. Palliat Med 2000;14:529–531

40. Fox PC, van der Ven PF, Baum BJ, Mandel ID. Pilocarpine for the treatment of xerostomia associated with salivary gland dysfunction. Oral Surg Oral Med Oral Pathol 1986;61:243–248

41. Chambers MS, Toth BB, Payne R, et al. Mutans streptococci and salivary flow rates in cancer patients attending a pain clinic [abstract]. J Dent Res 1997;76:358

42. Chambers MS, Martin C, Toth BB, et al. Assessment of functional improvement in cancer patients with oral pilocarpine as treatment for analgensia-induced xerostomia [abstract]. Support Care Cancer 1997;5:164

43. Chambers MS, Toth BB, Martin C, et al. Assessment of salivary flow improvement in cancer patients with oral pilocarpine as treatment for analgesia-induced xerostomia [abstract]. J Clin Oncol 1997;16:50a

44. Chambers MS, Keene HJ, Toth BB, et al. Mutans streptococci in xerostomic cancer patients after pilocarpine therapy: a pilot study. Oral Surg Oral Med Oral Pathol 2005;99:180–184

45. Wiseman LR, Faulds D. Oral pilocarpine: a review of its pharmacological properties and clinical potential in xerostomia. Drugs 1995;49:143–155

46. Atkinson JC, Baum BJ. Salivary enhancement: current status and future therapies. J Dent Educ 2001;65:1096–1101

47. al-Hashimi I. The management of Sjogren's syndrome in dental practice. J Am Dent Assoc 2001;132:1409–1417; quiz 1460–1401

48. Chambers MS, Posner MR, Jones CU, Weber RS, Vitti R. Two phase III clinical studies of cevimeline for post-radiation xerostomia in patients with head and neck cancer. Presented at the American Society of Clinical Oncology (ASCO), Orlando, FL, 2005

49. Orban B, Sicher H. The Oral Mucous Membrane. In: Orban B, ed. Oral Histology and Embryology. St. Louis: CV Mosby, 1953:211–262

50. Scully C, Epstein J, Sonis ST. Oral mucositis: a challenging complication of radiotherapy, chemotherapy, and radiochemotherapy: part 1, pathogenesis and prophylaxis of mucositis. Head Neck 2003;25:1057–1070

51. Toth BB, Martin JW, Fleming TJ. Oral and dental care associated with cancer therapy. Cancer Bull 1991;43:397–402

52. Parulekar W, Mackenzie R, Bjarnason G, Jordan RC. Scoring oral mucositis. Oral Oncol 1998;34:63–71

53. Sonis ST, Fazio RC, Fang L. Principles and Practice of Oral Medicine. Philadelphia: WB Saunders, 1984

54. Chambers MS. Xerostomia and its role in mucositis: complications and management. Paper presented at the Ninth International MASCC Symposium [abstract], 1997

55. Toth BB, Frame RT. Dental oncology: the management of disease and treatment-related oral/dental complications associated with chemotherapy. Curr Probl Cancer 1983;7:7–35

56. Kostler WJ, Hejna M, Wenzel C, Zielinski CC. Oral mucositis complicating chemotherapy and/or radiotherapy: options for prevention and treatment. CA Cancer J Clin 2001;51:290–315

57. Toth BB, Martin JW, Fleming TJ. Oral complications associated with cancer therapy. An M. D. Anderson Cancer Center experience. J Clin Periodontol 1990;17(7 pt 2):508–515

58. Bergmann OJ. Oral infections and septicemia in immunocompromised patients with hematologic malignancies. J Clin Microbiol 1988;26:2105–2109

59. Greenberg MS, Cohen SG, McKitrick JC, Cassileth PA. The oral floor as a source of septicemia in patients with acute leukemia. Oral Surg Oral Med Oral Pathol 1982;53:32–36

60. Sonis ST. Mucositis as a biological process: a new hypothesis for the development of chemotherapy-induced stomatotoxicity. Oral Oncol 1998;34:39–43

61. WHO Handbook of Reporting the Results of Cancer Treatment. Albany, NY: WHO Offset Publications, Geneva, 1979

62. Cancer Therapy Evaluation Program. Common Toxicity Criteria, 1998

63. Sonis ST, Eilers JP, Epstein JB, et al. Validation of a new scoring system for the assessment of clinical trial research of oral mucositis induced by radiation or chemotherapy. Mucositis Study Group. Cancer 1999;85:2103–2113

64. LeVeque FG, Parzuchowski JB, Farinacci GC, et al. Clinical evaluation of MGI 209, an anesthetic, film-forming agent for relief from painful oral ulcers associated with chemotherapy. J Clin Oncol 1992;10:1963–1968

65. Pfeiffer P, Madsen EL, Hansen O, May O. Effect of prophylactic sucralfate suspension on stomatitis induced by cancer chemotherapy. A randomized, double-blind cross-over study. Acta Oncol 1990;29:171–173

66. Epstein J, Ransier A, Lunn R, Spinelli J. Enhancing the effect of oral hygiene with the use of a foam brush with chlorhexidine. Oral Surg Oral Med Oral Pathol 1994;77:242–247

67. Loprinzi CL, Cianflone SG, Dose AM, et al. A controlled evaluation of an allopurinol mouthwash as prophylaxis against 5-fluorouracil-induced stomatitis. Cancer 1990;65:1879–1882

68. Wadleigh RG, Redman RS, Graham ML, Krasnow SH, Anderson A, Cohen MH. Vitamin E in the treatment of chemotherapy-induced mucositis. Am J Med 1992;92:481–484

69. Mills EE. The modifying effect of beta-carotene on radiation and chemotherapy induced oral mucositis. Br J Cancer 1988;57:416–417

70. Bleyer WA. New vistas for leucovorin in cancer chemotherapy. Cancer 1989;63(6 suppl):995–1007

71. Gordon B, Spadinger A, Hodges E, Ruby E, Stanley R, Coccia P. Effect of granulocyte-macrophage colony-stimulating factor on oral mucositis after hematopoietic stem-cell transplantation. J Clin Oncol 1994;12:1917–1922

72. Trotti A, Garden AS, Warde P, et al. A multinational, randomized phase III trial of iseganan HCl oral solution for reducing the severity of oral mucositis in patients receiving radiotherapy for head-and-neck malignancy. Int J Radiat Oncol Biol Phys 2004;58:674–681

73. Everett ED, Hirschmann JV. Transient bacteremia and endocarditis prophylaxis. A review. Medicine (Baltimore) 1977;56:61–77

74. Sickles EA, Greene WH, Wiernik PH. Clinical presentation of infection in granulocytopenic patients. Arch Intern Med 1975;135:715–719

75. Pizzo PA. Management of fever in patients with cancer and treatment-induced neutropenia. N Engl J Med 1993;328:1323–1332

76. Hickey AJ, Toth BB, Lindquist SB. Effect of intravenous hyperalimentation and oral care on the development of oral stomatitis during cancer chemotherapy. J Prosthet Dent 1982;47:188–193

77. Kaminsky SB, Gillette WB, O'Leary TJ. Sodium absorption associated with oral hygiene procedures. J Am Dent Assoc 1987;114:644–646

26

Osteoradionecrosis

Mark S. Chambers,

Peter J. Gerngross,

Caroline E. Fife,

Jack W. Martin,

John W. Werning,

William Mendenhall, and

Adam S. Garden

Osteoradionecrosis (ORN) is one of the most serious late complications of radiation therapy (RT) in the head and neck region. Patients who are afflicted with ORN frequently suffer from severe chronic pain, nonhealing intraoral wounds that impair masticatory function and prevent the use of dentures, orocutaneous fistulas that persistently drain, and pathologic fracture. As a consequence, patients who suffer from these sequelae are subjected to costly, time-consuming treatment that has limited proven efficacy. Unfortunately, few well-designed prospective research investigations have been conducted in this area, and widely accepted evidence-based guidelines for the diagnosis, prevention, and management of ORN have not been established. This chapter reviews our present understanding of osteoradionecrosis, and highlights the controversies that will only be resolved by the performance of insightfully designed clinical trials.

◆ Definition

There is no universally accepted definition for ORN, and several clinical definitions have been proposed in the peer-reviewed literature.[1] ORN can be defined as a condition in which irradiated, devitalized bone becomes exposed through a wound in the overlying mucosa or skin that is not due to tumor recurrence and that persists without healing for 3 to 6 months.[2] Marx and Johnson[3] in 1987 defined ORN as "an exposure of irradiated bone which fails to heal without intervention." However, some authors contend that ORN can exist in the presence of intact mucosa, whereas others have suggested that ORN can heal spontaneously.[4,5] This lack of consensus regarding the definition of ORN prevents accurate characterization of the incidence and types of ORN, and impairs our ability to evaluate responses to treatment using standardized criteria.

◆ Incidence and Risk Factors

The published incidence of ORN following irradiation of the maxilla or mandible ranges from 2 to 30%.[4,6–9] A better estimation of the risk of developing ORN, however, may be provided by evaluating the predisposing factors for ORN that have been established.

Irradiation of the Mandible

The overwhelming majority of oral cavity ORN involves the mandible. During RT for oral cancer and oropharyngeal cancer, the mandible is more commonly located within the field of irradiation than the maxilla.[10–12] However, the reported incidence of maxillary ORN is only 2.7% following RT for nasopharyngeal carcinoma that includes the maxilla within the field of irradiation, so other factors must be involved that place the mandible at particularly high risk.[7] Differences in the blood supply and anatomic structure of the mandible and maxilla are believed to account for this disparity in predilection. For example, histopathologic studies have documented radiation-induced obliteration of the inferior alveolar artery, which is the primary vascular supplier of the mandibular body, where most cases of ORN arise.[10,13]

Radiation Therapy

The mode of RT that is administered is an established risk factor for ORN. Brachytherapy has typically been associated with a higher incidence of ORN than external beam RT, but most cases of ORN that result from external beam RT tend to be more severe.[14] ORN develops in about 8.5 to 10% of patients treated with brachytherapy.[15,16] Because brachytherapy demonstrates a steep dose falloff phenomenon around the radioactive implant, the detrimental effects are usually localized to the region of the implant. In contrast, the damage caused by external beam RT tends to be more uniformly distributed within the irradiation field, including the contralateral mandible.[14] Store and colleagues[17] from Norway compared the effect of external beam RT (mean dose, 72 Gy) to external beam RT in combination with interstitial iridium 192 (^{192}Ir) implantation. The patients in the combined therapy group received an average brachytherapy dose of 44.6 Gy at an average rate of 0.83 Gy/hr, and a mean total radiation dose of 95.5 Gy (range, 81.9 to 135 Gy). Computed tomography demonstrated lingual cortical defects of the mandible in all of the patients who received external beam RT in combination with brachytherapy, and buccal cortical defects in 30% of cases. Lingual cortical defects corresponding to the site of ^{192}Ir implantation were identified in 52% of these patients. All of the patients who received external beam RT alone had defects of the lingual and buccal cortices, and 50% manifested alterations of the contralateral mandible. Notani et al[14] from Japan have correspondingly found that ORN induced by brachytherapy was usually more amenable to conservative therapy than ORN induced by external beam RT, and that successful management was directly related to the severity of ORN.

The relationship between the dose of RT and ORN has been the subject of some research investigation. At doses of less than 50 Gy, ORN is uncommon. The risk of ORN increases as the radiation dose increases above 50 Gy to a rate that is nearly 10 times greater than the risk associated with doses less than 50 Gy.[18–22] The severity and likelihood of healing with conservative treatment also diminishes with increasing dose.[18] An increased fraction dose has also been shown to increase the probability of injury.[6,12] In fact, decreasing the fraction dose appears to lower the risk of ORN, despite the delivery of higher total radiation doses. Glanzmann and Gratz[6] from Zurich found that as the mandibular dose per fraction (DPF) was decreased, the rate of ORN correspondingly decreased even though the total mandibular dose (TMD) increased: a DPF of 2 to 2.22 Gy (one fraction per day) and a TMD of 66 to 79.7 Gy resulted in an ORN rate of 24.8%; a DPF of 1.8 to 1.9 Gy (one fraction per day) and a TMD of 69 to 75.6 Gy resulted in an ORN rate of 19.6%; and a DPF of 1.2 Gy (two fractions per day), TMD of 75.2 to 82 Gy, with or without concomitant cisplatin led to an ORN rate of 2.2%.

The impact of fractionation regimens on the risk of developing ORN is unclear. The hyperfractionated irradiation group reported by Glanzmann and Gratz reported a lower rate of ORN than those treated with conventional fractionation protocols. A lower rate of ORN was also noted in the Continuous Hyperfractionated Accelerated Radiotherapy (CHART) study that compared 54 Gy in 36 fractions over 12 consecutive days (three daily fractions of 1.5 Gy) against conventional therapy using 66 Gy in 33 fractions over 6.5 weeks.[23] On the other hand, Niewald and colleagues[11] found that hyperfractionated external beam RT with 1.2 Gy twice a day resulted in a 22.9% rate of ORN, whereas treatment with 2 Gy once per day led to ORN in only 8.6% of the treated patients. Low-dose ^{192}Ir brachytherapy that is delivered at rates higher than 0.5 to 0.55 Gy/hr has been shown to significantly increase the risk of ORN.[16,24]

Trauma

Tissue breakdown usually occurs following some form of soft tissue trauma. Thorn et al[10] found that tooth extractions initiated ORN in 55% of the patients evaluated, whereas traumatic injury from other oral surgical procedures and removable dental prostheses accounted for an additional 16%. Twenty-nine percent of the cases were reportedly secondary to "spontaneous" tissue breakdown, which raises the possibility that unappreciated soft tissue trauma may have nevertheless occurred.[10] Marx and Johnson[3] found that spontaneous tissue breakdown occurred in 39% of ORN cases, and that such an occurrence was associated with RT doses exceeding 70 Gy, or when RT was performed in combination with surgery. Mandibular resective procedures such as marginal mandibulectomy and mandibulotomy that are located within the field of postoperative RT have also been associated with the development of ORN.[25]

Dental extractions have frequently been implicated as the inciting traumatic event that initiates the cascade associated with ORN. Beumer and colleagues[26] noted a 14.1% rate of radiation-induced bone necrosis associated with preradiation dental extractions that were mostly performed less than 14 days before the initiation of RT. The same investigators also documented a 22% rate of ORN that was precipitated by postirradiation dental extractions.[27] Most other investigators, however, have documented lower rates of ORN in association with dental extractions.[28] According to pooled data from the peer-reviewed literature since 1968 that evaluated 11,077 irradiated patients, the incidence of postextraction ORN is 5.4%.[18]

Patient-Related Variables

Poor dental hygiene and periodontal bone loss due to periodontitis are associated with an increased risk of ORN.[11,29–31] Periodontal disease results in the formation of periodontal pockets that provide a selective survival advantage to the colonization of virulent bacterial pathogens, which lead to persistent periodontal inflammation and progressive alveolar bone loss. Endodontic pathology also predisposes patients to ORN following RT.[32] The risk of ORN is significantly lower in edentulous patients.[3,27] Other risk factors include alcohol and tobacco use, primary tumor size and location, and the proximity of the tumor to bone.[6,29–31]

◆ Pathogenesis

The pathophysiologic events that lead to ORN remain a subject of contentious debate. Prior to 1983, trauma such as tooth extraction was considered a portal of entry for oral bacteria to infect the underlying bone, leading to "radiation osteomyelitis."[33] At that time, ORN was thought to arise from sequential injuries caused by radiation, trauma, and infection. In 1983, however, Marx[34] contended that ORN was a problem of wound healing rather than of infection, and proposed that ORN resulted from the following sequence of events:

1. Radiation
2. Hypoxic-hypovascular-hypocellular tissue
3. Tissue breakdown
4. Nonhealing wound

Microorganisms, according to Marx, were only contaminants rather than a source of infection. These conclusions were derived, in large part, from bacterial and fungal cultures of the exposed bone surface and the deeper medullary bone. Although bacteria were found on the exposed surface of more than two thirds of the bone specimens, none of the specimens harbored bacteria within the medullary space.

The belief that ORN was a form of aseptic necrosis rather than osteomyelitis resulted in a paradigm shift that was embraced by most clinicians. As a consequence, the importance of antimicrobial therapy was challenged, and the door to other forms of treatment was opened. Most investigations of treatment for ORN after 1983 evaluated the efficacy of therapy based on the presumption that bacterial infection was not a contributing factor. Recent evidence from Norwegian investigators, however, have documented the presence of bacteria within deep medullary bone specimens of patients with ORN using DNA–DNA hybridization as well as electron microscopy.[35,36] Between seven and 15 bacterial species were identified in each of 12 consecutive ORN specimens, including *Actinomyces* species, *Porphyromonas gingivalis*, and *Fusobacterium nucleatum*. Although these findings need to be verified by independent investigators, the term *infected osteoradionecrosis* has resurfaced in the peer-reviewed literature in 2006.[37]

Marx's observation that tissue perfusion progressively diminishes with time has been corroborated by other researchers who have confirmed that intramandibular oxygen tension is lower in ORN-afflicted regions, and radiation-induced obliteration of the inferior alveolar artery and branches of the facial artery occur in association with ORN.[13,38] These progressive, irreversible changes to the tissue vasculature correspondingly lead to a progressive increase in risk of ORN that is permanent and unalterable.

In the absence of compelling evidence to the contrary, the pathophysiologic mechanism advocated by Marx has remained as the most plausible explanation for ORN. This conceptualization went largely unchallenged until French investigators contended that ORN may develop from a radiation-induced "fibroatrophic process."[39] This theory, which was initially used to explain the events associated with radiation-induced fibrosis (RIF) of soft tissues, postulates that histopathologic alterations occur in the following sequence: (1) endothelial cell destruction; (2) excessive production of disorganized extracellular matrix and activated fibroblasts (myofibroblasts); and (3) friable, hypovascular, hypocellular tissue that contains few fibroblasts and a dense extracellular matrix (fibroatrophy).[39,40] Although

these investigators agree that vascular damage and hypoxia contribute to early histopathologic alterations, they believe that free radicals (e.g., reactive oxygen species) and cytokines such as TGF-β1 also play an important role in the pathogenesis of fibroatrophic tissue and ORN. The fibroatrophic theory suggests that, in contrast to the pathogenic mechanism presented by Marx, radiation-induced tissue alterations may be partially reversed by antioxidant therapy.

Additional insight into the pathogenesis and treatment of ORN may be provided by investigative work on the mechanism of bisphosphonate-induced necrosis. The bisphosphonates, which are commonly used to manage bone metastases and osteoporosis, are capable of inducing osteonecrosis of the mandible as well as the maxilla.[37,41,42] Their therapeutic effect is based on the ability to inhibit osteoclasts as well as angiogenesis, and these traits form the basis for two competing theories regarding the pathogenic mechanism of bisphosphonate-induced osteonecrosis, both of which differ from those purported for ORN. The leading theory suggests that the osteoclast-inhibiting effect results in cessation of bone remodeling and turnover, whereas the competing theory suggests that inhibition of endothelial cell proliferation leads to avascular necrosis.[41] In ORN, vessel obliteration is secondary to radiation-induced endarteritis that is followed by hyalinized vessel narrowing, whereas the bisphosphonates appear to directly inhibit endothelial function.[43] Ironically, one of the bisphosphonates was used to potentiate the effects of antioxidant therapy for ORN in a recent phase II trial.[44]

◆ Clinical Presentation

The onset of osteoradionecrosis most frequently occurs within 2 years of RT, but this complication can develop within a few months to several years later.[45,46] In their retrospective review of 536 patients with ORN, Marx and Johnson[3] noted that trauma-induced ORN tended to develop either within the first 3 to 6 months after RT (type I), or 2 years or longer following RT (type II). Type I injuries were always associated with surgical insult, whereas type II injuries may also develop from more trivial forms of trauma to injury-prone hypovascular, hypocellular, hypoxic tissue. Marx noted that 84% of the trauma-induced cases were associated with tooth removal. Spontaneous ORN rarely developed more than 24 months following RT. The lingual cortex of the premolar, molar, and retromolar trigone regions are the most vulnerable regions of the mandible.[10,13]

The diagnosis of ORN is based on clinical signs and symptoms of ulceration or necrosis of the mucosa with exposure of necrotic bone that persists for more than 3 months.[5] Pain is the most common presenting symptom in these patients, but some cases of ORN can be asymptomatic.[10] Bony sequestra may be present, and orocutaneous fistulization or pathologic fracture may also develop. A variety of scoring systems have been developed to grade the severity of mandibular ORN and to assess the response to treatment (**Tables 26–1** to **26–4**).[2,4–6,14] A clinical staging system

Table 26–1 Clinical Staging of Osteoradionecrosis (ORN) by Store and Boysen

Stage	Event
0	Mucosal defects only
I	Radiologic evidence of bone necrosis with intact mucosa
II	Radiologic evidence of bone necrosis with denuded bone
III	Exposed radionecrotic bone along with orocutaneous fistulas

From Store G, Boysen M. Mandibular osteoradionecrosis: clinical behavior and diagnostic aspects. Clin Otolaryngol Allied Sci 2000;25:378–384.

Table 26–2 Clinical Staging of ORN by Schwartz and Kagan

Stage	Event
I	Minimal soft tissue ulceration, superficial necrosis of exposed mandibular bone
II	Localized mandibular involvement, with necrosis of exposed cortical bone and a portion of the underlying medullary bone
	Division A: Soft tissue ulceration is minimal
	Division B: There is soft tissue necrosis, including orocutaneous fistulization
III	Diffuse involvement of the mandible, with full thickness involvement of a segment of bone, including the lower border; pathologic fracture may occur
IIIA	Soft tissue ulceration is minimal
IIIB	There is soft tissue necrosis, including orocutaneous fistulization

From Schwartz HC, Kagan AR. Osteoradionecrosis of the mandible: scientific basis for clinical staging. Am J Clin Oncol 2002;25:168–171.

was also recently developed for maxillary ORN that is based on the experience with RT for nasopharyngeal carcinoma in Taiwan.[7]

Computed tomography (CT) demonstrates osseous abnormalities such as cortical disruption and loss of trabeculation. Soft tissue thickening is also frequently seen, which must be differentiated from recurrent tumor. Visualization of cortical defects distant from the location of the original tumor, however, increases the probability that ORN is the diagnosis.[47] Magnetic resonance imaging (MRI) exhibits cortical destruction and marked contrast enhancement of osteoradionecrotic bone marrow.[48] The sensitivity of bone scintigraphy for the presence of ORN approaches 100%, but the specificity is only approximately 60%.[49] Panoramic radiography and other forms of plain radiography frequently fail to correlate with the clinical signs and symptoms of ORN.[5,10]

◆ Prevention of Osteoradionecrosis

General Considerations

A thorough pretreatment dental evaluation that includes radiographic evaluation with panoramic radiographs and, when indicated, periapical films, should be routinely performed prior to the initiation of surgery or RT. Dental treatment is focused on eliminating infection and preventing the necessity for invasive dental procedures following the initiation of cancer treatment.[41] Basic periodontal therapy

for the removal of plaque and calculus are performed, and endodontic therapy is completed. Caries control is achieved, and patients are instructed in methods of optimizing plaque control as well as the importance of complying with the recommended fluoride regimen. Teeth with a periodontally or endodontically questionable prognosis should be extracted to avoid complications following RT. Impacted teeth that are completely covered by bone or soft tissue should be left undisturbed, whereas those with an oral communication must be considered for extraction if they are at future risk for infection.[41] Invasive dental care should be performed at least 2 weeks before initiation of RT to optimize tissue healing. Care must be taken to handle the bone and soft tissues in an atraumatic manner, and the mucosa should be meticulously closed, avoiding undue soft tissue tension.[50] A simple forceps extraction with minimal mucoperiosteal flap elevation and minimal alveoloplasty is preferable. Prophylactic antibiotic coverage is generally not required for noninvasive dental procedures in the absence of other indications such as valvular heart disease. If antibiotics are desired for invasive dental procedures, penicillin remains the antibiotic of choice. Clindamycin by itself is not recommended because of its lack of activity against *Eikenella corrodens* and actinomyces. Metronidazole can be used in combination with erythromycin or a quinolone in patients who have a penicillin allergy.[41]

Table 26–3 Clinical Staging of ORN by Glanzmann and Gratz

Grade	Event
1	Bone exposure without signs of infection and persisting for at least 3 months
2	Bone exposure with signs of infection or sequester and without the signs of grade 3–5
3	Bone necrosis treated with mandibular resection
4	Bone necrosis with persisting problems despite mandibular resection
5	Death due to osteoradionecrosis

From Glanzmann C, Gratz KW. Radionecrosis of the mandible: a retrospective analysis of the incidence and risk factors. Radiother Oncol 1995;36:94–100.

Table 26–4 Clinical Staging of ORN by Notani et al

Grade	Event
I	ORN confined to the alveolar bone
II	ORN limited to the alveolar bone and/or the mandible above the level of the mandibular alveolar canal
III	ORN that extends to the mandible under the level of the mandibular alveolar canal *and* ORN with a skin fistula and/or a pathologic fracture

From Notani K, Yamazaki Y, Kitada H, et al. Management of mandibular osteoradionecrosis corresponding to the severity of osteoradionecrosis and the method of radiotherapy. Head Neck 2003;25:181–186.

Comprehensive dental care should be continued following completion of treatment, and the importance of lifelong preventive dental therapy must be emphasized.

Dental Extractions Before Radiation Therapy

The relationship between dental disease and ORN following RT was appreciated by clinicians in the 1960s, influencing the development of recommendations for evaluation and management of the dentition prior to the initiation of RT.[51] The adoption of a systematic approach to dental care in combination with the introduction of high-energy RT in the mid- to late 1960s reduced the incidence of ORN after preradiation dental extractions to 4.4%.[18] There is evidence that aggressive preventive dental care in combination with extractions performed by experienced oral and maxillofacial surgeons results in even lower rates of bone necrosis.[18]

A consensus report in 1990 from the National Cancer Institute recommended a minimum time of 2 weeks between extractions and the initiation of RT to allow for adequate healing of the extraction site.[52] Marx and Johnson[3] recommend extraction 21 days before RT whenever possible. Clinicians at Memorial Sloan-Kettering Cancer Center (MSKCC) strive to extract teeth 14 to 21 days before the onset of RT.[53] Investigators from The University of Texas M. D. Anderson Cancer Center (MDACC) documented a 3.6% rate of ORN when impacted third molars were extracted an average of 32.4 days prior to irradiation.[54]

The necessity for antibiotics at the time of preirradiation extraction is controversial, and their efficacy has not been evaluated in prospective fashion. Prophylactic antibiotic coverage was implemented by Oh and colleagues[54] from MDACC, achieving the results mentioned above. On the other hand, antibiotics are not routinely administered for dental extractions at MSKCC, where a 2% rate of ORN was documented following 951 dental extractions on 187 patients. Even though many clinicians often use prophylactic antibiotic coverage as a conservative and inexpensive preventive measure, its role has not been established as the standard of care.

Dental Extractions After Radiation Therapy

Minimal investigation has been undertaken regarding treatment approaches that could reduce the incidence of ORN in patients who undergo postirradiation dental extractions. Based on research evidence that hyperbaric oxygen (HBO) may be an effective treatment for established ORN, Marx and colleagues[9] conducted a randomized prospective clinical trial to determine whether HBO could reduce the development of ORN in patients who underwent postirradiation extractions. Patients received either HBO therapy or penicillin during the perioperative period, and were evaluated for the presence of exposed bone that had failed to heal 6 months following extraction. Patients who were treated with penicillin had a 29.9% of ORN, whereas those who received HBO had a 5.4% rate of ORN ($p = .005$). These findings have influenced many clinicians to routinely treat irradiated patients with HBO when tooth extraction is necessary.

The role for HBO in this setting, however, has been disputed by others. The findings reported by Marx et al have not been replicated, and the 29.9% rate of ORN that was reported for patients in the penicillin arm was unusually high in comparison to the 5.4% incidence of postextraction ORN published in the peer-reviewed literature between 1968 and 1992.[18] Sulaiman et al[53] from MSKCC believe that these findings are questionable and do not advocate its routine use. They reported a 2% rate of ORN in 107 patients (7 received HBO) who had 330 teeth extracted in the irradiation field. As a consequence, HBO at MSKCC is used as an adjunctive measure following clinical evaluation that designates a patient to be at unusually high risk for radiation-induced bone complications.

The economic impact of administering prophylactic HBO therapy to every patient who requires postirradiation extractions has also been evaluated. Clayman[18] from Henry Ford Hospital estimated that two of 100 patients would benefit from HBO therapy at a cost of $1.5 million (in 1997). Furthermore, a 98% rate of osseointegration 5 years after implantation into mandibles that were irradiated a median of 13 months earlier without the use of HBO has been documented.[56] These findings mandate the need for additional prospective research to define the role that prophylactic HBO and other forms of treatment play in prevention for these patients.

◆ Treatment of Osteoradionecrosis

Conservative Therapy

Conservative management of ORN with antibiotics, debridement, and irrigation can be performed as initial treatment for early-stage ORN. Limited research exists to substantiate its efficacy, however. At the Princess Margaret Hospital, local irrigation, systemic antibiotics, oral hygiene instruction, and the avoidance of irritants such as tobacco, alcohol, or denture use in combination with sequestrectomy led to complete healing in 48% of the patients with ORN.[1] The relationship between treatment response and the severity of ORN, however, was not assessed. The use of ultrasound in combination with local debridement and metronidazole has also been reported.[57] Most institutions have reported the use of conservative measures in combination with other treatments such as HBO or surgery, precluding evaluation of their true efficacy.

Hyperbaric Oxygen Therapy and Surgery

Hyperbaric oxygen—100% oxygen at two to three times the atmospheric pressure at sea level—is capable of markedly increasing the oxygen tension in tissue.[58] By increasing the partial pressure of oxygen within tissues, HBO may be able to counter the effects of local hypoxia, promoting collagen formation and angiogenesis.[59] Hyperbaric oxygen also restores defenses against infection that are impaired by local hypoxia, including bacterial phagocytosis.[60,61] The transmucosal oxygen tension of gingiva significantly increases following five 90-minute treatments at 2.4 ATA (atmosphere absolute), and higher oxygen tension is attained with 30 treatments.[62] Recent measurements of the oxygen partial pressure of cancellous mandibular bone demonstrated a partial pressure of 71.4 mm Hg in healthy bone versus 32.3 mm Hg in osteoradionecrotic bone.[38] These findings bolster the rationale for using HBO to treat ORN.

The current HBO protocol is based on the Wilford Hall protocol originally advocated by Marx, with some modification[55,63]:

Stage I   Perform 30 HBO treatments (one treatment per day, Monday to Friday) to 2.4 atmospheres for 90 minutes breathing 100% oxygen. The patient is closely monitored to for decreased bone exposure, granulation tissue covering exposed bone, resorption of nonviable bone, and absence of inflammation and infection. For patients who respond favorably, treatment is continued to a total of 40 or more treatments. For patients who are not responsive, advance to stage II treatment.

Stage II   Perform transoral sequestrectomy with attempted primary wound closure followed by continued HBO to a total of 40 treatments. If wound dehiscence occurs, advance patients to stage III treatment. Patients who present with orocutaneous fistula, pathologic fracture, or resorption to the inferior border of the mandible, advance to stage III treatment immediately after the initial 30 treatments.

Stage III   Perform transcutaneous mandibular resection, wound closure, and mandibular fixation with an external fixator, maxillomandibular fixation, or reconstruction plating, followed by an additional 10 to 20 postoperative HBO treatments.

Stage IIIR   Perform mandibular reconstruction 10 weeks after successful resolution of mandibular ORN. Complete 10 to 20 additional postoperative HBO treatments. Marx advocated the use of autogenous cancellous bone within a freeze-dried allogeneic bone carrier. The advent of free tissue transfer, however, frequently allows for reconstruction at the time of resection, integrating stage IIIR into stage III.

Marx used his original protocol to successfully treat 58 patients with refractory osteoradionecrosis, documenting resolution for 15% of the patients in stage I, 14% in stage II, and 70% in stage III.[55] He established four criteria for resolution: (1) freedom from pain; (2) retention or reconstruction of mandibular continuity; (3) restoration of mandibular function and wearing of prosthodontic appliances, if needed; and (4) maintenance of intact mucosa over all bone for the length of follow-up (minimum of 18 months).

Other investigators have subsequently reported their experience with HBO in an attempt to define the type of ORN abnormalities that respond to treatment as well as the treatment effect that can be expected.[14,19,45,64–67] Notani et al,[14] for example, evaluated the efficacy of antibiotics, curettage, debridement, and small sequestrectomy with or without HBO as a form of conservative therapy for ORN. Patients who had less extensive mandibular necrosis were more likely to respond to conservative therapy, whereas greater degrees of mandibular necrosis required extensive sequestrectomy or mandibulectomy. Epstein and colleagues[45] from British Columbia combined conservative measures (alcohol and tobacco cessation, dental care, 1.5%

hydrogen peroxide and chlorhexidine oral rinses, oral antibiotics) with HBO and surgery, achieving mucosal and cutaneous coverage in 69% of the treated patients, and meeting Marx's criteria for resolution in 50%.

Most investigators acknowledge that severe ORN with large areas of exposed necrotic bone, fistula formation, or loss of mandibular continuity (fracture) cannot be effectively treated solely with HBO, and surgical intervention is usually required.[14,45,67,68] Complete resection of necrotic bone should be followed by closure or reconstruction with vascularized tissue. Microvascular reconstruction of large soft tissue or bony defects is the treatment of choice, providing healthy, well-vascularized tissue that can support osseointegrated implants and functional dental prostheses.[50,69–71] Other forms of nonvascularized reconstruction such as cancellous bone grafting provide inferior results.[72]

Critics of HBO contend that its use is empirical and most reports of its efficacy are anecdotal in nature.[2] Schwartz and Kagan[2] argue that "most cases can be managed successfully without HBO." Investigators from Austria have published findings that demonstrated a 65% success rate with HBO versus a 100% success rate following debridement, clindamycin, and partial mandibulectomy in patients with severe ORN.[73] Their conclusion that HBO should not be used as treatment for severe HBO, however, does not appear to contradict the treatment philosophy of most investigators, including Marx, because HBO is frequently used in conjunction with surgical intervention to address severe ORN. Recently, a randomized, placebo-controlled, double-blind clinical trial that evaluated HBO was terminated because patients in the HBO arm demonstrated worse outcomes than the placebo arm.[74] Only 68 patients were enrolled, which has become a source of criticism, because a sample size of 222 patients was originally estimated to detect a 20% difference between the two treatment arms.[75] Critics also make the point that the criteria used to establish a diagnosis of ORN in this investigation may have led to the inclusion of patients who do not have ORN.[76] It is relevant to note that one of the authors is a proponent of the fibroatrophic process as the likely pathogenic process involved in ORN.[44]

Feldmeier et al[77] performed a systematic review of the literature reporting the application of hyperbaric oxygen prevention and treatment of delayed radiation injuries. Of the 74 articles reviewed, 67 noted positive outcomes in response to treatment with the negative papers primarily related to neurologic injury. Bennett et al[78] published an evidence-based review in collaboration with the Cochrane Group. They reviewed a total of 103 articles, of which 6 were randomized controlled trials. The Cochrane group concluded that HBOT is associated with improved outcome in late radiation tissue injury of the head and neck and that HBOT reduced the chance of ORN following tooth extraction in irradiated field.

Antioxidant Therapy

Based on the theory that the fibroatrophic process plays an important role in the pathogenesis of osteoradionecrosis, a phase II trial recently evaluated the treatment efficacy of pentoxifylline and α-tocopherol (vitamin E) in 18 patients with ORN.[44] Clodronate, a bisphosphonate that inhibits bone resorption, was also administered to the patients with severe ORN. Complete mucosal healing was achieved in 16 patients, and the remaining two patients exhibited a 75% response at 6 months. These investigators suggest that tissue healing may represent partial reversal of the alterations that occur in irradiated tissue. Additional investigation is necessary to compare the efficacy of this treatment approach to other more established forms of treatment such as HBO.

◆ Conclusion

The pathogenesis of osteoradionecrosis has not been clearly elucidated, and there is no consensus regarding the best clinical definition of osteoradionecrosis. Furthermore, none of the proposed staging systems has been sufficiently validated as predictors of outcome following treatment, and recommendations for the prevention and management of ORN have not been widely adopted. For example, oral and maxillofacial surgeons from Hirosaki University in Japan state that "the management of ORN appears to differ from hospital to hospital,"[71] and a recent survey of oral and maxillofacial surgeons from the United Kingdom found that one third of the respondents never referred irradiated patients who required mandibular molar extractions for HBO.[79] Efforts to establish guidelines for treatment have also been undermined by growing skepticism regarding the efficacy of hyperbaric oxygen therapy, and some investigators question the scientific rationale upon which this treatment modality has been based for more than two decades.[53,80] It is hoped that this state of controversy will inspire funding agencies to support research efforts so that clinically efficacious, evidence-based methods of prevention and treatment are eventually established.

References

1. Wong JK, Wood RE, McLean M. Conservative management of osteoradionecrosis. Oral Surg Oral Med Oral Pathol Oral Radiol Endod 1997; 84:16–21

2. Schwartz HC, Kagan AR. Osteoradionecrosis of the mandible: scientific basis for clinical staging. Am J Clin Oncol 2002;25:168–171

3. Marx RE, Johnson RP. Studies in the radiobiology of osteoradionecrosis and their clinical significance. Oral Surg Oral Med Oral Pathol 1987; 64:379–390

4. Store G, Boysen M. Mandibular osteoradionecrosis: clinical behaviour and diagnostic aspects. Clin Otolaryngol Allied Sci. 2000; 25:378–384

5. Epstein JB, Wong FL, Stevenson-Moore P. Osteoradionecrosis: clinical experience and a proposal for classification. J Oral Maxillofac Surg 1987;45:104–110

6. Glanzmann C, Gratz KW. Radionecrosis of the mandible: a retrospective analysis of the incidence and risk factors. Radiother Oncol 1995; 36:94–100

7. Cheng SJ, Lee JJ, Ting LL, et al. A clinical staging system and treatment guidelines for maxillary osteoradionecrosis in irradiated nasopharyngeal carcinoma patients. Int J Radiat Oncol Biol Phys 2006; 64:90–97

8. Teng MS, Futran ND. Osteoradionecrosis of the mandible. Curr Opin Otolaryngol Head Neck Surg 2005;13:217–221

9. Marx RE, Johnson RP, Kline SN. Prevention of osteoradionecrosis: a randomized prospective clinical trial of hyperbaric oxygen versus penicillin. J Am Dent Assoc 1985;111:49–54

10. Thorn JJ, Hansen HS, Specht L, Bastholt L. Osteoradionecrosis of the jaws: clinical characteristics and relation to the field of irradiation. J Oral Maxillofac Surg 2000;58:1088–1093

11. Niewald M, Barbie O, Schnabel K, et al. Risk factors and dose-effect relationship for osteoradionecrosis after hyperfractionated and conventionally fractionated radiotherapy for oral cancer. Br J Radiol 1996;69:847–851

12. Withers HR, Peters LJ, Taylor JM, et al. Late normal tissue sequelae from radiation therapy for carcinoma of the tonsil: patterns of fractionation study of radiobiology. Int J Radiat Oncol Biol Phys 1995;33: 563–568

13. Bras J, de Jonge HK, van Merkesteyn JP. Osteoradionecrosis of the mandible: pathogenesis. Am J Otolaryngol 1990;11:244–250

14. Notani K, Yamazaki Y, Kitada H, et al. Management of mandibular osteoradionecrosis corresponding to the severity of osteoradionecrosis and the method of radiotherapy. Head Neck 2003;25:181–186

15. Bachaud JM, Delannes M, Allouache N, et al. Radiotherapy of stage I and II carcinomas of the mobile tongue and/or floor of the mouth. Radiother Oncol 1994;31:199–206

16. Lozza L, Cerrotta A, Gardani G, et al. Analysis of risk factors for mandibular bone radionecrosis after exclusive low dose-rate brachytherapy for oral cancer. Radiother Oncol 1997;44:143–147

17. Store G, Evensen J, Larheim TA. Osteoradionecrosis of the mandible: comparison of the effects of external beam irradiation and brachytherapy. Dentomaxillofac Radiol 2001;30:114–119

18. Clayman L. Clinical controversies in oral and maxillofacial surgery. Part two. Management of dental extractions in irradiated jaws: a protocol without hyperbaric oxygen therapy. J Oral Maxillofac Surg 1997;55: 275–281

19. Hart GB, Mainous EG. The treatment of radiation necrosis with hyperbaric oxygen (OHP). Cancer 1976;37:2580–2585

20. Kumar HS, Bihani V, Kumar V, Chaudhary RK, Kumar L, Punia DP. Osteoradionecrosis of mandible in patients treated with definitive radiotherapy for carcinomas of oral cavity and oropharynx: a retrospective study. Indian J Dent Res 1992;3:47–50

21. Bedwinek JM, Shukovsky LJ, Fletcher GH, Daley TE. Osteonecrosis in patients treated with definitive radiotherapy for squamous cell carcinomas of the oral cavity and naso- and oropharynx. Radiology 1976; 119:665–667

22. Morrish RB Jr, Chan E, Silverman S Jr, Meyer J, Fu KK, Greenspan D. Osteonecrosis in patients irradiated for head and neck carcinoma. Cancer 1981;47:1980–1983

23. Dische S, Saunders M, Barrett A, Harvey A, Gibson D, Parmar M. A randomized multicentre trial of CHART versus conventional radiotherapy in head and neck cancer. Radiother Oncol 1997;44:123–136

24. Fujita M, Hirokawa Y, Kashiwado K, et al. An analysis of mandibular bone complications in radiotherapy for T1 and T2 carcinoma of the oral tongue. Int J Radiat Oncol Biol Phys 1996;34:333–339

25. Wang CC, Cheng MH, Hao SP, Wu CC, Huang SS. Osteoradionecrosis with combined mandibulotomy and marginal mandibulectomy. Laryngoscope 2005;115:1963–1967

26. Beumer J III, Harrison R, Sanders B, Kurrasch M. Preradiation dental extractions and the incidence of bone necrosis. Head Neck Surg 1983; 5:514–521

27. Beumer J III, Harrison R, Sanders B, Kurrasch M. Postradiation dental extractions: a review of the literature and a report of 72 episodes. Head Neck Surg 1983;6:581–586

28. Epstein JB, Rea G, Wong FL, Spinelli J, Stevenson-Moore P. Osteonecrosis: study of the relationship of dental extractions in patients receiving radiotherapy. Head Neck Surg 1987;10:48–54

29. Murray CG, Herson J, Daly TE, Zimmerman S. Radiation necrosis of the mandible: a 10 year study. Part I. Factors influencing the onset of necrosis. Int J Radiat Oncol Biol Phys 1980;6:543–548

30. Murray CG, Herson J, Daly TE, Zimmerman S. Radiation necrosis of the mandible: a 10 year study. Part II. Dental factors; onset, duration

and management of necrosis. Int J Radiat Oncol Biol Phys 1980;6:549–553

31. Kluth EV, Jain PR, Stuchell RN, Frich JC Jr. A study of factors contributing to the development of osteoradionecrosis of the jaws. J Prosthet Dent 1988;59:194–201

32. Seto BG, Beumer J III, Kagawa T, Klokkevold P, Wolinsky L. Analysis of endodontic therapy in patients irradiated for head and neck cancer. Oral Surg Oral Med Oral Pathol 1985;60:540–545

33. Meyer I. Infectious diseases of the jaws. J Oral Surg 1970;28:17–26

34. Marx RE. Osteoradionecrosis: a new concept of its pathophysiology. J Oral Maxillofac Surg 1983;41:283–288

35. Store G, Eribe ER, Olsen I. DNA–DNA hybridization demonstrates multiple bacteria in osteoradionecrosis. Int J Oral Maxillofac Surg 2005;34:193–196

36. Store G, Olsen I. Scanning and transmission electron microscopy demonstrates bacteria in osteoradionecrosis. Int J Oral Maxillofac Surg 2005;34:777–781

37. Hansen T, Kunkel M, Weber A, James Kirkpatrick C. Osteonecrosis of the jaws in patients treated with bisphosphonates: histomorphologic analysis in comparison with infected osteoradionecrosis. J Oral Pathol Med 2006;35:155–160

38. Maurer P, Meyer L, Eckert AW, Berginski M, Schubert J. Measurement of oxygen partial pressure in the mandibular bone using a polarographic fine needle probe. Int J Oral Maxillofac Surg 2006;35:231–236

39. Delanian S, Lefaix JL. Mature bone necrosis: from recent pathophysiological aspects to a new therapeutic action [in French]. Cancer Radiother 2002;6:1–9

40. Delanian S, Lefaix JL. The radiation-induced fibroatrophic process: therapeutic perspective via the antioxidant pathway. Radiother Oncol 2004;73:119–131

41. Marx RE, Sawatari Y, Fortin M, Broumand V. Bisphosphonate-induced exposed bone (osteonecrosis/osteopetrosis) of the jaws: risk factors, recognition, prevention, and treatment. J Oral Maxillofac Surg 2005;63:1567–1575

42. Melo MD, Obeid G. Osteonecrosis of the jaws in patients with a history of receiving bisphosphonate therapy: strategies for prevention and early recognition. J Am Dent Assoc 2005;136:1675–1681

43. Fournier P, Boissier S, Filleur S, et al. Bisphosphonates inhibit angiogenesis in vitro and testosterone-stimulated vascular regrowth in the ventral prostate in castrated rats. Cancer Res 2002;62:6538–6544

44. Delanian S, Depondt J, Lefaix JL. Major healing of refractory mandible osteoradionecrosis after treatment combining pentoxifylline and tocopherol: a phase II trial. Head Neck 2005;27:114–123

45. Epstein J, van der Meij E, McKenzie M, Wong F, Lepawsky M, Stevenson-Moore P. Postradiation osteonecrosis of the mandible: a long-term follow-up study. Oral Surg Oral Med Oral Pathol Oral Radiol Endod 1997;83:657–662

46. Store G, Larheim TA. Mandibular osteoradionecrosis: a comparison of computed tomography with panoramic radiography. Dentomaxillofac Radiol 1999;28:295–300

47. Hermans R, Fossion E, Ioannides C, Van den Bogaert W, Ghekiere J, Baert AL. CT findings in osteoradionecrosis of the mandible. Skeletal Radiol 1996;25:31–36

48. Store G, Smith HJ, Larheim TA. Dynamic MR imaging of mandibular osteoradionecrosis. Acta Radiol 2000;41:31–37

49. Bachmann G, Rossler R, Klett R, Rau WS, Bauer R. The role of magnetic resonance imaging and scintigraphy in the diagnosis of pathologic changes of the mandible after radiation therapy. Int J Oral Maxillofac Surg 1996;25:189–195

50. Hao SP, Chen HC, Wei FC, Chen CY, Yeh AR, Su JL. Systematic management of osteoradionecrosis in the head and neck. Laryngoscope 1999;109:1324–1327

51. Maccomb WS. Necrosis in treatment of intraoral cancer by radiation therapy. Am J Roentgenol Radium Ther Nucl Med 1962;87:431–440

52. Zlotolow IM. General considerations in prevention and treatment of oral manifestations of cancer therapies. In: Berger AM, Portenoy RK, Weissman DE, eds. Principles and Practice of Supportive Oncology. Philadelphia: Lippincott-Raven, 1998:237

53. Sulaiman F, Huryn JM, Zlotolow IM. Dental extractions in the irradiated head and neck patient: a retrospective analysis of Memorial Sloan-Kettering Cancer Center protocols, criteria, and end results. J Oral Maxillofac Surg 2003;61:1123–1131

54. Oh HK, Chambers MS, Garden AS, Wong PF, Martin JW. Risk of osteoradionecrosis after extraction of impacted third molars in irradiated head and neck cancer patients. J Oral Maxillofac Surg 2004;62:139–144

55. Marx RE. A new concept in the treatment of osteoradionecrosis. J Oral Maxillofac Surg 1983;41:351–357

56. Wagner W, Esser E, Ostkamp K. Osseointegration of dental implants in patients with and without radiotherapy. Acta Oncol 1998;37:693–696

57. Harris M. The conservative management of osteoradionecrosis of the mandible with ultrasound therapy. Br J Oral Maxillofac Surg 1992;30:313–318

58. Tibbles PM, Edelsberg JS. Hyperbaric-oxygen therapy. N Engl J Med 1996;334:1642–1648

59. Marx RE, Ehler WJ, Tayapongsak P, Pierce LW. Relationship of oxygen dose to angiogenesis induction in irradiated tissue. Am J Surg 1990;160:519–524

60. Mader JT, Brown GL, Guckian JC, Wells CH, Reinarz JA. A mechanism for the amelioration by hyperbaric oxygen of experimental staphylococcal osteomyelitis in rabbits. J Infect Dis 1980;142:915–922

61. Knighton DR, Halliday B, Hunt TK. Oxygen as an antibiotic: a comparison of the effects of inspired oxygen concentration and antibiotic administration on in vivo bacterial clearance. Arch Surg 1986;121:191–195

62. Thorn JJ, Kallehave F, Westergaard P, Hansen EH, Gottrup F. The effect of hyperbaric oxygen on irradiated oral tissues: transmucosal oxygen tension measurements. J Oral Maxillofac Surg 1997;55:1103–1107

63. Chambers MS, Toth BB, Martin JW, Fleming TJ, Lemon JC. Oral and dental management of the cancer patient: prevention and treatment of complications. Support Care Cancer 1995;3:168–175

64. Mounsey RA, Brown DH, O'Dwyer TP, Gullane PJ, Koch GH. Role of hyperbaric oxygen therapy in the management of mandibular osteoradionecrosis. Laryngoscope 1993;103:605–608

65. David LA, Sandor GK, Evans AW, Brown DH. Hyperbaric oxygen therapy and mandibular osteoradionecrosis: a retrospective study and analysis of treatment outcomes. J Can Dent Assoc 2001;67:384

66. Aitasalo K, Niinikoski J, Grenman R, Virolainen E. A modified protocol for early treatment of osteomyelitis and osteoradionecrosis of the mandible. Head Neck 1998;20:411–417

67. Wood GA, Liggins SJ. Does hyperbaric oxygen have a role in the management of osteoradionecrosis? Br J Oral Maxillofac Surg 1996;34:424–427

68. Koka VN, Deo R, Lusinchi A, Roland J, Schwaab G. Osteoradionecrosis of the mandible: study of 104 cases treated by hemimandibulectomy. J Laryngol Otol 1990;104:305–307

69. Shaha AR, Cordeiro PG, Hidalgo DA, et al. Resection and immediate microvascular reconstruction in the management of osteoradionecrosis of the mandible. Head Neck 1997;19:406–411

70. Chang DW, Oh HK, Robb GL, Miller MJ. Management of advanced mandibular osteoradionecrosis with free flap reconstruction. Head Neck 2001;23:830–835

71. Kobayashi W, Kobayashi M, Nakayama K, Hirota W, Kimura H. Free omental transfer for osteoradionecrosis of the mandible. Int J Oral Maxillofac Surg 2000;29:201–206

72. Jisander S, Grenthe B, Salemark L. Treatment of mandibular osteoradionecrosis by cancellous bone grafting. J Oral Maxillofac Surg 1999;57:936–942

73. Maier A, Gaggl A, Klemen H, et al. Review of severe osteoradionecrosis treated by surgery alone or surgery with postoperative hyperbaric oxygenation. Br J Oral Maxillofac Surg 2000;38:173–176

74. Annane D, Depondt J, Aubert P, et al. Hyperbaric oxygen therapy for radionecrosis of the jaw: a randomized, placebo-controlled, double-blind trial from the ORN96 study group. J Clin Oncol 2004;22:4893–4900

75. Mendenhall WM. Mandibular osteoradionecrosis. J Clin Oncol 2004;22:4867–4868

76. van Merkesteyn R, Bakker DJ. Comment on "Hyperbaric oxygen therapy for radionecrosis of the jaw: a randomized, placebo-controlled, double-blind trial from the ORN96 study group" [letter to the editor]. J Clin Oncol 2005;23:4465–4466

77. Feldmeier JJ, Hampson NB. A systematic review of the literature reporting the application of hyperbaric oxygen prevention and treatment of delayed radiation injuries: an evidence based approach. UHM 2002;29:4–30.

78. Bennett MH, et al. Hyperbaric oxygen therapy for late radiation tissue injury. The Cochrane Database of Systematic Reviews 2005, Issue 3. Art. No.: CD005005, pub 2.

79. Kanatas AN, Lowe D, Harrison J, Rogers SN. Survey of the use of hyperbaric oxygen by maxillofacial oncologists in the UK. Br J Oral Maxillofac Surg 2005;43:219–225

80. Assael LA. New foundations in understanding osteonecrosis of the jaws [editorial]. J Oral Maxillofac Surg 2004;62:125–126

27

Speech and Swallowing Following Treatment for Oral Cancer

Jan S. Lewin

The impact of oral cavity cancer and its treatment on speech and swallowing function can be significant. Patients with oral cancer experience functional disabilities associated with the tumor itself as well as treatment-related morbidity, both of which may have long-term deleterious effects on speech and swallowing. Depending on the size and location of the tumor and the therapeutic approach selected, the abilities to masticate, formulate, manipulate, and propel the food bolus through the oral cavity to elicit the pharyngeal swallow and final transit of the bolus to the stomach may be impaired. Furthermore, alterations in oral structures with resultant limitations in movement also affect articulation and speech production, often resulting in severely reduced intelligibility. Because impairments in oral function often lead to loss of social acceptance and worse quality of life, the sequelae associated with choosing a particular cancer therapy must be weighed against the desire to preserve function, physical appearance, and quality of life. This chapter addresses the impact of surgery, radiation therapy (RT), and chemotherapy on the functional outcomes of speech and swallowing, and reviews current evidence-based treatment strategies directed toward the rehabilitation and restoration of specific functional deficits.

◆ Normal Speech and Swallowing

Speech and swallowing are highly complex processes that depend on a series of physiologic events and interactions among the oral cavity, oropharynx, and larynx. The sequence of motor events involved in swallowing is fairly predictable, although investigators have shown that the relative timing of these events varies, depending on the size and consistency of the bolus of food or liquid being swallowed.[1–3] The act of swallowing can be divided into four stages: oral preparatory, oral, pharyngeal, and esophageal. Each stage depends on intact neurologic function and a coordinated succession of interactive movements. Thus, any structural or neurologic alteration that disrupts these patterns affects to some extent both speech and swallowing.

Before a swallow is initiated, oral preparation of the bolus is necessary. This requires a smoothly coordinated transition between bolus mastication by the teeth that chew food mixed with saliva, and the tongue, which gathers and forms the bolus into a cohesive, manageable bolus that can be transported posteriorly through the oral cavity into the pharynx. This triggers a swallow, mostly in the area of the faucial arches, initiating the pharyngeal stage of swallowing. Although propulsion of the bolus by the tongue is a clear indication that the swallow has begun, other less obvious events in the oral cavity must occur with precision and speed to ensure safe and efficient transit to the pharynx. From the moment that material is placed in the mouth until the bolus is swallowed, a labial seal ensures that no food or liquid spills from the mouth. During this time, the nasal airway must be open to permit breathing. The bolus must be held between the tongue and the anterior hard palate prior to the pharyngeal swallow. The movements of the tongue control the bolus as they contain and seal it against the lateral alveolus, or floor of mouth, and then lateralize and masticate it in concert with the movements of the mandible and teeth, propelling the bolus posteriorly in a stripping motion to the pharynx.

During the oral preparatory stage, the tongue may also subdivide the food after chewing, partitioning it and allowing only a portion to be swallowed at one time, holding the rest for subsequent swallows. Adequate contraction of the buccal musculature closes off the lateral sulcus and prevents the loss of the food into the buccal recesses between the mandible and cheek. If there is no active chewing during oral preparation, the soft palate is lowered and pulled anteriorly to seal off the oral cavity from the pharynx.[4] During active chewing, however, the soft palate is not pulled down and forward, and some material may spill over the base of tongue. Such spillage is normal during active chewing but should not occur when the bolus is held in the mouth before the actual swallow.[5] The pharyngeal swallow is rarely triggered in response to premature spillage unless the bolus begins to enter the larynx, which usually occurs when the oral stage, the second stage of the swallow, is not properly initiated.[6]

The oral stage is initiated when the tongue begins to move the bolus posteriorly in an anterior and posterior rolling or stripping action. A central groove is formed in the tongue, which acts as a ramp to help move the bolus through the oral cavity. In fact, correct re-creation of this groove is believed to be essential in the fabrication of palatal augmentation prostheses for patients who have undergone substantial tongue resections to enable the transit of food within the mouth. Adequate oral tongue pressure and strength are critical to efficient propulsion of the bolus without leaving residue behind as the bolus moves through the oral cavity and pharynx. The oral stage of the swallow typically lasts less than 1.5 seconds, increasing slightly as bolus viscosity increases.[7]

The pharyngeal swallow is triggered when sensory receptors in the oropharynx and tongue are stimulated, sending sensory information to the cerebral cortex and brainstem. The actions of the oral cavity structures propel the bolus posteriorly until they stimulate the area between the anterior faucial arches and the point where the tongue base crosses the lower rim of the mandible, at which time the oral stage of the swallow ends, and the pharyngeal swallow begins.[8] Initiation of the pharyngeal phase requires the presence of food as well as the onset of pharyngeal and laryngeal activity that protects the airway. These protective events precede posterior tongue propulsion and are associated with oral cavity activity. Clinicians who treat cancer of the oral cavity should have a thorough understanding of these events, because different therapeutic options likely have variable impact on posttreatment functioning.

Speech production and intelligibility similarly depend on a highly precise sequence of rapidly changing vocal tract shapes or configurations caused by the coordinated movements of the articulators of the oral cavity, namely, the lips, tongue, and soft palate. The place of articulatory contact may be bilabial, with primarily anterior contact for such sounds as p, b, and m; or it may be velar, which is necessary to produce k and g. Whether the sound is nasal or voiced depends on the degree of coarctation imposed on the vocal tract by valving action from the velum, which requires the soft palate to be lowered for the production of such nasal consonants as m and n. In contrast, laryngeal valving requires the opening or closing of the vocal folds to produce the voiced distinction between p and b, t and d, and k and g. In this case, the articulatory contact remains the same for each pair of consonants, but the activation of vibration or sound production makes the distinction. In the case of vowels, tongue shape and height become the key determinants of vocal production and distinction. Thus, any insult to the oral cavity from oral cancer or its treatment will affect speech production and, ultimately, conversational intelligibility.

◆ Functional Outcomes After Surgery

In general, the severity of speech and swallowing deficits following surgery for the management of oral cancer is closely associated with the *size* of the surgical defect that is created by the cancer resection. Reconstruction with adynamic bulky flaps that overfill the surgical defect tends to limit movement and reduce sensation. Primary closure frequently preserves postoperative function in many of these patients.[9,10] The *type* of surgical defect that is created by cancer resection also variably impacts the ultimate functional outcome. The functional deficits that can be expected from different types of surgical defects are reviewed here in detail.

Mandibular Resection

Oral cavity malignancies that extend into the mandible usually require composite resections of bone and soft tissue. Although speech and swallowing deficits associated with mandibular resection are usually relatively minor after surgical reconstruction, severe deformities may result in substantial deficits of deglutition, mastication, speech, and salivary retention. Although mandibular reconstruction has been shown to markedly improve masticatory function and dental rehabilitation, its impact on speech and swallowing efficiency is less predictable.[11] Continuity of the mandible should be maintained after surgical resection to preserve the balance and symmetry of mandibular function during mastication. The horizontal orientation of mandibular bone provides a platform for the soft tissues that enhances control and stability during speech and swallowing. The mandible, in conjunction with the lips, teeth, and buccal cavity, contributes to the articulation of some sounds and helps to prevent the anterior loss of food during the oral preparatory phase of swallowing. The extent of resection of the mandible, floor of mouth, and tongue dictates the degree of speech and swallowing impairment that will be encountered. Patients who have undergone a marginal mandibulectomy with resection of a portion of the floor of the mouth with primary closure should have little change in swallowing function if the remaining tongue is mobile, and mandibular contour has been preserved. In this situation, the mobile tongue can effectively propel the bolus during the oral stage of swallowing.[12]

The musculature that forms the floor of the mouth extends from the body of the mandible posteriorly to the hyoid bone, which also suspends the larynx. Movements in one of these structures can result in movements of the other structures that are attached to the hyoid bone. Patients who have had resection of the suprahyoid musculature tend to aspirate during swallowing because of the loss of elevation and the anterior tilting action of the larynx that normally protects the airway during swallowing. Although most patients have minimal swallowing dysfunction after mandibulectomy, surgical disruption of the muscular connections between the mandible and the hyolaryngeal complex in some patients can lead to considerable functional morbidity.

Mandibular resection also frequently leads to sensory alterations if inferior alveolar nerve transection occurs. The lower lip becomes permanently insensate, which reduces the strength of the labial seal. This alteration can interfere with the production of sounds that require oral air implosion or bilabial or labiodental articulatory placement, such as p, b, f, and v, because of air escape and sound distortion. An insensate lower lip and the resultant weak labial seal are extremely disturbing to patients because they are unable to prevent loss of food from the oral cavity while eating. Leakage due to oral incompetence is typically worse when the food consistency is less viscous, and drinking from a cup or straw is also more challenging. Lower lip anesthesia is also accompanied by proprioceptive deficits, which further exacerbate the patient's oral incompetence.

Mandibular resection is often associated with masticatory dysfunction that results from asymmetry and misalignment of the mandible, resulting in malocclusion. Masticatory function is also a product of the number of natural teeth that can be preserved as well as the quality of prosthetic dental restoration that is possible.

Therapy for patients with impaired mandibular function may include exercises to improve buccal tension that alternate between rounding and stretching the lips. Range-of-motion exercises are often helpful in improving the range of lateral mandibular movements. Changes in head position and placement of food on the better-functioning side may be helpful. In some cases, oral prostheses or adaptive devices may help to further strengthen the masticatory and perioral musculature.

Tongue Resection

The isolated resection of lingual tissue typically impacts only the oral phase of swallowing, and the degree of dysfunction is related to the extent and location of tongue resection. However, the tongue also plays a critical role in the pharyngeal phase of swallowing, and dysfunction during this phase can develop following surgery that alters the posterior oral tongue or base of tongue. The severity of speech and swallowing dysfunction usually parallel each other. If the tongue is sutured to the floor of mouth or buccal mucosa, mobility and range of motion of the tongue may be severely limited, causing severe speech and swallowing deficits.

Reconstruction of the tongue poses a variety of reconstructive challenges. The defect must be filled with an adequate volume of soft tissue that prevents pooling, preserves mobility, and restores the shape and volume of the remaining tongue. Achievement of these goals retains residual function and avoids overcorrection with excessive tissue bulk that can negatively impact articulation and oral swallowing.

Partial tongue resections involving as much as half of the oral tongue that are closed primarily frequently manifest good postoperative swallowing outcomes.[10] Adequate swallowing function after more extensive resection of the tongue is also possible. The degree of postoperative speech and swallowing impairment is often more reliant on the quality of the reconstruction than the extent of the resection. In fact, some patients who have undergone total glossectomy are able to speak and swallow better than many patients who have undergone composite reconstruction of the tongue, floor of mouth, and mandible.[11] However, it is also important to realize that successful reconstructive surgery does not predict functional success.

In situations where the tongue is minimally affected by surgery, swallowing and speech deficits are usually mild and temporary, and are often associated with postoperative edema. Oral transit may be slow, triggering of the swallow may be difficult, and speech may be slurred. Exercises that stress lingual range of motion and control help to expedite the return of swallowing function in the first 3 to 4 weeks postoperatively.[13] In most cases, the extent of tongue resection does not substantially affect long-term swallowing unless at least half of the tongue has been excised. Similarly, patients in whom at least half of the tongue has been preserved do not benefit from palatal augmentation prostheses.[14]

The tongue is the primary structure responsible for the production of most vowel and consonant sounds that are used in conversational speech. The tongue assumes three basic positions to convey most consonants: tongue-tip elevation (t, d, n, l, s, z, sh, ch, and zh), tongue-tip protrusion (th), and posterior-tongue elevation (k, g, ng). The production of vowel sounds depends on changes in the anterior-posterior and superior-inferior positions of the tongue. Surgical alterations of the tongue and oral cavity can change characteristics of vocal tract resonance such as pitch, nasality, and vocal quality. Although residual tongue structure and lingual mobility are essential to intelligibility, some patients are still able to produce intelligible speech despite the loss of the majority of their tongue.[15] Mechanisms for articulatory compensation may include exaggeration of labial, dental, pharyngeal, and laryngeal movements. Pharyngeal widening may be used for the articulation of high vowel sounds (i, e, and u) and a narrowing or compression of the pharynx for low vowel sounds (a and o).[16] Modifications of pitch, intonation, loudness, and vocal quality are also integral components of speech rehabilitation. Patients should be encouraged to maximize the use of nonverbal communication techniques that optimize understanding of the communicative intent.

Generally, resections of the oral cavity that preserve sensorimotor innervation in combination with reconstructions that allow the residual tongue to remain mobile result in better swallowing function and speech production. It is particularly important to preserve optimal function of the tongue base. Innervated cutaneous free flaps have been used in an attempt to restore normal lingual sensation, but the degree of functional recovery associated with sensate flap reconstructions requires further evaluation. Initial reports have suggested that sensate flaps may not significantly improve speech and swallowing.[17]

Palate Resection

The hard and soft palates are the key structures that contribute to the perception of nasal resonance. The hard palate comprises the roof of the mouth as well as the floor of the nose and the maxillary sinuses. The soft palate functions to seal the nasopharynx by making contact with the posterior pharyngeal wall, preventing nasal regurgitation during swallowing and air escape through the nasal cavity during speech production. The soft palate is also an integral component of the velopharyngeal mechanism. Occasionally, patients with normal swallowing function cannot maintain contact between the soft palate and base of tongue, which may result in the loss of a portion of the bolus over the tongue base with foods that require chewing. However, premature loss of food during swallows of liquids or foods with soft paste consistencies (such as pudding) is abnormal.[18]

Hard palate resections that result in oronasal fistulas are usually addressed at the time of surgery with a prosthetic obturator. Generally, patients who have undergone partial resection of the soft palate cannot be easily obturated and are therefore more difficult to rehabilitate than patients who have undergone total resection. Patients who have undergone total soft palate resection and who are adequately obturated usually swallow and speak with little difficulty.

◆ Functional Outcomes After Radiation Therapy

RT produces tissue changes that affect speech and swallowing immediately following treatment and that result in long-term adverse consequences. In general, RT has a more deleterious effect on swallowing than on speech.[19] RT frequently results in pain symptomatology that exacerbates swallowing problems and limits the patient's ability to maintain oral intake. The addition of chemotherapy is believed to exacerbate these effects. Furthermore, the cumulative adverse impact of RT on function can rival or exceed the sequelae from surgery.

The acute tissue reaction to RT follows a dose–response phenomenon. Early in the course of RT, changes in taste usually occur in concert with the development of tissue edema and erythema. Patients who receive oral irradiation experience mucositis and xerostomia that ultimately reduce lingual speed, slow the transit of food through the oral cavity, produce aberrant tongue movements, and slow the swallow reflex. These patients also experience difficulties with mastication and with formation and control of the bolus during the oral preparatory phase of the swallow, which in turn impairs the timing and coordination of the swallow. Patients often report clumsiness or slowness associated with articulatory precision and oral coordination, resulting in slurring of speech and reduced intelligibility. Xerostomia is associated with a decrease in salivary flow, and the saliva becomes thick, tenacious, ropy, and virtually impossible to swallow. The effects of xerostomia tend to be the most disturbing of all radiation sequelae because no effective management approach is available. The various medications, saliva substitutes, and oral rinses that are available do not provide permanent relief for these sequelae, and the associated side effects are often equally intolerable. Dietary modification that maximizes hydration and facilitates eating and swallowing to maintain daily caloric and nutritional requirements may be the best management strategy. Acidic and sharp-edged foods and extremely hot or cold foods should be avoided. Patients undergoing RT tend to develop aversions to foods with a particular taste or texture that may not necessarily resolve after the completion of RT.

Impairments in speech and swallowing that occur immediately following irradiation tend to resolve in concert with the resolution of treatment-induced edema and mucositis. Patients often report that they are able to speak with greater intelligibility and swallow more normally at this time. However, it is not uncommon for patients to experience functional deterioration several months to years after the completion of RT. These changes have been attributed to radiation-induced fibrosis, which can reduce the range of tongue, jaw, pharyngeal wall, and laryngeal motion, resulting in considerable functional impairment.[20]

Studies comparing swallowing function in patients at 6 months after RT with patients at 10 years after RT have shown similar disorders in swallowing. Thus, it is critical that irradiated patients are routinely referred for swallowing and speech intervention. The early institution of exercise protocols that are designed to strengthen and increase range of motion, precision, muscle elasticity, and mobility are associated with global improvements in oropharyngeal swallowing.[21,22]

◆ Conclusion

Patients who have received treatment for oral cancer and who develop functional impairment of speech and swallowing pose a variety of complex challenges to speech pathologists and other rehabilitation specialists, mandating the need to approach their issues from a multidisciplinary perspective. Early referral to a speech pathologist with expertise in rehabilitation after treatment for oral malignancy is critical to achieve a successful functional outcome. Patients should have the opportunity to meet with each member of the interdisciplinary team before head and neck cancer treatment is initiated. Baseline measurements of pretreatment speech and swallowing function are essential so that subsequent reassessment allows for the comparison of posttreatment outcomes with pretreatment status. Pretreatment counseling about expected posttreatment changes helps patients to maintain realistic expectations about their functional recovery, and they should be active participants in an aggressive rehabilitation program.

References

1. Kahrilas PJ, Logemann JA. Volume accommodation during swallowing. Dysphagia 1993;8:259–265
2. Kahrilas PJ, Lin S, Chen J, Logemann JA. Oropharyngeal accommodation to swallow volume. Gastroenterology 1996;111: 297–306
3. Logemann JA, Kahrilas PJ, Cheng J, et al. Closure mechanisms of laryngeal vestibule during swallow. Am J Physiol 1992;262(2 pt 1): G338–G344
4. Robbins J, Logemann JA, Kirshner H. Velopharyngeal activity during speech and swallowing in neurologic disease. Paper presented at the

American Speech-Language-Hearing Association annual meeting, Toronto, 1982

5. Palmer JB, Rudin NJ, Lara G, Crompton AW. Coordination of mastication and swallowing. Dysphagia 1992;7:187–200

6. Pouderoux P, Logemann JA, Kahrilas PJ. Pharyngeal swallowing elicited by fluid infusion: role of volition and vallecular containment. Am J Physiol 1996;270(2 pt 1):G347–G354

7. Logemann JA. Introduction: definitions and basic principles of evaluation and treatment of swallowing disorders. In: Berman D, ed. Evaluation and Treatment of Swallowing Disorders. Austin: Pro-Ed, 1998:1–11

8. Robbins J, Hamilton JW, Lof GL, Kempster GB. Oropharyngeal swallowing in normal adults of different ages. Gastroenterology 1992;103:823–829

9. Logemann JA, Pauloski BR, Rademaker AW, et al. Speech and swallow function after tonsil/base of tongue resection with primary closure. J Speech Hear Res 1993;36:918–926

10. McConnel FM, Pauloski BR, Logemann JA, et al. Functional results of primary closure vs flaps in oropharyngeal reconstruction: a prospective study of speech and swallowing. Arch Otolaryngol Head Neck Surg 1998;124:625–630

11. Allison GR, Rappaport I, Salibian AH, et al. Adaptive mechanisms of speech and swallowing after combined jaw and tongue reconstruction in long-term survivors. Am J Surg 1987;154:419–422

12. Ridley MB. Effects of surgery for head and neck cancer. In: Sullivan PA, Guilford AM, eds. Swallowing Intervention in Oncology. San Diego: Singular Publishing Group, 1999:84–85

13. Logemann JA. Swallowing disorders after treatment for oral and oropharyngeal cancer. In: Berman D, ed. Evaluation and Treatment for Oral and Oropharyngeal Cancer. Austin: Pro-Ed, 1998:251–279

14. Logemann JA, Bytell DE. Swallowing disorders in three types of head and neck surgical patients. Cancer 1979;44:1095–1105

15. LaBlance GR, Kraus K, Steckol KF. Rehabilitation of swallowing and communication following glossectomy. Rehabil Nurs 1991;16:266–270

16. Weber RS, Ohlms L, Bowman J, Jacob R, Goepfert H. Functional results after total or near total glossectomy with laryngeal preservation. Arch Otolaryngol Head Neck Surg 1991;117:512–515

17. Urken ML, Biller HF. A new bilobed design for the sensate radial forearm flap to preserve tongue mobility following significant glossectomy. Arch Otolaryngol Head Neck Surg 1994;120:26–31

18. Logemann JA. Disorders of deglutition. In: Berman D, ed. Evaluation and Treatment of Swallowing Disorders. Austin: Pro-Ed, 1998:89

19. Pauloski BR, Logemann JA, Rademaker AW, et al. Speech and swallowing function after oral and oropharyngeal resections: one-year follow-up. Head Neck 1994;16:313–322

20. Pauloski BR, Rademaker AW, Logemann JA, Colangelo LA. Speech and swallowing in irradiated and nonirradiated postsurgical oral cancer patients. Otolaryngol Head Neck Surg 1998;118:616–624

21. Lazarus CL, Logemann JA, Pauloski BR, et al. Swallowing disorders in head and neck cancer patients treated with radiotherapy and adjuvant chemotherapy. Laryngoscope 1996;106(9 pt 1):1157–1166

22. Lazarus CL. Effects of radiation therapy and voluntary maneuvers on swallow functioning in head and neck cancer patients. Clin Commun Disord 1993;3:11–20

28

Temporomandibular Disorder and Orofacial Pain

Henry A. Gremillion,
Franklin Dolwick, and
John W. Werning

Patients who have been successfully treated for oral cancer frequently redirect their concerns toward treatment-related issues that have adversely impacted their quality of life. Reconstructive surgery, osseointegrated implants, and prosthodontic therapy improve quality of life by providing predictable, measurable improvements in facial appearance and masticatory function. An understanding of the etiology and natural history of xerostomia and osteoradionecrosis has guided the application of intensity-modulated radiation therapy and pretreatment dental care to minimize the development of these complications. In contrast, the relationship between cancer treatment and the subsequent development of orofacial pain or temporomandibular dysfunction remains poorly defined, and limited options are available for its prevention and management. As a result, symptomatic patients are often treated with generic therapeutic modalities that inconsistently alleviate symptomatology and do not address the underlying etiology because objective diagnostic criteria and formal treatment guidelines have not been established. Physicians who treat patients for oral cancer must be familiar with the evaluation and management of patients with temporomandibular disorder and facial pain so that appropriate therapy is administered, and referral to dental professionals with special expertise in the management of orofacial pain can be expedited. This chapter reviews the normal anatomy and function of the masticatory system, and provides an overview of the diagnosis and management of temporomandibular disorder (TMD) and orofacial pain in the head and neck cancer patient.

◆ Normal Temporomandibular Joint Anatomy and Function

The temporomandibular joint (TMJ) is a bilateral synovial joint that is encapsulated by loose areolar connective tissue laterally, anterolaterally, and medially (**Fig. 28–1**). The posterior boundary is formed by the dynamic, vascular retrodiskal tissues. The anteromedial boundary is delineated by the superior belly of the lateral pterygoid muscle as it inserts into the articular disk and the mandibular condylar neck. The TMJ is divided internally by a biconcave fibrocartilaginous articular disk into superior and inferior compartments. The unique anatomy of the TMJ allows for the complex ginglymoarthrodial (hinging-gliding) movement necessary for optimum masticatory system function. Rotation or hinge movement occurs in the lower joint space, whereas translatory movement takes place in the upper joint space.

Several ligaments support the TMJ and passively restrict its border movements. The entire TMJ is encompassed by the capsular ligament, which extends from the neck of the condyle superiorly to articular surfaces of the mandibular fossa and articular eminence of the temporal bone. This ligament retains synovial fluid within the joint and resists medial, lateral, or inferior forces that tend to separate the articular surfaces. The capsular ligament also has proprioceptors that provide feedback regarding joint movement and position. The medial and lateral diskal ligaments, which are located within the TMJ deep to the capsular ligament, attach the articular disk to the medial and lateral poles of the condyle, respectively, and divide the joint into superior and inferior joint spaces. A third ligament, the temporomandibular ligament, limits the degree of rotational (hinging) movement of the condyle, so that no more than 20 to 25 mm of interincisal opening can be achieved without translation (gliding) of the condyle downward and forward across the surface of the articular eminence. The structural integrity of these ligaments is essential to the maintenance of normal TMJ function.[1]

The articular disk is composed of avascular, noninnervated fibrocartilage that is interposed between the condyle and the temporal bone. At rest with the mouth closed, the center of the disk should contact with the descending slope of the

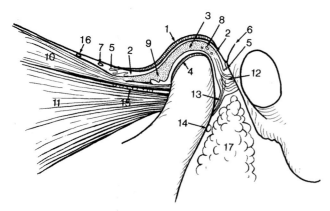

Figure 28–1 Parasagittal cut through the middle of the temporomandibular joint (TMJ), angled 25 degrees toward the anterior. 1, articular surface of glenoid fossa; 2, superior cavity; 3, disk (avascular); 4, articular surface of condyle; 5, synovial membranes; 6, squamotympanic suture; 7, masseteric nerve; 8, vascular knee of meniscus; 9, pes meniscus; 10, superior head of lateral pterygoid; 11, inferior head of lateral pterygoid; 12, superior stratum of bilaminar zone of meniscus; 13, inferior stratum of bilaminar zone of meniscus; 14, auriculotemporal nerve; 15, blood vessels; 16, posterior deep temporal nerve; 17, parotid gland. (From Mahan PE, Alling CC III, eds. Facial Pain, 3rd ed. Philadelphia: Lea & Febiger, 1991, with permission from Lippincott Williams & Wilkins.)

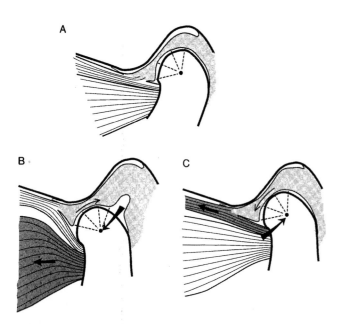

Figure 28–2 Relationship between the mandibular condyle, interarticular disk, and articular eminence during opening and closing of the mouth. The dotted lines represent the attachment of the articular disc at the lateral aspect of the temporomandibular joint condyle. **(A)** Condyle in fossa with mouth closed and both heads of lateral pterygoid muscle relaxed. **(B)** During mouth opening, the inferior head of the lateral pterygoid muscle is contracting (*shaded area*), pulling the condyle down the eminence. Because the superior head is not contracting, the disk rotates backward on the condyle. **(C)** During mouth closing, the superior head is contracting (in the active state) while it lengthens, because the condyle is translating back up into the glenoid fossa. This eccentric contraction serves to rotate the disk forward on the condyle during mouth closure to its normal position in the fossa. (From Mahan PE, Alling CC III, eds. Facial Pain, 3rd ed. Philadelphia: Lea & Febiger, 1991, with permission from Lippincott Williams & Wilkins.)

articular eminence superiorly, and with the anterior articular surface of the condyle inferiorly. During translation, maintenance of the proper position of the disk is reliant on normal disk morphology and interarticular pressure, structural integrity of the ligaments, and the contractile forces of the lateral pterygoid muscle. The lateral pterygoid muscle is composed of two heads that have antagonistic functions.[1–3] The *inferior* portion inserts on the neck of the condyle, and bilateral contraction pulls the mandibular condyles down the articular eminence, protruding the mandible. The *superior* portion inserts on the anteromedial region of the TMJ capsule, the disk, and the neck of the condyle. The resting muscle tone of the superior head maintains the disk in its anterior location within the mandibular fossa (**Fig. 28–2A**). During mouth opening (condylar translation), the inferior head contracts, pulling the condyle down the eminence, whereas the superior head does not contract, allowing the disk to slide posterior to the condyle (**Fig. 28–2B**). During mouth closure, the superior head contracts, which rotates the disk forward into its normal position within the mandibular fossa (**Fig. 28–2C**).

The TMJ receives sensory innervation from the auriculotemporal nerve and other branches of the mandibular portion of the trigeminal nerve (V3). The anteromedial aspect of the TMJ also receives innervation from branches of the maxillary division (V2).[4] The TMJ capsule also contains mechanoreceptors (Golgi tendon organs, pacinian corpuscles) and nociceptors.[5] Neuropeptides such as substance P and calcitonin gene-related peptides have been localized to the TMJ region.[6] Additional research is necessary to characterize how these neural pathways and neurotransmitters mediate pain transmission from the temporomandibular region.

◆ Clinical Examination

Because treatment for an underlying temporomandibular disorder frequently differs from therapy for treatment-induced injuries, patients should undergo evaluation prior to surgery or radiation therapy (RT) to determine whether temporomandibular pathology or other causes of orofacial pain are present. Otherwise, assessment following cancer treatment may preclude the clinician from distinguishing between a preexisting disorder and treatment-related pathologic changes.

A comprehensive physical examination of the patient includes inspection, palpation, auscultation, and measurement of the mandibular range of motion. Additionally, a thorough evaluation of the patient's occlusal function and masticatory functional ability is required. The patient's face should be evaluated for atrophy, hypertrophy, signs of infection or trauma (swelling, redness), deformity, and asymmetry.

The TMJ should be evaluated for tenderness by palpating laterally while at rest and posterolaterally during mandibular opening. Palpation pressure should be approximately 3 to 5 lb/in^2 (just enough to blanch the nail bed). Pain upon loading of the TMJ may be evaluated by gentle manipulation that seats the condyle superiorly and anteriorly, a maneuver that loads both TMJ complexes simultaneously.

The patient's biting on two stacked tongue blades that are placed between the most posterior occluding teeth unilaterally serves to load the contralateral joint. Joint sounds and their location during opening, closing, and excursive movements of the mandible may be detected with a stethoscope. It must be kept in mind that joint sounds such as clicking are a common finding in the general population and may not be related to the patient's chief pain concern. After each phase of the TMJ examination, the patient is asked to rate the level of pain experienced as follows: no pain, mild, moderate, or severe. The clinician should also ask the patient whether or not the pain experienced during the evaluation duplicates the symptomatology. Patterns of referred pain should also be documented.

Physiologic mandibular motion results from sensorimotor innervation that gives rise to a complex array of coordinated movements that occur between bilaterally normal TMJs and the masticatory musculature. Clinicians must understand normal TMJ anatomy and function as well as the relationship between masticatory muscular and temporomandibular function to appropriately assess for pathologic alterations in biomechanics. The examiner should note whether the line of vertical opening is straight and smooth, or deviates with jerky movements. The normal adult range of painless opening is 35 to 50 mm measured between the incisor teeth (interincisal distance), and overbite (the overlapping vertical distance between the incisal edges of opposing upper and lower incisors when the posterior teeth are in occlusion) is also measured. The normal range of protrusive and lateral movement is greater than or equal to 7 mm.

Palpation of the masticatory and cervical musculature is also performed to document areas of tenderness, taut bands, myofascial trigger points, and patterns of referred pain. Once again, the patient is asked to rate the level of pain and to describe whether the pain experienced upon palpation is similar to the presenting pain concern. Direct palpation of the lateral pterygoid muscle is not possible, so provocation testing is recommended. This can be accomplished by asking the patient to open slightly and protrude the mandible against firm, gentle resistance provided by placement of the clinician's fingers against the patient's chin. The clinician is cautioned not to distalize the mandible (forces directed posteriorly) due to the potential for compression of vascularized, innervated retrodiskal tissue.

Occlusal evaluation is accomplished through static and dynamic assessment. When the mandible is closed so that the teeth are in full occlusion, the relationship of the teeth is termed the maximum intercuspal position (ICP). The relationship of the teeth in the maximum intercuspal position is noted, and wear facets, fractures, mobility patterns, and migration of teeth are recorded. Occlusal relationships should also be recorded with the mandible in centric relation, which is a reproducible mandibular position where the condyles are located in the most superoanterior position within the articular fossae with the articular disks properly interposed.[1] Because occlusal relationships with the condyles in the centric relation position may differ from the occlusal relationships in ICP, deviations from centric relation occlusion to intercuspal position should be documented. In addition, contact between posterior cuspal inclines and anterior incisal edges during lateral excursion and anterior protrusion, respectively, should be recorded.

◆ Temporomandibular Disorder

Temporomandibular disorder (TMD) encompasses a group of conditions that affect the temporomandibular joint, the muscles of mastication, or associated structures, and is the most common non-odontogenic cause of masticatory system dysfunction.[1,7,8] Approximately 10 million Americans suffer from TMD-related complaints each year.[9,10] The conditions that constitute TMD are categorized as either arthrogenous TMD or myogenous TMD.

Arthrogenous Temporomandibular Disorder

Intracapsular pathology within the TMJ is classified as arthrogenous TMD. The most common sign of an arthrogenous TMD is TMJ clicking, although its presence does not consistently signify the presence of degenerative changes within the TMJ. General population-based studies have found that click-like sounds can be heard in approximately 50% of those studied.[11] An investigation with magnetic resonance imaging (MRI) found that joints with displacement of the articular disk were present in 25% of asymptomatic volunteers with no joint sounds versus 86% of patients with TMD ($p = .001$).[12] Several authors have attempted to correlate the number and timing of joint clicks that can be heard during mandibular motion with a continuum of progressive degenerative changes within the TMJ.[1,3] However, there is currently no convincing evidence that the development of, or changes in, TMJ clicking represents progressive joint degeneration.[13–15] Arthralgia is variably present in patients with arthrogenous TMD. Most degenerating joints tend to eventually become nonpainful, although approximately one sixth of these individuals experience long-term pain symptomatology.[15,16] Intracapsular TMD may develop from traumatic injuries such as hyperextension associated with intubation or forceful manipulation of the mandible during a surgical procedure. Clinicians must be able to recognize the presence of these conditions prior to radiation or surgical treatment to facilitate prompt referral, diagnosis and management, and to prevent the exacerbation of a preexisting arthrogenous TMD by RT or surgery.

Intracapsular Disorders

Synovitis, capsulitis, and retrodiskitis are defined as an inflammation of the synovial lining, capsular, and retrodiskal tissues of the TMJ, respectively. This inflammatory condition may be due to infection, systemic disease (i.e., autoimmune conditions), articular surface degeneration, or trauma (acute or chronic). Diagnostic criteria include (1) localized TMJ pain that is exacerbated by function, particularly with superior or posterior loading or palpation; and (2) the absence of extensive osteoarthritic changes on radiographic imaging. Other clinical findings that may be present include localized TMJ pain at rest, limited range of motion

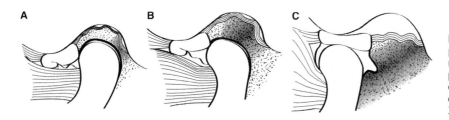

Figure 28–3 Biomechanics of the temporomandibular joint. Disk displacement with reduction. This condition is associated with reciprocal clicking (joint sounds on opening and closing). (Adapted from Okeson JP. Management of Temporomandibular Disorders and Occlusion, 3rd ed. St. Louis: Mosby-Year Book, 1993, with permission from Elsevier.)

secondary to pain, fluctuating swelling (due to joint effusion) that decreases the ability to occlude on the ipsilateral posterior teeth, and otalgia.

Internal derangement is defined as a disturbed arrangement of intracapsular joint parts causing interference with smooth joint movement. Internal derangements of the TMJ include elongation, tear, or rupture of the capsule or ligaments, resulting in alterations in disk position or morphology. The potential for these conditions to develop from acute trauma to the TMJ such as surgical manipulation is significant.

Disk displacement with reduction is associated with an abrupt alteration or interference of the structural relationship between the articular disk and the condyle during mandibular translation with mouth opening or closing (**Fig. 28–3**). Diagnostic criteria include (1) reproducible clicks that usually occur at variable positions during opening and closing mandibular movements, (2) soft tissue imaging (e.g., MRI) that reveals a displaced articular disk that reduces during jaw opening, and (3) hard tissue imaging that demonstrates the absence of extensive degenerative bone changes. Pain, when present, is precipitated by joint movement. A deviation of the mandible during opening typically coincides with a click, and momentary episodic disruptions in smooth jaw movements can occur during mouth opening.

Disk displacement without reduction (closed lock) is an altered or misaligned disk-condyle structural relationship that is maintained during mandibular translation (**Fig. 28–4**). Clinically, the patient presents with (1) persistent, marked limitations of mouth opening (<35 mm); (2) a history of sudden onset; (3) mandibular deflection to the affected side on mouth opening; (4) severely limited movement to the contralateral side; (5) soft tissue imaging that reveals a displaced disk without reduction upon opening; and (6) hard tissue imaging that reveals no evidence of extensive osteoarthritic changes. This condition may be painful or nonpainful, although pain may be precipitated by forced mouth opening. The patient may confirm a history of clicking that ceased with the onset of "locking." It is possible for gradual resolution of limited mouth opening to occur over time.

In contrast, TMJ dislocation (open lock, subluxation) is a condition in which the condyle is positioned anterior to the articular eminence and is unable to return to a closed position (**Fig. 28–5**). The cause of subluxation is usually not pathologic (there is no internal derangement), and it can spontaneously occur when the mouth is opened excessively wide (e.g., a yawn), or can result from forced mouth opening (e.g., during a dental procedure). The dislocation may be momentary or prolonged. Diagnostic criteria include (1) inability to close the mouth without a specific manipulative maneuver, (2) radiographic evidence revealing the condyle well beyond the articular eminence, and (3) pain associated with the dislocation with variable levels of pain after the episode.

Osteoarthritis (primary) is a degenerative condition of the joint characterized by deterioration and abrasion of the articular tissue with concomitant remodeling of the underlying subchondral bone due to a prior event (acute or repetitive) or disease that overloaded the joint remodeling mechanism. It is associated with pain during function, point tenderness upon palpation of the temporomandibular joint, limited range of motion with mandibular deviation to the affected side on opening, and crepitus or multiple joint noises. Hemarthrosis of the TMJ may occur with forceful mandibular manipulation such as may be associated with surgical procedures or intubation.

Myogenous Temporomandibular Disorder

Muscle-related signs and symptoms are also very common in the general population and in patient-based studies. In fact, conditions involving the masticatory musculature (extracapsular disorders) constitute the most common subgroup of TMD.[7,17] Individuals demonstrate variations in muscle anatomy, biomechanics, and fiber type and composition that differentially predispose a subset to muscle fatigue and discomfort. Moreover, excessive function resulting from parafunctional habits such as clenching or bruxism tends to exacerbate muscular fatigue and discomfort.

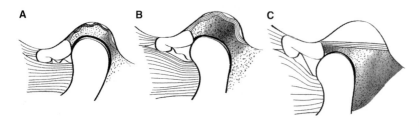

Figure 28–4 Biomechanics of the temporomandibular joint. Disk displacement without reduction, or closed lock. (Adapted from Okeson JP. Management of Temporomandibular Disorders and Occlusion, 3rd ed. St. Louis: Mosby-Year Book, 1993, with permission from Elsevier.)

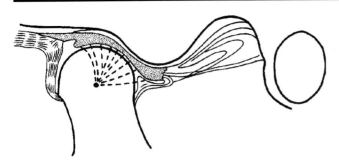

Figure 28–5 Condylar subluxation/dislocation. The condyle achieves a position anterior and superior to the articular eminence at maximum opening. (From Mahan PE, Alling CC III, eds. Facial Pain, 3rd ed. Philadelphia: Lea & Febiger, 1991, with permission from Lippincott Williams & Wilkins.)

Extracapsular Disorders

Myositis is inflammation of a muscle usually due to local causes such as infection or injury. Localized myositis (delayed-onset muscle soreness) is clinically expressed as increased pain with mandibular movement that occurs following prolonged or unaccustomed use (up to 48 hours afterward). The hallmarks of generalized myositis include pain (usually acute), tenderness over the entire region of the muscle, increased pain with mandibular movement, moderate to severely limited range of motion due to pain and swelling, and onset following injury or infection.

Protective muscle splinting is defined as restricted or guarded mandibular movement that results from co-contraction of muscles to avoid pain that is initiated by movement. Characteristics of protective muscle splinting include (1) severe pain with function (not at rest), (2) markedly limited range of motion without a significant increase in passive stretch, and (3) a history of some insult or injury to the area. The pain associated with a neoplastic process or treatment has great potential for initiating muscle splinting, which may have additive effects on the patient's global pain and dysfunction. Tumor extension or surgical resection can result in muscle splinting secondary to stimulation of sensory fibers that stimulate the maxillary and mandibular divisions of the trigeminal nerve, which transmit impulses to the principal sensory trigeminal nucleus in the pons and rostrally to the somatosensory cortex, where pain is registered (deep pain input). Some impulses are also transmitted to the trigeminal motor nucleus with activation of the efferent portion of the tonic reflex arc, leading to increased tonus of the muscles of mastication.[18]

Myospasm is an involuntary, sudden tonic contraction of a muscle that is associated with acute pain, continuous muscle contraction (fasciculation), altered mandibular posture, and increased electromyographic (EMG) activity at rest. Muscle spasm of the masticatory musculature is relatively rare and typically occurs in response to trauma (e.g., surgery, tumor invasion) or pain in the masticatory region or in contiguous structures, resulting in *trismus*.

Myofascial pain is defined as a regional, dull, aching muscle pain with the presence of localized sites of tenderness (trigger points) in muscle, tendon, or fascia. Patients present with a history that may include pain with function (chewing, talking), parafunctional habits (bruxism, clenching), postural

dysfunction, tension headaches, ear signs and symptoms (otalgia, tinnitus, fullness, disequilibrium), or toothache-like pain (endodontic tests are normal). Clinical findings include (1) limited interincisal opening, which is increased with passive stretch by >4 mm; (2) alterations in mandibular range of motion; (3) dull/aching pain (may be generalized or localized); (4) tenderness of the masticatory muscles; and (5) trigger points with referred pain to other sites. Palpation of trigger points may produce autonomic symptoms and secondary hyperalgesia in the area of referred pain. Myofascial pain is the most commonly experienced myogenous pain other than intermittent postexercise related phenomena. It may result from excessive contraction associated with clenching, bruxism, or excessive stretching or mouth opening (e.g., endotracheal intubation).

Contracture (chronic trismus, muscle fibrosis, muscle scarring) is chronic resistance of a muscle to passive stretch as a result of fibrosis of the supporting tendons, ligaments, or muscle fibers themselves. This condition may be reversible (myostatic contracture) or irreversible (myofibrotic contracture). Clinical characteristics include (1) limited range of mandibular motion (hypomobility), (2) unyielding firmness on passive stretch, and (3) a history of trauma or infection. Fibrosis followed by scar contracture may arise in the muscles of mastication or the muscles of facial expression after irradiation or surgery, resulting in trismus.

◆ Etiology and Management of Temporomandibular Disorder

The causative factors that lead to TMD include (1) trauma, (2) occlusal factors, (3) emotional stress, (4) deep pain input, and (5) parafunctional activity.[1] Examples of definitive treatment for TMD that is caused by each of these factors include, respectively, (1) avoidance or prevention of trauma (soft mouth guards for contact sports); (2) occlusal therapy (acrylic appliance therapy, occlusal adjustment via selective grinding or restorative dentistry); (3) therapy to reduce emotional stress (counseling, biofeedback, behavioral modification); (4) identification and management of sources of deep pain input (cervical myalgia, neoplasm); and (5) minimization of parafunctional activity (patient education, occlusal appliance therapy). Nonspecific supportive therapies that treat symptoms include analgesics (acetaminophen), nonsteroidal (ibuprofen, naproxen) and steroidal antiinflammatory medications, anxiolytics (diazepam, clonazepam), muscle relaxants (metaxalone, cyclobenzaprine), antidepressants (selective serotonin reuptake inhibitors), and local anesthetics.[1] The administration of supportive (symptomatic) therapy and definitive cause-specific therapy requires accurate diagnosis and identification of the initiating factors as well as any perpetuating factors that prevent resolution or exacerbate the progression of TMD.

The coexistence of more than one TMD may contribute to a particular patient's clinical picture, requiring the application of multimodality therapy. For example, acute mandibular trauma that results in hemarthrosis, capsular and intracapsular ligamentous injury, and articular disk trauma will also

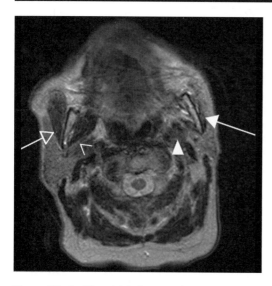

Figure 28–6 T2-weighted magnetic resonance image (MRI) that demonstrates denervation atrophy of the left masseter (*arrow*) and medial pterygoid muscle (*arrowhead*) in a patient with oral cancer. The high signal intensity of the atrophied muscles represents fatty replacement. The cross-sectional muscle area of the right masseter (*open arrow*) and medial pterygoid muscles (*open arrowhead*) is normal. The high signal intensity within the mandible represents the marrow space, which is surrounded by cortical bone (low signal intensity). The other MRIs demonstrated enlargement of the left foramen ovale, consistent with retrograde perineural tumor invasion.

result in deep pain that initiates protective muscle splinting, or protective co-contraction. In this case, the clinical picture is a consequence of overlapping arthrogenous and myogenous TMDs, and therapy must be tailored to address the patient's symptoms as well as any inciting factors.

◆ Malignant Neoplasms and Temporomandibular Disorder

Patients with head and neck cancer can present with orofacial pain or signs and symptoms suggestive of TMD.[19–21] Investigators from the University of Washington documented four patients with malignant neoplasms who were initially diagnosed with a TMD, leading to a delay in diagnosis ranging from 1.5 to 8 years.[22] Perineural invasion from cancer of the oral cavity or pharynx may result in referred pain to the temporomandibular region, and denervation atrophy of the masticatory muscles due to V3 involvement can occur as a consequence of direct invasion from the oral cavity or oropharynx into the infratemporal fossa.[23] Retrograde perineural invasion from the inferior alveolar nerve can also lead to pain or denervation atrophy (**Fig. 28–6**). Sensory deficits such as hypesthesia or paresthesia occasionally develop in combination with motor deficits.[24] Limitations of mandibular motion may also develop from tumor infiltration into the pterygoid or temporalis muscles.[19,25,26]

Differentiation between a malignant process and a nonneoplastic orofacial pain disorder or TMD can usually be achieved through careful clinical assessment. A comprehensive examination of the mucosal surfaces of the oral cavity and pharynx should be routinely conducted at the time of initial presentation. A low threshold should be maintained for atypical signs and symptoms or unusual examination findings. Cutaneous sensory loss, focal motor denervation, or palpable intraoral or preauricular masses should elevate the concern about a neoplasm. Radiographic imaging is an invaluable tool that should be employed whenever clinical findings provide an inconsistent picture.

◆ Trismus

Trismus is broadly defined as the presence of restricted mandibular opening, regardless of etiology. Unfortunately, there is a lack of consensus regarding the degree of restricted mouth opening that establishes the diagnosis of trismus. A systematic review of the peer-reviewed literature documented a range of values from 20 to 40 mm of mouth opening.[27] Causes of trismus can be categorized as congenital, traumatic, neoplastic, neuromuscular, reactive, psychogenic, or drug-induced. Trismus can be an acute (myospasm) or chronic (contracture or muscle fibrosis) manifestation of myogenous TMD. The recent onset of trismus in a patient with a malignancy of the oral cavity or pharynx is suggestive of pterygoid muscle invasion.[19,25,26] Treatments for oral cancer are also frequent causes of trismus as a result of reactive, traumatic, or neuromuscular alterations of the masticatory apparatus. Significant impairment in mandibular function is perceived by patients with cancer of the oral cavity or oropharynx who demonstrate less than 35 mm of mandibular opening.[28] These patients manifest difficulties with eating and oral hygiene, and dental care delivery is also less feasible.[29] The following section reviews some of the most important causes of treatment-induced trismus and other disorders involving the temporomandibular region.

◆ Temporomandibular Disorder and Orofacial Pain Following Oral Cancer Therapy

Surgery

Soft tissue fibrosis following the resection of tumors involving the buccal mucosa, retromolar trigone, or tonsillar fossa can result in surgically induced trismus. Contracture may occur if the resection included violation of the masseter, temporalis, or pterygoid musculature. However, limitations in mouth opening can develop from more superficial resections of the buccal soft tissues in the absence of masticatory muscle injury if significant fibrosis occurs.[30]

Performance of a mandibulotomy involves lateral rotation of the divided mandible to gain access into the oral cavity and oropharynx for resection and reconstruction. Because lateral rotation of the mandible is not a physiologic position, stretching or tearing of the ligaments of the TMJ, which were intended to passively restrict physiologic border movements, is possible. Although the positional relationship between the condyle, disk, and glenoid fossa with the mandible in a lateralized position has not been characterized, the likelihood that pathologic interarticular pressure could result in direct trauma to these structures exists. Postoperative malocclusion resulting from imprecise repositioning and plate fixation of the mandible may also result in myogenous pain.

Only a few investigators have attempted to characterize the relationship between mandibulotomy and TMD. A retrospective investigation from the University of Pittsburgh evaluated 23 patients who underwent mandibulotomy (mean duration of follow-up, 24 months).[31] A median mandibular opening distance of 45 mm (range, 10–65 mm) was documented, and only one patient was reported to have trismus, with mandibular opening of 10 mm. Mediolateral deviation during opening also occurred (median, 3.3 mm; range, 0–11 mm). Seventeen percent of the patients reported pain in the TMJ region. Investigators from the University of Pennsylvania reported that trismus did not develop in 30 patients who underwent midline mandibulotomy (mean duration of follow-up, 28 months), although measurements of mandibular opening were not recorded and orofacial pain was not assessed. None of the patients in either study had postoperative malocclusion.

Mandibulectomy or posterior tooth extractions that alter the occlusal vertical dimension can result in pathologic forces within the TMJ that lead to bony remodeling.[32–34] The functional impact of mandibulectomy with loss of mandibular continuity was also evaluated by the investigators from the University of Pittsburgh in 39 patients (mean duration of follow-up, 48 months). Most of these patients received a soft tissue reconstruction, so the findings do not apply to patients who have reestablishment of mandibular continuity with a bridging reconstruction plate or osseous reconstruction (e.g., fibula free flap). Thirteen percent of the patients complained of temporomandibular pain symptomatology. A median mandibular opening distance of 51.5 mm (range, 30–75 mm) was documented, whereas the median mediolateral deviation upon opening was 10 mm (range, 0–25 mm). The authors reported that trismus did not occur in any of these patients, and postoperative malocclusion was present in one patient.

The retrospective nature of these studies provides limited insight into the relationship between mandibular surgery and orofacial pain or TMD. Prospective evaluation that includes objective baseline assessments of temporomandibular function and occlusion as well as subjective evaluation using validated survey instruments is necessary, and the impact of radiation therapy or reconstructive surgery with flaps must also be considered.

There are only limited data pertaining to masticatory performance following mandibulotomy or mandibulectomy. Marunick et al[35,36] prospectively evaluated masticatory performance preoperatively and postoperatively by asking patients to chew Frito corn chips (Frito-Lay, Dallas TX), and analyzing particle size following 15 or 30 chewing strokes. Postoperative masticatory performance scores were adversely affected by tooth loss and surgery, whereas prosthodontic rehabilitation following surgery improved masticatory performance. Larger prospective investigations are required to clarify the impact that different surgical procedures can have on masticatory function.

Radiation Therapy

Orofacial pain and TMD following radiation therapy for cancer of the oral cavity, pharynx, or parotid gland has been extensively documented.[37–41] Trismus and pain can also occur following intensity-modulated radiation therapy.[40,42] In a recent review of 849 patients treated for nasopharyngeal cancer, trismus developed in 12% of the patients at a median duration of 35 months following treatment.[41] The frequency and severity of impairment is directly related to the dose of radiation administered, and irradiation of the pterygoid musculature appears to be a more critical factor than irradiation of the TMJ.[37,41] In a prospective evaluation of 24 patients with nasopharyngeal cancer who were treated with external beam radiation to a total dose of 68.4 to 70.2 Gy, maximal interincisal distance decreased by 2.4% per month during the 9 months following irradiation.[38] Mouth opening continued to decrease by 0.2% per month 12 to 24 months following treatment and 0.1% per month 24 to 48 months following treatment. Goldstein et al[37] prospectively evaluated the effects of external beam radiation in 58 patients treated for head and neck cancer by measuring mouth opening (maximal vertical dimension) and through use of the Helkimo Masticatory Dysfunction Index (HMDI), which assesses the range of jaw movement, TMJ function, pain on mandibular movement, pain on palpation of the masticatory muscles, and TMJ pain. Measurements were obtained 6 to 12 months after completion of RT. These results were correlated with the RT doses to the TMJ and the pterygoid muscles for each patient. Mouth opening decreased in 86% of the patients. Larger decrements in mouth opening were directly associated with increasing radiation doses to either the TMJ or the pterygoid muscles. However, greater decreases in mandibular dysfunction, as measured by the HMDI, were observed secondary to irradiation of the pterygoid muscles than irradiation of the TMJ.

Radiation-induced fibrosis (RIF) is the primary cause of trismus that develops following radiation therapy (RT).[43,44] RIF is a form of late radiation toxicity that typically evolves over the course of months to years as a consequence of gradually diminishing vascular supply.[45] An investigation that used serial computed tomography demonstrated that RT resulted in decrements in the cross-sectional muscle area of the masseter and medial pterygoid muscles at rates of 3.9% and 2.3% per year, respectively. Histologically, RIF is characterized by the presence of inflammatory cells, atypical fibroblasts, and large quantities of various extracellular matrix components.[46] Cytokines such as transforming growth factor-β (TGF-β) and platelet-derived growth factor are produced in response to radiation, with TGF-β acting as the primary modulator of fibrogenesis.[47]

◆ Management of Temporomandibular Disorder Caused by Surgery or Radiation

The relative impact of surgery or RT on posttreatment symptoms and function cannot be accurately assessed unless an adequate pretreatment clinical evaluation was also conducted. Proper diagnostic assessment that differentiates between arthrogenous TMD and myogenous TMD and its causes provides important prognostic information and allows the implementation of cause-specific therapy.

Myogenous TMD may be effectively managed using pharmacotherapeutic approaches. The administration of centrally acting skeletal muscle relaxants in combination with an analgesic agent can reduce muscle spasm and pain that may also allow the patient to comfortably increase mandibular opening. Centrally acting muscle relaxants such as Soma® and Flexeril® diminish the output of nerve impulses to voluntary muscle and are pharmacologically similar to sedative-hypnotics and antianxiety agents that act as mild sedatives. Diazepam, an anxiolytic, potentiates the action of γ-aminobutyric acid (GABA), which mediates presynaptic and postsynaptic inhibition in the central nervous system and is an effective skeletal muscle relaxant when used at low doses (2 mg four times a day). Baclofen (Lioresal®), a muscle relaxant, can also effectively relieve postradiation contracture by decreasing the frequency and severity of muscle spasm. Baclofen exerts its effects on GABA receptors, depressing excitatory synaptic transmission in the spinal trigeminal nucleus.[48]

Surgically induced fibrosis can be minimized following resection of buccal tissues that do not extend to the masseter muscle by skin graft placement. If tumor resection can be achieved without performing a mandibulotomy, the risk of intracapsular injury may be reduced, although trauma during excessive, prolonged mouth opening is also possible. When mandibulotomy is performed, lateral mandibular rotation should be gently performed so that ligamentous injury and pathologic interarticular forces are minimized. Precise mandibular reapproximation following resection is critical so that the preoperative occlusion is perfectly reproduced. If mandibular resection results in loss of mandibular continuity, restoration of continuity should be achieved via osseous microvascular reconstruction. Mandibular reconstruction must also reestablish the premorbid mandibular arch form to ensure that the physiologic positional relationship among the condyle, disk, and glenoid fossa at rest remains undisturbed (**Fig. 28–2A**), and normal shifts in the condyle-disk-glenoid fossa relationship are able to occur during the process of translation and mouth closure. Alterations in condylar position may lead to intracapsular pathology as well as extracapsular symptomatology secondary to asymmetric masticatory muscle loading, potentially resulting in myospasm or myofascial pain.

A variety of methods have been used to mechanically increase mandibular opening in patients with trismus.[49] Tongue blades can be serially wedged between stacked tongue blades that have been inserted between the upper and lower teeth. Therabite® (Atos Medical AB, Horby, Sweden) has been shown to significantly increase the interincisal opening in patients with RIF when compared with the use of tongue blades.[50] A surgically placed modified distraction device has also been used to correct RIF by stretching fibrotic soft tissue.[51] Such mechanical methods should also have applicability in patients with trismus resulting from surgically induced fibrosis. Although physical rehabilitation appears to be an essential component of posttreatment management, mandibular range of motion exercises performed concurrently with RT can be employed to prevent RIF.[52] Coronoidectomy with detachment of the temporalis insertion followed by aggressive postsurgical physical therapy generally improves reductions in mandibular opening that have occurred secondary to fibromyositis of the temporalis muscle and is the procedure of choice. Braun[53] reported that patients who had a postsurgical opening of less than 30 mm did not improve unless professionally guided physiotherapy was undertaken.

Other approaches to the management of RIF in the head and neck region have been investigated. Impedance-controlled microcurrent therapy resulted in subjective improvements in trismus in 62% of evaluated patients.[44] A growing body of evidence supports a role for pentoxifylline (PTX) in the treatment of RIF. PTX, which is used in the treatment of peripheral vascular disease, has been shown to result in measurable improvements in extremity range of motion and postirradiation fibrosis involving the neck, chest wall, and pelvis.[54,55] A prospective investigation of PTX for the treatment of RIF in patients who were treated for head and neck cancer documented decreased rates of soft tissue necrosis and fibrosis.[56] A prospective investigation that evaluated the efficacy of PTX in the treatment of trismus resulting from RIF has also been published.[43] Treatment with PTX at a dose of 400 mg three times daily for 8 weeks resulted in a mean increase in mandibular opening of 4 mm ($p = .023$). The addition of α-tocopherol (vitamin E) has been shown to augment the treatment effect in some studies.[55] The precise mechanism by which PTX reduces RIF is unknown. PTX improves tissue oxygenation and microcirculation by increasing oxygen release from red blood cells, increasing red cell deformability, and decreasing blood viscosity.[57] The drug also manifests immunomodulatory properties, which may include downregulation of TGF-β.[58]

◆ Conclusion

The impact that TMD has on the quality of life of patients treated for head and neck cancer is significantly underestimated. Surgery and RT can lead to various intracapsular and extracapsular disorders that, if properly diagnosed, can be treated with definitive cause-specific therapy and supportive symptom-reducing therapy. Evaluation of temporomandibular and masticatory function prior to cancer treatment is critical to appreciate the relative impact of treatment on posttreatment function and symptomatology. Clinicians who treat head and neck cancer should understand the principles of evaluation and management of TMD and orofacial pain so that prompt diagnosis is made and referral to a dentist with expertise in the management of TMD can be expedited. The development and refinement of validated measures of temporomandibular function in patients treated for head and neck cancer, and prospective investigation of novel therapeutic approaches for treatment-induced TMD are essential to improve the diagnostic assessment and care of these patients.

References

1. Okeson JP. Management of Temporomandibular Disorders and Occlusion, 5th ed. Philadelphia: Mosby, 2003

2. Mahan PE, Wilkinson TM, Gibbs CH, Mauderli A, Brannon LS. Superior and inferior bellies of the lateral pterygoid muscle EMG activity at basic jaw positions. J Prosthet Dent 1983;50:710–718

3. Mahan PE, Alling CCI. Temporomandibular joint anatomy, function, and pathofunction. In: Mahan PE, Alling CCI, eds. Facial Pain, 3rd ed. Philadelphia: Lea & Febiger, 1991:198–217

4. Davidson JA, Metzinger SE, Tufaro AP, Dellon AL. Clinical implications of the innervation of the temporomandibular joint. J Craniofac Surg 2003;14:235–239

5. Wink CS, Onge MS, Zimmy ML. Neural elements in the human temporomandibular articular disc. J Oral Maxillofac Surg 1992;50:334–337

6. Kido MA, Kiyoshima T, Kondo T, et al. Distribution of substance P and calcitonin gene-related peptide-like immunoreactive nerve fibers in the rat temporomandibular joint. J Dent Res 1993;72:592–598

7. Dworkin SF, Huggins KH, LeResche L, et al. Epidemiology of signs and symptoms in temporomandibular disorders: clinical signs in cases and controls. J Am Dent Assoc 1990;120:273–281

8. Lipton JA, Ship JA, Larach-Robinson D. Estimated prevalence and distribution of reported orofacial pain in the United States. J Am Dent Assoc 1993;124:115–121

9. National Institutes of Health Technology Assessment Conference Statement. Management of temporomandibular disorders. J Am Dent Assoc 1996;127:1595–1606

10. Slavkin HC. A lifetime of motion: temporomandibular joints. J Am Dent Assoc 1996;127:1093–1098

11. Wabeke KB, Spruijt RJ. On Temporomandibular Joint Sounds: Dental and Psychological Studies. Amsterdam: University of Amsterdam, 1994

12. Ribeiro RF, Tallents RH, Katzberg RW, et al. The prevalence of disc displacement in symptomatic and asymptomatic volunteers aged 6 to 25 years. J Orofac Pain 1997;11:37–47

13. Nikerson JW, Boering G. Natural course of osteoarthrosis as it relates to internal derangement of the temporomandibular joint. Oral Maxillofac Surg Clin North Am 1989;1:1–19

14. de Bont LG, Dijkgraaf LC, Stegenga B. Epidemiology and natural progression of articular temporomandibular disorders. Oral Surg Oral Med Oral Pathol Oral Radiol Endod 1997;83:72–76

15. de Leeuw R, Boering G, Stegenga B, de Bont LG. Clinical signs of TMJ osteoarthrosis and internal derangement 30 years after nonsurgical treatment. J Orofac Pain 1994;8:18–24

16. Toller PA. Osteoarthrosis of the mandibular condyle. Br Dent J 1973; 134:223–231

17. Schiffman EL, Fricton JR, Haley DP, Shapiro BL. The prevalence and treatment needs of subjects with temporomandibular disorders. J Am Dent Assoc 1990;120:295–303

18. Kveton JF, Pillsbury HC. "How I do it"–head and neck. A targeted problem and its solution. Breaking trismus to facilitate drainage of peritonsillar abscess. Laryngoscope 1980;90(11 pt 1):1892–1893

19. Cohen SG, Quinn PD. Facial trismus and myofascial pain associated with infections and malignant disease: report of five cases. Oral Surg Oral Med Oral Pathol 1988;65:538–544

20. Christiansen EL, Thompson JR, Appleton SS. Temporomandibular joint pain/dysfunction overlying more insidious diseases: report of two cases. J Oral Maxillofac Surg 1987;45:335–337

21. Orlean SL, Robinson NR, Ahern JP, Mallon CF, Blewitt G. Case report. Carcinoma of maxillary sinus manifested by temporomandibular joint pain dysfunction syndrome. J Oral Med 1966;21:127–131

22. Mostafapour SP, Futran ND. Tumors and tumorous masses presenting as temporomandibular joint syndrome. Otolaryngol Head Neck Surg 2000;123:459–464

23. Ariji Y, Fuwa N, Tachibana H, Ariji E. Denervation atrophy of the masticatory muscles in a patient with nasopharyngeal cancer: MR examinations before and after radiotherapy. Dentomaxillofac Radiol 2002;31:204–208

24. Carter RL, Pittam MR, Tanner NSB. Pain and dysphagia in patients with squamous carcinomas of the head and neck: the role of perineural spread. J R Soc Med 1982;75:598–606

25. Hauser MS, Boraski J. Oropharyngeal carcinoma presenting as an odontogenic infection with trismus. Oral Surg Oral Med Oral Pathol 1986;61:330–332

26. Ariji Y, Fuwa N, Toyama M, Katoh M, Gotoh M, Ariji E. MR features of masticatory muscles in adenoid cystic carcinoma involving the masticator space. Dentomaxillofac Radiol 2004;33:345–350

27. Dijkstra PU, Kalk WWI, Roodenburg JLN. Trismus in head and neck oncology: a systematic review. Oral Oncol 2004;40:879–889

28. Dijkstra PU, Huisman PM, Roodenburg JLN. Criteria for trismus in head and neck oncology. Int J Oral Maxillofac Surg 2006;35:337–342; Epub 2005 Nov 8

29. Eanes WC. A review of the considerations in the diagnosis of limited mandibular opening. Cranio 1991;9:137–144

30. Beekhuis GJ, Harrington EB. Trismus. Etiology and management of inability to open the mouth. Laryngoscope 1965;75:1234–1258

31. Christopoulos E, Carrau R, Segas J, Johnson JT, Myers EN, Wagner RL. Transmandibular approaches to the oral cavity and oropharynx: a functional assessment. Arch Otolaryngol Head Neck Surg 1992;118: 1164–1167

32. Pirttiniemi P, Kantomaa T, Salo L, Tuominen M. Effect of reduced articular function on deposition of type I and type II collagens in the mandibular condylar cartilage of the rat. Arch Oral Biol 1996;41: 127–131

33. Sim Y, Carlson DS, McNamara JA Jr. Condylar adaptation after alteration of vertical dimension in adult rhesus monkeys, Macaca mulatta. Cranio 1995;13:182–187

34. Rashed MZ, Sharawy MM. Histopathological and immunocytochemical studies of the effect of raised occlusal vertical dimension on the condylar cartilage of the rabbit. Cranio 1993;11:291–296

35. Marunick M, Mahmassani O, Siddway J, Klein B. Prospective analysis of masticatory function following lateral mandibulotomy. J Surg Oncol 1991;47:92–97

36. Marunick MT, Mathes BE, Klein BB. Masticatory function in hemimandibulectomy patients. J Oral Rehabil 1992;19:289–295

37. Goldstein M, Maxymiw WG, Cummings BJ, Wood RE. The effects of antitumour irradiation on mandibular opening and mobility: a prospective study of 58 patients. Oral Surg Oral Med Oral Pathol Oral Radiol Endod 1999;88:365–373

38. Wang CJ, Huang EY, Hsu HC, Chen HC, Fang FM, Hsiung CY. The degree and time-course assessment of radiation-induced trismus occurring after radiotherapy for nasopharyngeal cancer. Laryngoscope 2005; 115:1458–1460

39. Karakoyun-Celik O, Norris CM, Tishler R, et al. Definitive radiotherapy with interstitial implant boost for squamous cell carcinoma of the tongue base. Head Neck 2005;27:353–361

40. Chao KS, Ozyigit G, Blanco AI, et al. Intensity-modulated radiation therapy for oropharyngeal carcinoma: impact of tumor volume. Int J Radiat Oncol Biol Phys 2004;59:43–50

41. Yeh SA, Tang Y, Lui CC, Huang YJ, Huang EY. Treatment outcomes and late complications of 849 patients with nasopharyngeal carcinoma treated with radiotherapy. Int J Radiat Oncol Biol Phys 2005; 62:672–679

42. Lee N, Xia P, Quivey JM, et al. Intensity-modulated radiotherapy in the treatment of nasopharyngeal carcinoma: an update of the UCSF experience. Int J Radiat Oncol Biol Phys 2002;53:12–22

43. Chua DTT, Lo C, Yuen J, Foo YC. A pilot study of pentoxifylline in the treatment of radiation-induced trismus. Am J Clin Oncol 2001;24: 366–369

44. Lennox A, Shafer JP, Hatcher M, Beil J, Funder SJ. Pilot study of impedance-controlled microcurrent therapy for managing radiation-induced fibrosis in head-and-neck cancer patients. Int J Radiat Oncol Biol Phys 2002;54:23–34

45. Bentzen SM, Thames HD, Overgaard M. Latent-time estimation for late cutaneous and subcutaneous radiation reactions in a single-follow-up clinical study. Radiother Oncol 1989;15:267–274

46. Brocheriou C, Verola O, Lefaix JL, Daburon F. Histopathology of cutaneous and subcutaneous irradiation-induced injuries. Br J Radiol Suppl 1986;19:101–104

47. Canney PA, Dean S. Transforming growth factor beta: a promoter of late connective tissue injury following radiotherapy? Br J Radiol 1990;63:620–623

48. Storer RJ, Akerman S, Goadsby PJ. GABA receptors modulate trigeminovascular nociceptive neurotransmission in the trigeminocervical complex. Br J Pharmacol 2001;134:896–904

49. Lund TW, Cohen JI. Trismus appliances and indications for use. Quintessence Int 1993;24:275–279

50. Buchbinder D, Currivan RB, Kaplan AJ, Urken ML. Mobilization regimens for the prevention of jaw hypomobility in the radiated patient: a comparison of three techniques. J Oral Maxillofac Surg 1993; 51:863–867

51. Nicholls DW, Lowe N. Use of a modified distraction appliance to treat radiation-induced trismus. J Oral Maxillofac Surg 2003;61:972–974

52. Jansma J, Vissink A, Spijkervet FK, et al. Protocol for the prevention and treatment of oral sequelae resulting from head and neck radiation therapy. Cancer 1992;70:2171–2180

53. Braun BL. The effect of physical therapy intervention on incisal opening after temporomandibular joint surgery. Oral Surg Oral Med Oral Pathol 1987;64:544–548

54. Okunieff P, Augustine E, Hicks JE, et al. Pentoxifylline in the treatment of radiation-induced fibrosis. J Clin Oncol 2004;22:2207–2213

55. Delanian S, Porcher R, Balla-Mekias S, Lefaix JL. Randomized, placebo-controlled trial of combined pentoxifylline and tocopherol for regression of superficial radiation-induced fibrosis. J Clin Oncol 2003;21:2545–2550

56. Aygenc E, Celikkanat S, Kaymakci M, Aksaray F, Ozdem C. Prophylactic effect of pentoxifylline on radiotherapy complications: a clinical study. Otolaryngol Head Neck Surg 2004;130:351–356

57. Ward A, Clissold SP. Pentoxifylline: a review of its pharmacodynamic and pharmacokinetic properties, and its therapeutic efficacy. Drugs 1987;34:50–97

58. Dezube BJ, Sherman ML, Fridovich-Keil JL, Allen-Ryan J, Pardee AB. Down-regulation of tumor necrosis factor expression by pentoxifylline in cancer patients: a pilot study. Cancer Immunol Immunother 1993;36:57–60

29

Chemoprevention

Sanjay R. Jain,
Fadlo R. Khuri, and
John W. Werning

Refinements in the treatment of patients with head and neck squamous cell carcinoma (HNSCC) have yielded minimal improvement in disease-specific survival during the past 30 years. As investigators continue to search for more effective ways to treat patients with head and neck cancer, it is essential to evaluate methods to prevent the development of HNSCC. Abstention from exposure to carcinogenic agents such as tobacco, alcohol, and betel nuts is the most rational approach to the prevention of cancer involving the upper aerodigestive tract. Continued smoking by patients who were previously treated for HNSCC has also been shown to adversely impact disease-free survival.[1] Chemoprevention, which is the administration of agents that block or reverse carcinogenesis, is an area of active investigation that has the potential to decrease the incidence of, and mortality associated with, HNSCC.[2] Chemoprevention has been successfully used to decrease the risk of breast cancer by the administration of tamoxifen, and research findings also suggest that chemoprevention with nonsteroidal antiinflammatory drugs or cyclooxygenase inhibitors may eventually play a role in reducing the risk of colon cancer.[3–5] This chapter reviews the principles of chemoprevention and the evidence supporting its role as a method to decrease cancer incidence in patients with oral premalignant lesions (OPLs) and in individuals at risk for second primary tumors (SPTs).

◆ Oral Premalignant Lesions

Oral leukoplakia and erythroplakia are surface manifestations of mucosal abnormalities that on histologic examination may demonstrate hyperplasia, hyperkeratosis, dysplasia, or carcinoma. An investigation of 257 patients with oral leukoplakia found that 18% of leukoplakic lesions progressed to invasive cancer within 7 years, and 36% of dysplastic lesions evolved into invasive malignant disease.[6] Erythroplakia is similarly associated with a 30 to 40% long-term risk of oral cancer.[7] The natural history of oral leukoplakia and erythroplakia is variable, and present diagnostic techniques are not able to consistently predict the likelihood of carcinogenic progression or regression within a particular lesion (see Chapter 4). A chemopreventive agent that disrupts carcinogenic progression in OPLs would markedly reduce the incidence of oral cancer.

◆ Second Primary Tumors

In the 1950s, Slaughter et al[8] observed that the normal-appearing mucosa surrounding oral squamous cell carcinoma demonstrated changes consistent with dysplasia. The concept of *field cancerization* provides a plausible explanation for the development of local recurrences following cancer treatment, as well as the increased risk of SPTs in patients who have been diagnosed with HNSCC. Field cancerization occurs in patients with carcinoma of the oral cavity, oropharynx, larynx, lung, and esophagus as a result of diffuse epithelial injury that is caused primarily by inhaled carcinogens. In patients who have been successfully treated for HNSCC, SPTs develop at a rate of 4 to 6% annually for at least 8 years after the original cancer was diagnosed, and the lifetime risk of a SPT is over 20%.[7,9,10] The process of field cancerization results from the accumulation of genetic alterations in injured epithelial cells that lead to carcinogenic progression from a normal cell to a cancer cell, a process that has been explained by a genetic progression model, the *theory of multistep carcinogenesis*. Disruption of carcinogenic progression by a chemopreventive agent could reduce local recurrence rates following cancer treatment and prevent the future development of topographically distinct squamous cell carcinomas in the head and neck region.

◆ The Theory of Multistep Carcinogenesis

According to the theory of multistep carcinogenesis, invasive cancer is associated with multiple genetic alterations that result from repeated exposure to carcinogens, leading to dysfunctional cellular growth, differentiation, and function. These genetic events occur early in the neoplastic process and continue to accumulate as the progression to cancer evolves (**Fig. 29–1**).[11,12] For example, the loss of tumor suppressor function has been associated with injuries to chromosome 3p, 6p, 9p, or 13q, and each of these genetic alterations has been implicated in different phases of the multistep carcinogenic process.[13–16] One molecular alteration that can result in the loss of tumor suppressor function is loss of heterozygosity (LOH). Because tumor suppressor genes are recessive, cells that contain one normal and one mutated gene (heterozygous) behave normally. However, deletion of the normal allele or the chromosome arm containing the normal allele can result in a loss of heterozygosity. LOH on chromosome 9p21–22, the locus of the tumor suppressor gene *p16/MTS1/CDKN2* that encodes for the cell-cycle regulator protein p16, can result in p16 inactivation.[17] LOH at 3p and 9p is frequently present in dysplastic lesions and is predictive of progression to invasive cancer.[18,19] Amplification of the 11q13 region is another frequent genetic alteration in head and neck cancer, and the cyclin D1 gene is thought to play a role in its amplification.[20] Cyclin D1 plays a role in G1-S transition, and abnormalities of cyclin D1 and p16 may work together in the carcinogenic process.[21] Mutations of the *p53* tumor suppressor gene on the short arm of chromosome 17 (17p) occur in more than 40% of HNSCC.[22] Wild-type p53 protein induces apoptosis or growth arrest at the G1 phase of the cell cycle, and alterations in p53 result in genomic instability.

A variety of other genetic events have been associated with the multistep carcinogenic process. The expression of RARβ, a retinoid receptor that modulates the effects of retinoids on cell growth and differentiation, decreases as dysplasia progresses to invasive carcinoma.[23–25] Elevated levels of transforming growth factor-α (TGF-α) and the dysregulated overexpression of epidermal growth factor receptor (EGFR) have been documented in HNSCC.[26–28] Both TGF-α and EGF are ligands that bind to the EGFR. The EGFR regulates cell growth, and its overexpression results in transforming potential.[29] Expression of TGF-α and the EGFR have also been associated with decreased disease-specific survival.[30] Cyclooxygenase-2 (COX-2), which is typically not detected in normal tissue, is expressed in HNSCC. COX-2 contributes to epithelial carcinogenesis by decreasing apoptosis, catalyzing the conversion of procarcinogens to carcinogens, stimulating the invasive phenotype of cancer cells,

enhancing the production of vascular growth factors that result in neoangiogenesis, and mediating cytokines involved in chronic inflammation.[31,32] These genetic alterations comprise some of the most important abnormalities associated with the proposed multistep carcinogenic process, providing the rationale for conducting clinical chemoprevention trials that target specific molecular abnormalities that contribute to carcinogenic progression.

◆ Potential Chemoprevention Agents

Vitamin A is a nonspecific term that includes preformed vitamin A (retinol, retinal, and retinyl esters) and provitamin A carotenoids (β-carotene and other carotenoids that are metabolic precursors of retinal). The retinoids, which include natural derivatives and synthetic analogues of vitamin A, and β-carotene, have received the most attention in clinical research as potential chemopreventive agents.[33]

Retinoids exert regulatory control over normal epithelial cell growth and differentiation, and various retinoids have demonstrated the ability to suppress or reverse epithelial carcinogenesis. There are two classes of retinoid receptors (RARs and RXRs), which are DNA-binding transcription factors that can activate or suppress gene expression, resulting in effects on cell growth, differentiation, and apoptosis.[33] During the carcinogenic progression from dysplasia to invasive carcinoma, there is a selective, stage-dependent loss of RARβ messenger RNA (mRNA) expression.[25] In one preclinical investigation, RARβ mRNA expression was detected in 72% of histologically normal and hyperplastic tissue adjacent to SCC, 56% of dysplastic tissue, and in only 35% of SCCs ($p < .05$).[34] Subsequent translational research detected RARβ mRNA expression in only 40% of OPLs versus 100% expression in normal controls.[25] These investigators also found that high-dose 13-*cis*-retinoic acid (13cRA), or isotretinoin, upregulated RARβ expression in oral premalignant tissue from 40 to 90%, and the upregulation was associated with a clinically measurable response ($p = .039$). Although 13cRA cannot bind directly to RARs, its isomer, all-*trans*-retinoic acid (ATRA), can bind directly to the RARβ promoter region. These results suggest that RARβ expression may be able to suppress carcinogenic progression, whereas loss of RARβ expression may enhance the progression of carcinogenesis. A defect in intracellular vitamin A metabolism that results in reduced levels of retinoic acid in premalignant cells has been associated with loss of RARβ expression.[35] The administration of pharmacologic doses of retinoids may be able to overcome this deficiency by upregulating RARβ and increasing tumor suppressor activity (**Fig. 29–2**).[33] Retinoids have also been shown to normalize the increased transcription rate of EGFR and TGF-α that has been associated with carcinogenic progression.[36,37] These mechanisms of action establish the basis for a molecular model of retinoid chemoprevention in the head and neck region.

Several other potential chemopreventive agents have been evaluated for clinical efficacy. Carotenoids such as β-carotene have been reported to demonstrate antioxidant activity, inhibit mutagenesis, and result in the regression of premalignant lesions. Vitamin E, or α-tocopherol (α-TF) also has

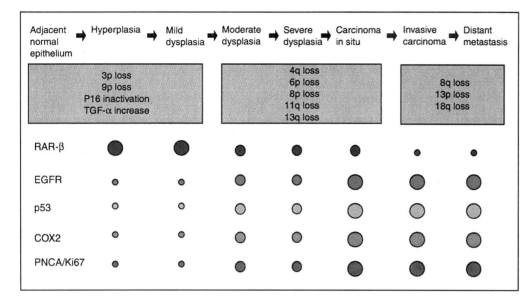

Figure 29–1 Multistep process of the development of head and neck squamous cell carcinoma (HNSCC). Changes in the diameter of each circle signify changes in expression. COX, cyclooxygenase; EGFR, epidermal growth factor receptor; PCNA, proliferating cell nuclear antigen; RAR, retinoic acid receptor; TGF-α, transforming growth factor-α. (From Rhee JC, Khuri FR, Shin DM. Advances in chemoprevention of head and neck cancer. Oncologist 2004;9: 302–311, with permission.)

antioxidant activity. The expression of mutated H-*ras* genes, which have been identified in 30% of cases of oral leukoplakia and 27 to 61% of HNSCCs, can be inhibited by farnesyl-transferase inhibitors.[38,39] Other potential chemopreventive agents that are under investigation include EGFR tyrosine kinase inhibitors, COX-2 inhibitors, and gene replacement therapy such as ONYX-015. These novel approaches to chemoprevention are also discussed in Chapter 30.

◆ Chemoprevention Research

General Considerations

Investigational new drugs such as chemopreventive agents must be evaluated in controlled clinical trials to assess their safety and efficacy before they can be used in the clinical setting. Phase I trials evaluate the safety and tolerability as well as the safe dosage range (a dose-ranging trial) of an experimental drug, typically in 20 to 80

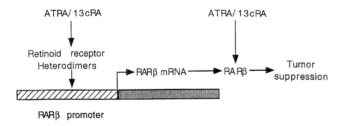

Figure 29–2 Molecular model of retinoid chemoprevention. ATRA, all-*trans*-retinoic acid; 13cRA, 13-*cis*-retinoic acid; RARβ, retinoic acid receptor-β. (From Mayne ST, Lippman SM. Retinoids, carotenoids, and micronutrients. In: DeVita VT, Hellman S, Rosenberg SA, eds. Cancer: Principles and Practice of Oncology, 6th ed. Philadelphia: Lippincott Williams & Wilkins, 2001, with permission.)

healthy subjects. Phase Ia trials test a single dose, whereas phase Ib trials evaluate the effects of multiple doses. Phase II trials are controlled clinical studies that test the efficacy and safety of the experimental drug for the treatment of a certain disease process (i.e., cancer) in 100 to 300 patients using the dosage information obtained from phase I trials. Phase IIa studies consist of only one arm, whereas phase IIb studies also have a control arm. Phase III trials compare the effectiveness of the study drug to the efficacy of other established treatments for a particular disease process in large numbers of subjects (1000–3000), monitor adverse effects and tolerability, and evaluate the overall benefit-risk relationship of the studied drug.

Phase III chemoprevention trials use cancer incidence as the primary end point, which may require thousands of subjects and several years to complete. The sample size, expense, and duration of follow-up that are necessary limit the number of chemopreventive agents and dosing regimens that can be tested. These limitations have stimulated interest in the development and validation of *intermediate end point biomarkers* that can be used to assess the efficacy of an intervention over shorter periods of time. In the retinoid oral premalignant model, RARβ and p53 have been most extensively studied as surrogate end points.

The *oral premalignancy model* is an excellent research model for head and neck clinical chemoprevention trials. OPLs are ideally suited to evaluate the efficacy of chemopreventive agents because oral leukoplakia and erythroplakia can be easily monitored clinically and histologically. Furthermore, the response of OPLs to treatment may be indicative of the response that occurs at other sites of epithelial injury in the aerodigestive tract. Consequently, the oral premalignancy model is frequently used in chemoprevention research.

Table 29–1 Grades of Adverse Events

Grade	Severity of Adverse Event (AE)
0	No AE or within normal limits
1	Mild AE
2	Moderate AE
3	Severe and undesirable AE
4	Life-threatening or disabling AE
5	Death related to AE

Data from Common Terminology Criteria for Adverse Events (CTCAE) v3.0: National Cancer Institute. https://webapps.ctep.nci.nih.gov/webobjs/ctc/webhelp/Grading_General_Characteristics.htm.

The toxicity of chemopreventive agents has been an important consideration in clinical chemoprevention trials that has precluded their use in the clinical setting. Ideally, a significant reduction in cancer incidence must be achieved with an agent that is tolerable and safe. Moreover, minimal toxicity is necessary to optimize compliance with the dosing regimen, because research suggests that chemoprevention requires long-term maintenance therapy. The National Cancer Institute has defined adverse events by using pathophysiologic, organ-specific criteria, and uses a scale from 0 to 5 to grade the severity of an adverse event (**Table 29–1**).[40] For example, common toxicity criteria have been established to define the severity of dermatitis at each grade.

Retinoid Clinical Trials

Oral Premalignant Lesions

In 1986, Hong et al[41] reported the results of a landmark double-blind placebo-controlled trial, which found that 3 months of high-dose 13cRA (2 mg/kg/d) resulted in partial reversal of OPLs in 67% of patients versus 10% in the placebo arm ($p = .0002$). Histologic reversal of dysplasia was also higher in the retinoid arm (54% vs. 10%, $p = .01$). Toxicity associated with retinoid treatment included cheilitis, dermatitis, hypertriglyceridemia, and conjunctivitis. Significant toxicity was associated with this short-term high-dose regimen, and more than 50% of the responders relapsed within 3 months after therapy was discontinued.[41]

To address the problems with toxicity and relapse, a phase IIb randomized trial was conducted in which all patients with oral leukoplakia initially received a 3-month induction course of 13cRA (1.5 mg/kg/d). Enrolled subjects that had stable or improved lesions were then randomized to receive either β-carotene (30 mg/d) or low-dose 13cRA (0.5 mg/kg/d) for 9 months as maintenance therapy. A clinical response occurred in 55% of the patients during the high-dose induction phase. The rate of progression during the maintenance phase was 55% in the β-carotene group versus only 8% in the retinoid group ($p < .001$), and minimal toxicity was documented during the maintenance phase.[42] Unfortunately, rates of malignant transformation following cessation of maintenance therapy were similar in both arms, suggesting that long-term maintenance therapy is required to prevent carcinogenic progression.

Vitamin A (retinol) administered at a dose of 200,000 IU/wk for 6 months resulted in a 57% rate of complete remission in a randomized controlled trial of smokeless tobacco users and betel nut chewers with oral leukoplakia.[43] The synthetic retinoid fenretinide 4-HPR has also been shown to effectively reverse OPLs.[44–46]

Second Primary Tumors

The success of retinoid therapy in the reversal of OPLs led to clinical trials of retinoids to evaluate their efficacy in the prevention of SPTs. In 1990, Hong et al[47] published the results of a phase III clinical trial in which 103 patients with stage I to IV HNSCC received either 50 to 100 mg/m^2/d 13cRA (>1 mg/kg/d) or placebo for 12 months. At a median follow-up of 32 months, the rate of SPT was 24% in the placebo group and only 4% in the 13cRA group ($p = .005$). At a median follow-up of 54.5 months, the rate of SPT development was 14% in the treatment group and 31% in the placebo group ($p = .04$).[48]

More recently, low-dose 13cRA was evaluated in a placebo-controlled double-blinded study of 1190 patients with stage I or II HNSCC. Patients were randomized to either 13cRA 30 mg/d or placebo for 3 years. The annual SPT was 4.7% in both arms, and there was no difference in disease-free survival or overall survival. However, disease-free survival was adversely impacted by continued smoking.[1,49]

In 2005, the results of another randomized, double-blinded placebo-controlled trial from Australia were reported.[50] In this three-armed study, 151 patients were randomized to receive one of the following: (1) 13cRA 1 mg/kg/d for 1 year followed by 13cRA 0.5 mg/kg/d for 2 years; (2) 13cRA 0.5 mg/kg/d for 3 years; or (3) placebo for 3 years. There was no significant difference in the rate of SPT development, disease recurrence or disease-free interval between the three arms. However, 66% of the patients failed to complete the entire course of therapy, and the small sample size may have limited the ability to detect a small but nevertheless a meaningful treatment effect.

A randomized trial from France that evaluated the chemopreventive efficacy of etretinate was also unable to detect a difference in the rate of SPT development. Unlike 13cRA, etretinate does not isomerize to ATRA and is not transcriptionally active, which may explain this negative result.[51]

Finally, a phase III trial known as Euroscan evaluated the efficacy of retinyl palmitate and *N*-acetylcysteine in preventing SPTs in 2592 patients who had been treated for early-stage HNSCC and non–small-cell lung cancer. No improvement in the rate of SPT development or survival was found.[52]

It seems that low-dose retinoids do not decrease the incidence of cancer, whereas high-dose retinoids are associated with significant toxicity. These limitations have prevented retinoids from becoming the standard of care for chemoprevention.

Nonretinoid Studies

Although β-carotene has shown some promise in several nonrandomized studies, the outcomes of placebo-controlled trials have not convincingly demonstrated a treatment effect. In 2001, for example, Mayne et al[53] reported the findings of a randomized, double-blinded, placebo-controlled trial that found no difference in the rates of local recurrence, mortality, or time to SPT development between the β-carotene group and the placebo group. Interest in further investigation of β-carotene for the chemoprevention of HNSCC has also diminished because of the findings from the Carotene and Retinol Efficacy Trial (CARET) and the Physicians' Health Study.[54,55] The CARET trial was a multicenter lung cancer prevention trial of β-carotene (30 mg/day) plus retinol (25,000 IU/day) versus placebo in asbestos workers and smokers. Lung cancer incidence *increased* by 28% [relative risk (RR), 1.28; 95% confidence interval (CI), 1.04–1.57)] and mortality rate was higher (RR, 1.17; 95% CI, 1.03–1.33) in the treatment arm. In the Physicians' Health Study of more than 22,000 male physicians, the rates of total cancer or lung cancer was not affected by the administration of β-carotene 50 mg every other day when compared with placebo.

Other agents, including selenium and α-TF (vitamin E) have inconsistently demonstrated chemopreventive efficacy, and additional placebo-controlled trials are needed. Treatment approaches that target specific molecular processes that have been associated with carcinogenic progression are also being investigated in phase I or II trials, including farnesyl transferase inhibitors, EGFR tyrosine kinase inhibitors, COX-2 inhibitors, and gene replacement therapy such as ONYX-015 (see Chapter 30).

◆ Biochemoprevention

In the ongoing search for the ideal chemoprevention regimen, combined therapy with interferon-α (IFN-α) has been investigated. In a prospective nonrandomized phase II

trial, patients with biopsy-proven dysplastic lesions of the oral cavity, oropharynx, and larynx were treated with 13cRA, α-TF, and IFN-α. α-TF decreases the toxicity of 13cRA and has a synergistic effect with retinoids. Although 50% of the patients with laryngeal dysplasia had a complete response at 12 months, patients with lesions of the oral cavity and oropharynx did not respond.[56]

This treatment combination was also used in a phase II trial of patients with locally advanced HNSCC. Patients received 13cRA 50 mg/m^2/d, α-TF 1,200 IU/d, and 3 million units/m^2 of IFN-α three times a week.[57] Long-term follow-up demonstrated 1-, 3-, and 5-year disease-free survival rates of 89%, 78%, and 74%, respectively.[58] Grade 3 toxicity occurred in less than 10% of the patients.

◆ Conclusion

Substantial research has shown that the incidence of squamous cell carcinoma of the head and neck can be decreased through reversal of the carcinogenic process in OPLs and at potential future sites of SPTs. However, additional clinical trials are necessary to elucidate the most efficacious, least toxic regimen for use in the clinical arena. It is hoped that the use of biomarkers as an intermediate end point in lieu of decreased cancer incidence as the definitive end point will facilitate the performance of clinical trials by decreasing cost, expediting results, and facilitating the testing of multiple different therapeutic combinations and dosing regimens.

References

1. Khuri FR, Kim ES, Lee JJ, et al. The impact of smoking status, disease stage, and index tumor site on second primary tumor incidence and tumor recurrence in the head and neck retinoid chemoprevention trial. Cancer Epidemiol Biomarkers Prev 2001;10:823–829

2. Lippman SM, Benner SE, Hong WK. Cancer chemoprevention. J Clin Oncol 1994;12:851–873

3. Fisher B, Costantino JP, Wickerham DL, et al. Tamoxifen for prevention of breast cancer: report of the National Surgical Adjuvant Breast and Bowel Project P-1 study. J Natl Cancer Inst 1998;90:1371–1388

4. Thun MJ, Namboodiri MM, Heath CW. Aspirin use and reduced risk of fatal colon cancer. N Engl J Med 1991;325:1593–1596

5. Steinbach G, Lynch PM, Phillips RK, et al. The effect of celecoxib, a cyclooxygenase-2 inhibitor, in familial adenomatous polyposis. N Engl J Med 2000;342:1946–1952

6. Silverman S Jr, Gorsky M, Lozada F. Oral leukoplakia and malignant transformation: a follow-up study of 257 patients. Cancer 1984;53:563–568

7. Vokes EE, Weichselbaum RR, Lippman SM, Hong WK. Head and neck cancer. N Engl J Med 1993;328:184–194

8. Slaughter DP, Southwick HW, Smejkal W. Field cancerization in oral stratified squamous epithelium: clinical implications of multicentric origin. Cancer 1953;6:963–968

9. Spitz MR, Fueger JJ, Beddingfield NA, et al. Chromosome sensitivity to bleomycin-induced mutagenesis, an independent risk factor for upper aerodigestive tract cancers. Cancer Res 1989;49:4626–4628

10. Lippman SM, Hong WK. Not yet standard: retinoids versus second primary tumors. J Clin Oncol 1993;11:1204–1207

11. Farber E. The multistep nature of cancer development. Cin Cancer Res 1984;44:4217–4223

12. Papadimitrakopoulou VA, Shin DM, Hong WK. Chemoprevention of head and neck cancer. In: Harrison LB, Session RB, eds. Head and Neck Cancer: A Multidisciplinary Approach, 2nd ed. Philadelphia: Lippincott Williams & Wilkins, 2004:985–1000

13. van der Riet P, Nawroz H, Hruban RH, et al. Frequent loss of chromosome 9p21–22 early in head and neck cancer progression. Cancer Res 1994;54:1156–1158

14. Okami K, Wu L, Riggins G, et al. Analysis of PTEN/MMAC1 alterations in aerodigestive tract tumors. Cancer Res 1998;58:509–511

15. Shao X, Tandon R, Samara G, et al. Mutational analysis of the PTEN gene in head and neck squamous cell carcinoma. Int J Cancer 1998;77:684–688

16. Yoo GH, Washington J, Oliver J, et al. The effects of exogenous p53 overexpression on HPV-immortalized and carcinogen transformed oral keratinocytes. Cancer 2002;94:159–166

17. Nawroz H, van der Riet P, Hruban RH, Koch W, Ruppert JM, Sidransky D. Allelotype of head and neck squamous cell carcinoma. Cancer Res 1994;54:1152–1155

18. Mao L, Lee JS, Fan YH, et al. Frequent microsatellite alterations at chromosomes 9p21 and 3p14 in oral premalignant lesions and their value in cancer risk assessment. Nat Med 1996;2:682–685

19. Partridge M, Pateromichelakis S, Phillips E, Emilion G, A'Hern R, Langdon JD. A case-control study confirms that microsatellite assay can identify patients at risk of developing oral squamous cell carcinoma within a field of cancerization. Cancer Res 2000; 60:3893–3898

20. Berenson JR, Yang J, Mickel RA. Frequent amplification of the bcl-1 locus in head and neck squamous cell carcinomas. Oncogene 1989; 4:1111–1116

21. Lukas J, Aagaard L, Strauss M, Bartek J. Oncogenic aberrations of p16INK4/CDKN2 and cyclin D1 cooperate to deregulate G1 control. Cancer Res 1995;55:4818–4823

22. Tominaga O, Hamelin R, Remvikos Y, Salmon RJ, Thomas G. p53 from basic research to clinical applications. Crit Rev Oncog 1992;3:257–282

23. Mangelsdorf DJ, Umesono K, Evans RM. The retinoid receptors. In: Sporn MB, Roberts AB, Goodman DS, eds. The Retinoids, 2nd ed. New York: Raven Press, 1994:319

24. Chambon P. The retinoid signaling pathway: molecular and genetic analyses. Semin Cell Biol 1994;5:115–125

25. Lotan R, Xu XC, Lippman SM, et al. Suppression of retinoic acid receptor-beta in premalignant oral lesions and its up-regulation by isotretinoin. N Engl J Med 1995;332:1405–1410

26. Carpenter G. Receptors for epidermal growth factor and other polypeptide mitogens. Annu Rev Biochem 1987;56:881–914

27. Grandis JR, Tweardy DJ. Elevated levels of transforming growth factor alpha and epidermal growth factor receptor messenger RNA are early markers of carcinogenesis in head and neck cancer. Cancer Res 1993;53:3579–3584

28. Shin DM, Ro JY, Hong WK, Hittelman WN. Dysregulation of epidermal growth factor receptor expression in premalignant lesions during head and neck tumorigenesis. Cancer Res 1994;54:3153–3159

29. Velu TJ, Beguinot L, Vass WC, et al. Epidermal-growth-factor-dependent transformation by a human EGF receptor proto-oncogene. Science 1987;238:1408–1410

30. Rubin Grandis J, Melhem MF, Gooding WE, et al. Levels of TGF-alpha and EGFR protein in head and neck squamous cell carcinoma and patient survival. J Natl Cancer Inst 1998;90:824–832

31. Masferrer JL, Leahy KM, Koki AT, et al. Antiangiogenic and antitumor activties of cyclooxygenase-2 inhibitors. Cancer Res 2000;60:1306–1311

32. Rhee JC, Khuri FR, Shin DM. Advances in chemoprevention of head and neck cancer. Oncologist 2004;9:302–311

33. Mayne ST, Lippman SM. Retinoids, carotenoids, and micronutrients. In: DeVita VT, Hellman S, Rosenberg SA, eds. Cancer: Principles and Practice of Oncology, 6th ed. Philadelphia: Lippincott Williams & Wilkins, 2001:575–590

34. Xu XC, Ro JY, Lee JS, Shin DM, Hong WK, Lotan R. Differential expression of nuclear retinoid receptors in normal, premalignant, and malignant head and neck tissues. Cancer Res 1994;54:3580–3587

35. Xu XC, Zile MH, Lippman SM, et al. Anti-retinoic acid (RA) antibody binding to human premalignant oral lesions, which occurs less frequently than binding to normal tissue, increases after 13-cis-RA treatment in vivo and is related to RA receptor beta expression. Cancer Res 1995;55:5507–5511

36. Rubin Grandis J, Zeng Q, Tweardy DJ. Retinoic acid normalizes the increased gene transcription rate of TGF-alpha and EGFR in head and neck cancer cell lines. Nat Med 1996;2:237–240

37. Song JI, Lango MN, Hwang JD, et al. Abrogation of transforming factor-alpha/epidermal growth factor receptor autocrine signaling by an RXR-selective retinoid (LGD 1069, Targretin) in head and neck cancer cell lines. Cancer Res 2001;61:5919–5925

38. Anderson JA, Irish JC, McLachlin CM, Ngan BY. H-ras oncogene mutation and human papillomavirus infection in oral carcinomas. Arch Otolaryngol Head Neck Surg 1994;120:755–760

39. Oku N, Shimada K, Itoh H. Ha-ras oncogene product in human oral squamous cell carcinoma. Kobe J Med Sci 1989;35:277–286

40. National Cancer Institute. Common Terminology Criteria for Adverse Events (CTCAE) v3.0. http://www.fda.gov/cder/cancer/toxicityframe.htm

41. Hong WK, Endicott J, Itri LM, et al. 13-cis-retinoic acid in the treatment of oral leukoplakia. N Engl J Med 1986;315:1501–1505

42. Lippman SM, Batsakis JG, Toth BB, et al. Comparison of low-dose isotretinoin with beta carotene to prevent oral carcinogenesis. N Engl J Med 1993;328:15–20

43. Stich HF, Hornby AP, Mathew B, Sankaranarayanan R, Nair MK. Response of oral leukoplakias to the administration of vitamin A. Cancer Lett 1988;40:93–101

44. Chiesa F, Tradati N, Marazza M, et al. Prevention of local relapses and new localisations of oral leukoplakias with the synthetic retinoid fenretinide (4-HPR): preliminary results. Eur J Cancer B Oral Oncol 1992;28B:97–102

45. Han J, Jiao L, Lu Y, Sun Z, Gu QM, Scanlon KJ. Evaluation of N-4-(hydroxycarbophenyl) retinamide as a cancer prevention agent and as a cancer chemotherapeutic agent. In Vivo 1990;4:153–160

46. De Palo G, Veronesi U, Marubini E, et al. Controlled clinical trials with fenretinide in breast cancer, basal cell carcinoma and oral leukoplakia. J Cell Biochem Suppl 1995;22:11–17

47. Hong WK, Lippman SM, Itri LM, et al. Prevention of second primary tumors with isotretinoin in squamous-cell carcinoma of the head and neck. N Engl J Med 1990;323:795–801

48. Benner SE, Pajak TF, Lippman SM, Earley C, Hong WK. Prevention of second primary tumors with isotretinoin in patients with squamous cell carcinoma of the head and neck: long-term follow-up. J Natl Cancer Inst 1994;86:140–141

49. Khuri FR, Lee JJ, Lippman SM, et al. Isoretinoin effects on head and neck cancer recurrence and second primary tumors. Proc Am Soc Clin Oncol 2003;22:359a

50. Perry CF, Stevens M, Rabie I, et al. Chemoprevention of head and neck cancer with retinoids: a negative result. Arch Otolaryngol Head Neck Surg 2005;131:198–203

51. Bolla M, Lefur R, Ton Van J, et al. Prevention of second primary tumours with etretinate in squamous cell carcinoma of the oral cavity and oropharynx: results of a multicentric double-blind randomised study. Eur J Cancer 1994;30A:767–772

52. van Zandwijk N, Dalesio O, Pastorino U, de Vries N, van Tinteren H. EUROSCAN, a randomized trial of vitamin A and N-acetylcysteine in patients with head and neck cancer or lung cancer. For the European Organization for Research and Treatment of Cancer Head and Neck and Lung Cancer Cooperative Groups. J Natl Cancer Inst 2000;92:977–986

53. Mayne ST, Cartmel B, Baum M, et al. Randomized trial of supplemental beta-carotene to prevent second head and neck cancer. Cancer Res 2001;61:1457–1463

54. Omenn GS, Goodman GE, Thornquist MD, et al. Effects of a combination of beta carotene and vitamin A on lung cancer and cardiovascular disease. N Engl J Med 1996;334:1150–1155

55. Hennekens CH, Buring JE, Manson JE, et al. Lack of effect of long-term supplementation with beta carotene on the incidence of malignant neoplasms and cardiovascular disease. N Engl J Med 1996;334:1145–1149

56. Shin DM, Wang ZK, Feng C, et al. Biochemopreventive combination (13-cis-retinoic acid, interferon-α2a and α-tocopherol) may have synergistic effects over single agents or 2-drug combinations in vitro culture of squamous cell carcinoma of the head and neck cells. Proc Am Assoc Cancer Res 2002;43:311a

57. Shin DM, Khuri FR, Murphy B, et al. Combined interferon-alpha, 13-cis-retinoic acid, and alpha-tocopherol in locally advanced head and neck squamous cell carcinoma: novel bioadjuvant phase II trial. J Clin Oncol 2001;19:3010–3017

58. Shin DM, Richards TJ, Seixas-Silva JA. Phase II trial of bioadjuvant therapy with interferon-alpha2a, 13-cis-retinoic acid, and alpha-tocopherol for locally advanced squamous cell carcinoma of the head and neck: long term follow-up. Proc Am Soc Clin Oncol 2003;22:1995a

30

Novel Therapeutics for Head and Neck Cancer

Edward S. Kim and

Alyssa G. Rieber

Head and neck squamous cell carcinoma (HNSCC) is the fifth most common cause of cancer and the sixth leading cause of cancer death worldwide. Approximately 40,400 new cases of HNSCC are diagnosed each year, and 12,300 cancer deaths are attributed to HNSCC in the United States annually.[1] Early-stage disease can usually be treated successfully with surgery or radiation therapy, whereas locally advanced disease typically requires multimodality therapy that may require surgical resection, radiation, chemotherapy, or a combination of these approaches. Despite significant improvements in diagnosis, local management, and chemotherapy of head and neck cancer, there has been no significant increase in long-term survival over the past 30 years, and advanced-stage disease (stage III and IV) has a cure rate of less than 30%.[2] Patients with recurrent or metastatic disease have a median survival of approximately 6 months, and randomized trials have not been able to demonstrate improved survival advantages when compared with treatment with cisplatin and infusional 5-fluorouracil (5-FU), the historical standard.[3,4] Several novel cytotoxic agents, including the taxanes paclitaxel and docetaxel, have been tested for efficacy in the therapy of recurrent or metastatic HNSCC. Although these agents have provided less toxic choices, treatment efficacy remains dismal.

As our insight into the pathogenesis of HNSCC evolves, the complex signaling that is necessary for carcinogenesis to occur becomes more clearly defined. Translational research has led to a new era in aerodigestive tract cancer therapeutics, and the development of several novel targeted therapies for the treatment of patients with HNSCC has provided the scientific community with renewed optimism that an impact on survival can be realized (**Table 30–1**). Although these therapeutic agents remain investigational, the successful development of rationally designed novel therapeutic agents for the treatment of other solid tumors, including gastrointestinal stromal tumors (e.g., Imatinib mesylate, Gleevac, Novartis Pharmaceuticals, Basel, Switzerland) and breast cancer (e.g., Trastuzumab, Herceptin, Genentech, San Francisco, CA) provides proof-of-principle that targeted therapy for HNSCC may be feasible. This chapter reviews some of the more promising novel biologic compounds for the treatment of HNSCC that target specific cellular domains.

◆ Epidermal Growth Factor Receptor

Overexpression of epidermal growth factor receptor (EGFR) has been observed in cancers of the breast, ovary, prostate, bladder, lung, brain, and pancreas.[5–12] In HNSCC, EGFR overexpression has been reported in about 90% of specimens and is associated with a poor prognosis.[12,13] The expression of EGFR or of transforming growth factor-α (TGF-α) has been associated with worse disease-free and disease-specific survival, and has independent prognostic significance.[13] Therefore, several strategies to block or downregulate EGFR have been developed to inhibit tumor proliferation and improve overall clinical outcome.[14]

Expression of EGFR appears to contribute to the growth and survival of tumor cells in addition to maintaining normal cellular function. The EGFR signal transduction pathways contribute to the development of malignancy by its effects on cell cycle progression and angiogenesis, inhibiting apoptosis, and by promoting tumor cell motility and metastases.[15–18]

Table 30–1 Potential Anticancer Agents that Modulate Specific Molecular Targets in Head and Neck Squamous Cell Carcinoma

Epidermal growth factor (EGFR)/cell growth regulation agents
  Monoclonal anti-EGFR antibodies
    Cetuximab (Erbitux)
  EGFR tyrosine kinase inhibitors
    Gefitinib (Iressa)
    Erlotinib (Tarceva)
    CI-1033
    PKI-166
Vascular endothelial growth factor (VEGF)/angiogenesis agents
  Monoclonal anti-VEGF antibodies
    Bevacizumab (Avastin)
    HuMV833
    DC101
    IMC-1C11
  VEGF receptor tyrosine kinase inhibitors
    ZD 6474
    SU 6668
    SU 5416
Gene replacement therapy
    ONYX-015
    Ad-p53
Farnesyl transferase inhibitors
    Lonafarnib
    BMS-214662
    Tipifarnib (Zarnestra)

Epidermal growth factor receptor (EGFR/erb-B1) is part of the erb-B family of receptor tyrosine kinases, which also include erb-B2/Her2-neu, erb-B3/Her3, and erb-B4/Her4.[19,20] EGFR is a transmembrane protein composed of a 1186–amino acid polypeptide chain with three distinct regions: an extracellular ligand-binding domain, a transmembrane lipophilic region, and an intracellular protein tyrosine kinase domain (**Fig. 30–1**).[20–22] Endogenous ligands to EGFR include EGF (TGF-α), heparin-binding EGF, amphiregulin, and betacellulin.[5] Erb-B family members can form homodimers or heterodimers upon ligand binding to the cytoplasmic domain of the receptors, which can lead to phosphorylation of the tyrosine residues and further activation of the downstream signal transduction pathways, including *ras*/mitogen-activated protein (MAP) kinase and phosphatidylinositol-3 kinase. The signal transduction pathway can lead to cell proliferation in tumor growth as well as progression of invasion and metastasis.[23–25]

Because of EGFR's important role in cell cycle progression and tumor cell proliferation, it is logical to hypothesize that combinations of anti-EGFR therapy with chemotherapy or radiation therapy could result in a synergistic antitumor effect by inhibiting various processes that contribute to tumor growth.[26,27] Numerous EGFR blockers have been investigated, including anti-EGFR monoclonal antibodies, tyrosine kinase inhibitors, ligand conjugates, immunoconjugates, and

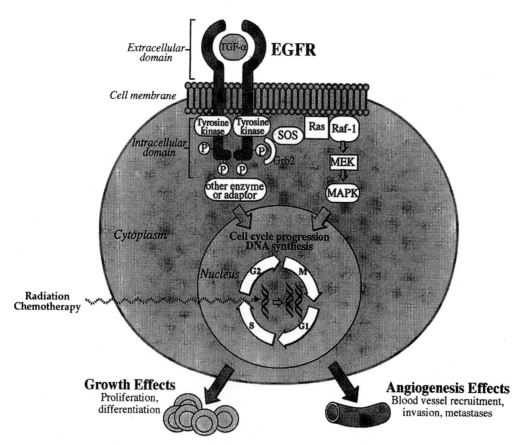

Figure 30–1 Schematic illustration of the epidermal growth factor receptor (EGFR) system, depicting EGFR, mitogen-activated protein kinase (MAPK), signal transduction cascade to the nucleus, and resultant stimulation of cell cycle machinery. TGF-α, transforming growth factor-α. (From Huang SM, Harari PM. Epidermal growth factor receptor inhibition in cancer therapy: biology, rationale and preliminary clinical results. Invest New Drugs 1999;17:260, with permission from Springer Science and Business Media.)

antisense oligonucleotides.[28] Anti-EGFR monoclonal antibodies target the extracellular domain and thus are able to effectively block the EGFR pathways in a highly specific manner. Small molecules such as the tyrosine kinase inhibitors, which target the intracellular tyrosine kinase signaling pathways, also inhibit the EGFR pathway.

Monoclonal Anti-EGFR Antibodies

Several monoclonal antibodies have been developed and are being tested in a variety of tumors, including HNSCCs. Anti-EGFR monoclonal antibodies appear to enhance the antitumor efficacy of chemotherapy agents such as cisplatin and doxorubicin by increasing the *in vitro* radiosensitivity of HNSCC cells.[29]

Cetuximab

Cetuximab (Erbitux; ImClone Systems, New York, NY; formerly IMC-225) is the most extensively studied anti-EGFR monoclonal antibody. Cetuximab is a chimeric monoclonal antibody directed against EGFR that competes for natural ligand-binding sites and causes receptor internalization and downregulation.[30] Mendelsohn and Baselga[31] proposed that the combination of anti-EGFR therapy and chemotherapy or radiation therapy might lead to synergistic antitumor activities by targeting various processes that contribute to tumor growth.

Therefore, many phase I studies of cetuximab were primarily in combination with chemotherapy or radiotherapy. They demonstrated acceptable toxicity profiles and many complete or partial responses.[32] Three phase I trials evaluated conventional dose-escalation of cetuximab in combination with cisplatin in 52 patients with advanced solid tumors expressing EGFR.[32] Thirteen head and neck patients were evaluated, with two partial tumor responses. Shin et al[33] evaluated 12 patients with recurrent or metastatic HNSCC with positive EGFR treated with cetuximab in combination with cisplatin. Major responses were observed in 67% of the patients, including two complete responses. The dose of cetuximab found to have the highest percentage of EGFR saturation in tumor tissue was found to be 400 mg/m^2 loading dose followed by 250 mg/m^2 weekly maintenance dose. The major toxicities are skin toxicity with acneiform rash and hypersensitivity reactions.[33,34]

Phase II studies[35–38] of cetuximab alone and in combination with chemotherapy in patients with progressive disease on platinum-based chemotherapy showed improved survival over historical controls. The median survival ranged from 5.2 to 6.1 months in the treated groups versus 3.4 months in the control group. Response rates in these patients treated with cetuximab either as monotherapy or in combination with a platinum-based agent were 10 to 14%. A phase III trial by Burtness et al[39] compared cisplatin/placebo to cisplatin/cetuximab in patients with metastatic or recurrent HNSCC. Preliminary results for 44 of 121 patients were reported in 2002. Response was significantly higher in the combination group compared with the cisplatin group (23.6% vs. 9.8%). The median overall survival for the entire group was 7.2 months, but there was a trend toward better 2-year overall survival in the combination group (15.6% vs. 9.2%). These results are promising for patients who previously had limited options after platinum-based chemotherapy had failed. Further studies of cetuximab monotherapy would help to determine whether cetuximab helps overcome platinum resistance or if cetuximab alone results in improved response and survival.

A phase I study of cetuximab with radiotherapy evaluated treatment-naive patients with locally advanced HNSCC. Sixteen patients received weekly cetuximab in combination with daily radiotherapy. Thirteen patients achieved complete remission and two had partial remissions. Follow-up data showed 65% 2-year disease-free survival.[40] A phase III study by Bonner et al[41,42] compared radiation therapy alone and in combination with cetuximab; 424 patients with no prior therapy for their locally advanced HNSCC were randomized to radiation alone or cetuximab with radiation. The combination arm had significantly improved 3-year survival of 55% versus 45%. Cetuximab was given weekly with radiotherapy. These studies are promising for the continued use of combination cetuximab and radiotherapy in treatment-naive patients. Based on this study, cetuximab has been approved for use in HNSCC. Further studies will assess its activity with chemotherapy and radiotherapy.

Epidermal Growth Factor Receptor Tyrosine Kinase Inhibitors

Inhibiting signal transduction via EGFR tyrosine kinase inhibition is a strategy that has shown promise in several clinical trials. The outcomes of investigations that have evaluated treatment with the tyrosine kinase inhibitors gefitinib, erlotinib, CI-1033, and PKI-166 are reviewed here.

Gefitinib

Gefitinib (Iressa, AstraZeneca UK, London, UK; formerly ZD 1839) is a selective EGFR tyrosine kinase inhibitor (TKI) that results in significant antitumor activity and minimal toxicity when used as monotherapy. Gefitinib also appears to potentiate the antitumor and apoptotic effects of cytotoxic agents such as the platinums and taxanes against several human tumor xenografts, including non–small-cell lung cancer (NSCLC), vulvar, and prostate cancer.[43,44] Preexposure of cells to gefitinib has been shown to enhance cisplatin-induced apoptosis in oral squamous cell carcinoma cell lines.[45] When combined with radiation, gefitinib demonstrates dose-dependent inhibition of cellular proliferation in human SCC cell lines grown in culture and inhibits tumor angiogenesis in tumor xenograft models in vivo.[46] Dose-related, mechanism-based toxicities have been common in the phase I trials and have been confined to the skin (rash or erythema) and gastrointestinal system (diarrhea, nausea, and vomiting); transient hepatic enzyme elevation has also occurred. The phase I dose-limiting toxicity (DLT) of gefitinib is diarrhea at 800 to 1000 mg/day.

In four phase I monotherapy trials, 252 patients were treated with dosages ranging from 50 to 1000 mg, at which DLT occurred. In the largest trials, eligible tumor types included NSCLC, hormone-refractory prostate, colorectal, ovarian, and head and neck cancer. None of these trials used tumor EGFR expression or overexpression as a criterion for eligibility, and most of the patients had received prior cancer treatment. Responses were primarily seen in patients with NSCLC. Although originally promising single-agent activity was observed in phase II trials, a randomized phase III study failed to demonstrate efficacy versus placebo in patients with NSCLC.[47] Gefitinib has been approved for patients with NSCLC who are refractory to platinum and docetaxel chemotherapy.

Investigators at the University of Chicago enrolled patients with recurrent or metastatic HNSCC who had received no more than one course of prior therapy in a study that evaluated single-agent gefitinib at a dose of 500 mg/d. Fifty-two patients were enrolled and 47 were assessable for response, with an observed response rate of 10.6% and a disease control rate of 53%. Median time to progression and survival were 3.4 and 8.1 months, respectively. The only grade 3 toxicity encountered was diarrhea in three patients. Performance status and development of skin toxicity were found to be strong predictors of response, progression, and survival. Other investigations of gefitinib in HNSCC are ongoing.[48]

Erlotinib

Erlotinib (Tarceva, Genentech Inc.; formerly OSI-774) is an oral, highly selective, reversible EGFR tyrosine kinase inhibitor. Extensive preclinical studies[49] demonstrated activity in solid tumors, including HNSCC, in combination with chemotherapy. Erlotinib was found to have an additive effect on antitumor therapy without increased toxicity. A phase I study[50] of erlotinib in solid tumors determined 150 mg/day as the maximum tolerated dose (MTD), with the dose-limiting toxicities of diarrhea and skin rash. One of three patients with HNSCC enrolled in the trial exhibited stable disease for 15 months.

One hundred fifteen patients with recurrent or metastatic HNSCC were enrolled in a multicenter phase II study[51] with single-agent erlotinib. Five patients (4.3%) achieved a partial response, and 44 patients (38.3%) had stable disease. The median overall survival was 6 months, and median progression-free survival was 9.6 weeks. Improved overall survival was demonstrated in the subgroup of patients who experienced at least grade 2 skin rashes ($p = .045$).

Other Tyrosine Kinase Inhibitors

CI-1033 (Pfizer, New York, NY) and PKI-166 (Novartis) are two more TKIs that target EGFR and its family of receptors. CI-1033 is an orally active 4-anilinoquinazoline that acts as a pan-erb-B tyrosine kinase inhibitor. In a phase I dose-escalation study in patients with advanced solid tumors, including 14 patients with HNSCC, the MTD was found to be 750 mg. DLTs included grade 3 nausea and diarrhea. The most common toxicities included acneiform rash, emesis and diarrhea, and reversible thrombocytopenia. One patient had a clinical response and 13 had stable disease.[52] This agent continues to be studied in both phase I and phase II settings.

PKI-166 is a selective inhibitor of the tyrosine kinase of EGFR and the erb-B2 receptor. A phase I study of oral PKI-166 treated 23 patients with advanced solid tumors at five different dose levels, ranging from 50 to 450 mg/d. All patients had failed prior treatment. The predominant tumor types included colorectal ($n = 7$), HNSCC ($n = 4$), and NSCLC ($n = 3$). No DLTs have been observed to date. Of 20 evaluable patients, no responses have been observed, but two patients have demonstrated stable disease. Patient accrual in this study will continue until the MTD has been defined.[53]

◆ Vascular Endothelial Growth Factor

Angiogenesis, the formation of new blood vessels from existing capillaries, plays an important role in the metastasis and growth of solid tumors.[54–56] Vascular endothelial growth factor (VEGF), its isoforms, and its receptor (VEGFR) have an important role in regulating angiogenesis.[57] VEGFR is a member of the receptor tyrosine kinase (RTK) family of growth-signal transducing proteins.[58] These transmembrane proteins transduce extracellular growth signals into intracellular growth responses by initiating various signaling cascades through the phosphorylation of tyrosine residues on specific cytosolic proteins.[59] VEGF binding to its receptor will lead to activation of several downstream signal transduction pathways, including phospholipase C, PI3K, and ras guanosine triphosphatase (GTPase) activating protein.[60]

Vascular endothelial growth factor receptor expression on the surface of endothelial cells appears to be regulated by hypoxia, similar to VEGF.[58] Isoforms of membrane-bound VEGFR have been identified, each with a distinct role in angiogenesis.[61] VEGFR-1, also known as Flt-1 (fms-like tyrosine kinase-1), has the highest binding affinity for VEGF-A, but does not have significant kinase activity. VEGFR-2, also known as KDR (kinase domain region) and Flk-1 (fetal liver kinase-1), are frequently associated with endothelial cell proliferation and chemotaxis. Expression of VEGFR-2 has been found in mammary, ovarian, lung, and glioma tissue, which suggests a role for VEGF in these malignancies that could be used as a potential therapeutic target.[62] VEGFR-3, also known as Flt-4, appears to primarily regulate lymphangiogenesis.[63]

Monoclonal Anti–Vascular Endothelial Growth Factor Antibodies

Bevacizumab [Avastin; Genentech (rhuMAb VEGF)] is a recombinant human monoclonal antibody that targets the VEGF protein and sequesters VEGF-A, inhibiting signal transduction. Both in vitro and in vivo data indicate that endothelial cell proliferation is inhibited and tumor growth is reduced with administration of this antibody.[64] It is the most widely studied VEGF agent and has been approved for use in colon cancer. The Eastern Cooperative Oncology Group has reported a survival advantage by adding 15 mg/kg bevacizumab to carboplatin and paclitaxel therapy in patients with advanced nonsquamous NSCLC.[65] A phase I study of bevacizumab in combination with 5-FU, hydroxyurea, and hyperfractionated split-course radiation in poor prognosis patients with HNSCC achieved a 75%

response rate, but with significant toxicities.[66] Other phase I and phase II studies of bevacizumab in combination with chemotherapy, radiation, and chemoradiation are underway.

Vascular Endothelial Growth Factor Receptor (VEGF-R) Tyrosine Kinase Inhibitors

ZD6474 (AstraZeneca) is an oral VEGFR-2 tyrosine kinase inhibitor (TKI). This compound has also shown activity against the EGFR tyrosine kinase region. Preclinical findings have demonstrated that ZD6474 inhibits the growth of prostate xenografts and induces tumor regression. Furthermore, tumor growth resumes with cessation of ZD6474; conversely, tumor regression can be reinduced upon reintroduction of ZD6474.[67] In an ongoing phase I dose-escalation study, 41 patients with various solid tumors have been treated with ZD6474.[68] Drug-related toxicity has been minimal, with only two grade 1 (facial flushing, facial rash) and one grade 2 (fatigue) adverse events reported. Stable disease has been documented in two patients (gastrointestinal stromal tumor, melanoma) after 56 days of treatment.

SU6668 (Pfizer) is an oral TKI with multiple receptor targets, including VEGF RTK as well as the basic fibroblast growth factor (bFGF) and platelet-derived growth factor (PDGF) RTKs. In preclinical studies, SU6668 inhibited the growth of various human tumor xenografts in athymic mice. Notably, A431 epidermoid tumor xenografts were eradicated in over 50% of the treated mice, and eradication persisted for at least 133 days following cessation of treatment.[69] Although clinical trials remain in the early stages, a phase I trial in 68 patients with various advanced tumors demonstrated that SU6668 is well tolerated at a wide range of dose levels ($100–2400$ mg/m^2/d). Only mild to moderate side effects occurred, including nausea, diarrhea, fatigue, and dyspnea.[70,71] Disease stabilization for more than 4 weeks was observed in 31 of 51 patients. Several studies are currently being conducted to identify prognostic features in patients most likely to respond to SU6668 therapy.

◆ Gene Replacement Therapy

Alcohol and tobacco use are associated with p53 mutations, which occur in 45 to 70% of HNSCC.[72,73] In tumors with a normal *p53* gene sequence, loss of p53 function can occur through p53 protein inhibition or degradation.[74,75] p53 is a multifunctional protein, which can be induced by DNA damage, and plays a significant role in the detection and repair of damaged DNA. p53 can also induce apoptosis or programmed cell death in severely damaged cells, and has been associated with both carcinogenesis and overall prognosis in HNSCC.[76] Thus, strategies targeting the *p53* gene and protein may halt or reverse the process of tumorigenesis and metastasis. Most investigative efforts have been directed toward strategies that utilize gene replacement therapy.

ONYX-015 (Onyx Pharmaceuticals, Emeryville, CA) is an E1B 55-kd gene-deleted replication-selective adenovirus that replicates and causes cytopathogenicity in certain cancer cells.[77,78] Although preclinical in vitro results have varied, clinical data with regard to safety and antitumor activity following intratumoral injection of ONYX-015 have been definitive. Selective intratumoral replication and tumor-selective tissue destruction of ONYX-015 have been documented in phase I and II clinical trials in patients with recurrent/refractory HNSCC.[79–81] However, durable responses and clinical benefit were seen in less than 15% of these end-stage patients. As predicted, p53 mutant tumors underwent necrosis at a higher rate than did tumors with a wild-type gene sequence (58% and 0%, respectively).[80] Both in vitro and nude mouse-human tumor xenograft studies have shown additive or potentially synergistic efficacy of ONYX-015 in combination with cisplatin-based chemotherapy compared with that of either ONYX-015 or chemotherapy alone, and ONYX-015 is able to enhance the efficacy of cisplatin both in p53 deficient and p53-functional tumor cells.[77] Sensitization of p53-functional tumor cells may involve expression of the adenovirus E1A gene product, which may play a role as a potent chemosensitizer, in the induction of high levels of p53 protein, or both.[78–82]

The results of a phase II multicenter trial of intratumoral ONYX-015 in combination with cisplatin and 5-FU in patients with recurrent HNSCC were published in 2000. In 2001, a phase II trial of ONYX-015 administered to patients with HNSCC at two different dose schedules (standard fractionation versus hyperfractionation) was reported.[83,84] Tumor responses and disease stabilization were observed in both groups. Systemic toxicity was similar, although injection site pain was more common with the hyperfractionated regimen (80% vs. 47%). Because of this adverse effect, a dose-escalation study of intravenous ONYX-015 has been conducted in patients with NSCLC.[85]

Gene replacement strategies have also been used to target *p53* mutations by using an adenovirus containing the wild-type *p53* gene (Ad-p53 or RPR-INGN-201; Introgen Therapeutics, Houston, TX). Ad-p53 is a vector system in which the wild-type *p53* gene is inserted into a first-generation adenoviral vector. In preclinical studies, Ad-p53 gene treatment induced apoptosis of cancer cells without affecting normal cells, and it was active against *p53* mutant cancer cells as well as cancer cells with a wild-type *p53* genomic sequence. Ad-p53 also reduced tumor growth in mouse xenograft models of HNSCC and other cancers.[86,87] Clayman et al[88] conducted a phase I trial of Ad-p53 gene transfer in patients with advanced recurrent HNSCC. Thirty-three patients received intratumoral injections of Ad-p53 at a dose of 1×10^{11} plaque-forming units (PFUs) three times a week, which consisted of one treatment course. Patients with resectable tumors received one full course of treatment followed by two additional administrations—one during surgery and one 72 hours after surgery. Patients with unresectable tumors received a course of treatment every 4 weeks. Both treatment regimens were well tolerated. The most common adverse effect was injection site pain, which was not related to the dose or the anatomic site of injection. Other common side effects included transient fever, headache, pain, and edema; these symptoms occurred mainly at doses of 1×10^{10} PFUs or greater. No allergic reactions or evidence of systemic hypersensitivity was observed. Two (11.8%) of 17 evaluable patients with unresectable disease at a dose of 1×10^{10} and 1×10^{11} PFUs had major responses, which were 7 weeks and 18 days in duration, respectively. Among resectable tumor patients, one patient had a pathologic complete response at the time of surgery and remained free of disease at 26 months from the initial treatment, and a second patient had no evidence of disease at 24 months. Ad-p53 was detected in blood, urine, and the sputum of patients, but viremic symptoms were not reported. Based on this promising initial data, clinical trials have been initiated (1) to evaluate Ad-p53 with cisplatin and 5-FU against cisplatin and 5-FU alone in patients with the recurrent or metastatic HNSCC, and (2) to evaluate the results of Ad-p53 administered by direct intratumoral injection versus methotrexate in patients with recurrent and/or metastatic HNSCC.

◆ Farnesyl Transferase Inhibitors

Data suggest that up to 27% of oral cavity cancers have mutations in the H-*ras* gene.[89] Farnesyl transferase inhibitors (FTIs) are a class of compounds that inhibit a critical enzymatic step in the constitutive expression of mutated *ras* genes.[90–93] FTIs appear to have extensive activity in preclinical studies utilizing HNSCC cell lines as well as in NSCLC cell lines.

A phase Ib randomized trial, which was designed to estimate the inhibition of farnesylation of two proteins (DNA-J and prelamin-A) by the FTI lonafarnib (Schering Plough, Kenilworth, NJ; formerly SCH66336) in vivo, enrolled patients who were scheduled for preoperative assessment. Patients were randomized to one of three dosing arms of orally administered lonafarnib (100, 200, and 300 mg twice a day) or to a fourth arm that received no treatment. DNA-J, a heat shock protein, and prelamin-A, typically found in tissue as lamin-A, were assayed following an 8- to 14-day treatment schedule. The phase I MTD for prolonged administration was found to be 200 mg twice a day. Preliminary data indicate successful inhibition of protein farnesylation in both proteins, with four patients experiencing significant tumor reduction. One patient who initially presented a large oral cavity tumor had only microscopic disease after 3 days of twice-daily lonafarnib at 300 mg.[94]

Preclinical data have indicated that the addition of FTIs to either paclitaxel or epothilones are able to overcome acquired resistance to these agents in a variety of cancer cell lines.[93] A phase I/II trial of lonafarnib in combination with paclitaxel has been conducted in patients with solid tumors, and a phase II dose of lonafarnib 100 mg po b.i.d. and paclitaxel 175 mg/m² was established.[95] Additionally, responses and disease stabilization were observed in HNSCC and NSCLC. The phase II study included only patients with NSCLC who failed treatment with a taxane.[96] Trials of lonafarnib in combination with chemotherapy that will enroll patients with NSCLC (phase III) and HNSCC (phase II) have been developed.

Other FTIs are under active investigation. Studies with BMS-214662 (Bristol-Myers Squibb, New York, NY) have demonstrated preferential cytotoxicity against nonproliferating cells. A phase I study in patients with solid tumors evaluated escalating doses of BMS-214662 followed by cisplatin 75 mg/m² given every 3 weeks. The MTD has not been established, but adverse events included nausea, vomiting, stomatitis, lethargy, and neutropenia.[97]

Tipifarnib (Zarnestra; Johnson and Johnson, Raritan, NJ; formerly R115777) is a nonpeptidomimetic, orally bioavailable imidazole, competitive FTI with in vitro and in vivo preclinical antitumor activity that has been shown to exert anticancer activity as a single agent and when combined with cytotoxic agents in humans. Tipifarnib has demonstrated minimal toxicity, with reversible myelosuppression being the most common DLT. Other adverse events associated with tipifarnib include rash, fatigue, mild nausea/vomiting, renal dysfunction, and peripheral neuropathy. Peripheral neuropathy, which was seen when tipifarnib was given continuously, has not been observed with the recommended dosing schedules.[98] Phase I studies of tipifarnib in combination with a variety of cytotoxic agents, including irinotecan, docetaxel, gemcitabine, and cisplatin, have been conducted or are underway.

◆ Other Biologic Strategies

Transforming Growth Factor-α Antisense Gene Therapy

Transforming growth factor-α (TGF-α) mRNA and protein are both overexpressed by HNSCCs as these substances are required for sustaining proliferation of cells in vitro. Liposome gene-mediated transfer into head and neck tumor cells resulted in inhibition of tumor growth and increased apoptosis with sustained effects up to a year. This strategy may prove useful by interfering with the autocrine signaling pathway of the TGF-α/EGFR ligand/receptor pair.[99]

13-*cis*-Retinoic Acid (13cRA)

13-*cis*-Retinoic acid (13cRA) has also been tested in both the treatment and adjuvant settings. A phase I/II study evaluated the combination of 13cRA, cisplatin, and ifosfamide in patients with advanced/recurrent HNSCC.[100] Patients received fixed doses of cisplatin (20 mg/m² for 5 days every 3 weeks) and 13cRA (0.5 mg/kg orally for 5 days a week) and escalating doses of ifosfamide (1000 to 1500 mg/m²). Fifty-two patients were enrolled in the phase I study, with the ifosfamide MTD of 1500 mg/m². The phase II study used cisplatin, 13cRA, and ifosfamide (1200 mg/m²), resulting in a response rate of 72%. The median time to progression was 10.4 months, and median overall survival was 12.95 months.

Retinoids and interferons, when combined, demonstrate synergistic effects in modulating proliferation, differentiation, and apoptosis. A phase II study tested the combination of interferon-α (IFN-α), 13cRA, and α-tocopherol (α-TF) as adjuvant treatment for the reduction of local-regional recurrence and second primary tumors in 45 patients who had been definitively treated for locally advanced HNSCC (24% stage III, 76% stage IV).[101] Patients were treated with IFN-α (3×10^6 IU/m², subcutaneous injection, three times a week), 13cRA (50 mg/m^2/d, orally), and α-TF (1200 IU/d, orally) for 12 months. Eighty-six percent of the patients completed the 12-month course of treatment. At a median of 24 months follow-up, the rate of local-regional recurrence was 9%, local-regional recurrence and distant metastases was 5%, and the rate of development of second primary tumors was 2% (nonaerodigestive tract). Median 1- and 2-year survival rates were 98% and 91%, with disease-free survival rates of 91% and 84%, respectively. This biologic combination was generally well tolerated and seems promising as adjuvant treatment for locally advanced HNSCC. A phase III study is ongoing, and if the results are positive, this approach will establish a new standard of care in definitively treated advanced HNSCC patients.

Other combinations of biologic agents are being explored in multiple settings. A phase I study of erlotinib (Tarceva) and bevacizumab (Avastin, or RhuMAb-VEGF) in HNSCC is currently ongoing. This study is based on another phase I study of this treatment combination in NSCLC, which demonstrated a 25% response rate in pretreated patients.[102]

◆ Conclusion

Novel therapeutic agents that target specific cellular domains are under active investigation as potential treatment options for patients with HNSCC. Cytotoxic agents have reached a plateau of efficacy, mandating the need to search for alternative therapeutic approaches that can be used alone or in combination with existing treatment options. The potential utility of targeted therapies in patients with advanced HNSCC could eventually lead to their integration into the treatment of early stage HNSCC.

References

1. Jemal A, Thomas A, Murray T, Thun M. Cancer statistics, 2002. CA Cancer J Clin 2002;52:23–47

2. Lamont EB, Vokes EE. Chemotherapy in the management of squamous-cell carcinoma of the head and neck. Lancet Oncol 2001;2:261–269

3. Jacobs C, Lyman G, Velez-Garcia E, et al. A phase III randomized study comparing cisplatin and fluorouracil as single agents and in combination for advanced squamous cell carcinoma of the head and neck. J Clin Oncol 1992;10:257–263

4. Forastiere AA, Metch B, Schuller DE, et al. Randomized comparison of cisplatin plus fluorouracil and carboplatin plus fluorouracil versus methotrexate in advanced squamous-cell carcinoma of the head and neck: a Southwest Oncology Group study. J Clin Oncol 1992;10:1245–1251

5. Salomon DS, Brandt R, Ciardiello F, et al. Epidermal growth factor–related peptides and their receptors in human malignancies. Crit Rev Oncol Hematol 1995;19:183–232

6. Gullick WJ. Prevalence of aberrant expression of the epidermal growth factor receptor in human cancers. Br Med Bull 1991;47:87–98

7. Lofts FJ, Gullick WJ. C-erbB2 amplification and overexpression in human tumors. In: Dickson RB, Lippman ME, eds. Genes, Oncogenes, and Hormones: Advances in Cellular and Molecular Biology of Breast Cancer. Boston: Kluwer Academic, 1991:161–179

8. Prewett M, Rockwell P, Rockwell RF, et al. The biologic effects of C225, a chimeric monoclonal antibody to the EGFR, on human prostate carcinoma. J Immunother Emphasis Tumor Immunol 1996;19:419–427

9. Bruns CJ, Harbison MT, Davis DW, et al. Epidermal growth factor receptor blockade with C225 plus gemcitabine results in regression of human pancreatic carcinoma growing orthotopically in nude mice by antiangiogenic mechanisms. Clin Cancer Res 2000;6:1936–1948

10. Fischer-Colbrie J, Witt A, Heinzl H, et al. EGFR and steroid receptors in ovarian carcinoma: comparison with prognostic parameters and outcome of patients. Anticancer Res 1997;17:613–620

11. Chow N-H, Liu H-S, Lee EI, et al. Significance of urinary epidermal growth factor and its receptor expression in human bladder cancer. Anticancer Res 1997;17:1293–1296

12. Ke LD, Adler-Storthz K, Clayman GL, et al. Differential expression of epidermal growth factor receptor in human head and neck cancers. Head Neck 1998;20:320–327

13. Rubin Grandis J, Melhem MF, Barnes EL, et al. Quantitative immuno-histochemical analysis of transforming growth factor-α and epidermal growth factor receptor in patients with squamous cell carcinoma of the head and neck. Cancer 1996;78:1284–1292

14. Modjtahedi H, Affleck K, Stubberfield C, et al. EGFR blockade by tyrosine kinase inhibitor or monoclonal antibody inhibits growth, directs terminal differentiation and induces apoptosis in human squamous cell carcinoma HN5. Int J Oncol 1998;13:335–342

15. de Jong JS, van Diest PJ, van der Valk P, et al. Expression of growth factors, growth-inhibiting factors, and their receptors in invasive breast cancer. II. Correlations with proliferation and angiogenesis. J Pathol 1998;184:53–57

16. Radinsky R, Risin S, Fan Z, et al. Level and function of epidermal growth factor receptor predict the metastatic potential of human colon carcinoma cells. Clin Cancer Res 1995;1:19–31

17. Nagane M, Coufal F, Lin H, et al. A common mutant epidermal growth factor receptor confers enhanced tumorigenicity on human glioblastoma cells by increasing proliferation and reducing apoptosis. Cancer Res 1996;56:5079–5086

18. Perrotte P, Matsumoto T, Inoue K, et al. Chimeric monoclonal antibody (Mab) C225 to the epidermal growth factor receptor (EGF-R) antibody inhibits angiogenesis in human transitional cell carcinoma (TCC) [abstract]. Proc Am Assoc Cancer Res 2000;41:3372

19. Carpenter G. Receptors for epidermal growth factor and other polypeptide mitogens. Annu Rev Biochem 1987;56:881–914

20. Carpenter G, Cohen S. Epidermal growth factor. J Biol Chem 1990;265:7709–7712

21. Harari PM, Huang SM. Modulation of molecular targets to enhance radiation. Clin Cancer Res 2000;6:323–325

22. Schlessinger J. The epidermal growth factor receptor as a multifunctional allosteric protein. Biochemistry 1988;27:3119–3123

23. Yarden Y, Ullrich A. Growth factor receptor tyrosine kinases. Annu Rev Biochem 1988;57:443–478

24. Thompson DM, Gill GN. The EGF receptor: structure, regulation and potential role in malignancy. Cancer Surv 1985;4:767–788

25. Shin DM, Ro JY, Hong WK, et al. Dysregulation of epidermal growth factor receptor expression in multistep process of head and neck tumorigenesis. Cancer Res 1994;54:3153–3159

26. Huang S-M, Bock JM, Harari PM. Epidermal growth factor receptor blockade with C225 modulates proliferation, apoptosis, and radiosensitivity in squamous cell carcinomas of the head and neck. Cancer Res 1999;59:1935–1940

27. Sartor C. Biological modifiers as potential radiosensitizers: targeting the epidermal growth factor receptor family. Semin Oncol 2000;27(suppl 11):15–20

28. He Y, Zeng Q, Drenning SD, et al. Inhibition of human squamous cell carcinoma growth in vivo by epidermal growth factor receptor antisense RNA transcribed from the U6 promoter. J Natl Cancer Inst 1998;90:1080–1087

29. Baselga J, Norton L, Masui H, et al. Antitumor effects of doxorubicin in combination with anti-epidermal growth factor receptor monoclonal antibodies. J Natl Cancer Inst 1993;85:1327–1333

30. Kim ES, Khuri FR, Herbst RS. Epidermal growth factor receptor biology (IMC-C225). Curr Opin Oncol 2001;13:506–513

31. Mendelsohn J, Baselga J. Status of epidermal growth factor receptor antagonists in the biology and treatment of cancer. J Clin Oncol 2003;21:2787–2799

32. Baselga J, Pfister D, Cooper MR, et al. Phase I studies of anti-epidermal growth factor receptor chimeric antibody IMC-C225 alone and in combination with cisplatin. J Clin Oncol 2000;18:904–914

33. Shin DM, Donato NJ, Perez-Soler R, et al. Epidermal growth factor receptor targeted therapy with C225 and cisplatin in patients with head and neck cancer. Clin Cancer Res 2001;7:1204–1213

34. Pomerantz RG, Grandis JR. The epidermal growth factor receptor signaling network in head and neck carcinogenesis and implications for targeted therapy. Semin Oncol 2004;31:734–743

35. Baselga J, Trigo JM, Bourhis J, et al. Phase II multicenter study of the antiepidermal growth factor receptor monoclonal antibody cetuximab in combination with platinum-based chemotherapy in patients with platinum-refractory metastatic and/or recurrent squamous cell carcinoma of the head and neck. J Clin Oncol 2005; 23:5568–5577

36. Herbst RS, Arquette M, Shin DM, et al. Phase II multicenter study of the epidermal growth factor receptor antibody cetuximab and cisplatin for recurrent and refractory squamous cell carcinoma of the head and neck. J Clin Oncol 2005;23:5578–5587

37. Trigo J, Hitt, R, Koralewski P, et al. Cetuximab monotherapy is active in patients (pts) with platinum-refractory recurrent/metastatic squamous cell carcinoma of head and neck (SCCHN): results of a phase II study [abstract]. J Clin Oncol 2004;22:488s(suppl)

38. Vermorken J, Bourhis J, Trigo J, et al. Cetuximab in recurrent/metastatic (R&M) squamous cell carcinoma of the head and neck (SCCHN) refractory to first-line platinum-based therapies. Presented at the American Society of Clinical Oncology (ASCO) annual meeting, 2005, abstract 5505

39. Burtness BA, Li Y, Flood W, et al. Phase III trial comparing cisplatin (C) + placebo (P) to C + anti-epidermal growth factor antibody (EGF-R) C225 in patients (pts) with metastatic/recurrent head & neck cancer (HNC) [abstract]. Proc Am Soc Clin Oncol 2002;21:226a

40. Robert F, Ezekiel MP, Spencer SA, et al. Phase I study of anti-epidermal growth factor receptor antibody cetuximab in combination with radiation therapy in patients with advanced head and neck cancer. J Clin Oncol 2001;19:3234–3243

41. Bonner JA, Giralt J, Harari PM, et al. Cetuximab prolongs survival in patients with locoregionally advanced squamous cell carcinoma of head and neck: A phase III study of high dose radiation therapy with or without cetuximab [abstract]. J Clin Oncol 2004;22:489a(suppl)

42. Bonner JA, Harari PM, Giralt J, et al. Radiotherapy plus cetuximab for squamous cell carcinoma of the head and neck. N Engl J Med 2006; 354:567–578

43. Sirotnak FM, Zakowski MF, Miller VA, et al. Efficacy of cytotoxic agents against human tumor xenografts is markedly enhanced by coadministration of ZD1839 (Iressa), an inhibitor of EGFR tyrosine kinase. Clin Cancer Res 2000;6:4885–4892

44. Baselga J, Averbuch SD. ZD1839 ("Iressa") as an anticancer agent. Drugs 2000;60(suppl 1):33–40

45. Al-Hazzaa AA, Bowen ID, Birchall MA, et al. p53-independent apoptosis induced by cisplatin and enhanced by the combination of cisplatin with ZD1839 (Iressa) an EGFR-TK inhibitor in an oral squamous cell carcinoma cell line [abstract]. Proceedings of the AACR-NCI-EORTC International Conference, 2001:348

46. Huang S, Harari PM. Modulation of radiation response and tumor-induced angiogenesis following EGFR blockade by ZD1839 (Iressa) in human squamous cell carcinomas [abstract]. Proceedings of the AACR-NCI-EORTC International Conference, 2001:259

47. Thatcher N, Chang A, Parikh P, et al. Gefitinib plus best supportive care in previously treated patients with refractory advanced non-small-cell lung cancer: results from a randomised, placebo-controlled, multicentre trial (Iressa Survival Evaluation in Lung Cancer). Lancet 2005;366:1527–1537

48. Cohen EE, Rosen F, Stadler WM, et al. Phase II trial of ZD1839 in recurrent or metastatic squamous cell carcinoma of the head and neck. J Clin Oncol 2003;21:1980–1987

49. Akita RW, Sliwkowski MX. Preclinical studies with Erlotinib (Tarceva). Semin Oncol 2003;30:15–24

50. Hidalgo M, Siu LL, Nemunaitis J, et al. Phase I and pharmacologic study of OSI-774, and epidermal growth factor receptor tyrosine kinase inhibitor, in patients with advanced solid malignancies. J Clin Oncol 2001;19:3267–3279

51. Soulieres D, Senzer NN, Vokes EE, et al. Multicenter phase II study of erlotinib, an oral epidermal growth factor receptor tyrosine kinase inhibitor, in patients with recurrent or metastatic squamous cell cancer of the head and neck. J Clin Oncol 2004;22:77–85

52. Zinner RG, Nemunaitis JJ, Donato NJ, et al. A phase I clinical and biomarker study of the novel pan-erbB tyrosine kinase inhibitor, CI-1033, in patients with solid tumors [abstract]. Proceedings of the AACR-NCI-EORTC International Conference, 2001:566

53. Papadimitrakopoulou VA, Murren JR, Fidler IJ, et al. A phase I dose-escalating study to evaluate the biological activity and pharmacokinetics of PKI166, a novel tyrosine kinase inhibitor, in patients with advanced cancers [abstract]. Proceedings of the AACR-NCI-EORTC International Conference, 2001:276

54. Griffioen AW, Molema G. Angiogenesis: potentials for pharmacologic intervention in the treatment of cancer, cardiovascular diseases, and chronic inflammation. Pharmacol Rev 2000;52:237–268

55. Hanahan D, Weinberg RA. The hallmarks of cancer. Cell 2000; 100:57–70

56. Denekamp J. Review article: angiogenesis, neovascular proliferation and vascular pathophysiology as targets for cancer therapy. Br J Radiol 1993;66:181–196

57. Fischer-Colbrie J, Witt A, Heinzl H, et al. EGFR and steroid receptors in ovarian carcinoma: comparison with prognostic parameters and outcome of patients. Anticancer Res 1997;17:613–620

58. Ferrara N. Molecular and biological properties of vascular endothelial growth factor. J Mol Med 1999;77:527–543

59. Millauer B, Wizigmann-Voos S, Schnurch H, et al. High affinity VEGF binding and developmental expression suggest FLK-1 as a major regulator of vasculogenesis and angiogenesis. Cell 1993; 72:835–846

60. Guo D, Jia Q, Song HY, et al. Vascular endothelial cell growth factor promotes tyrosine phosphorylation of mediators of signal transduction that contain SH2 domains. Association with endothelial cell proliferation. J Biol Chem 1995;270:6729–6733

61. Waltenberger J, Claesson Welsh L, Siegbahn A, et al. Different signal transduction properties of KDR and Flt1, two receptors for vascular endothelial growth factor. J Biol Chem 1994;269:26988–26995

62. Millauer B, Longhi MP, Plate KH, et al. Dominant-negative inhibition of Flk-1 suppresses the growth of many tumor types in vivo. Cancer Res 1996;56:1615–1620

63. Kukk E, Lymboussaki A, Taira S, et al. VEGF-C receptor binding and pattern of expression with VEGFR-3 suggests a role in lymphatic vascular development. Development 1996;122:3829–3837

64. DeVore RF, Fehrenbacher RS, Herbst RS, et al. A randomized phase II trial comparing rhumab VEGF (recombinant humanized monoclonal antibody to vascular endothelial cell growth factor) plus carboplatin/paclitaxel (CP) to CP alone in patients with stage IIIB/IV NSCLC [abstract]. Proc Am Soc Clin Oncol 2000;19:485a

65. Sandler A, Gray R, Brahmer J, et al. Randomized phase II/III Trial of paclitaxel (P) plus carboplatin (C) with or without bevacizumab (NSC # 704865) in patients with advanced non-squamous non-small cell lung cancer (NSCLC): An Eastern Cooperative Oncology Group (ECOG) Trial E4599 [abstract]. Proc Am Soc Clin Oncol 2005;23:4

66. Gustin DM, Winegarden J, Haraf D, et al. Phase I study of bevacizumab, fluorouracil, hydroxyurea and radiotherapy (B-FHX) for patients with poor prognosis head and neck cancer. Proceedings of the American Association for Cancer Research (AACR), 2nd ed. Washington, DC, July 11–14, 2003

67. Wedge SR, Ogilvie DJ, Dukes M, et al. VEGF receptor tyrosine kinase inhibitors as potential anti-tumor targets [abstract]. Proceedings of the American Association for Cancer Research (AACR) 2000;41:566

68. Basser R, Hurwitz H, Barge A, et al. Phase I pharmacokinetic and biological study of the angiogenesis inhibitor, ZD6474, in patients with solid tumors [abstract]. Proc Am Soc Clin Oncol 2001;20:396

69. Laird AD, Vajkoczy P, Shawver LK, et al. SU6668 is a potent antiangiogenic and antitumor agent that induces regression of established tumors. Cancer Res 2000;60:4152–4160

70. Rosen LS, Rosen PJ, Kabbinavar F, et al. Phase I experience with SU6668, a novel multiple receptor tyrosine kinase inhibitor in patients with advanced malignancies [abstract]. Proc Am Soc Clin Oncol 2001;20:383

71. Rosen L, Hannah A, Rosen P, et al: Phase I experience oral SU006668, a novel multiple receptor tyrosine kinase inhibitor in patients with advanced malignancies [abstract]. Clin Cancer Res 2000;6:458(suppl)

72. Boyle JO, Hakim J, Koch W, et al. The incidence of p53 mutations increases with progression of head and neck cancer. Cancer Res 1993;53:4477–4480

73. Brennan JA, Boyle JO, Koch WM, et al. Association between cigarette smoking and mutation of the p53 gene in squamous cell carcinoma of the head and neck. N Engl J Med 1995;332:712–717

74. Werness BA, Levine AJ, Howley PM. Association of human papillomavirus type 16 and 18 E6 proteins with p53. Science 1990;248:76–79

75. Gillison ML, Koch WM, Capone RB, et al. Evidence for a causal association between human papillomavirus and a subset of head and neck cancers. J Natl Cancer Inst 2000;92:709–720

76. Cabelguenne A, Blons H, de Waziers I, et al. p53 alterations predict tumor response to neoadjuvant chemotherapy in head and neck

squamous cell carcinoma: a prospective series. J Clin Oncol 2000;18:1465–1473

77. Bischoff JR, Kirn DH, Williams A, et al. An adenovirus mutant that replicates selectively in p53-deficient human tumor cells. Science 1996;274:373–376

78. Lowe SW, Ruley HE, Jacks T, et al. p53-dependent apoptosis modulates the cytotoxicity of anticancer agents. Cell 1993;74:957–967

79. Lowe SW, Bodis S, McClatchey A, et al. p53 status and the efficacy of cancer therapy in vivo. Science 1994;266:807–810

80. Sanchez-Prieto R, Quintanilla M, Cano A, et al. Carcinoma cell lines become sensitive to DNA-damaging agents by the expression of the adenovirus E1A gene. Oncogene 1996;13:1083–1092

81. Lowe SW, Ruley HE. Stabilization of the p53 tumor suppressor is induced by adenovirus 5 E1A and accompanies apoptosis. Genes Dev 1993;7:535–545

82. Barker DD, Berk AJ. Adenovirus proteins from both E1B reading frames are required for transformation of rodent cells by viral infection and DNA transfection. Virology 1987;156:107–121

83. Khuri FR, Nemunaitis J, Ganly I, et al. A controlled trial of intratumoral ONYX-015, a selectively-replicating adenovirus, in combination with cisplatin and 5-fluorouracil in patients with recurrent head and neck cancer. Nat Med 2000;6:879–885

84. Nemunaitis J, Khuri F, Ganly I, et al. Phase II trial of intratumoral administration of ONYX-015, a replication-selective adenovirus, in patients with refractory head and neck cancer. J Clin Oncol 2001;19:289–298

85. Nemunaitis J, Cunningham C, Buchanan A, et al. Intravenous infusion of a replication-selective adenovirus (ONYX-015) in cancer patients: safety, feasibility and biological activity. Gene Ther 2001; 8:746–759

86. Horio Y, Hasegawa Y, Sekido Y, et al. Synergistic effects of adenovirus expressing wild-type p53 on chemosensitivity of non-small cell lung cancer cells. Cancer Gene Ther 2000;7:537–544

87. Ishida S, Yamashita T, Nakaya U, et al. Adenovirus-mediated transfer of p53-related genes induces apoptosis of human cancer cells. Jpn J Cancer Res 2000;91:174–180

88. Clayman GL, El-Naggar AK, Lippman SM, et al. Adenovirus-mediated p53 gene transfer in patients with advanced recurrent head and neck squamous cell carcinoma. J Clin Oncol 1998;16:2221–2232

89. Glisson S, Huber J, Gaugler M, et al. Smokeless tobacco induced oral cavity tumors in Kentucky have a high incidence of H-ras mutations. American Society of Clinical Oncology (ASCO), vol 17, 1998

90. Chou TC. The median-effect principle and the combination index for quantitation of synergism and antagonism. In: Chou T-C, Rideout DC (eds). Synergism and Antagonism in Chemotherapy. San Diego: Academic, 1991:61–102

91. Lebowitz PF, Davide JP, Prendergast GC. Evidence that farnesyltransferase inhibitors suppress Ras transformation by interfering with Rho activity. Mol Cell Biol 1995;15:6613–6622

92. Sepp-Lorenzino L, Ma Z, Rands E, et al. A peptidomimetic inhibitor of farnesylprotein transferase blocks the anchorage-dependent and -independent growth of human tumor cell lines. Cancer Res 1995;55:5302–5309

93. Moasser MM, Sepp-Lorenzino L, Kohl NE, et al. Farnesyl transferase inhibitors cause enhanced mitotic sensitivity to taxol and epothilones. Proc Natl Acad Sci U S A 1998;95:1369–1374

94. Kies MS, Clayman GL, El-Naggar AK, et al. Induction therapy with SCH 66336, a farnesyltransferase inhibitor, in squamous cell carcinoma (SCC) of the head and neck [abstract]. Proc Am Soc Clin Oncol 2001;20:896

95. Kim ES, Glisson BS, Meyers ML, et al. A phase I/II study of the farnesyl transferase inhibitor (FTI) SCH66336 with paclitaxel in patients with solid tumors [abstract]. Proc Am Assoc Cancer Res 2001; 20:2629

96. Kim ES, Kies MS, Fossella FV, et al. A phase I/II study of farnesyl transferase inhibitor (FTI) SCH66336 (lonafarnib) with paclitaxel in taxane-refractory/resistant patients with non-small cell lung cancer: final report [abstract]. Proc Am Assoc Cancer Res 2002

97. Mackay HJ, Hoekstra R, Eskens F, et al. A phase I dose escalating study of BMS-214662 in combination with cisplatin in patients with advanced solid tumours [abstract]. Proc Am Soc Clin Oncol 2001; 20:315

98. Nakagawa K, Yamamoto N, Nishio K, et al. A phase I, pharmacokinetic (PK) and pharmacodynamic (PD) study of the farnesyl transferase inhibitor (FTI) R115777 in Japanese patients with advanced non-hematological malignancies [abstract]. Proc Am Soc Clin Oncol 2001;20:317

99. Endo S, Zeng Q, Burke NA, et al. TGF-alpha antisense gene therapy inhibits head and neck squamous cell carcinoma growth in vivo. Gene Ther 2000;7:1906–1914

100. Recchia F, Lalli A, Lombardo M, et al. Ifosfamide, cisplatin, and 13-cis retinoic acid for patients with advanced or recurrent squamous cell carcinoma of the head and neck: a phase I–II study. Cancer 2001;92:814–821

101. Shin DM, Khuri FR, Murphy B, et al. Combined interferon-alpha, 13 cis-retinoic acid, and alpha-tocopherol in locally advanced head and neck squamous cell carcinoma: novel bioadjuvant phase II trial. J Clin Oncol 2001;19:3010–3017

102. Mininberg ED, Herbst RS, Henderson T, et al. PhaseI/II study of the recombinant humanized monoclonal anti-VEGF antibody bevacizumab and the EGFR-TK inhibitor erlotinib in patients with recurrent non-small cell lung cancer (NSCLC) [abstract]. Proc Am Soc Clin Oncol 2003

31

Medical/Legal Issues

Richard E. Anderson

Despite remarkable advances in scientific knowledge, medicine remains more art than science. As our understanding increases, the complexity of biologic systems is revealed to be ever greater. Sophisticated new treatments are developed to harness the therapeutic implications of this knowledge, and patient expectations continue to rise. We have made manifest progress in lengthening the average life span, in treating certain forms of cancer, in reducing the ravages of stroke and coronary artery disease, and in surgical technique and reconstructive potential. Nonetheless, most medical progress is incremental, and outcomes for individual patients remain unpredictable. Unfortunately, the tide of litigation against doctors in the United States has risen even faster than medical progress.

◆ Overview of Malpractice Litigation

Approximately one of every six practicing physicians in the United States faces a malpractice claim every year. In high-risk specialties such as obstetrics, orthopedics, trauma surgery, and neurosurgery, there is one claim for each doctor every 2.5 years.[1] In otolaryngology, the frequency of malpractice claims is 0.153.[2] This means that about 15% of otolaryngologists report a claim every year. Therefore, the average otolaryngologist reports about one malpractice claim every 6 years. Seventy to 80% of all cases are found to be without merit.[1,2] Nonetheless, the legal defense of each case is costly. Nationally, these litigation expenses averaged $22,967 per defendant in 1999.[1] Cases that go all the way through trial before a defense verdict cost

an average of $85,718 per defendant.[3] A single national physician-owned insurer, the Doctors' Company, has spent more than $400 million in legal fees defending claims that ultimately were shown to be without merit.[1]

Coupled with this very high level of frequency, there has been a dramatic increase in severity. Severity is defined as the cost of the average claim, but by extension refers to the range of potential verdicts. The *median* cost of the average jury verdict in malpractice claims doubled to over $1 million between 1997 and 2000.[4] The average medical malpractice jury verdict exceeded $3 million in 2002.[5] Approximately 8% of all malpractice claims now involve indemnities of $1 million or more.[1]

The range of outlier claims has increased even more. In 2000, Texas recorded a $268 million malpractice verdict, and several other states have experienced verdicts in excess of $100 million. Though the threat of an appeal forces plaintiff's attorneys to settle some of these larger awards for less than the amount of the full jury verdict, these judgments set the bar for settlement negotiations in cases where liability is present. Moreover, physicians feel increased pressure to settle claims with doubtful liability when the potential damages could exceed their insurance coverage.

The product of frequency and severity can be used to create an index of specialty relativity. If we arbitrarily set internal medicine as 1.0, then neurosurgery has a relativity of 6.5. This means, in an actuarial model, the average neurosurgeon would pay a malpractice insurance premium 6.5 times that of the average internist. For otolaryngology, excluding facial cosmetic surgery, the figure is 1.65 (**Fig. 31–1**).

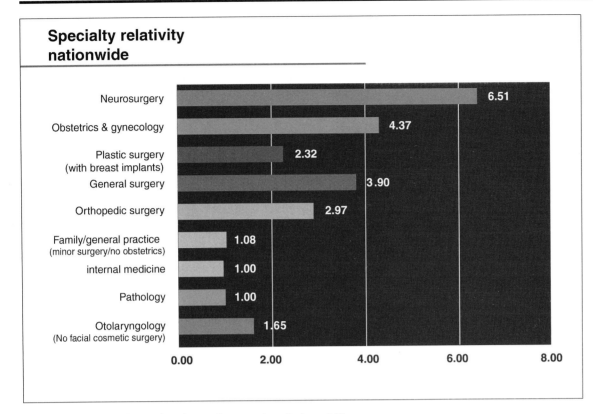

Figure 31–1   Index of specialty relativity for several medical specialties.

◆ Historical Antecedents

Medical liability claims were fairly uncommon until the 1970s, when the first antecedent of today's crises occurred. Nearly 80% of California's malpractice claims for the first 75 years of the century were filed between 1970 and 1975.[6] This unexpected tide of litigation led most commercial insurance companies to conclude that the practice of medicine was uninsurable, and they refused to provide malpractice coverage at any price. This resulted in skyrocketing insurance rates by the remaining companies and a "crisis of availability" that left many physicians unable to find coverage at any price. The medical community responded emergently. Doctors contributed their own funds as capital to support the efforts of their state medical and hospital associations, among others, to start as many as 100 provider-owned specialty carriers across the country. These mutual or reciprocal insurers, owned by the policyholders themselves, now insure more than 60% of American physicians.

The creation of physician-owned insurers was the product of necessity, but became feasible only after the passage of seminal tort reforms in California. California's Medical Injury Compensation Reform Act of 1975 has four principal provisions:

1. Noneconomic (pain and suffering) damages are capped at $250,000.
2. The collateral source rule prevents duplicate recovery of damages that have already been indemnified. For example, the plaintiff cannot recover a second time for the cost of health care that has already been paid for by health insurance.
3. A periodic payments rule allows indemnity to be paid out over the intended length of the compensation rather than as a lump sum. For example, a $30 million verdict intended to cover an expected life span of 30 years might be paid out at $1 million per year for 30 years.
4. There is a limitation on the contingency fee charged by the plaintiff's attorney. Under this sliding scale, an attorney winning a million-dollar case could charge no more than $221,000 plus expenses. On the other hand, the plaintiff's attorney would still keep 40% of a $50,000 award.

◆ The Second Wave of Litigation

A second crisis emerged in the early 1980s, again brought on by sharp increases in both frequency and severity. States like California and Nebraska, having passed necessary reforms a decade earlier, experienced no crisis. States that had failed to pass effective tort reforms experienced significant increases in the volume and cost of litigation. By this time, physician-owned insurers and returning commercial carriers had sufficiently adapted to the medical-legal environment to continue to offer coverage, albeit with sharp increases in premiums. This crisis was primarily about affordability rather than availability. The health care system was able to accommodate this increase in litigation because physicians and hospitals began to assign the cost of some of these premium escalations to patients in the form of fees for service.

◆ Cancer Litigation

Allegations of malpractice involving cancer are probably the most common category of litigation in the United States. Of these, the majority involves putative delays in diagnosis. There are several reasons for this[7]:

1. Cancer is a common disease that will affect one in every four Americans. Fifty to 60% of these cases will be fatal, so the consequences of a delay may be serious.
2. Few diagnoses evoke the kind of visceral fear that cancer does. Frightened patients may focus on the medical process rather than the cancer itself as the offending entity.
3. The public has been educated to place a very high value on early detection, so it is easy to believe that any delay in diagnosis can have dire consequences.
4. Patients frequently detect the index sign or symptom, and these individuals are particularly aware of delays in properly addressing their concern.

Most cancers are readily detectable once the physician is determined to make a definitive diagnosis. However, the presenting signs and symptoms are often protean and suggest a broad differential diagnosis that includes many conditions encountered in daily clinical practice. To avoid missing a diagnosis, physicians must maintain a high index of suspicion, and exclude malignant disease with certainty. For example, otolaryngologists often encounter nonspecific complaints such as fever, night sweats, pruritus, pain, cough, hoarseness, and lymphadenopathy, or isolated abnormal laboratory values in the complete blood count, serum alkaline phosphatase, lactic dehydrogenase, calcium, or sedimentation rate. Such complaints or findings often pose a dilemma for the treating physician that requires further investigation to exclude malignancy.

Frequently, the differential diagnosis in these situations can be broad, and delays in diagnosis may occur for a variety of reasons:

1. Routine assumption of benign etiology: It is easy to attribute hoarseness or cough to an upper respiratory tract infection.
2. Acceptance of a sign or symptom as a diagnosis: For example, it is common to make a diagnosis of anemia without defining the etiology. This is, at best, an incomplete diagnosis. Even iron-deficiency anemia, which is a diagnosis, is incomplete unless the source of the iron deficit is identified.
3. Overreliance on indirect means of diagnosis: This potentially serious error may occur when physicians accept radiographic studies as definitive. A negative x-ray often does not definitively exclude cancer, and an abnormal x-ray alone is usually insufficient to confirm a new diagnosis of cancer. All new diagnoses of malignant disease should be *confirmed histologically where possible.*
4. Failure to mandate adequate follow-up: It is important that patients with indeterminate findings be followed until a definitive diagnosis can be made. Physicians must be diligent in insisting on necessary evaluation.

Because the physician is assumed to have superior knowledge, courts may not exonerate a doctor for a delayed diagnosis when the patient fails to appear for appointments. It may be necessary to prove the patient understood the potential implications of the behavior and the physician has made a reasonable effort to see that necessary evaluation is undertaken. This begins by confirming that ordered tests were actually completed. In many cases, a follow-up visit for a repeat examination of a borderline physical finding or repeat discussion of symptoms will be the difference between making a diagnosis and missing it.

5. Failure to review laboratory and x-ray reports: This oversight can be fatal. A regrettably common example is the failure to act on a chest x-ray reporting a new coin lesion. In some cases, the report is filed in the patient's chart before being initialed by the physician. In others, the finding is not immediately communicated to the patient and is forgotten until the disease is advanced.

◆ Malpractice Litigation in Otolaryngology

The risk profile of otolaryngology is intermediate when compared with other specialties. As a surgical subspecialty, it is not surprising that most claims arise in the operating room, but delays in diagnosis make up the preponderance of the remaining litigation. A review of 100 consecutive closed claims in otolaryngology was undertaken at the Doctors Company, a national physician-owned malpractice insurer that covers 360 otolaryngologists.[2] The claims occurred between 1995 and 2002. Indemnity was paid in 25% of the cases, meaning the plaintiff received nothing 75% of the time. This approximates the company experience for all claims. Indemnities ranged from $4500 to $900,000. Of these, eight were $100,000 or higher, with two above $500,000. The average paid claim was just over $150,000, compared with $173,000 for the average paid claim company-wide. It is of interest that there were no indemnities in excess of $1 million. Nationally, approximately 8% of all paid claims today exceed that figure.[1]

Although the series of 100 paid claims for otolaryngology is the largest one available, we should not overgeneralize from this sample. It was accrued over 7 years, a period in which severity was increasing at an especially high rate in the latest years and may underestimate the cost of today's liabilities. Nonetheless, these data are consistent with the intermediate position of otolaryngology along the medical liability spectrum.

A closer look at these claims showed that 50% were operative complications of noncosmetic surgery. An additional 29% represented alleged poor outcomes of cosmetic surgery. Twelve percent involved delays in diagnosis. Of these 12 cases, 5 involved delays in the diagnosis of cancer, 3 of which resulted in death. Overall, 9 of the 100 claims involved the death of the patient (**Fig. 31–2**).

Of the noncosmetic surgery operative complications, there were nine involving tonsillectomy, nine involving septoplasty, and nine involving sinus surgery. Interestingly, none

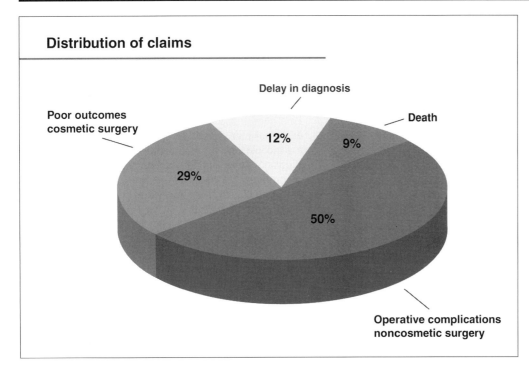

Figure 31–2   The distribution of 100 consecutive paid claims for otolaryngologists.

involved laryngectomy or radical neck dissection and only two involved parotidectomy. Head and neck cancer surgery may have a lower risk profile than more common procedures in the specialty, though proof would require a careful correlation with the number of procedures that are performed. This would be consistent with risk assessment in specialties like medical oncology or radiation oncology. Patients are generally well aware of the serious nature of their disease, informed consent is undertaken more rigorously because of the potentially damaging consequences of therapy, and perfect outcomes are not expected. Cancer specialists are also generally spared the litigation that surrounds the diagnostic process, because the cancer is at least overtly suspected prior to referral. In this context, it is notable that five of 12 cases (42%) of delayed diagnosis involved cancer. This is consistent with the fact that the patient is usually aware of the index signs and symptoms of cancer of the head and neck such as hoarseness or a neck mass, making them more cognizant of delays in diagnosis.

Longitudinal reviews of jury verdicts involving cancer of the oral cavity[8] and larynx[9] have been undertaken. Lydiatt[9] identified 50 cases involving cancer of the oral cavity between 1984 and 2000. The average age of these plaintiffs was 47, whereas the median age for patients with oral cancer in the United States is greater than 60. Younger plaintiffs more frequently alleged misdiagnosis, won a higher percentage of their suits (60%), and received higher average awards ($755,824) than the older cohort. Eighty-six percent of the cases alleged delay in diagnosis. When the delay was 3 months or less, the defense won 86% of the verdicts. This figure fell to 40% for longer delays. For cancer of the larynx, the picture was generally similar. Twenty-three recorded jury verdicts involving laryngeal cancer were identified

between 1976 and 1997. Eighty-three percent involved delays in diagnosis. Hoarseness was present in 53%, and 16% had a mass in the neck. Indemnity was paid just over half the time and was more likely in younger patients. General practitioners were the target defendants in about half of these cases. The findings of both of these series are consistent with the observation that most cancer litigation revolves around the diagnostic, rather than the treatment, process. Schuring[10] found that 20% of *all* suits against otologists are for failure to diagnose cancer.

Litigation involving head and neck cancer appears to be *relatively* uncommon, especially considering the extent of surgical intervention sometimes necessary for treatment. Some of the reasons for this have already been discussed. It is clear that delays in diagnosis are more likely to result in litigation, especially in the patient who presents for evaluation of a specific cancer-related complaint. Most otolaryngologists are quite familiar with diagnostic paradigms for their specialty. Moreover, the diagnostic tools are usually in the hands of the physician, who frequently does not rely on additional outside consultation. This unfortunately makes the physician's liability relatively clear when the diagnostic process fails.

Although contemporary reviews have detected few claims involving informed consent for cancer surgery, the allegation is common in other areas of otolaryngology, especially for elective or cosmetic surgery. In the future, however, we may anticipate more litigation alleging loss of opportunity for voice preservation when laryngectomy is recommended without discussion of organ-sparing alternatives, or when delays in diagnosis make laryngectomy the only appropriate therapy. This type of litigation has already appeared in breast cancer cases where allegations involving lost opportunity for breast conservation are increasingly common.

Overall, there can be no doubt that the tide of litigation is increasing. This means that issues that have rarely been litigated in the past, such as lost opportunity for organ preservation and adverse outcomes involving even the most complex cases, are more likely to result in litigation. In addition, there is more litigation in areas already heavily contested, such as delayed diagnosis cases alleging ever-shorter periods of delay.

◆ Risk Management

There are no certain pathways to preventing litigation, in part because a significant percentage of the litigation is without merit. The notion that malpractice suits are directed only at "bad" doctors is not supportable. In high-risk specialties such as neurosurgery, virtually all practitioners have already been sued, and on average half of neurosurgeons will report a malpractice claim every year.[2] The situation is not much better in several other specialties including obstetrics, orthopedics, and emergency medicine. The authors of the Harvard Medical Practice Study could find no correlation between the outcome of a malpractice lawsuit and the presence or absence of medical negligence. The only variable that correlated with suit outcome was the degree of injury. Patients with severe injury, *regardless of cause*, are more likely to be indemnified.[11] In addition, we know that 70 to 80% of all malpractice claims are closed with no indemnity payment.[1,2]

Nonetheless, there are several things that can be done to reduce the likelihood of a suit. The most obvious is maintaining excellent communication with patients. This extends beyond a good bedside manner, though that is still important, to careful informed consent, thorough family discussions, and careful ascertainment of test results and follow-up responsibilities. The maintenance of excellent medical records is also of paramount importance. Most attorneys will argue that if it isn't written down, it didn't happen. Illegible records are not only problematic in court, they are also likely to be too brief for an adequate medical defense. Typed records are clearly preferable, but the next major step forward will be the electronic medical record. It has the potential to reduce common causes of malpractice litigation, such as unreviewed laboratory tests and x-rays, missed follow-up appointments, incomplete documentation, and overlooked drug allergies. In the absence of a national standard for such records and the high cost of adopting currently available alternatives, it will be some time before such a system is widely available.

Lydiatt[8] has drawn from the experience in delayed diagnosis of breast cancer to offer the following guidelines for the evaluation of oral cancer:

1. Patients' statements that something is different must be heeded.
2. A firm diagnosis must be made for any abnormality, or the patient must have referral or follow-up.
3. Cancer must be considered in all patients with symptoms, irrespective of age.
4. Patients with neck masses must be followed to resolution or diagnosis.
5. All follow-up should be directed so that definitive diagnosis is made within 3 months.
6. Patients, dentists, and physicians must understand that repeated examinations may be necessary to arrive at a diagnosis.
7. Fine-needle aspiration, tissue biopsy, or radiographic examinations cannot be considered definitive if they are inconsistent with the clinical examination.
8. Biopsy of any suspicious lesion should be performed.
9. A complete history must be taken.
10. Maintain close communication with the patient's other health care providers.
11. Primary care physicians and dentists must screen for oral cancer.

It is important to avoid disparaging remarks about prior care. Physicians should not make inadvertent negative comments about aspects of a patient's history, try to interpret equivocal studies, comment about the appearance of a scar, or opine about how a problem could have been approached differently. A lack of first-hand knowledge regarding the circumstances that were originally presented to the physician frequently prevents anyone else from making firm conclusions regarding the quality of care that was delivered. On the other hand, blatant errors should not be hidden from the patient, and the treating physician should continue to be the patient's advocate.

Direct doctor-to-doctor communication can be equally problematic. It is critical that referring physicians forward complete medical records to consultants, and consultants should provide a detailed report of their findings to the referring physician. Lack of communication frequently leads to poorly coordinated care and, occasionally, missed diagnoses.

Doctor-to-patient conversations should be clear and well documented. This is especially important for phone calls, which are frequently not documented. In this case, a court is left to choose between conflicting verbal accounts provided by the doctor and the patient. Follow-up care presents a similar problem. Recommendations regarding follow-up care and evaluation should be clearly documented, and an effort should be made to contact the noncompliant patient. Although this may seem an unfair burden on the physician in an era of patient autonomy, the effort is well rewarded when it results in improved outcomes and prevents an undeserved lawsuit.

Finally, otolaryngologists follow patients long-term for a variety of specific specialty-related problems, such as cancer and chronic sinusitis. Patients tend to rely on these regular encounters for comprehensive medical care, neglecting visits to primary care physicians for the purpose of general prevention and screening. Although there should be no expectation that tests such as mammograms and prostate examinations should be requested by otolaryngologists, it is prudent for the specialist to remind patients that other aspects of their medical care continue to require attention, even when the focus of their concern is on a serious illness such as malignancy.

References

1. Harming Patient Access to Care: Implications of Excessive Litigation. Subcommittee on Health, Committee on Energy and Commerce, U.S. House of Representatives, 107th Congress, 2nd session. Washington, DC: U.S. Government Printing Office, 2002:160

2. The Doctors Company data on file, 2002

3. Physician Insurers Association of America. PIAA Data Sharing Project, May 2002

4. Bagin G. Medical Malpractice Verdict and Settlement Study Released. Horsham, PA: Jury Verdict Research, 2002

5. Jury Verdict Research. Benfield Healthcare Region Report on Medical Professional Liability Insurance/Reinsurance Industry Review, July 28, 2003

6. American Medical Association. Professional Liability in the 1980s. AMA

7. Anderson R. Delayed Diagnosis of Cancer. The Doctors Company Sourcebook, May

8. Lydiatt DD. Cancer of the oral cavity and medical malpractice. Laryngoscope 2002;112:816–819

9. Lydiatt DD. Medical malpractice and cancer of the larynx. Laryngoscope 2002;112:445–448

10. Schuring AG. Defensive otology. Am J Otol 1993;14:515–516

11. Weiler PC, Hiatt HH, Newhouse JP, Johnson WG, Brennan TA, Leape LL. A Measure of Malpractice. Cambridge, MA: Harvard University Press, 1993

Index

Note: Page numbers followed by *f* and *t* indicate figures and tables, respectively.